Bovine Medicine

Bovine Medicine

Editor: Katie Stevens

STATES
ACADEMIC PRESS
www.statesacademicpress.com

States Academic Press,
109 South 5th Street,
Brooklyn, NY 11249, USA

Visit us on the World Wide Web at:
www.statesacademicpress.com

ISBN: 978-1-63989-084-2 (Hardback)

Cataloging-in-Publication Data

Bovine medicine / edited by Katie Stevens.
p. cm.
Includes bibliographical references and index.
ISBN 978-1-63989-084-2
1. Cattle--Diseases. 2. Veterinary medicine. 3. Animals--Diseases. I. Stevens, Katie.
SF961 .B68 2022
636.208 96--dc23

Table of Contents

Preface

Bovine medicine is a sub-discipline of veterinary medicine which deals with the prevention, diagnosis and treatment of disease, disorder and injury in bovines. The bovine family includes domestic cattle, African buffalo, water buffalo, four-horned and spiral-horned antelopes, and bison. They are raised as livestock for the production of milk and meat. Diseases like blackleg, blue tongue, bovine tuberculosis and bovine spongiform encephalopathy (BSE) are some of the prominent diseases amongst bovines. Infected bovines can be a risk factor for transmission to humans through the production of milk and meat. Therefore, bovine medicine is of paramount significance to prevent and control such diseases and their transmission. The topics included in this book on bovine medicine are of utmost significance and bound to provide incredible insights to readers. It is compiled in such a manner, that it will provide in-depth knowledge about the theory and practice of bovine medicine. Researchers and students in this field will be assisted by this book.

The researches compiled throughout the book are authentic and of high quality, combining several disciplines and from very diverse regions from around the world. Drawing on the contributions of many researchers from diverse countries, the book's objective is to provide the readers with the latest achievements in the area of research. This book will surely be a source of knowledge to all interested and researching the field.

In the end, I would like to express my deep sense of gratitude to all the authors for meeting the set deadlines in completing and submitting their research chapters. I would also like to thank the publisher for the support offered to us throughout the course of the book. Finally, I extend my sincere thanks to my family for being a constant source of inspiration and encouragement.

Editor

1

Differential intracellular calcium influx, nitric oxide production, ICAM-1 and IL8 expression in primary bovine endothelial cells exposed to nonesterified fatty acids

Anitsi Loaiza[1], María D. Carretta[1], Anja Taubert[2], Carlos Hermosilla[2], María A. Hidalgo[1] and Rafael A. Burgos[1*]

Abstract

Background: Nonesterified fatty acids (NEFAs) are involved in proinflammatory processes in cattle, including in the increased expression of adhesion molecules in endothelial cells. However, the mechanisms underlying these effects are still unknown. The aim of this study was to assess the effects of NEFAs on the intracellular calcium ($Ca^{2+}{}_i$) influx, nitric oxide production, and ICAM-1 and IL-8 expression in primary bovine umbilical vein endothelial cells (BUVECs).

Results: Myristic (MA), palmitic (PA), stearic (SA), oleic (OA) and linoleic acid (LA) rapidly increased $Ca^{2+}{}_i$. The calcium response to all tested NEFAs showed an extracellular calcium dependence and only the LA response was significantly inhibited until the intracellular calcium was chelated. The EC_{50} values for MA and LA were 125 μM and 37 μM, respectively, and the MA and LA effects were dependent on calcium release from the endoplasmic reticulum stores and on the L-type calcium channels. Only the calcium response to MA was significantly reduced by GW1100, a selective G-protein-coupled free fatty acid receptor (GPR40) antagonist. We also detected a functional FFAR1/GPR40 protein in BUVECs by using western blotting and the FFAR1/GPR40 agonist TAK-875. Only LA increased the cellular nitric oxide levels in a calcium-dependent manner. LA stimulation but not MA stimulation increased ICAM-1 and IL-8-expression in BUVECs. This effect was inhibited by GW1100, an antagonist of FFAR1/GPR40, but not by U-73122, a phospholipase C inhibitor.

Conclusions: These findings strongly suggest that each individual NEFA stimulates endothelial cells in a different way, with clearly different effects on intracellular calcium mobilization, NO production, and IL-8 and ICAM-1 expression in primary BUVECs. These findings not only extend our understanding of NEFA-mediated diseases in ruminants, but also provide new insight into the different molecular mechanisms involved during endothelial cell activation by NEFAs.

Keywords: Nonesterified fatty acid, Primary bovine endothelial cell, Interleukin 8, Intercellular adhesion molecule 1, Calcium flux

Background

The levels of nonesterified fatty acids (NEFAs) in bovine plasma increase during transition periods, such as after calving and during early lactation [1]. During these stages, a negative energy balance is generated, which is mainly characterized by an increased release of NEFAs from adipose tissues into the plasma [2]. Elevated plasma NEFA concentrations have recently been related to the incidence of metabolic and infectious bovine diseases, including fatty hepatitis, metabolic ketosis, mastitis, and endometritis, which cause high economic losses to the cattle industry worldwide [2, 3]. Therefore, NEFAs directly affect tissue/organ functions, and even more importantly, indirectly affect the bovine innate immune system, as previously reported [4].

Endothelial cells are highly immunoreactive cells that synthesize a broad spectrum of chemokines, cytokines, and adhesion molecules, and therefore play an active

* Correspondence: rburgos1@uach.cl
[1]Instituto de Farmacología, Facultad de Ciencias Veterinarias, Universidad Austral de Chile, Valdivia, Chile
Full list of author information is available at the end of the article

part in early proinflammatory reactions [5]. Consistent with this, the exposure of primary bovine aortic endothelial cells (BAECs) to a mixture of NEFAs for 24 h altered their membrane phospholipid profile, increasing the stearic acid concentration and reducing the polyunsaturated fatty acid concentrations [6]. In the same study, 0.75 mM NEFA increased the expression of the proinflammatory cytokines interleukin 6 (IL-6) and IL-8, and the adhesion molecules intercellular adhesion molecule 1 (ICAM-1) and vascular cell adhesion molecule 1 (VCAM-1) in BAECs [6], which interact with other immunocompetent cells, such as neutrophils. Although the effects of NEFAs on bovine leukocytes and endothelial cells have been examined previously [1, 7, 8], the exact molecular mechanisms are still poorly understood.

It has long been accepted that the hydrophobic nature of lipids allows them to activate cells after they enter them, e.g., through membrane transport mechanisms [9, 10]. However, a G-protein-coupled free fatty acid receptor known as GPR40 or free fatty acid receptor 1 (FFAR1) has recently been described [11]. This novel free fatty acid receptor recognizes saturated and unsaturated medium- and long-chain fatty acids, and the human, rat, and mouse isoforms of FFAR1/GPR40 have been described [11, 12]. Recently, the effects of FFAR1/GPR40 agonists, such as oleic acid (OA) and linoleic acid (LA), have been demonstrated in epithelial mammary cells [13] and neutrophils [14, 15]. Consequently, primary bovine tissues are thought to be susceptible to NEFA exposure primarily *via* the corresponding bovine free fatty acid receptor 1 (bFFA1R/bGPR40). Based on this evidence, we evaluated whether different types of NEFAs can rapidly modify the intracellular calcium response in primary bovine endothelial cells exposed to single fatty acids and to study in more detail the molecular mechanisms involved in this endothelial activation.

Results

Acute treatment with NEFAs does not affect the viability of primary bovine umbilical vein endothelial cells (BUVECs)

Cells exposed to 300 μM LA, palmitic acid (PA), OA, myristic acid (MA), or stearic acid (SA) showed no significant difference in the propidium iodide signal for 15 min when compared with untreated cells (basal condition) (see Additional file 1). Similar results were observed in BUVECs exposed to 1 % vehicle (DMSO or ethanol) for the same period. Therefore, exposure to 300 μM of each fatty acid did not increase BUVEC death any more than Triton X-100 treatment, used as the positive control. We demonstrated that 0.3 mM EGTA, 50 μM BAPTA-AM or each NEFA plus EGTA or BAPTA did not affect the viability of BUVECs (see Additional file 1). These results clearly demonstrate that these fatty acid concentrations and exposure time have no toxic effects on BUVECs.

NEFAs increase the intracellular calcium influx in BUVECs

The intracellular calcium response in primary bovine endothelial cells was evaluated in BUVECs exposed acutely to different NEFAs for 100 s. The calcium signal increased quickly after stimulation with 300 μM MA, PA, SA, or OA, with similar kinetics, and the intracellular calcium levels reached a new steady state (Fig. 1a–d, black traces). In contrast, LA caused a slow but constant increase in intracellular calcium (Fig. 1e). To identify the roles of intracellular and extracellular calcium, we used the well-known calcium-chelating agents BAPTA-AM and EGTA. Incubation with BAPTA-AM reduced the slope of calcium increase by more than 50 % in all cases, except for LA (see Additional file 2). However, this did not affect the area under the curve (AUC) of calcium flux (Fig. 1f–i). Moreover, the BAPTA-AM treatment significantly reduced the area under the curve (AUC) only in cells previously exposed to LA (Fig. 1j). The latter suggests that the increase in calcium induced by LA is dependent on intracellular and extracellular calcium mobilization. In our experiments, the NEFA-mediated increase in calcium was significantly inhibited in the presence of EGTA (as illustrated in Fig. 1a–e, light gray traces; Fig. 1f–j), suggesting that the increase in calcium in the whole experiment is mainly depended on calcium influx.

Mechanisms of MA and LA effects on intracellular calcium release in BUVECs

We investigated the potential differential responses of BUVECs to MA and LA, exemplary for saturated and unsaturated NEFAs, respectively. To investigate the mechanism of the calcium increase, we first constructed dose–response curves of the calcium signal after stimulation with MA and LA, and obtained half-maximal effective concentrations (EC_{50}) of 125 and 37 μM, respectively (Fig. 2a, d). We then used concentrations close to the EC_{50} values to assess the mechanisms involved in calcium flux. Upon stimulation with 100 μM MA, BUVECs showed a rapid increase in calcium, which decreased until a new steady state was reached after 30 s (Fig. 2b, inset). In contrast, stimulation with 30 μM LA caused a sustained increase in calcium within the first 100 s (see Fig. 2e, inset), and a steady state was observed after stimulation for 200 s (data not shown).

To evaluate whether FFAR1/GPR40 actively participates in the calcium increase induced by MA or LA, we used its antagonist GW1100, as previously reported [16]. The response produced by 100 μM MA was inhibited by 59 % by 10 μM GW1100 (see Fig. 2c). This was also observed when other saturated fatty acids were used in our in vitro bovine endothelial cell system, and GW1100 inhibited 66 and 63 % of the calcium response induced by 300 μM PA and SA, respectively (see Additional file 3). In

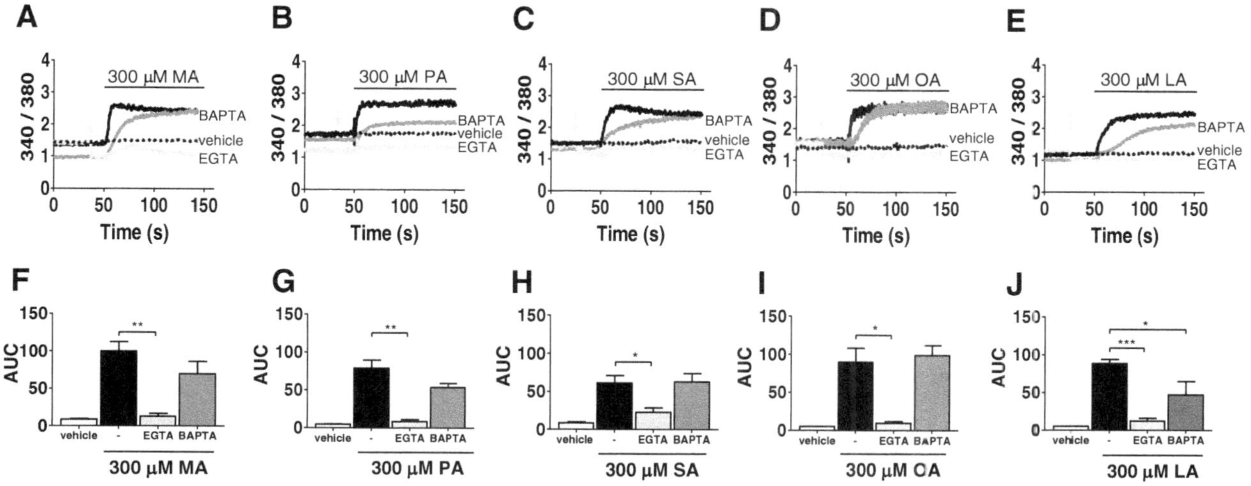

Fig. 1 Intracellular calcium increases caused by NEFAs are dependent on extracellular calcium. **a**–**e** Time courses of representative Fura-2 ratio signals in at least three assays, caused by 300 μM of each NEFA in BUVEC cells. Each NEFA was added at 50 s during a 100 s period (*black line*). Suspended cells were exposed to each NEFA in HBSS, without or with pretreatment with 50 μM BAPTA-AM or calcium-free HBSS/0.3 mM EGTA (*black, dark grey,* and *light grey traces*, respectively). Before fatty acid exposure, EGTA was added at the *light grey arrow*. BUVECs were also exposed to only to the vehicle control at 50 s (*dotted traces*). Ethanol (1 %) was used as the vehicle for MA and SA. DMSO (1 %) was used as the vehicle for PA, OA, and LA. **f**–**j** AUCs for NEFAs in HBS buffer (*black bars*), calcium-free buffer with 0.3 mM EGTA (*light grey bars*), or after BAPTA treatment (*dark grey bars*). AUC of vehicle alone, 1 % ethanol or 1 % DMSO (white bars). The data are expressed as the means ± SEM of at least three experiments. $^{*}p < 0.05$, $^{**}p < 0.01$, $^{***}p < 0.005$

contrast, the calcium influx response to 30 μM LA was not affected by GW1100 (Fig. 2f), and a similar response was observed when OA was used as the unsaturated fatty acid (see Additional file 3).

To assess the role of the G-protein $G\alpha_{i/o}$, phospholipase C (PLC), and the inositol triphosphate (IP_3) receptors/calcium-operated channels induced by MA and LA, we used pertussis toxin (PTX) [17], U73122 [18], and 2-APB [19–21], respectively. We demonstrated that preincubation with 100 ng/ml PTX for 16 h did not inhibit the calcium influx induced either by MA or LA fatty acids in BUVECs, which suggests that $G\alpha_{i/o}$ does not participate in this type of response. The mobilization of calcium by LA was reduced by 4 μM U73122, but the effect of MA was not affected by treatment with the PLC inhibitor. 2-APB (100 μM) reduced both the MA- and LA-mediated increases in calcium by 25 and 23 %, respectively (see Fig. 2c and f).

There is some evidence that fatty acids can directly and indirectly activate the L-type calcium channels (LTCCs) in HEK293, COS-7 and rat insulinoma INS-1E cells in vitro [22, 23]. However, the participation of LTCCs in the calcium increase induced by MA or LA in BUVECs has not been evaluated. Therefore, we investigated whether these channels participate in the calcium increase induced by MA or LA stimulation. Our results show that the LTCC blocker nifedipine (20 μM) inhibited the increases in calcium induced by MA and LA by 45 and 22 %, respectively (Fig. 2c and f). These results suggest that LTCCs participate in the increases in calcium caused by saturated and unsaturated fatty acids in BUVECs.

FFAR1/GPR40 expression and activity

To examine FFAR1/GPR40 protein expression in BUVECs, we used western blotting and immunofluorescence assays directed against the conserved epitope of bovine GPR40, as described elsewhere [14]. An immunoblotting analysis of the total protein extracts of BUVECs showed a band with an apparent molecular size of 23-kDa, lower than expected but similar to that observed in LoVo cells, which were used as the positive control, as suggested by the manufacturer of the anti-GPR40 antibody (Fig. 3a). The same antibody was used for the immunofluorescence assays of BUVECs, which detect the internal region of human GPR40, and therefore the intracellular and plasma membrane distribution (Fig. 3b). To confirm that the FFAR1/GPR40 protein is in its active form in BUVECs, we also measured the calcium signal separately with two known FFAR1/GPR40 agonists, TAK-875 [24] and GW9508 [16]. TAK-875 increased the intracellular calcium in a dose-dependent manner (Fig. 3c, d), whereas GW9508 did not change the calcium signal at either low (10, 50 μM) or high concentrations (100 μM; data not shown).

LA increases nitric oxide (NO) production

To assess whether NEFAs affect NO production in the endothelium, we exposed BUVECs to MA, SA, PA, OA,

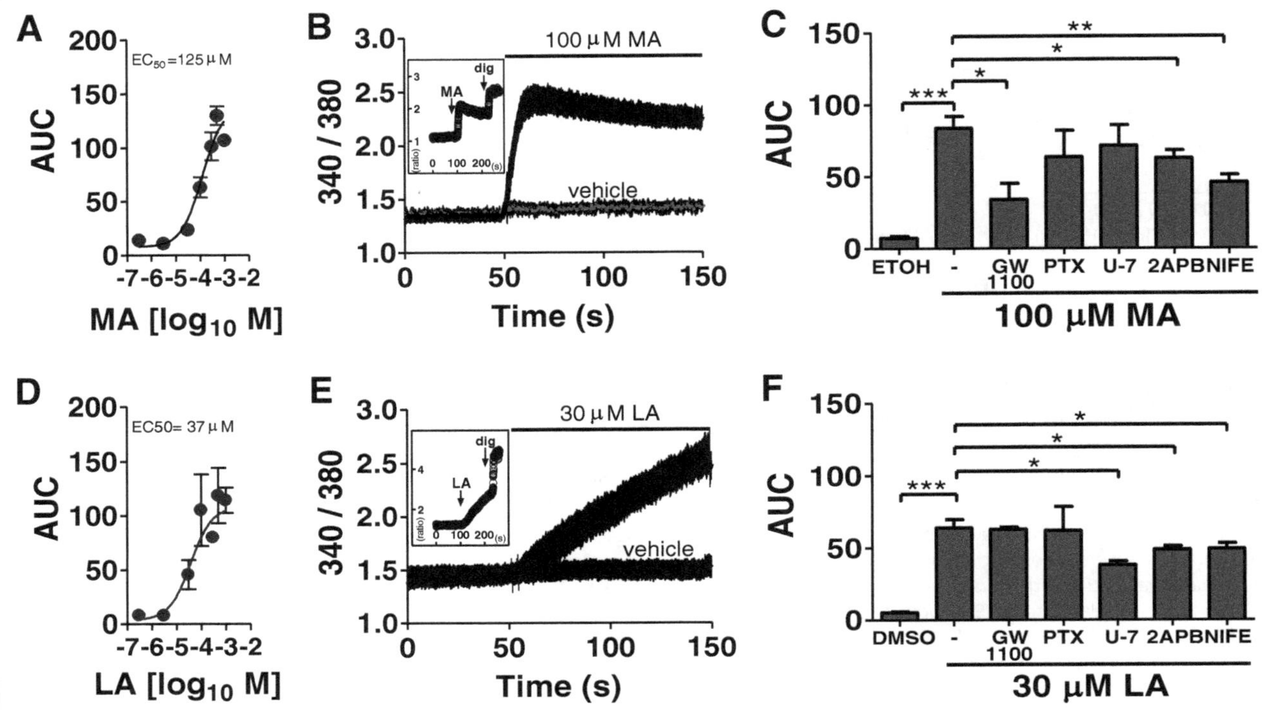

Fig. 2 Signaling routes of the calcium responses caused by MA and LA in BUVECs. **a** and **d** Dose–response of calcium signaling induced by myristic acid (MA) or linoleic acid (LA). The area under the curve (AUC) calculated for the first 100 s of the Fura-2/AM time course. **b** and **e** Average time courses for the Fura-2 ratio in BUVECs exposed to 100 μM MA in ethanol or 30 μM LA in 1 % DMSO. Graph inset: whole time course of the Fura-2/AM ratio after exposure to 100 μM MA before the addition of 132 μM digitonin (dig) (representative assay). **c** and **f** Calcium response in cells triggered by 1 % ethanol or 1 % DMSO, 100 μM MA or 30 μM LA alone or after preincubation with 100 μM 2-APB, 10 μM GW1100, 4 μM U73122 (U7), or 20 μM nifedipine (NIFE) for 15 min. Cells were incubated for 16 h with 100 ng/ml pertussis toxin (PTX) before MA or LA supplementation. The data are expressed as the means ± SEM of at least three independent experiments. $^{*}p < 0.05$, $^{**}p < 0.01$, $^{***}p < 0.005$

or LA and evaluated the cells for NO production using DAF-FM signals. Only LA significantly increased the DAF-FM fluorescence intensity in BUVEC monolayers. As illustrated in Fig. 4a, the DAF-FM signal increased approximately 1.5-fold in LA-exposed BUVECs compared with the signal in cells treated with vehicle (DMSO). The increase in NO induced by LA was reduced by 25 % when the cells were treated with 100 μM L-NAME, a potent endothelial nitric oxide synthase (eNOS) inhibitor (Fig. 4c). This indicates that LA activates eNOS in primary bovine endothelial cells. Treatment with BAPTA, EGTA, or BAPTA plus EGTA reduced the increase in NO induced by LA by 50, 91, and 86 %, respectively (Fig. 4b). In contrast, neither 4 μM U73122, 10 μM GW1100, 100 μM 2-APB, 20 μM nifedipine, nor 100 ng/ml PTX reduced the LA-mediated increase in NO (data not shown).

LA but not MA increases ICAM-1 and IL-8 mRNA expression

Because only LA effectively increased eNOS activity in BUVECs, we tested whether LA also affects ICAM-1 or IL-8 expression. Only LA induced the expression of ICAM-1 and IL-8 mRNAs in BUVECs, and LA-induced IL-8 expression was significantly inhibited by GW1100. However, the expression of ICAM-1 was not reduced by treatment with the FFAR1/GPR40 antagonist (Fig. 5).

Discussion

The NEFA levels in blood plasma are particularly elevated during the transition period in dairy cattle, when lipids are strongly mobilized from the adipose tissues to the bloodstream, with plasma concentrations increasing from the basal level of 0.1 mM to 0.7–2 mM [1, 25–27]. Until now, the involvement of G-coupled fatty acid receptors, such as FFAR1/GPR40, in the NEFA-mediated calcium response in primary endothelial cells has been unclear. This study has demonstrated that single NEFAs alone, at low concentrations of 0.3 mM, increase the intracellular calcium response in primary bovine endothelial cells, inducing different molecular pathways involved in the endothelial cell activation process. In naturally occurring acute systemic coliform mastitis linoleic acid and oleic acid were the most abundant NEFA, suggesting that specific fatty acids can be involved in inflammation and innate immunity, and to be relevant as risk factors during the transition period [28].

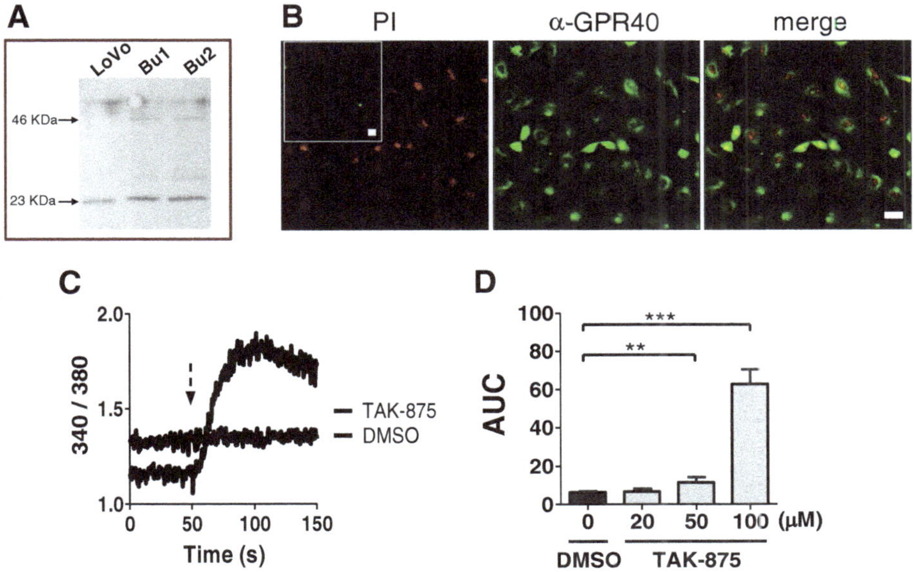

Fig. 3 Protein expression and functional detection of FFAR1/GPR40 in BUVEC monolayers. **a** Western blot of bovine FFAR1/GPR40. Total protein extract from LoVo cells was used as the positive control for two BUVEC isolates. 50 μg of total protein was loaded onto a 6 % polyacrylamide gel. **b** FFAR1/GPR40 immunofluorescence. *Left image*, nuclear signals of cells incubated with propidium iodide (PI); inset image: only the secondary antibody was used, as the negative control, bar = 20 μm. *Middle image*, FFAR1/GPR40 detected with rabbit anti-GPR40 antiserum and an anti-rabbit IgG secondary antibody. *Right image*, nuclear signals and GPR40 images are superimposed, bar = 20 nm. **c** Representative time course of the Fura-2/AM ratio in BUVECs exposed to 1 % DMSO or 100 μM TAK-875 at the time indicated by the arrow. **d** Cells were exposed to DMSO or TAK-875. The area under the curve (AUC) was calculated during the first 100 s after exposure to the stimulus. The data are expressed as the means ± SEM of at least three independent experiments. $^{**}p < 0.01$, $^{***}p < 0.005$

Different studies have reported the potency with which MA and LA bind to human FFAR1/GPR40 in transfected CHO and HEK293 cells by measuring the calcium signal. For MA, a EC_{50} value has been described in these cells, close to 7 μM, but for LA, the EC_{50} values ranged from 1.8 to 6.6 μM [11, 12]. In contrast, the EC_{50} values for MA and LA were 30.3 and 38.4 μM, respectively, in a reporter cell line based on HeLa cells transfected with hGPR40 [29]. These results are quite similar to those observed in the present study, especially regarding the stimulatory potency of LA. Because many of the effects of NEFAs on primary bovine endothelial cells could be attributed to bGPR40, including increased intracellular calcium influx, the presence of this specific NEFA receptor was assessed in BUVECs in this study. We detected FFAR1/GPR40 expression in BUVECs, and also evaluated its effect on the calcium flux using the agonist TAK-875 in our in vitro primary bovine endothelial cell system. There is some evidence that FFAR1/GPR40 is expressed in bovine cells and bovine FFAR1/GPR40 has been shown to share 84 % nucleotide sequence identity with the human isoform [13, 14]. Previous studies have examined the expression of GPR40 in endothelial cells from monkey brain tissues [30], neuromicrovascular cells from rodent tissues [31], and human cardiac endothelial cells [32]. To the best of our knowledge, this work is the first to report the expression of GPR40 in primary bovine endothelial cells.

Our data also suggest that the MA-mediated increase in calcium occurs when MA binds to bGPR40, because it was clearly inhibited by GW1100, a potent FFAR1/GPR40 antagonist. In contrast, the increase in calcium induced by LA does not involve this receptor, according to our antagonist experiments. We also observed that IP_3 receptors/calcium-operated channels and LTCCs seem to participate in the cellular responses to MA and LA, respectively. Others have shown, that OA increased the calcium signal in HEK 293 cells transiently transfected with the α1 subunits of the LTCCs [23]. The pathway of calcium entry *via* the LTCCs induced by NEFAs is evidently cell-type dependent. LTCCs were also associated with the increase in calcium mediated by FFAR1/GPR40 activation that was induced by the saturated fatty acid PA in rat β-cell line INS-1E [22], by the unsaturated fatty acid OA in islet β-cells from rats [33], and by LA in primary cultured chicken hepatocytes [34]. Our examination of the cellular calcium flux suggests that MA, but not LA, recognizes FFAR1/GPR40 in BUVECs. The *CACNA2D1* gene encodes the alpha 2/delta subunit which is an accessory part of the voltage-gated calcium channel family (e.g., LTCC) and considered to be an important candidate protein influencing bovine mastitis

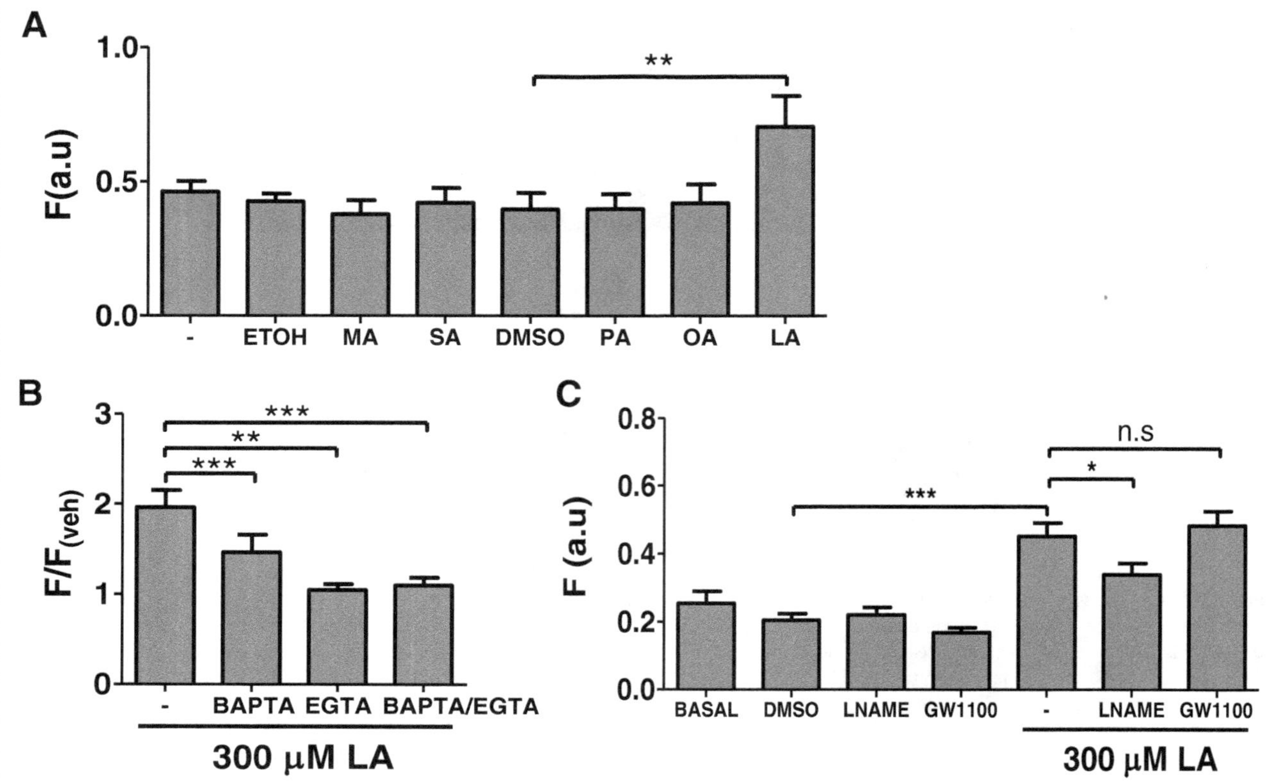

Fig. 4 NEFA effects on nitric oxide production in BUVECs. **a** Basal DAF fluorescence (–), and after treatment with 0.1 % ethanol, 300 μM myristic acid (MA), 300 μM stearic acid (SA), 0.1 % DMSO (D), 300 μM palmitic acid (PA), 300 μM oleic acid (OA), or 300 μM linoleic acid (LA) for 5 min at 37 °C. **b** DAF fluorescent signal after incubation with 300 μM LA for 5 min, normalized to the signal without fatty acids. The cells were incubated with BAPTA, EGTA, or BAPTA + EGTA before treatment with LA. **c** Effect of L-NAME and GW1100 on the LA-induced increase in the DAF signal. Basal fluorescence. DAF fluorescence is expressed in arbitrary units (a.u.). Each bar represents the mean ± SEM of at least three independent experiments. $^*p < 0.05$, $^{**}p < 0.01$, $^{***}p < 0.005$

[35]. Although many publications have reported LTCC activity in bovine immune cells, there is not yet any evidence that these channels are expressed in bovine endothelial cells. In the present study, nifedipine affected BUVECs, suggesting the participation of LTCCs. It has also been recently demonstrated that the increase in calcium caused by endothelin-1 is LTCC-dependent in cultured bovine corneal endothelial cells [36].

We also evaluated the NO response in NEFA-exposed bovine endothelium, because NO is a well-known indicator of inflammation [37]. All NEFAs were evaluated, but only LA increased NO in the endothelial cells. This response was dependent on both calcium and eNOS. There is evidence that eNOS activity is dependent on Ca^{2+}/calmodulin [38], and it is probable that the increase in NO is a secondary effect after the interaction of eNOS with Ca^{+2}/calmodulin. Both NO and eNOS actively participate in the regulation of vascular tone and are therefore important intracellular enzymes, especially in microvascular hyperpermeability [39]. There is some evidence that increased levels of NO in endothelial cells produce proinflammatory profiles, which might lead to metabolic diseases. LA induces reactive oxygen species (ROS) and the overproduction of NO after an increase in calcium, causing peroxynitration in endothelial cells [40]. NF-κB, a crucial transcription factor, is then activated by peroxynitrite, a potent oxidative agent, inducing the expression of adhesion molecules [40] and chemokines, such as IL-8 [41]. We also demonstrated that LA, but not MA, induces ICAM-1- and IL-8-expression, suggesting an active role for NO in this response. In bovine endothelial cell cultures, high concentrations of total NEFAs might increase ICAM-1 mRNA and protein expression [6]. The LA-induced adhesion molecules and chemokines may participate in leukocyte-endothelial cell interactions, facilitating transendothelial migration [42], and may play a role in the onset of a proinflammatory process during the transition period in dairy cattle. Massive lipid mobilization leading to an increase in plasma NEFAs is observed in cows around parturition, causing an increased incidence of metabolic and infectious diseases, including laminitis, endometritis, and mastitis

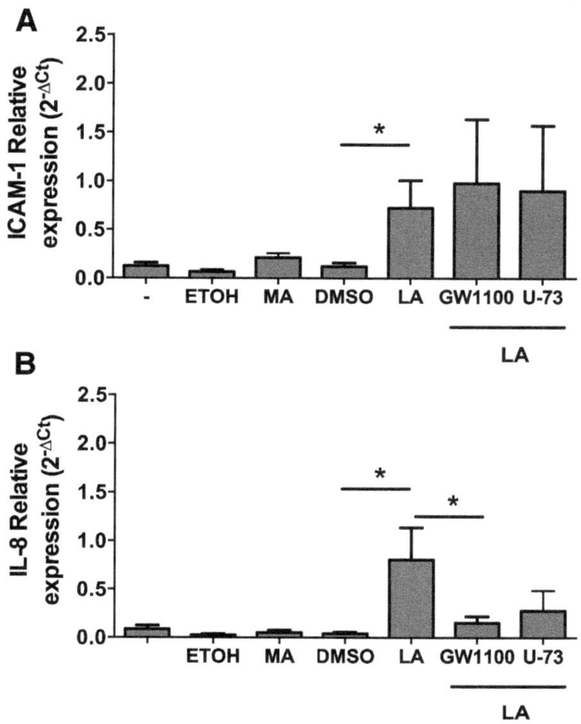

Fig. 5 NEFA effects on ICAM-1 and IL-8 expression in BUVECs. Cells were treated with 0.1 % ethanol, 300 μM myristic acid (MA), 0.1 % DMSO, 300 μM oleic acid (OA), or 300 μM linoleic acid (LA) for 3 h and their RNAs were then isolated. Some cells were treated with 10 μM GW1100 or 4 μM U73122 (U-73) for 30 min before the LA treatment. The expression of ICAM-1 and IL-8 was analyzed with real-time PCR using specific primers. Relative abundance = $2^{-\Delta Ct}$, where ΔCt = cycle treshold ICAM-1 or Ct IL-8 minus cycle treshold SDHA. The data are expressed as the means ± SEM of three experiments. *$p < 0.05$

[1–4]. The exposure of bovine endothelial cells to NEFAs increases the expression of the proinflammatory cytokines IL-6 and IL-8 and the adhesion molecules ICAM-1 and VCAM-1 [6]. It has also been postulated that the excessive accumulation of NEFAs during chronic inflammatory responses might increase TNFα, IL-6, and IL-1β expression by activating NF-κB in adipocytes and macrophages. These cytokines are thought to link the metabolic state and the inflammatory response, usually in the postpartum period within the uteri of cows [3, 4].

There is evidence that endothelial calcium participates in the transendothelial lymphocyte migration caused by ICAM-1 [43]. Moreover, an intracellular calcium increase has been related with ICAM-1 expression in HUVEC [44]. However, in BUVECs, intracellular calcium increase could be not directly associated with the expression of ICAM-1 or IL-8. Consistently with these assumption MA increased calcium flux was not sufficient to increase the expression of these molecules and the inhibition of PLC did not reduce the expression of ICAM-1 and IL-8 induced by LA. Our data also demonstrate that the individual NEFAs have different effects on endothelial cell activity and diverse mechanisms of action. LA induces the expression of ICAM-1 independently of FFAR1/GPR40 or PLC activity, although the expression of IL-8 is associated with the activation of FFAR1/GPR40 in BUVECs. In contrast, our results showed that NO was induced by LA, in a rather G-protein-coupled-receptor-independent process. There is some evidence that these receptors need not bind to a G-protein in the presence of high agonist concentrations, which thereby alternatively activate the ERK/MAPK pathway [45]. It has been suggested that LA activates the phosphoinositide 3-kinase, ERK1/2, and p-38 MAPK pathways in vascular endothelial cells [46]. In our laboratory, we have recently shown that the increase in NO caused by LA is p38-dependent (unpublished data). For this reason, it is possible that LA activates FFAR1/GPR40 or another receptor in a G-protein-independent manner. For instance, we cannot exclude the possibility that the GPR120 receptor recognizes LA by another mechanism [16, 47], or that LA is recognized by GPR84, a medium-chain fatty acid receptor [48], or CD36, a fatty acid transporter protein [49, 50]. Only CD36 expression has been demonstrated in endothelial cells [51]. It has also been proposed that LA mobilizes intracellular calcium *via* an LA metabolite that induces intracellular mitochondrial calcium fluxes [52].

Conclusions

We have demonstrated for the first time in primary bovine endothelial cells that GPR40 is involved in the increase in calcium induced by MA, and conversely, that the LA calcium flux is not associated with this receptor. We have also demonstrated the participation of IP_3 receptors/calcium-operated channels and LTCCs in the cellular responses to MA and LA. We observed FFAR1/GPR40 expression in the bovine endothelium and confirmed its activity using its agonist, TAK-875. Only LA increased NO levels, and this was independent of FFAR1/GPR40. Only LA induced the expression of ICAM-1 and IL-8, and this phenomenon is a FFAR1/GPR40- dependent cellular process. These results indicate that the responses of endothelial cells to individual NEFAs are highly variable. Recently, it has been demonstrated that there is an association of LA enhancement in plasma and milk in naturally occurring acute systemic coliform mastitis [52]. Therefore, the increase in total NEFAs that is described as risk factor for the onset of pro-inflammatory process that occur during transition periods in cattle, should be revised carefully in the future. Further studies are required to determine whether other individual NEFAs participate in the bovine proinflammatory responses in vivo during the transition period and in other NEFA-dependent disorders in cattle.

Methods

Fatty acids

We used those fatty acids that have shown changes during transition period [1]. Myristic and stearic acids were purchased from Sigma Chemical Co. (St. Louis, MO, USA) and suspended in 100 % analytical-grade ethanol (Merck, Germany). Palmitic, oleic, and linoleic acids (Sigma Chemical Co. USA) were prepared in 100 % DMSO (Sigma Chemical Co. USA). Stocks of single fatty acids were prepared at concentrations of 300 mM, protected from light, and stored at −20 °C. To estimate the calcium dose responses, the fatty acids were diluted to the indicated concentrations, with the vehicle maintained at 1 % DMSO or 1 % ethanol to avoid a possible dilution effect of vehicles. Because 300 μM concentrations of all fatty acids were used in the NO experiments, 0.1 % DMSO or 0.1 % ethanol were used as the vehicles. Neither the DMSO nor ethanol concentration used for the calcium and NO assays affected the viability of BUVECs during period of exposure. The working stocks of fatty acids were maintained at 37 °C and were protected from light before to use.

Cell culture

Primary BUVECs were isolated from bovine umbilical cords according to Hermosilla et al. [53]. All bovine umbilical cords were obtained as part of natural parturition procedures at the Clinic for Obstetrics and Gynaecology and Andrology of Large and Small animals, Faculty of Veterinary Medicine, Justus Liebig University Giessen, Germany therefore no intervention was made or ethic approval was requested.

Briefly, the umbilical veins were isolated from the umbilical cords of calves born by cesarean section and kept at 4 °C in sterile 0.9 % Hanks balanced salt solution HBSS–HEPES buffer (w/v; pH 7.4; Gibco, USA) supplemented with 1 % penicillin (v/v; 500 U/ml) and streptomycin (v/v; 500 μg/ml, Sigma-Aldrich) until use. Under sterile conditions, one end of each umbilical cord vein was clamped shut, and 0.025 % collagenase type II (w/v; Worthington Biochemicals Corporation, USA) in Puck's saline A solution (PSA; Gibco, USA) was gently infused into the vein lumens. After the remaining open ends of the umbilical veins were clamped, they were incubated at 37 °C in 5 % CO_2 for 20 min. The umbilical veins were then gently massaged and unclamped, and the resulting collagenase solutions were collected individually in 50 ml plastic tubes (Nunc, USA) containing 1 ml of fetal calf serum (FCS; Gibco) to inactivate the collagenase. The umbilical vein lumens were then washed twice with RPMI 1640 culture medium (Gibco). The washes were pooled, centrifuged (400 × *g*, 10 min), resuspended in complete endothelial cell growth medium (ECGM; PromoCell, Germany), plated in 25 cm^2 plastic tissue culture flasks (Nunc), and incubated at 37 °C in 5 % CO_2. The BUVEC monolayers were fed complete ECGM one day after isolation and then every 2–3 days thereafter. The purity of BUVEC was at least 97 % and characterized by their typical cobblestone morphology and by the incorporation assay of Dil-Ac-LDL (dioactecyltetramethyl-indocarbocyanine perchlorate acetylated low-density lipoprotein) as described elsewhere, [54]. The cells were used for the NEFA experiments after 1–6 passages in vitro.

BUVEC cultures were fed three times a week with modified ECGM culture medium: 70 % M199 (Gibco) with 30 % complete ECGM supplemented with epithelial and endothelial growth factors, heparin (all from PromoCell), 2 mM glutamine, 2 % FCS, 100 U/ml penicillin, and 100 μg/ml streptomycin sulfate (HyClone, Thermo Scientific, USA). The cells were maintained at 37 °C in a 5 % CO_2 atmosphere.

Intracellular calcium measurement

For the NEFA experiments, BUVEC monolayers were trypsinized with 0.25 % trypsin/EDTA (Gibco) from plastic tissue culture plates (Life Technologies, USA), and 5×10^6 cells/ml were suspended and incubated for 30 min at 37 °C in HEPES-buffered saline (HBS) buffer (concentrations in mM: 150 NaCl, 5 KCl, 1 $CaCl_2$, 1 $MgCl_2$, 20 HEPES, 5 glucose, pH 7.4), supplemented with 10 μM Fura-2-AM and 0.02 % Pluronic F-127 (Invitrogen, Molecular Probes, USA). The unincorporated dye was removed twice with HBS buffer washes. The cells (250,000 cells/ml) were stored in HBS at 4 °C, and then prewarmed for 5 min at 37 °C. Fluorescence intensities were detected every 0.2 s at 509 nm emission and 340/380 nm dual-wavelength excitation in an LS55 spectrofluorometer (PerkinElmer Life Science, USA). The time course of FURA-2/AM in BUVECs was recorded as the ratio of the fluorescent signals without stimulus for 50 s and during exposure to each fatty acid for 100 s. The area under curve (AUC) of calcium flux was calculated for the 100 s of NEFA exposure after background subtraction. The slopes of the increase in the calcium signal caused by fatty acids were calculated with a linear regression adjusted to the first 8 s of the fluorescent signal ratio (340/380) under basal and BAPTA-AM conditions.

NO measurement

Cells were trypsinized, as described above, seeded in a 96-well plate at a density of 20,000 cell/well, and cultured with 100 μl of ECGM-supplemented medium (PromoCell). On day 3, the cells were washed gently once with HBS and incubated for 20 min at room temperature with 5 μM DAF-FM and 0.02 % pluronic acid (Invitrogen, Molecular Probes, USA). The unincorporated dye was removed by washing once with HBS. When the cells were pretreated before fatty acid exposure, they were incubated for 15 min. The cells were then incubated with different NEFAs in the absence and presence of different treatments for 5 min at 37 °C. The DAF-FM signals were then detected with a fluorescence multiplate reader (Varioskan®, Thermo Scientific) at 480 nm excitation/520 nm emission with light detection for 800 ms.

To assess the roles of intracellular and extracellular calcium in the calcium flux and NO production in BUVECs, the cells were incubated for 30 min with 50 μM BAPTA/AM at 37 °C, then washed, and maintained in HBS. For the EGTA treatment, the cells were treated with HEPES-buffered saline without calcium, and EGTA (0.3 mM) was added just before measurement [55].

Immunoblotting

BUVECs were lysed with a previously described method [53], and 50 μg of total protein was loaded onto a 12 % polyacrylamide gel and transferred to a nitrocellulose membrane at 100 mA for 1 h. The nitrocellulose membrane was incubated with blocking buffer for 1 h, and probed overnight at 4 °C with 0.001 μg/μl anti-human-GPR40 antiserum prepared in a rabbit (Abcam, USA). The membrane was washed three times in Tris-buffered saline and then exposed to 1:5000 anti-rabbit-IgG antibody conjugated with horseradish peroxidase (Cell Signaling) for 1 h at room temperature. Blocked antibody solutions were prepared with 1 % fat-free milk phosphate-buffered saline (PBS)–Tween 0.1 % (PBST), and signals were detected with an enhanced chemiluminescence system.

Indirect immunofluorescence

Cells were grown on 12 mm glass coverslips, fixed with 4 % paraformaldehyde (Merck), permeabilized with 100 μM digitonin (Sigma-Aldrich). They were incubated with 0.010 μg/μl anti-GPR40 antiserum (Abcam, USA) overnight at room temperature, and then with 0.4 μg/μl Alexa-Fluor-488-conjugated anti-rabbit IgG antibody (Calbiochem, USA) for 1 h at room temperature. The anti-GPR40 antiserum was raised against the human epitope, but this particular peptide region is conserved in bovine species, as the predictive sequence indicates [13]. This antibody has been used successfully in our laboratory, as described elsewhere [14]. The blocking and antibody solutions were prepared with 1 % BSA–PBST (Sigma-Aldrich). Cell nuclei were stained with 0.1 μg/μl propidium iodide (Invitrogen, Molecular Probes, USA) diluted in PBS. The images were obtained on a Fluoview SV1000® confocal microscope (Olympus) (Centre of Scientific Studies, Valdivia, Chile) equipped with a digital camera.

Cell death assay

Cells were seeded in 96-well plates at 20,000 cells/ml, and on day 3, were washed gently with HBS before exposure to NEFAs for 15 min at 37 °C. As the positive control for cell death, cells were treated with 0.2 % Triton X-100 diluted in HBS at 37 °C for 15 min. BUVECs were treated with different single NEFAs (300 μM LA, PA, OA, MA, or SA), Triton X-100, or 1 % vehicle (DMSO or ethanol). The cells were then incubated with 5 μM propidium iodide (Molecular Probes, Invitrogen) in HBS for 15 min. The propidium iodide signals were detected with a fluorescence multiplate reader (Varioskan®, Thermo Scientific) at 530 nm excitation/620 nm emission.

NEFA effects on adhesion molecule expression in BUVECs

To determine the effects of NEFAs on the expression of adhesion molecules, confluent BUVEC monolayers were treated with 300 μM MA or vehicle (0.1 % ethanol), or 300 μM OA, 300 μM LA, or vehicle (0.1 % DMSO) for 3 h and their total RNA was then isolated. In another set of experiments, BUVECs were preincubated with 10 μM GW1100 or 4 μM U73122 for 30 min before LA treatment.

RNA isolation and RT–PCR analysis

Total RNA was isolated from BUVECs with the E.Z.N.A Total RNA Kit® (Omega Bio-Tek, Norcross, GA, USA), according to the manufacturer's instructions. The samples were treated with ribonuclease-free deoxyribonuclease I (Turbo DNA-free Kit, Ambion, UK) to remove any genomic DNA, and the RNA was quantified with a NanoDrop 2000 spectrophotometer (Thermo Fisher Scientific). For cDNA synthesis, 200 ng of RNA was reverse transcribed in the presence or absence of M-MLV reverse transcriptase (Promega). The PCR reaction was performed with Maxima SYBR Green/ROX qPCR Master Mix and 1 μL of cDNA. The primers for ICAM-1 and IL-8 used in this study were designed previously [15, 53]. SDHA cDNA was also amplified as the housekeeping control [56].

Statistical analysis

The results are illustrated in bar graphs as the means ± SEM of at least four independent experiments. Student's *t* test or one-way analysis of variance and Dunnett's multiple comparison test were performed with a significance level of 5 %, using GraphPad Prism for Mac OS X (ver. 5.0; GraphPad Software, USA).

Additional files

Additional file 1: NEFA treatment did not affect BUVEC cell viability. Cells were incubated for 15 min in the presence of HBS alone (basal), 0.3 mM EGTA (in HBS), solvent (DMSO or ethanol), 300 μM of each fatty acid or 300 μM fatty acid plus EGTA. In other experimental set, cells also were incubated for 30 min with 50 μM BAPTA-AM in HBS and then exposed to each fatty acid for 15 min. Afterwards, the cells were exposed to propidium iodide in HBS for 15 min. The signals of the incorporated propidium iodide were detected with a fluorescence multiplate reader in arbitrary units of fluorescence. Each bar represents the mean ± SEM of at least three independent experiments. Myristic acid (MA), palmitic acid (PA), stearic acid (SA), linoleic acid (LA), oleic acid (OA). $^{**}p < 0.05$ compared with basal.

Additional file 2: Effects of BAPTA and EGTA treatments on the slope of the Fura-2/AM signal in cells treated with myristic acid (MA) palmitic acid (PA), stearic acid (SA), linoleic acid (LA), or oleic acid (OA). Data are means ± standard deviations; NS: not significant.

Additional file 3: Effect of GW110 on the increase in the area under curve of Fura-2/AM, induced with myristic acid (MA) palmitic acid (PA), stearic acid (SA), linoleic acid (LA), or oleic acid (OA). Data are means ± standard deviations; NS: not significant.

Abbreviations
BAPTA-AM: 1,2-Bis(2-aminophenoxy)ethane-N,N,N',N'-tetraacetic acid tetrakis(acetoxymethyl ester); BSA: bovine serum albumin; BUVEC: bovine umbilical vein endothelial cells; DMSO: dimethyl sulfoxide; EGTA: ethylene glycol-bis-(2-aminoethyl)-N,N,N', N'- tetraacetic acid; eNOS: endothelial nitric oxide synthase; ETOH: ethanol; FFAR1: free fatty acid receptor 1; GPR40: G protein-coupled receptor 40; HBS: HEPES buffered saline; HBSS: Hank's balanced salt solution; ICAM-1: intercellular adhesion molecule 1; IL-8: interleukin 8; LA: linoleic acid; LTCC: L-type of calcium channels; MA: myristic acid; NEFA: non-esterified fatty acid; NO: nitric oxide; OA: oleic acid; PA: palmitic acid; PTX: Pertuxis toxin; SA: stearic acid; VCAM-1: vascular cell adhesion molecule 1.

Competing interests
The authors declare that they have no competing interests.

Authors' contributions
AL took part in all the experiments, MDC helped to carry out RT-PCR experiments, RBA and MAH helped to write the manuscript. RBA and AL designed all the experiments. AT and CH participated in the BUVEC isolation, cell culture and helped in RT-PCR. All authors have read and approved the final manuscript.

Acknowledgements
This work was supported by FONDECYT grants 3120255, 1120718, 1151047 and FONDEF IDeA grant ID14I10050. The authors would like to thank Felipe Barros for granting access to the confocal microcopy unit in the CECS, Valdivia, Chile, and Francisco Morera for substantial discussions and encouraging words in developing this research.

Author details
[1]Instituto de Farmacología, Facultad de Ciencias Veterinarias, Universidad Austral de Chile, Valdivia, Chile. [2]Institute of Parasitology, Faculty of Veterinary Medicine, Justus Liebig University Giessen, Giessen, Germany.

References

1. Contreras GA, O'Boyle NJ, Herdt TH, Sordillo LM. Lipomobilization in periparturient dairy cows influences the composition of plasma nonesterified fatty acids and leukocyte phospholipid fatty acids. J Dairy Sci. 2010;93(6):2508–16.
2. Contreras GA, Sordillo LM. Lipid mobilization and inflammatory responses during the transition period of dairy cows. Comp Immunol Microbiol Infect Dis. 2011;34(3):281–9.
3. LeBlanc SJ. Interactions of metabolism, inflammation, and reproductive tract health in the postpartum period in dairy cattle. Reprod Domest Anim. 2012;47:18–30.
4. Sordillo LM, Raphael W. Significance of metabolic stress, lipid mobilization, and inflammation on transition Cow disorders. Vet Clin North Am Food Anim Pract. 2013;29(2):267–78.
5. Cook-Mills JM, Deem TL. Active participation of endothelial cells in inflammation. J Leukoc Biol. 2005;77(4):487–95.
6. Contreras GA, Raphael W, Mattmiller SA, Gandy J, Sordillo LM. Nonesterified fatty acids modify inflammatory response and eicosanoid biosynthesis in bovine endothelial cells. J Dairy Sci. 2012;95(9):5011–23.
7. Lacetera N, Scalia D, Franci O, Bernabucci U, Ronchi B, Nardone A. Short communication: effects of nonesterified fatty acids on lymphocyte function in dairy heifers. J Dairy Sci. 2004;87(4):1012–4.
8. Scalia D, Lacetera N, Bernabucci U, Demeyere K, Duchateau L, Burvenich C. In vitro effects of nonesterified fatty acids on bovine neutrophils oxidative burst and viability. J Dairy Sci. 2006;89(1):147–54.
9. Hajri T, Abumrad NA. Fatty acid transport across membranes: relevance to nutrition and metabolic pathology. Annu Rev Nutr. 2002;22:383–415.
10. Kremmyda LS, Tvrzicka E, Stankova B, Zak A. Fatty acids as biocompounds: their role in human metabolism, health and disease - a review. Part 2: fatty acid physiological roles and applications in human health and disease. Biomed Pap. 2011;155(3):195–218.
11. Itoh Y, Kawamata Y, Harada M, Kobayashi M, Fujii R, Fukusumi S, Ogi K, Hosoya M, Tanaka Y, Uejima H, et al. Free fatty acids regulate insulin secretion from pancreatic beta cells through GPR40. Nature. 2003;422(6928):173–6.
12. Briscoe CP, Tadayyon M, Andrews JL, Benson WG, Chambers JK, Eilert MM, Ellis C, Elshourbagy NA, Goetz AS, Minnick DT, et al. The orphan G protein-coupled receptor GPR40 is activated by medium and long chain fatty acids. J Biol Chem. 2003;278(13):11303–11.
13. Yonezawa T, Haga S, Kobayashi Y, Katoh K, Obara Y. Unsaturated fatty acids promote proliferation via ERK1/2 and Akt pathway in bovine mammary epithelial cells. Biochem Bioph Res Co. 2008;367(4):729–35.
14. Hidalgo MA, Nahuelpan C, Manosalva C, Jara E, Carretta MD, Conejeros I, Loaiza A, Chihuailaf R, Burgos RA. Oleic acid induces intracellular calcium mobilization, MAPK phosphorylation, superoxide production and granule release in bovine neutrophils. Biochem Bioph Res Co. 2011;409(2):280–6.
15. Mena J, Manosalva C, Ramirez R, Chandia L, Carroza D, Loaiza A, Burgos RA, Hidalgo MA. Linoleic acid increases adhesion, chemotaxis, granule release, intracellular calcium mobilisation, MAPK phosphorylation and gene expression in bovine neutrophils. Vet Immunol Immunopathol. 2013;151(3–4):275–84.
16. Briscoe CP, Peat AJ, McKeown SC, Corbett DF, Goetz AS, Littleton TR, McCoy DC, Kenakin TP, Andrews JL, Ammala C, et al. Pharmacological regulation of insulin secretion in MIN6 cells through the fatty acid receptor GPR40: identification of agonist and antagonist small molecules. Br J Pharmacol. 2006;148(5):619–28.
17. Bokoch GM, Katada T, Northup JK, Hewlett EL, Gilman AG. Identification of the predominant substrate for ADP-ribosylation by islet activating protein. J Biol Chem. 1983;258(4):2072–5.
18. Bleasdale JE, Thakur NR, Gremban RS, Bundy GL, Fitzpatrick FA, Smith RJ, Bunting S. Selective inhibition of receptor-coupled phospholipase C-dependent processes in human platelets and polymorphonuclear neutrophils. J Pharmacol Exp Ther. 1990;255(2):756–68.
19. Bishara NB, Murphy TV, Hill MA. Capacitative Ca(2+) entry in vascular endothelial cells is mediated via pathways sensitive to 2 aminoethoxydiphenyl borate and xestospongin C. Br J Pharmacol. 2002;135(1):119–28.
20. Bootman MD, Collins TJ, Mackenzie L, Roderick HL, Berridge MJ, Peppiatt CM. 2-aminoethoxydiphenyl borate (2-APB) is a reliable blocker of store-operated Ca2+ entry but an inconsistent inhibitor of InsP3-induced Ca2+ release. FASEB J. 2002;16(10):1145–50.
21. Putney JW. Pharmacology of Store-operated Calcium Channels. Mol Interv. 2010;10(4):209–18.
22. Shapiro H, Shachar S, Sekler I, Hershfinkel M, Walker MD. Role of GPR40 in fatty acid action on the beta cell line INS-1E. Biochem Bioph Res Co. 2005;335(1):97–104.

23. Tian YR, Corkey RF, Yaney GC, Goforth PB, Satin LS, de Vargas LM. Differential modulation of L-type calcium channel subunits by oleate. Am J Physiol Endoc M. 2008;294(6):E1178–86.
24. Negoro N, Sasaki S, Mikami S, Ito M, Suzuki M, Tsujihata Y, Ito R, Harada A, Takeuchi K, Suzuki N, et al. Discovery of TAK-875: a potent, selective, and orally bioavailable GPR40 agonist. Acs Med Chem Lett. 2010;1(6):290–4.
25. Douglas GN, Rehage J, Beaulieu AD, Bahaa AO, Drackley JK. Prepartum nutrition alters fatty acid composition in plasma, adipose tissue, and liver lipids of periparturient dairy cows. J Dairy Sci. 2007;90(6):2941–59.
26. Leroy JLMR, Vanholder T, Mateusen B, Christophe A, Opsomer G, de Kruif A, Genicot G, Van Soom A. Non-esterified fatty acids in follicular fluid of dairy cows and their effect on developmental capacity of bovine oocytes in vitro. Reproduction. 2005;130(4):485–95.
27. Melendez P, Marin MP, Robles J, Rios C, Duchens M, Archbald L. Relationship between serum nonesterified fatty acids at calving and the incidence of periparturient diseases in Holstein dairy cows. Theriogenology. 2009;72(6):826–33.
28. Mavangira V, Gandy JC, Zhang C, Ryman VE, Daniel Jones A, Sordillo LM. Polyunsaturated fatty acids influence differential biosynthesis of oxylipids and other lipid mediators during bovine coliform mastitis. J Dairy Sci. 2015;98(9):6202–15.
29. Kotarsky K, Nilsson NE, Flodgren E, Owman C, Olde B. A human cell surface receptor activated by free fatty acids and thiazolidinedione drugs. Biochem Bioph Res Co. 2003;301(2):406–10.
30. Ma D, Lu L, Boneva NB, Warashina S, Kaplamadzhiev DB, Mori Y, Nakaya MA, Kikuchi M, Tonchev AB, Okano H, et al. Expression of free fatty acid receptor GPR40 in the neurogenic niche of adult monkey hippocampus. Hippocampus. 2008;18(3):326–33.
31. Honore JC, Kooli A, Hamel D, Alquier T, Rivera JC, Quiniou C, Hou X, Kermorvant-Duchemin E, Hardy P, Poitout V, et al. Fatty acid receptor Gpr40 mediates neuromicrovascular degeneration induced by transarachidonic acids in rodents. Arterioscl Throm Vas. 2013;33(5):954–U202.
32. Lu ZY, Li YC, Jin JF, Zhang XM, Hannun YA, Huang Y. GPR40/FFA1 and neutral sphingomyelinase are involved in palmitate-boosted inflammatory response of microvascular endothelial cells to LPS. Atherosclerosis. 2015;240(1):163–73.
33. Fujiwara K, Maekawa F, Yada T. Oleic acid interacts with GPR40 to induce Ca2+ signaling in rat islet beta-cells: mediation by PLC and L-type Ca2+ channel and link to insulin release. Am J Physiol Endocrinol Metab. 2005;289(4):E670–677.
34. Suh HN, Huong HT, Song CH, Lee JH, Han HJ. Linoleic acid stimulates gluconeogenesis via Ca2+/PLC, cPLA(2), and PPAR pathways through GPR40 in primary cultured chicken hepatocytes. Am J Physiol Cell Ph. 2008;295(6):C1518–27.
35. Deb R, Singh U, Kumar S, Kumar A, Singh R, Sengar G, Mann S, Sharma A. Genotypic to expression profiling of bovine calcium channel, voltage-dependent, alpha-2/delta subunit 1 gene, and their association with bovine mastitis among Frieswal (HFX Sahiwal) crossbred cattle of Indian origin. Anim Biotechnol. 2014;25(2):128–38.
36. Hong SJ, Wu KY, Wang HZ, Fong JC. Change of cytosolic Ca2+ mobility in cultured bovine corneal endothelial cells by endothelin-1. J Ocul Pharmacol Th. 2003;19(1):1–9.
37. Torreilles J. Nitric oxide: One of the more conserved and widespread signaling molecules. Front Biosci. 2001;6:D1161–72.
38. Fleming I, Busse R. Signal transduction of eNOS activation. Cardiovasc Res. 1999;43(3):532–41.
39. Sanchez FA, Rana R, Gonzalez FG, Iwahashi T, Duran RG, Fulton DJ, Beuve AV, Kim DD, Duran WN. Functional Significance of Cytosolic Endothelial Nitric-oxide Synthase (eNOS) REGULATION OF HYPERPERMEABILITY. J Biol Chem. 2011;286(35):30409–14.
40. Saraswathi V, Wu GY, Toborek M, Hennig B. Linoleic acid-induced endothelial activation: role of calcium and peroxynitrite signaling. J Lipid Res. 2004;45(5):794–804.
41. Kofler S, Nickel T, Weis M. Role of cytokines in cardiovascular diseases: a focus on endothelial responses to inflammation. Clin Sci (Lond). 2005;108(3):205–13.
42. Lawson C, Wolf S. ICAM-1 signaling in endothelial cells. Pharmacol Rep. 2009;61(1):22–32.
43. Etienne-Manneville S, Manneville JB, Adamson P, Wilbourn B, Greenwood J, Couraud PO. ICAM-1-coupled cytoskeletal rearrangements and transendothelial lymphocyte migration involve intracellular calcium signaling in brain endothelial cell lines. J Immunol. 2000;165(6):3375–83.
44. Barnett Jr CC, Moore EE, Silliman CC, Abdalla EK, Partrick DA, Curley SA. Cytosolic phospholipase A(2)-mediated ICAM-1 expression is calcium dependent. J Surg Res. 2001;99:307–10.
45. Sun Y, McGarrigle D, Huang XY. When a G protein-coupled receptor does not couple to a G protein. Mol Biosyst. 2007;3(12):849–54.
46. Hennig B, Lei W, Arzuaga X, Das Ghosh D, Saraswathi V, Toborek M. Linoleic acid induces proinflammatory events in vascular endothelial cells via activation of PI3K/Akt and ERK1/2 signaling. J Nutr Biochem. 2006;17(11):766–72.
47. Watson SJ, Brown AJH, Holliday ND. Differential signaling by splice variants of the human free fatty acid receptor GPR120. Mol Pharmacol. 2012;81(5):631–42.
48. Wang JH, Wu XS, Simonavicius N, Tian H, Ling L. Medium-chain fatty acids as ligands for orphan G protein-coupled receptor GPR84. J Biol Chem. 2006;281(45):34457–64.
49. Gaillard D, Laugerette F, Darcel N, El-Yassimi A, Passilly-Degrace P, Hichami A, Khan NA, Montmayeur JP, Besnard P. The gustatory pathway is involved in CD36-mediated orosensory perception of long-chain fatty acids in the mouse. FASEB J. 2008;22(5):1458–68.
50. Ozdener MH, Subramaniam S, Sundaresan S, Sery O, Hashimoto T, Asakawa Y, Besnard P, Abumrad NA, Khan NA. CD36-and GPR120-mediated Ca2+ signaling in human taste Bud cells mediates differential responses to fatty acids and is altered in obese mice. Gastroenterology. 2014;146(4):995–U544.
51. Kerkhoff C, Sorg C, Tandon NN, Nacken W. Interaction of S100A8/S100A9 - Arachidonic acid complexes with the scavenger receptor CD36 may facilitate fatty acid uptake by endothelial cells. Biochemistry. 2001;40(1):241–8.
52. Zhao YF, Wang L, Qiu JH, Zha DJ, Sun Q, Chen C. Linoleic acid stimulates [Ca2+]i increase in Rat pancreatic beta-cells through both membrane receptor- and intracellular metabolite-mediated pathways. Plos One. 2013;8(4):e60255.
53. Hermosilla C, Zahner H, Taubert A. Eimeria bovis modulates adhesion molecule gene transcription in and PMN adhesion to infected bovine endothelial cells. Int J Parasitol. 2006;36(4):423–31.
54. Taubert A, Hermosilla C. Bovine recombinant IFNgamma induces endothelial cell gene transcription of immunoregulatory molecules and upregulates PMN and PBMC adhesion on bovine endothelial cells. Vet Res Commun. 2008;32(1):35–47.
55. Sandoval AJ, Riquelme JP, Carretta MD, Hancke JL, Hidalgo MA, Burgos RA. Store-operated calcium entry mediates intracellular alkalinization, ERK1/2, and Akt/PKB phosphorylation in bovine neutrophils. J Leukocyte Biol. 2007;82(5):1266–77.
56. De Ketelaere A, Goossens K, Peelman L, Burvenich C. Technical note: validation of internal control genes for gene expression analysis in bovine polymorphonuclear leukocytes. J Dairy Sci. 2006;89(10):4066–9.

2

Prevalence of Bovine Viral Diarrhoea Virus (BVDV), Bovine Herpes Virus 1 (BHV 1), Leptospirosis and Neosporosis, and associated risk factors in 161 Irish beef herds

Damien Barrett[1*], Mervyn Parr[4], John Fagan[2], Alan Johnson[3], Jamie Tratalos[6], Francis Lively[7], Michael Diskin[5] and David Kenny[4]

Abstract

Background: There are limited data available, in Ireland or elsewhere, to determine the extent of exposure to various endemic diseases among beef cows and factors associated with exposure to causative pathogens. The objectives of this study were to determine the herd and within herd prevalence of Bovine Viral Diarrhoea Virus (BVDV), Bovine Herpes Virus 1 (BHV-1), Leptospirosis and Neosporosis in a large scale study of commercial beef herds on the island of Ireland, and to examine herd level factors associated with exposure to these pathogens in these herds.

Results: The average number of cows tested per herd was 35.5 (median 30). Herd level seroprevalence to Bovine Herpesvirus-1(BHV-1), Bovine Viral-Diarrhoea Virus (BVDV), Leptospirosis and Neosporosis was 90%, 100%, 91% and 67%, respectively, while the mean within herd prevalence for the these pathogens was 40%, 77.7%, 65.7% and 5.7%, respectively. The study confirms that the level of seroconversion for the four pathogens of interest increases with herd size. There was also evidence that exposure to one pathogen may increase the risk of exposure to another pathogen.

Conclusions: Herd level seroprevalences were in excess of 90% for BVDV, BHV-1 and Leptosporosis. Larger herds were subject to increased exposure to disease pathogens. This study suggests that exposure to several pathogens may be associated with the further exposure to other pathogens.

Keywords: Beef cow herds, BVDV, BHV-1, Neosporosis, Leptospirosis, Herd size, Pathogen associations

Background

In recent years, the issue of herd health and, in particular, infectious disease has received increasing prominence as a potential factor influencing reproductive efficiency in Ireland and elsewhere. However, despite its obvious critical importance, there are limited published data available, to quantify the influence of various endemic diseases on beef cow and herd fertility. Reproductive performance in beef cow herds is related to several management, physiological and disease factors [1, 2]. The current level of reproductive performance in Irish beef cow herds leave considerable room for improvement in achieving more efficient, sustainable and profitable beef cow beef production [3]. There is a need to establish the prevalences of the most significant infectious diseases associated with impaired reproductive performance.

Numerous bacterial, viral and protozoan pathogens have been associated with infertility and abortion in cattle. BVDV, BHV-1, *Leptospira interrogans* hardjo-bovis

* Correspondence: Damien.barrett@agriculture.gov.ie
[1]Department of Agriculture, Food and the Marine, SAT Division, Admin Building, Backweston, Celbridge, Co. Kildare, Ireland
Full list of author information is available at the end of the article

and *Neospora caninum* are four of the most significant pathogens associated with infertility and abortion in Irish cattle. While non-infectious agents probably contribute more to overall reproductive wastage in cattle, there is limited information on the extent and importance of infectious disease on reproductive performance in Irish beef cow herds.

BVDV is a pestivirus which is endemic in the cattle population of several countries and is responsible for a wide range of clinical syndromes, amongst which are immunosuppression and early embryonic death [4]. In recent years, several countries including the Republic of Ireland and Northern Ireland have initiated national BVD eradication schemes. Data from the national BVD eradication scheme in the Republic of Ireland (initiated in 2012) reveal the presence of one or more BVD virus positive animals is 8.74%, 5.96% and 3.311%, 2.38% of beef herds for the years 2013, 2014, 2015 and 2016, respectively (Graham, personal communication). A recent study showed BVDV seroprevalence of 98% in Irish beef cow beef herds [5]. Furthermore, in a study commissioned by Animal Health Ireland prior to the launch of a national BVD eradication scheme, BVDV was estimated to cost the Irish beef cow industry between €32 and €41 per cow per year [6].

Bovine herpes virus 1 (BHV-1) is associated with clinical syndromes such as rhinotracheitis, pustular vulvovaginitis and balanoposthitis, abortion, infertility, conjunctivitis and encephalitis in cattle [7, 8]. It establishes latent lifelong infection and becomes reactivated during periods of immunosuppression, induced by stressful incidents, resulting in virus excretion when infection becomes re activated [9]. Two recent studies conducted on Irish beef [10, 11] and dairy herds [11] both reported herd level seroprevalence of BHV-1 to be approximately 75% and that this was consistent throughout the country.

Leptospirosis is a bacterial disease of cattle that is characterised by reproductive failure in the form of abortions, stillbirths and birth of weak calves. It is also a zoonotic disease. In cattle, the leptospires of most interest are interrogans hardjo-bovis and -prajitno genotypes (i.e. sub-serovars). A number of studies have reported reduced conception rates in seropositive dairy cows [12, 13].A previous study of Irish beef cow herds has shown that 82% of herds were seropositive for leptospirosis, with 40% of cows within those herds seropositive for leptospirosis [14].

Abortions due to *Neospora caninum* typically occur during the early second trimester, but may occur throughout gestation. A number of authors have suggested that cattle infected with the parasite are two to 12 times more likely to abort compared with uninfected cattle [15, 16]. These can be sporadic, endemic or epidemic-abortions [17]. In a large scale Canadian study, cows seropositive for Neosporosis were 1.43 times more likely to be culled for reproductive inefficiency than seronegative cows [18]. A recent Australian study of Neosporosis in beef cow herds reported that calving rates were 10.4% lower in herds that had one or more animals positive for Neosporosis [19] As far as the authors of this paper are aware, this is the first serological survey for Neosporosis in Irish beef cow herds.

The objectives of this study were to (i) determine the herd and within herd prevalence of BVDV, BHV-1, Leptospirosis and Neosporosis in a large cohort of commercial beef herds on the island of Ireland, and (ii) examine herd level factors associated with exposure to these pathogens in these herds.

Methods

Herd selection and sampling method

In all, 6049 cows in 161 beef cow herds from across the island of Ireland were sampled in this study. Of these, 156 were commercial beef cow herds, including 25 participating in national extension programmes. The remaining five herds were located on state owned research facilities. Blood sampling took place once for each herd over the summer months of either 2014 or 2015, and only spring calving cows within the herds were sampled. Data on herd vaccination and mineral supplementation policies were gathered at the time of sampling.

Ethical statement on blood sampling

All experimental procedures involving animals were licensed by the Irish Health Products Regulatory Authority (HPRA). Protocols were conducted in accordance with the Cruelty to Animals Act (Ireland 1876, as amended by European Communities regulations 2002 and 2005) and the European Community Directive 86/609/EC and were sanctioned by the Teagasc Animal Ethics Committee. Blood samples were collected via the coccygeal vessel into 10 ml non additive containers (Becton Dickenson Vacutainer Systems, Plymouth, UK) for serological analysis.

Laboratory processing

Sera were centrifuged and aliquots for each test were partitioned into serum vials and frozen at −20 °C pending analysis. Sera were screened using commercially available ELISA kits for BVDV, BHV-1, Leptospirosis and Neosporosis in Department of Agriculture, Food and the Marine Regional Veterinary Laboratory service (RVL). In each case the tests were carried out according to the manufacturer's instructions.

For herds where IBR vaccination was reported, the kit used for BHV-1 was the IDEXX IBR gE kit (IDEXX, Maine, USA). The manufacturer's report a sensitivity of

98.41% and a specificity of 99.76%. The cut off for a positive sample was an SN (sample to negative control ratio) value of <0.6.

In herds that did not declare an IBR vaccination policy the testing kit used for BHV-1 was the IDEXX IBR gB X3 (IDEXX, Maine, USA). The cut off for a positive sample for this kit was >55% blocking. The manufacturer's report a sensitivity of 100% and a specificity of 99.8%.

The kit used for BVDV antibody was the Svanovir BVD – Ab Bovine Virus Diarrhoea Virus antibody Test (Boehringer Ingelheim Svanova, Uppsala, Sweden). The cut off for a positive result was a PP (percent positivity) value >35. The manufacturer's report a sensitivity of 100% and a specificity of 98.2%.

The kit used for Leptospirosis antibody was the PrioCHECK *L.hardjo* antibody kit (Thermofischer, Massachusetts, USA). The manufacturer's report a sensitivity of 99% and a specificity of 85%. The cut off for a positive sample was a PP (percent positivity) value of >45%.

The kit used for Neosporosis antibody was the IDEXX Neospora antibody kit (IDEXX, Maine, USA). The manufacturer's report a sensitivity of 97.56% and a specificity of 98.53%. The cut off for a positive sample was a S/P (sample to positive ratio) value of >0.4.

Herd level BVDV status

The herd level BVDV status for each of the Republic of Ireland herds ($n = 139$) was accessed from the Irish Cattle Breeding Federation (ICBF) database for the years 2013, 2014 and 2015. This information was not available for the herds located in Northern Ireland.

Data management and analysis

Data were collated on Microsoft Excel spreadsheets (Microsoft Corporation, Redmond, WA, USA). Details of the herd demographics for Republic of Ireland herds are presented in Table 1. Only serological data and vaccination history were available for Northern Ireland herds. Each farmer was asked to complete a short questionnaire on vaccination and mineral supplementation practices in their herd. The vaccination status of the herd was based on the recall of the owner when completing the questionnaire at the time of sampling. We therefore cannot be certain that vaccinations were carried out in full compliance with the manufacturers' instructions. However, where the farmer reported using a BVDV or Leptospirosis vaccine, these herds were removed from the analysis, in order to ensure, in as much as possible, that the analysis only related to naturally occurring infections. In the case of IBR / BHV-1, only marker vaccines have been available in the Republic of Ireland since 2005, and herds using IBR vaccination were tested with the marker vaccine test kit. Both marker and conventional vaccines are available for purchase in Northern Ireland and this may account for some of the seroconversion seen in the NI herds, as the tests we had available could not differentiate between seroconversion due to natural infection and seroconversion due to the use of a non-marker vaccine.

Herd level registration and movement data were obtained from the Irish Department of Agriculture, Food and the Marine's Animal Identification and Movement (AIM) database and the following variables were calculated for each herd: herd size, number of cows, overall mortality rate, calf mortality up to 30 days of age, calves per cow per year and purchase rate. These variables and herd level prevalence of the various serological tests were calculated and entered into the spreadsheet, in addition to herd vaccination history. Statistical analysis was carried out using Stata 14 (StataCorp LP, Texas, USA). A descriptive statistical analysis of the data was initially conducted. In order to examine the potential for regional differences the herds were divided into seven geographical regions (Fig. 1) as described by Ryan et al. [14].

Relationship between pathogen and within herd seroprevalence

A univariate linear regression analysis was initially carried out using a range of herd level statistics downloaded from the AIM system and with the herd prevalence of

Table 1 Mean and median total herd size, number of cows, overall mortality rate, calf mortality rate up to 30 days, the number of calves per cow per year and purchase rate among Republic of Ireland herds in the study

Region	Herd Size		No cows		Mortality Rate		Calf Mortality rate up to 30 days		Calves per cow per year		Purchase rate	
	Mean	Median	Mean	Median	Mean	Median	Mean	Median	Mean	Median	Mean	Median
1	88	79	46.9	41.5	5.3	5.4	2.8	2	0.98	1	16.2	16.6
2	78	67	33.9	32.5	4.2	3.1	2.2	2	0.87	0.97	17.5	13.8
3	190	134	74.5	54	4.5	3.6	4.9	4.23	0.85	0.99	15.8	15.6
4	131	116	42.7	43	3.4	2.1	4.1	3.3	0.93	1	26.7	13.5
5	158	136	58.4	49	3.6	3.3	4.6	3.6	0.95	1	20.5	16.3
6	172	135	57.4	53.5	3	2.9	3.4	2.9	0.86	1	15.9	13.1
Overall	145	114	53.8	46	3.7	3.2	3.7	2.7	0.9	1	18.6	13.85

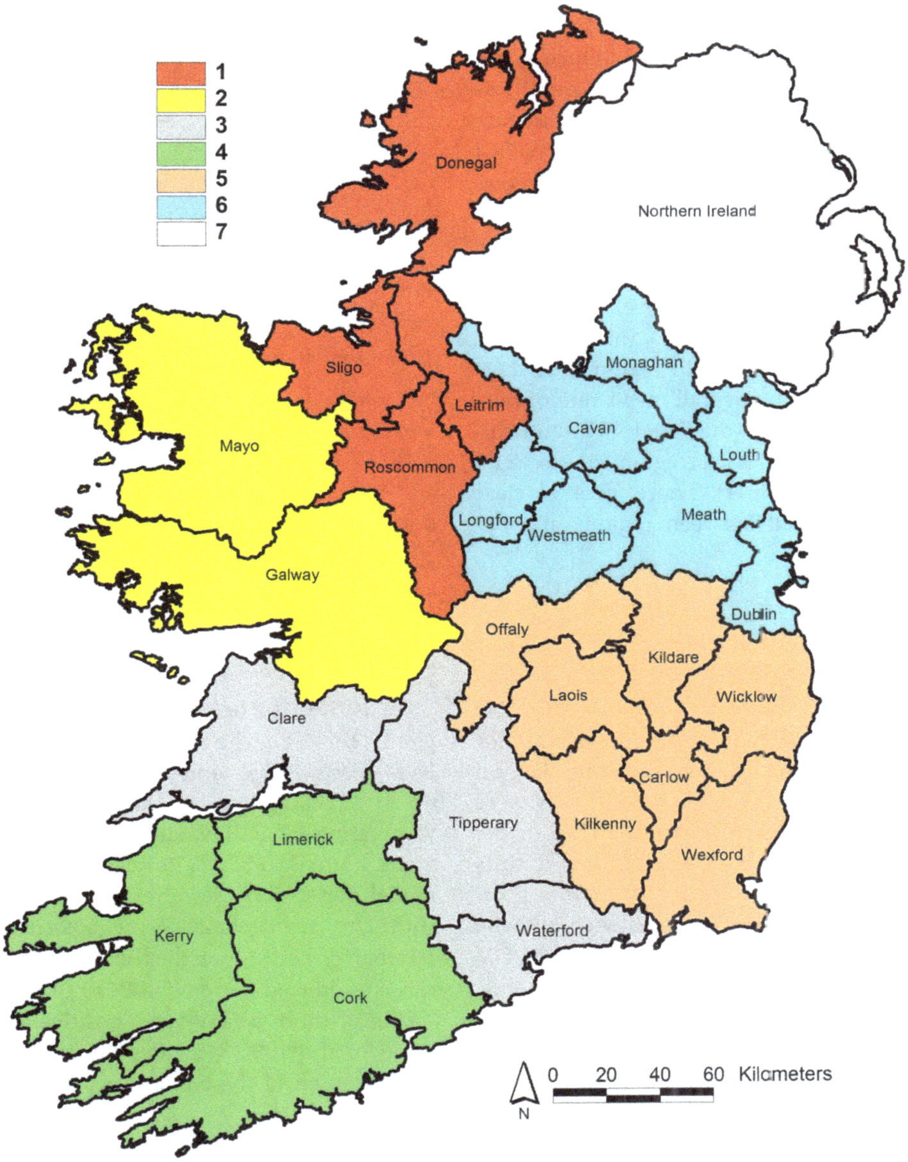

Fig. 1 Geographical spread of the regions employed in the study

each pathogen as the dependent variable of interest. Variables with a *P* value less than 0.2 were then considered for inclusion in a multivariate linear regression model for each pathogen (Tables 4, 6 and 9 and 11). Variables with a P value >0.05 were removed from the model in a stepwise fashion, until the variables remaining in the final model all reached a *P* value <0.05. For Leptospirosis and BVDV data from only non-vaccinating herds were included in the statistical model.

Logistic regression for BVD eradication scheme herd status

In order to identify independent variables for inclusion in a multivariate model for BVDV, univariate logistic regressions was calculated. The dependent variable was the disclosure of BVDV positive calves in the course of the national BVDV eradication scheme, from the inception of the scheme until 2015. Variables with a *P* value less than 0.2 were considered for inclusion in the multivariate model. Variables with a P value >0.05 were removed from the model in a stepwise fashion, until the variables remaining in the final model had a P value <0.05, as outlined for the linear regression analysis above.

Results

There were 14, 18, 16, 17, 48, 26 and 22 herds in Regions 1 to 7 respectively. The mean total herd size was 145.0, which varied from 82.4 (median 70.0) in Region 1 to 172.0 (median 135.0) in Region 4 (Table 1). The mean number of calves born per herd (which was a proxy for the number of breeding cows in the herd) was 53.8 overall (median 46), and similar to the herd size varied from 33.9 (median 36.0) (Region 1) up to 58.4 (median 49.0) (Region 3). The average number of cows tested per herd was 35.5 (median 30). The mean level of overall herd mortality was 3.7% (median 3.2%), ranging from 4.7% (median 3.8%) % in Region 1 to 3.0% (median 2.9%) in region 4. Although the mean level of calf mortality up to 30 days of age was also 3.7% (median 2.7%), this ranged from 2.4% (median 2%) in region 1, to 4.6% (median 3.6%) in region 3. The overall mean rate of purchases into the herds was 18.6, (median 13.85), and this varied from 15.9 (median 13.1) (region 4) to 21.4 (median 16.6) (region 1) (Table 1). There were no clear geographic patterns observed between regions and between herds.

Table 3 A linear regression model of BHV-1sero prevalence with Neospora within herd prevalence, the disclosure of BVD virus positive animals in the herd, herd size, the number of animals dead per year, mortality rate, mortality rate up to 30 days as predictors which fit

	Coef.	Std. Err.	t	P > t	95% Conf. interval	
Neospora within herd sero prevalence	0.852	0.369	2.11	0.022	0.123	1.562
Disclosure of BVD virus positive animals in herd	11.466	5.249	2.18	0.031	1.083	21.851
Herd Size	0.139	0.049	2.84	0.05	0.042	0.236
Overall mortality	−2.416	0.977	−2.47	0.015	−4.350	−0.483
Mortality rate	3.716	1.325	2.80	0.006	1.095	6.337
Mortality rate up to 30 days of age	−0.186	0.076	−2.45	0.015	−0.337	−0.036
Intercept	15.654	6.649	2.35	0.020	2.501	28.807

Number of observations =139
F (6,132) = 4.3
Prob >F = 0.0005
R-square = 0.1636
Adj R- squared = 0.1256
Root MSE = 27.85

Seroprevalence data

For BHV-1, the herd seroprevalence was 90% overall (Table 2, and this ranged from 76% in region 3 to 100% in Region 7. The mean within herd seroprevalence for BHV-1was 39.8%, and ranged from 11.1% in the Region 2 up to 45.5% in Region 7. Overall, 18% of herds were vaccinating for IBR, and this ranged from 11.5% in the Republic of Ireland to 45.5% in Northern Ireland. Results from the multivariate regression model indicated a positive association between BHV-1 seroprevalence and the herd prevalence of Neosporosis, the disclosure of BVDV positive animals within the BVD eradication scheme, herd size, and mortality rate (all age groups) (Table 3). There was a negative association between BHV-1 seroprevalence and calf mortality up to 30 days of age as well as with overall herd mortality.

Table 2 Herd sero prevalence and the percentage of herds vaccinating for BHV-1, the mean and median number of cows tested per herd, and the mean and median within herd BHV-1 sero prevalence

Region	% BHV-1 vaccination	BHV 1 Herd sero prevalence	BHV-1Within Herd Prevalence	
			Mean	Median
1	0	90	49.2	54.8
2	11.1	83	18.6	10.6
3	12.5	94	48.2	46.3
4	11.8	76	30.6	26.9
5	8.8	94	44.1	48.2
6	25.0	96	36.1	33.1
7	45.5	100	52.3	44.5
Overall	18.0	90	39.79	38.1

For BVDV, the herd seroprevalence was 100% in all regions (Table 4). The mean within herd seroprevalence of BVDV was 77.7%, and ranged from 42.8% in Region 2 up to 88.3% in Region 7. Overall, 32.3% of herds were vaccinating for BVDV, and this ranged from 23.5% in regions 4 and 5 to 57.1% in Region 1. The linear regression model for BVDV seroprevalence, showed associations with the seroprevalence of Neosporosis, the overall number of cattle that died in the herd in 2014, and the calves produced per cow in 2014 (Table 5).

One or more BVDV virus positive animals were found in 46 of the 139 (34%) Republic of Ireland herds since the inception of the compulsory BVD programme in the

Table 4 The herd sero prevalence for BVDV, the mean and median within herd BVDV sero prevalence, percentage of herds vaccinating for BVD, and the percentage of herds where a BVDV animal was disclosed

Region	BVDV Herd Sero prevalence	BVDV Within Herd Sero prevalence		% BVD vaccination	% herds with BVD virus positive calves
		Mean	Median		
1	100	71.7	68	57.1	50
2	100	42.8	37.7	38.9	28
3	100	87.8	93.7	25.0	50
4	100	81	98.1	23.5	18
5	100	69.3	72.9	23.5	23
6	100	80.5	88.4	32.5	35
7	100	88.3	96	36.4	NA
Overall	100	77.7	85.2	32.3	34

Table 5 A linear regression model of BVDV sero prevalence with Neospora canium within herd prevalence, the number of animals dead per year, and calves per cow per year as predictors which fit

	Coef.	Std. Err.	t	P > t	95% Conf. interval	
Neospora within herd sero prevalence	0.807	0.402	2.01	0.048	0.008	1.606
Overall mortality	1.550	0.561	2.76	0.007	0.435	2.665
Calves per cow per year	−30.431	13.401	−2.27	0.026	−57.059	−3.804
Intercept	93.377	12.341	7.57	0.000	68.856	117.898

Number of observations =93
F (3,89) = 4.50
Prob >F = 0.0055
R-square = 0.1317
Adj R- squared = 0.1025
Root MSE = 23.47

Republic of Ireland (Table 4). The annual incidence of herds where BVDV positive animals were founded for 2013, 2014 and 2015 were 12.2%, 7.9% and 9.3%. The disclosure of BVD virus positive animals was associated with increasing herd size and increasing BHV-1seroprevalence (Table 6).

For Leptospirosis, the overall herd seroprevalence was 91%, and this ranged from 80% in Region 1 to 100% in Region 7 (Table 7). The mean within herd seroprevalence of leptospirosis was 65.7%, and ranged from 43.4% in Region 4 up to 73.3% in Region 6. Overall, 47.2% of herds were vaccinating for Leptospirosis, and this ranged from 23.5% in Regions 4 to 78.6% in Region 1. There was an association between the use of BVDV vaccine in the herd, the herd size and the purchasing patterns, particularly in 2014 and the Leptospirosis seroprevalence in the Leptospirosis linear regression model (Table 8).

For Neosporosis, the herd prevalence was 67% overall, and this ranged from 44% in Region 2 to 85% in Region 6 (Table 9). The mean within herd seroprevalence of Neosporosis was 5.7%, and ranged from 2.2% in Region 2 up to 7.4% in Region 1. Linear regression revealed a negative association between Neosporosis and both (i) the disclosure of BVDV positive animals in the herd during the BVDV eradication scheme and (ii) herd BHV-1seroprevalence (Table 10).

Table 6 The presence of BVD virus positive animals in the herd logistic regression model

	Odds ratio	Std. Err.	z	P > z	95% Conf. interval	
No cows in herd	1.025	0.010	2.62	0.009	1.006	1.045
BHV-1herd sero prevalence	1.013	0.006	2.02	0.044	1.000	1.026
Intercept	0.118	0.056	−4.51	0.000	0.046	0.298

No of observations =139
LR chi 2 (2) = 12.98
Prob > chi 2 = 0.0015
Pseudo R 2 = 0.0735
Log likelihood = −81.755

Table 7 Herd seroprevalence and within herd sero prevalence and percentage of herds vaccinating for Leptospirosis

Region	Herd Sero Prevalence	Within Herd Sero Prevalence		% Leptosporisis vaccination
		Mean	Median	
1	80	79.2	77.7	78.6
2	83	70.4	81.4	50.0
3	94	68.2	68.3	31.3
4	88	43.4	45.9	23.5
5	94	72.6	83.3	52.9
6	96	73.3	78.6	45.0
7	100	60.7	72.2	50.0
Overall	91	65.7	75.4	47.2

Discussion

This study describes the herd level characteristics of a large scale study of over 6000 beef cows from 161 herds and is the first study of its kind to be conducted across the island of Ireland. The serological sampling and analysis for the four pathogens of interest was carried out specifically for the purposes of the study. To the knowledge of the authors, no previous study has concurrently examined multiple pathogens in the same beef cows, which facilitates the study of potential associations amongst these pathogens on economically important outcomes at herd level. As part of our study we combined seroprevalence data, a targeted brief herd questionnaire, data on the BVDV status of each herd from the ICBF database, and animal identification and movement data (AIM data) for the first time within an Irish context. This is one of the first studies in Europe to integrate data from the national cattle identification and movement database with disease prevalence data, to

Table 8 A linear regression model of leptosporosis sero prevalence with number of cattle purchased in marts and herd size as predictors which fit

	Coef.	Std. Err.	t	P > t	95% Conf. interval	
Herd vaccinating BVD	27.979	12.373	2.26	0.027	3.293	52.664
No of mart purchases in 2014	0.247	0.081	3.03	0.003	0.084	0.041
Herd size	0.093	0.029	3.21	0.002	0.035	0.151
Intercept	44.929	5.013	8.96	0.000	34.928	54.93

Number of observations =73
F (3,69) = 9.92
Prob >F = 0.000
R-squared = 0.3013
Adj R- squared = 0.2709
Root MSE = 23.942

Table 9 Herd and within herd seroprevalences for Neospora canium

Region	Neospora herd sero prevalence	Within Herd Prevalence	
		Mean	Median
1	60	7.4	6.6
2	44	2.2	0
3	75	4.5	2.05
4	76	6.2	3.3
5	71	6	3.9
6	85	5.9	5
7	55	6.9	2.45
Overall	67	5.7	3.7

identify risk factors associated with the occurrence of BHV-1, BVDV, Leptospirosis and Neosporosis.

Increasing herd size emerged as a factor associated with seroconversion to BHV-1, BVDV and Leptospirosis, and the disclosure of BVDV positive animals. Herd size has previously been documented as a significant risk factor associated with exposure to these pathogens in Ireland [5, 11, 14, 20]. Similar experiences have been documented internationally for several pathogens. Increasing herd size increases the probability of an individual animal becoming exposed to pathogens and becoming a carrier animal, and is a well recognised risk factor for the occurrence of disease. Larger herds are likely to have management practices which could predispose them to exposure to the pathogens. Additionally the purchase of animals into the herd is often required to achieve increased herd size but this too is an acknowledged risk factor associated with exposure to pathogens.

There were numerous associations identified between the pathogens under investigation. For example, the seroprevalence of BHV-1was associated with the seroprevalence of Neosporosis, and the disclosure of BVDV

Table 10 A linear regression model of Neospora caninum sero prevalence with BHV-1sero prevalence and the disclosure of BVD virus positive calves as predictors which fit

	Coef.	Std. Err.	t	P > t	95% Conf. interval	
BHV-1Herd sero prevalence	0.045	0.018	2.45	0.016	0.008	0.082
Disclosure of BVD virus positive animals in herd	−2.355	1.171	−2.01	0.046	−4.671	−0.040
Intercept	4.531	0.907	5.00	0.000	2.739	6.325

Number of observations =139
F (2,136) = 4.18
Prob >F = 0.0173
R-squared = 0.0579
Adj R- squared = 0.044
Root MSE = 6.357

positive calves in the herd. Indeed, the role of co-infection has been previously described by Van Leeuwen et al. [15], where cows seropositive for Bovine Leukaemia Virus (BLV) were 1.5 times more likely to be seropositive for Neosporosis than BLV seronegative cows. Another possible explanation is that infection with one of the pathogens could facilitate infection with another. The role of BVDV, in particular, as an immunosuppressive agent is well documented [4].

BHV-1

In addition to herd size and associations with other pathogens increased BHV-1 seroprevalence was associated with increased overall herd mortality rates. Previous studies have reported herd level seroprevalences of 77% and 74% in Northern Ireland and the Republic of Ireland, respectively [5, 20]. The 90% BHV-1 herd prevalence reported in the present study would indicate that BHV-1 is endemic in the Irish cattle population. The level of herd prevalence described here is probably related to the relatively large size of the participating herds. An earlier study also found a significant association between BHV-1 seroprevalence and herd size in Ireland [11]. Previous studies have reported IBR vaccine usage of 1.8% and 11% in the Republic of Ireland and Northern Ireland respectively [11, 20]. The comparable levels of IBR vaccination in the present study, were 11.5% and 45.5% respectively, which is a marked increase on the previous studies by Cowley et al., [11, 20]. This may reflect a greater awareness of animal health issues among the owners of our study herds employed here, which included research herds and herds participating in Knowledge Transfer demonstration programmes.

BVDV seroprevalence

Previous studies have described herd level seroconversion to BVDV in excess of 98% in both the Republic of Ireland and Northern Ireland [5, 20]. Similar levels of herd seroconversion to BVDV have been reported in England and Wales [21]. In our study 32% of herds were vaccinated for BVD, which is substantially greater than the rates of 2.2% in the Republic of Ireland and 16% in Northern Ireland reported in studies of beef herds [5, 20]. We found evidence of an association between seroprevalence of both BVDV and Neosporosis. BVDV seroprevalence was also positively associated with the total herd mortality (2014) in the herd. There was a negative association between the calves produced per cow per year (2014) and increased BVDV seroprevalence in the herd. Both of these findings are not unexpected as BVDV infection is associated with increased calf morbidity, increased mortality as well as early embryonic death [22], which would decrease the number of calves per cow per year.

Disclosure of BVD virus positive calves

The disclosure of BVDVpositive calves was related to the seroprevalence of BHV-1and herd size. One third of the Republic of Ireland study herds participating in the national BVD eradication scheme reported one or more BVD virus positive calves in the initial 3 years of the scheme [23]. The disclosure of BVDV positive calves in many of the herds in this study could account for the high levels of herd and within herd seroconversion observed. Herd size was a significant risk factor in this study which is consistent with previous Irish reports [24]. It is of note that the disclosure of BVDV positive calves in the herds in this study was consistently higher than herds in the general population as recorded as part of the Irish national BVD eradication scheme [23].

Leptospirosis seroprevalence

In addition to herd size, the seroprevalence of Leptospirosis was associated with the level of livestock mart purchases in 2014. It is difficult to determine the significance of this, as it was only found to reach statistical significance in 2014. This association is likely to be biosecurity related, and was associated with movement of animals between holdings and spread within holdings.

In this study there was evidence of seroconversion among 90% of non-vaccinating herds, which was greater than the 82% herd level seroprevalence described in a previous Irish study of beef cow herds [14] (Table 7). The mean within herd seroprevalence was 75%, which was almost twice the rate of the 40% seroprevalence described by Ryan et al., [14]. That study concluded it was likely that there were carrier animals actively transmitting leptospires at the seroprevalences described in their study. They also described a regional effect in relation to Leptospirosis seroprevalence, although no such pattern was observed in our study. They also reported a positive association between herd seroprevalence and herd size. Previously, Leptospirosis was described as independent of region and rainfall [25]. A previous UK study has described a 24.2% seroprevalence in beef herds [26]. The high within herd seroprevalence in our study is probably related to the fact that beef calves spend relatively more time in contact with adult cows than do dairy calves and there is consequently a greater risk of exposure to carrier animals in the herd. In addition, this contact is greater during winter housing, where calves tend to be kept on creep areas and are able to enter a pen of calved cows, some of which may be carriers. In this study, almost half of herds (47%) were vaccinating for Leptospirosis, which is substantially greater than the 3% described by Ryan et al., [14].

Neospora seroprevalence

The herd seroprevalence for Neosporosis of 67% reported here is almost identical to that of a similar study in Australian beef cow herds [19], which also reported a within herd seroprevalence similar to our findings. The within-herd prevalence of Neosporosis was relatively low compared to the other three pathogens studied, which probably reflects the fact that transmission of Neosporosis, is, for the most part vertical [27]. A previous US study found prevalence was lower among beef cows grazed on pasture as opposed to housed cows [28]. This might suggest that horizontal transmission, or exposure from a point source, could account for herds with a higher within herd seroprevalence. Exposure to *Neospora caninum* has previously been associated with the presence of dogs and wild canine species such as foxes on the farm [15, 16]. In our study, participants were not asked about the presence of dogs on the farm, but it is worthy of further consideration. The seroprevalence of Neosporosis was associated with the seroprevalence of BHV-1and the disclosure of BVDV positive animals in the herd. Seroconversion to Neosporosis has also previously been linked to the presence of BVDV exposure in herds [15].

The farmers that participated in our study volunteered to do so and were not evenly distributed across the island of Ireland. Region did not emerge as a significant variable in any of the multivariate analyses and the disease prevalences in the various regions were broadly similar. While this study may not be representative of beef cow herds overall, participating herds came from a wide range of sizes, which enabled us to adequately investigate the effect of herd size.

While there are few perfect serological tests available, the tests that were used in this study were of a high sensitivity and specificity. We are confident that the tests BHV-1, BVDV and Letporosis provided areflection of the sero status of the animals tested. However, given the dynamics of the host parasite interaction and the characteristics of neospora serological tests, it is probable that the Neospora ELISA underestimated the true prevalence of Neosporosis in the cows tested [29].

The level of seroconversion to BHV-1in Northern Ireland may have been over estimated, as conventional non marker BHV-1vaccines are still available on the market there. For this reason, data from herds located in Northern Ireland were not included in the linear model, and the BHV 1seroprevelance in the various regions was calculated individually as we avoided using a cumulative figure so as to prevent any one region biasing the overall results.

Seroconversion is a reflection of historic exposure to a particular pathogen, and is not necessarily an accurate reflective of infection status of an individual animal. However, a high herd seroprevalence, especially among younger animals in a herd, may be suggestive of active infection in that herd. This study was herd based and could not take account of the age of the animals within those herds. The issue of individual animal factors will be addressed in a parallel piece of research (Parr et al., unpublished). Only seropositive animals were included in calculating the herd seroprevalence, and animals with an inconclusive test result were treated as seronegative as this was a herd level based study.

Vaccine usage was much higher among herds in this study than in previous studies. This may be a reflection of the targeted nature of participant selection, whereas previous studies selected herds randomly. The farmers in our study volunteered for inclusion and were therefore likely to be more motivated than the general population.

Conclusions

Our findings support those of several previous studies that as herds increase in size there is increased exposure to pathogens. Consequently farmers with larger herds need to be aware that they must increase their efforts to avoid the introduction and spread of pathogens to their herds, to establish the health status of their herds and determine what mitigation measures are required to address those diseases.

This study has also shown that exposure to several pathogens is associated with exposure to other pathogens. This suggests that there is a common factor common to the exposure among these herds, which is likely to be related to biosecurity. This also indicates that biosecurity needs greater attention in larger herds.

Abbreviations

AIM: Animal Identification and Movement database; BHV-1: Bovine Herpes Virus - 1; BLV: Bovine Leukaemia Virus; BVD(V): Bovine Viral Diarrhoea (Virus),; HPRA: Health Products Regulatory Authority; IBR: Infectious Bovine Rhinotracheitis; ICBF: Irish Cattle Breeding Federation

Acknowledgements

The authors wish to acknowledge Peter Doolan and Federico Randi for assistance in sampling the herds. We wish to thank staff in the Sligo, Athlone and Limerick RVLs for logging in samples, aliquoting samples and serological testing.

Funding

This project was funded by a Dept of Agriculture, Food and the Marine FIRM grant.

Authors' contributions

DB drafted the manuscript and oversaw the design and operation of the serological testing. MP led the herd selection in the Republic of Ireland, on farm serological sampling and data gathering and assisted in the drafting of the manuscript. JF oversaw the BVDV serological testing. AJ oversaw the BHV-1, Leptospirosis and Neosporosis serological testing. JT interrogated the bovine registration and movement database for all the Republic of Ireland herds. FL oversaw the serological testing and herd recruitment in Northern Ireland. MD participated in the study design. DK led the grant application to fund the project, oversaw study design and assisted in drafting the manuscript. All authors were given the opportunity to review and comment on the manuscript. All authors read and approved the final manuscript.

Ethics approval

All experimental procedures involving animals were licensed by the Irish Health Products Regulatory Authority (HPRA). Protocols were conducted in accordance with the Cruelty to Animals Act (Ireland 1876), as amended by European Communities regulations 2002 and 2005) and the European Community Directive 86/609/EC and were sanctioned by the Teagasc Animal Ethics Committee. Informed verbal consent was obtained from the owners of the cattle sampled for this study, in accordance with the licensing protocols, which were overseen by the Teagasc Animal Ethics Committee.

Consent for publication

Not applicable.

Competing interests

The authors declare that they have no competing interests.

Author details

[1]Department of Agriculture, Food and the Marine, SAT Division, Admin Building, Backweston, Celbridge, Co. Kildare, Ireland. [2]Department of Agriculture, Food and the Marine, Athlone RVL, Co. Westmeath, Athlone, Ireland. [3]Department of Agriculture, Food and the Marine, Limerick RVL, LimerickCo. LimerickIreland. [4]Teagasc, Grange, Dunsany, Trim, Co. Meath, Ireland. [5]Teagasc, Mellows College, Athenry, Co. Galway, Ireland. [6]Centre for Veterinary Epidemiology and Risk Analysis, University College Dublin, Belfield, Dublin 4, Ireland. [7]Agri-Food and Biosciences Institute, 18a Newforge Lane, Belfast, Co Antrim BT9 5PX, Northern Ireland.

References

1. Perry GA, Dalton JC, Geary TW. Management factors influencing fertility in beef cattle breeding programmes. Boise: Proceedings, Applied Reproductive Strategies in Beef Cattle-Northwest; 2011.
2. Diskin MG, Kenny DA. Optimising reproductive performance of beef cows and replacement heifers. Animal Suppl. 2014;1:27–39. https://doi.org/10.1017/S175173111400086X. Epub 7 Apr 2014
3. McHugh N, Cromie AR, Evans RD, Berry DP. Validation of national genetic evaluations for maternal beef cattle traits using Irish field data. J Animal Sci. 2014;92:1423–32.
4. Baker JC. The clinical manifestations of bovine viral diarrhea infection. Vet Clin North Am Food Anim Pract. 1995;11:425–45.
5. Cowley DJ, Clegg TA, Doherty ML, More SJ. Bovine viral diarrhoea virus seroprevalence and vaccination usage in dairy and beef herds in the Republic of Ireland. Irish Vet J. 2012;65(1):16.
6. Stott AW, Humphry RW, Gunn GJ , Higgins I, Hennessy T, O'Flaherty J, Graham DA. Predicted costs and benefits of eradicating BVDV from Ireland. Irish VetJ. 2012;65 https://doi.org/10.1186/2046-0481-65-12.
7. Straub O. BHV-1 infections, relevance and spread in Europe. Comp Immunol Microbiol Infect Dis. 1991;14:175–86.
8. Nandi S, Kumar M, Manohar M, Chauhan RS. Bovine herpes virus infections in cattle. Anim Health Res Rev. 2009;10:85–98.
9. Givens MD, Marley MSD. Infectious causes of embryonic and fetal mortality. Therio. 2008;66:648–54.
10. O'Grady L, O'Neill R, Collins D, Clegg T, More S. Herd and within-herd BoHV-1 prevalence among Irish beef herds submitting bulls for entry to a performance testing station. Irish Vet J. 2008;61:809–15.
11. Cowley DJ, Clegg TA, Doherty ML, More SJ. Aspects of bovine herpesvirus 1 in dairy and beef herds in the Republic of Ireland. Acta Vet Scand. 2011;53:40. https://doi.org/10.1186/1751-0147-53-40.

12. Dhaliwal GS, Murray RD, Dobson H, Montgomery J, Ellis WA. Reduced conception rates in dairy cattle associated with serological evidence of Leptospira Interrogans serovar hardjo infection. Vet Rec. 1996;139:110–4.
13. Guitian J, Thurmond MC, Hietala SK. Infertility and abortion among first-lactation dairy cows seropositive or seronegative for Leptospira Interrogans serovar hardjo. J Amer Vet Med Assoc. 1999;215:515–8.
14. Ryan EG, Leonard N, O'Grady L, More SJ, Doherty ML. Seroprevalence of Leptospira Hardjo in the Irish suckler cattle population. Irish V J. 2012;65:8.
15. VanLeeuwen JA, Haddad JP, Dohoo IR, Keefe GP, Tiwari A, Scott HM. Risk factors associated with Neospora caninum seropositivity in randomly sampled Canadian dairy cows and herds. Prev Vet Med. 2010;93:129–38.
16. Moloney BJ, Heur C, Kirkland PD. Neospora caninum in beef herds in new South Wales, Australia.2. Analysis of risk factors. Aust Vet J. 2017;95:101–9.
17. Dubey JP. Review of Neospora caninum and neosporosis in animals. Kor J Parasit. 2003;41:1–16.
18. Tiwari A, VanLeeuwen JA, Dohoo IR, Stryhn H, Keefe GP, Haddad JP. Effects of seropositivity for bovine leukemia virus, bovine viral diarrhoea virus, Mycobacterium Avium subspecies paratuberculosis and Neospora caninum on culling in dairy cattle in four Canadian provinces. Vet Micro. 2005;109:147–58.
19. Moloney BJ, Kirkland PD, Heur C. Neospora caninum in beef herds in new South Wales, Australia. 1: seroprevalence study. Aust Vet J. 2017;95:72–9.
20. Cowley DJB, Graham DA, Guelbenzu M, Doherty ML, More SJ. Aspects of bovine herpesvirus 1 and bovine viral diarrhoea virus herd-level seroprevalence and vaccination in dairy and beef herds in Northern Ireland. I Vet J. 2014;67:18.
21. Paton DJ, Christiansen KH, Alenius S, Cranwell MP, Pritchard GC, Drew TW. Prevalence of antibodies to bovine virus diarrhea virus and other viruses in bulk tank milk in England and Wales. Vet Rec. 1998;142:385–91.
22. Lanyon SR, Hill FI, Reichel MP, Brownlie J. Bovine viral diarrhoea: pathogenesis and diagnosis. Vet J. 2014;199:201–9. https://doi.org/10.1016/j.tvjl.2013.07.024.
23. Anon. AHI BVD programme results 2013–2016. 2017 http://animalhealthireland.ie/?page_id=229. Accessed 27 Jan 2017.
24. Graham DA, Clegg TA, Lynch M, More SJ. Herd-level factors associated with the presence of bovine viral diarrhoea virus in herds participating in the voluntary phase of the Irish national eradication programme. Prev Vet Med. 2013;112:99–108. https://doi.org/10.1016/j.prevetmed.2013.07.011.
25. Ellis WA. Bovine leptospirosis in the tropics: prevalence, pathogenesis and control. Prev Vet Med. 1984;2:411–21.
26. Pritchard DG, Allsup NJ, Penycott TW, Stebbings D. A survey of Leptospiral agglutinating antibody in beef and dairy cattle in Herefordshire, England. Isr J Vet Med. 1987;43:342–3.
27. Schares G, Peters M, Wurm R, Barwald A, Conraths FJ. The efficiency of vertical transmission of Neospora caninum in dairy cattle analysed by serological techniques. Vet Parasitol. 1998;31:87–98.
28. Sanderson MW, Gay JM, Baszler TV. Neospora caninum seroprevalence and associated risk factors in beef cattle in the northwestern United States. Vet Parasitol. 2000;90:15–24.
29. Guido S, Katzer F, Nanjiani I, Milne E, Innes EA. Serology-based diagnostics for the control of bovine neosporosis. Trends in Parasitol. 2016;32:131–43.

3

A strategy to estimate the rate of recruitment of inflammatory cells during bovine intramammary infection under field management

J. Detilleux

Abstract

Background: In most infectious diseases, among which bovine mastitis, promptness of the recruitment of inflammatory cells (mainly neutrophils) in inflamed tissues has been shown to be of prime importance in the resolution of the infection. Although this information should aid in designing efficient control strategies, it has never been quantified in field studies.

Methods: Here, a system of ordinary differential equations is proposed that describes the dynamic process of the inflammatory response to mammary pathogens. The system was tested, by principal differential analysis, on 1947 test-day somatic cell counts collected on 756 infected cows, from 50 days before to 50 days after the diagnosis of clinical mastitis. Cell counts were log-transformed before estimating recruitment rates.

Results: Daily rates of cellular recruitment was estimated at 0.052 (st. err. = 0.005) during health. During disease, an additional cellular rate of recruitment was estimated at 0.004 (st. err. = 0.001) per day and per bacteria. These estimates are in agreement with analogous measurements of in vitro neutrophil functions.

Conclusions: Results suggest the method is adequate to estimate one of the components of innate resistance to mammary pathogens at the individual level and in field studies. Extension of the method to estimate components of innate tolerance and limits of the study are discussed.

Keywords: Principal differential analysis, Ordinary differential equation, Cell recruitment rate, Bovine mastitis, Resistance, Tolerance

Background

Mastitis remains a major challenge to the dairy industry. Mastitis is characterized by the invasion of the udder by bacteria, their multiplication in the milk-producing tissues, and the production of inflammatory mediators. In response to mediators, inflammatory cells (mainly neutrophils) are recruited from the circulation into the lumen of the alveolus, thus increasing somatic cell counts (SCC) and decreasing the quantity and quality of mastitis milk. Within the gland, neutrophils will phagocyte and destroy invading pathogens. This process is characteristic of the innate immune response to many infectious pathogens.

One control strategy consists of increasing the resistance (host's ability to reduce parasite establishment) of animals to udder pathogens, either therapeutically or by selection [1]. Mechanisms behind the cow's ability to resist to mastitis pathogens include traits that reduce pathogen transmission (resistance to infection or "direct" resistance) and pathogen growth rate once infection has occurred (resistance to disease or "indirect" resistance). Different methods have already proven their efficacy in increasing cow's "direct" resistance, including dry cow antibiotic therapy [2] and vaccination [3]. A contributor to the level of "indirect" resistance is the establishment of a "healthy" immune response in which the infected cow clears the

Correspondence: jdetilleux@ulg.ac.be
Fundamental and Applied Research for Animals and Health, Sustainable Animal Production, Faculty of Veterinary Medicine, University of Liège, Quartier Vallée 2, Avenue de Cureghem, 6, 4000 Liège, Belgium

infection and returns to pre-infection status [4]. Among the many components of this healthy immune response, the promptness of the recruitment of blood inflammatory cells in mammary tissues and milk has been shown to be of paramount importance [5–7] but, to the author's best knowledge, has never been quantified on cows clinically infected under natural conditions.

Ordinary differential equations (ODEs) have been proposed to study the dynamic process of the inflammatory response, including the cell recruitment [8–11]. However, estimation of ODE parameters from complex real data can be difficult, ODEs may not have analytic solutions and numerically solving ODEs can be computationally expensive. Also, stationary confounder effects may not always be included in ODEs and this can be a problem in situations where noise levels are high and the number of data points is low [12].

Here, principal differential analysis (PDA) is proposed to estimate ODE parameters. In this methodology, observed measurements are fitted empirically using spline functions which are then differentiated with respect to time to obtain time-derivative curves. Next, these curves are substituted into the ODEs that can be solved using least-square methods so estimates of the parameters can be obtained [13]. This method has the advantages of being conceptually simpler and more practical than sophisticated numerical methods for solving ODEs by iterative numerical integration. Initials conditions and boundary value need not be known and PDA does not require uniformly sampled data [13]. Missing data can be handled and parameters of interest may be adjusted for known confounders. However, poor splines fit can result in misleading time-derivative information which can lead to poor parameter estimates.

The goal of this study is to test the practicality of PDA in estimating the rate of recruitment of inflammatory cells as an indicator of "indirect" resistance in cows with clinical mastitis.

Methods

To reach this goal, the following procedure was followed (Fig. 1). In the first step, a system of ODEs was proposed to represent the theoretical interaction between inflammatory cells and bacteria during mastitis (model [1]) and to obtain their "model predictions". In the second step, these predictions (= simulated dataset 1) and SCS collected at specific points in time in cows clinically infected (= observed dataset 2) were smoothed with cubic spline models and variable knots (= models [2]). In step 3, time derivatives of models [2] were computed (= models [3]). Finally, in step 4, rates of recruitment were estimated via a linear regression (= models [4a, 4b]) on these time derivatives. All computations were done on SAS 9.1. To achieve normality of distribution, concentrations in all models were expressed under the log scale as it is done routinely.

Mathematical simulation of an inflammatory response during mastitis

The model [1] obeyed key biological characteristics observed within an infected udder:

$$\begin{aligned} dx/dt_i &= \gamma x - \omega\ x\ y \\ dy/dt_i &= \upsilon\ (y_0 - y) + \beta\ xy \end{aligned} \tag{1}$$

where x (t_i) symbolizes the bacterial and y (t_i) the somatic cell concentrations at a particular point in time (t_i = 0, 1, 2, ..., 100 time-units; i = 1, 2, 3, ..., 101). At start, the concentrations are x_0 and y_0. Across time, the bacterial concentration is controlled by the multiplication rate (γ) and the rate at which each inflammatory cell kills bacteria (ω). This last parameter is a first indicator of the level of resistance of the cow. If the animal is insufficiently resistant, ω is low and its inflammatory cells cannot successfully kill bacteria. This is observed in animals with inherited disorders of phagocytic cells [14] and in cows during the peri-parturient period [15]. During health, the concentration of inflammatory cells is controlled by the first term of the second equation where υ is the rate at which cells are recruited and removed in the absence of infection. So, even in the absence of bacteria, there is a standing stock of cells ready to attack. During mastitis, an extra-concentration of activated cells is recruited at a rate β. This is a second indicator of the level of resistance of the host and the indicator of interest in this study. Indeed, an infected host is not very resistant when β is low because activated somatic cells cannot migrate towards the site of infection. This is observed in diseases such as the bovine leukocyte adhesion deficiency syndrome [16].

Initial values were set at x_0 = 2 and y_0 = 10, and a range of values, from 0.001 to 0.50, were set for the different rates in model [1]. Because it is deterministic, the model

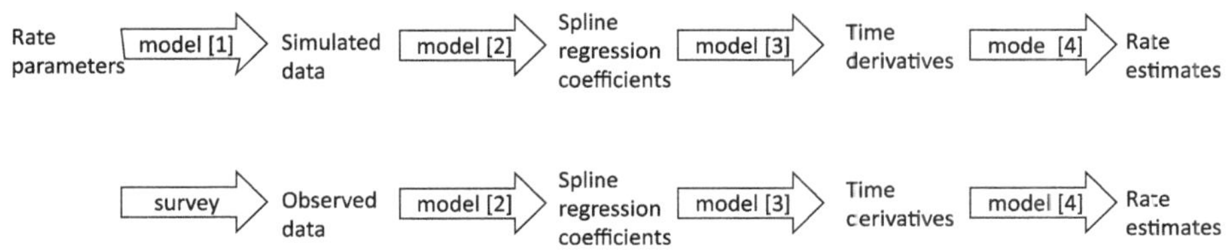

Fig. 1 Methodology

doesn't take into account the discreteness of the populations and their random fluctuations so extinction is not possible. Indeed, as the number of cells decreased, the assumption of continuous cell populations is no longer valid and oscillations may occur [17]. As a solution, a threshold of 0.01 was introduced below which the bacterial population is considered extinct, alike in [10].

The system accepts two equilibria, one in the absence and one in the presence of infection. The linear stability of these equilibria was determined by evaluating the characteristic equation (s) of the Jacobian. The equilibrium is stable when all eigenvalues of its Jacobian matrix have negative real parts; it is unstable if at least one eigenvalue has positive real part [18].

Simulated and observed datasets

Two datasets were used for the second step of the procedure. The simulated dataset (dataset 1) consisted of the values of the concentrations of bacteria (x (t_i)) and inflammatory cells (y (t_i)) obtained with [1]. Simulation steps were executed for a period of 100 time-units or until the infection dies out.

The second dataset (dataset 2) came from a survey of 31 commercial dairy farms conducted between January 2008 and December 2011 in the Walloon region of Belgium (Additional file 1)[19]. Herds were enrolled in the regional dairy herds recording system from which test-day somatic cell scores or SCS (i.e., the log-transform of SCC; denoted s (t_i)) were obtained. Farmers recorded 756 mastitis cases and 1947 SCS values were used in the analyses. Other information included year of calving, parity, days in milk, and number of days between successive events. Clinical mastitis was diagnosed by the breeder when milk from one or more glands was abnormal in color, viscosity, or consistency, with or without accompanying heat, pain, or redness. Only the first mastitis case per parity was considered. Data were collected from 50 days before up to 50 days after the date of mastitis detection. Lactation must include at least two months of lactation. No information was available on bacterial concentrations.

Cubic Spline models

For the second step of the analysis, records from both datasets were fitted with cubic splines and variable knots:

$$U(t_i) = g_0 + g_1 t_i + g_2 t_i^2 + g_3 t_i^3 + \Sigma_i h_i (t_i - k_i)^3 d_i + e(t_i) \quad (2)$$

for i = 1, 2, ... 100. The variables U (t_i) are either x (t_i) and y (t_i) (dataset 1) or s (t_i) (dataset 2) measured at time t_i where t_i is, for dataset 1, the time since infection (t_i = 1, 2,.., 100) and, for dataset 2, the number of days elapsed between the date of milk recording and the date of the case occurrence (t_i = −50 to +50 days). Parameters g_0, g_1, g_2, g_3 and h_i are regression coefficients. The knots k_i can be any value of t_i and the dummy variable d_i = 0 if $t_i \le$ ki and d_i = 1 if $t_i > k_i$. Besides effects in [2], the model for dataset 2 included fixed effects of parity (1, 2, ≥3), days in milk (1, 2 ..., 300) and herd-year-season (1, 2 ..., 174) when the case was observed. These last effects are known factors affecting test-day milk yield and SCS (e.g., [20]). Cubic B-splines are the most frequently chosen spline to fit biological systems because they ally simplicity and biological signification and estimates tend to have high variance when the order of the spline gets larger (e.g., [21]).

Statistically significant knots were selected in a stepwise manner. The final model contained only variables with F-statistics for entry and staying in the model significant at the 0.15 level. The selection stopped at a local minimum of the predicted residual sum of squares (PRESS) criterion. The e (t_i) were assumed normally and independently distributed with E (e (t_i)) = 0 and var. (e (t_i)) = σ_e^2. Estimated values of U (t_i) (= $\hat{U}$ (t_i)) and of regression coefficients (= $\hat{h}$ and $\hat{g}$) were obtained by minimizing the squared differences between U (t_i) and $\hat{U}$ (t_i). Differences between U (t_i) and $\hat{U}$ (t_i) and R^2 values (called R1 values in the following text) were used to evaluate the fit of the model.

Estimation of rates of recruitment

For both datasets and after stepwise selection, time derivatives (step 3) were computed as:

$$d\hat{U}(t_i)/dt_i = \hat{g}_1 + 2\,\hat{g}_2 t_i + 3\hat{g}_3 t_i^2 + 3\Sigma_p \hat{h}_p (t_p - k_p)^2 d_p \quad (3)$$

For $\hat{U}(t_i) = \widehat{x(t_i)}$, $\widehat{y(t_i)}$ and $\widehat{s(t_i)}$ with i = 1, 2, ... 100; p indexes the significant segments (p = 1, ... ≤100); $\hat{g}$ and $\hat{h}$ are the ordinary least-squares estimates obtained for the regression coefficients in [2]. Differences between dU_i (model [1]) and $d\hat{U}_i$ (model [3]) were computed.

Finally (step 4), the derivatives were regressed on each system of ODE Eqs. For dataset 1 (model [4a]),

$$\begin{aligned} d\hat{x}/dt_i &= \gamma\ x - \omega\ x\ y \\ d\hat{y}/dt_i &= \upsilon\ (y_0 - y) + \beta\ x\ y, \end{aligned} \quad (4a)$$

and for dataset 2 (model [4b]),

$$\begin{aligned} dz/dt_i &= \gamma\ z - \omega\ zy \\ ds/dt_i &= \upsilon\ (s_0 - s) + \beta\ zs. \end{aligned} \quad (4b)$$

The R^2 values (called R2 values in the following text) were computed to assess the fit of the models in estimating ODE rate parameters. In dataset 2, no information was available on bacterial concentrations necessary to solve model [4b]. As an alternative and to prove the concept of the proposed methodology, they were replaced by z. The values of z were simulated thanks to the first equation of [4b] (dynamics similar to [4a]) with $\gamma = 0.1$ and the value of ω that gave the highest R2.

Results

Mathematical simulation of an inflammatory response during mastitis

The ODE equations (model [1]) reproduced qualitatively outcomes that can be realistically observed during a healthy response to infection (i.e., scenario 'a' in Fig. 2). Such a response is characterized by the following steps. Firstly, bacteria multiply (i.e., $x(t_i)$ increases) which is followed by an increase in the concentration of inflammatory cells (i.e., $y(t_i)$ increases). Next, bacteria are killed and their concentrations decrease. At the end of the infection episode, both cell concentrations return to pre-infection values. In scenarios 'b' and 'c', the increase in $x(t_i)$ is depressed when compared to scenario 'a' because recruitment rates are different (They were set at 0.01, 0.025, and 0.05 cells/time units in scenario a, b, and c, respectively). Peaks for $y(t_i)$ were at the 24, 19 and 12 time units since infection in scenario 'a', 'b' and 'c', respectively. That is, peaks in cell concentrations occurred faster for higher recruitment rates. Values for the other parameters were unchanged in all three scenarios (i.e., $\omega = 0.01$, $\gamma = 0.3$, $\upsilon = 0.05$).

The system accepts two equilibria. The first one occurs in the absence of infection for $(x_i; y_i) = (0; y_0)$, i.e. no bacteria and concentration of resident phagocytic cells (y_0). The equilibrium is stable if $\omega y_0 > \gamma$ and all eigenvalues of the Jacobian matrix are negative. When $\omega y_0 > \gamma$, the rate at which resident cells kill bacteria is greater than their multiplication rate (γ) so bacterial concentration decreases immediately after invasion. When $\omega y_0 < \gamma$, it is the reverse: Bacteria multiply and colonize the udder. In the presence of infection, a second equilibrium may occur for $(x; y) = (\upsilon/\beta\,(1 - (\omega y_0/\gamma)); \gamma/\omega)$. At this equilibrium, one of the eigenvalue of the Jacobian matrix is zero and one can't tell whether the equilibrium point is stable or not.

Principal differential analysis

In Table 1, one can find some parameter values used to simulate records of dataset 1. Whatever the chosen parameter values, fits of the cubic splines to data (model [2]), and fits of the linear regressions to time derivatives (model [4a]), were excellent. Indeed, R1 and R2 values were above 95% and estimates were close to their corresponding parameter values (see Table 1 for different simulations).

Regarding observed SCS in dataset 2, SCS data were from cows in parity 1 (33%), parity 2 (23%) and parity 3 (44%). Mastitis cases were reported all along the lactation period, with the highest frequencies in the second (11.77%) and third (12.30%) month in lactation. Parity, days in milk and herd-year-season affected significantly SCS. The SCS means were highest in parity ≥3 and in the third month in milk, they decreased across calendar year and were the lowest in winter as compared to summer. Means of observed (s (ti)) and estimated ($s(t_i)$) values and cubic splines are depicted in Fig. 3. The cubic splines are $s(t_i)$ values adjusted for the effects of parity, days in milk and herd-year-season. Standard errors varied from 0.19 to 0.52 for s (ti) and from 0.16 to 0.41 for $s(t_i)$. The R1 value was 58.23%. Location of the three knots in the cubic spline was at 14 days before, 12 days after and 27 days after diagnosis of clinical mastitis.

In eq. [(4b)], the value of $\omega = 0.007$ gave the best R2 (39.03%). Estimate of s_0 is 3.84 (st. err. = 0.70), estimate of υ is 0.0522 (st. err. = $0.50\ 10^{-3}$) and estimate of β is 0.0039 (st. err. = $0.112\ 10^{-3}$). All are significantly different from null ($p < 0.05$).

Discussion

Once a cow is infected with mammary pathogens, its immune system mounts a response to them. This response is orchestrated by a hierarchically organized set of molecular, cellular and organismal networks, including the massive influx of inflammatory cells and the killing of bacteria. Although simple, equations in model [1] were able to

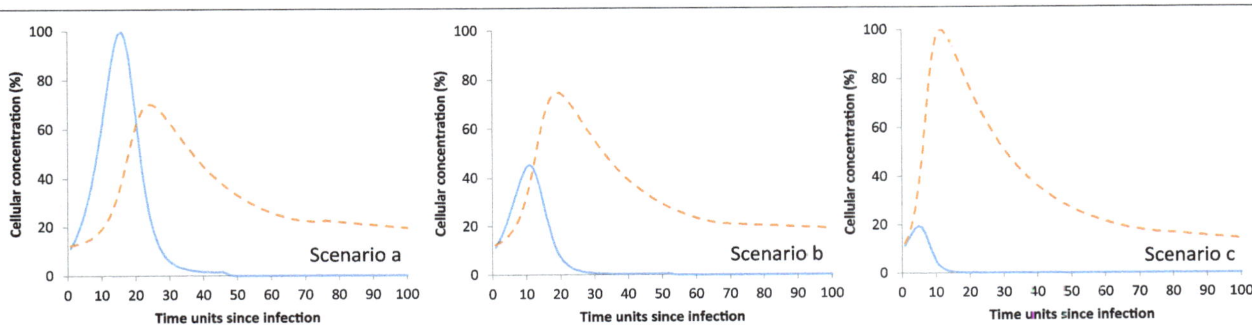

Fig. 2 Percentages of the maximum values for y_i (dotted line) and x_i (plain line) simulated for $i = 1$ to 100 time units since nfection and with increasing extra-migration rates when going from scenario 'a' to 'c'

Table 1 Model parameters values (E), their estimates (Ê) and standard errors (in parentheses) for 10 different simulations

Simulation		Multiplication rate (□)	Killing rate (□)	Migration rate during health (□)	Extra-migration rate during infection (□)
1	E	0.10	0.01	0.05	0.10
	Ê	0.10 (3.19 10^{-4})	0.01 (2.44 10^{-4})	0.05 (9.66 10^{-4})	0.10 (0.001)
2	E	0.01	0.01	0.01	0.01
	Ê	0.01 (8.21 10^{-5})	0.01 (8.21 10^{-5})	0.01 (8.21 10^{-5})	0.01 (8.21 10^{-5})
3	E	0.10	0.10	0.10	0.10
	Ê	0.10 (1.95 10^{-4})	0.10 (1.95 10^{-4})	0.10 (1.95 10^{-4})	0.10 (1.95 10^{-4})
4	E	0.15	0.15	0.15	0.15
	Ê	0.15 (0.0014)	0.15 (0.0014)	0.15 (0.0014)	0.15 (0.0014)
5	E	0.10	0.10	0.10	0.10
	Ê	0.10 (1.08 10^{-4})	0.10 (1.08 10^{-4})	0.10 (1.08 10^{-4})	0.10 (1.08 10^{-4})
6	E	0.50	0.50	0.50	0.50
	Ê	0.38 (0.026)	0.38 (0.026)	0.38 (0.026)	0.38 (0.026)
7	E	0.10	0.10	0.10	0.10
	Ê	0.101 (2.92 10^{-4})	0.101 (2.92 10^{-4})	0.101 (2.92 10^{-4})	0.101 (2.92 10^{-4})
8	E	0.15	0.15	0.15	0.15
	Ê	0.14 (0.0039)	0.14 (0.0039)	0.14 (0.0039)	0.14 (0.0039)
9	E	0.15	0.15	0.15	0.15
	Ê	0.1467 (0.0014)	0.1467 (0.0014)	0.1467 (0.0014)	0.1467 (0.0014)
10	E	0.15	0.15	0.15	0.15
	Ê	0.149 (5.44 10^{-4})	0.149 (5.44 10^{-4})	0.149 (5.44 10^{-4})	0.149 (5.44 10^{-4})

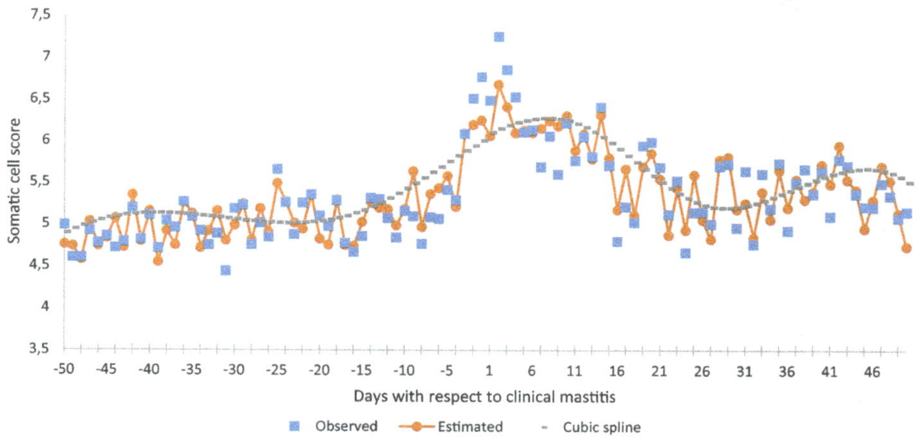

Fig. 3 Means of observed and estimated somatic cell scores for 50 days before to 50 days after clinical mastitis. Standard errors are omitted for clarity of the plot

produce realistic outcomes after intramammary infection [9, 10], as shown in Fig. 2. Using data simulated with model [1], it was verified that PDA (models [2] to [4]) were adequate to estimate parameters of model [1]. Indeed, it fits data almost perfectly as shown in Table 1. This motivates the application of the method to data collected on clinically infected cows (i.e., observed dataset 2). There, the fit was poorer (R1 = 58.23%; R2 = 39.03%). One explanation for this lower fit is that SCS modelled in dataset 2 are only a substitute of the concentrations of phagocytic cells modelled in dataset 1. This last information is often lacking in field studies although, during mastitis, over 90% of the somatic cells are blood neutrophils migrating into the milk [7].

Another explanation is linked to the fact that bacterial concentrations were not observed but simulated using a fixed bacterial growth rate ($\gamma = 0.1$). Such information is also often lacking in field studies. Estimates in model [4b] were also not adjusted for the differences that exist between immune responses caused by different bacterial species and strains [22]. Note however that all mastitis cases were suspected to be due to major pathogens, mainly *E. coli* (discussed below). Also, ranking may still be legitimate if we accept that higher killing rates against bacteria that multiply at a rate of 0.1 will also be higher against bacteria that multiply at higher rates.

A third explanation for the poorer fit in observed than simulated data is that ODEs are a simplified version of reality based on various assumptions. For example, it was assumed that a constant proportion of bacterial load was killed by cells at a rate ω, the time needed to process bacteria was negligible and phagocytic cells did not become "satiated". Another assumption was that concentration of newly migrating cells increased monotonically with concentrations of somatic cells and of bacteria already present in the gland. We may partially accept these assumptions. For example, it was observed in the in vitro study by Li et al. (2004) that rate of bacterial killing of human neutrophils mixed with *S. epidermidis* was only dependent upon the concentration of neutrophils (constant ω). It was also reported that neutrophilic recruitment during mastitis is initiated by inflammatory mediators released from tissue-resident leukocytes when they come into contact with pathogens [6, 23]. This means that a minimum concentration of somatic cells is necessary to initiate the response, which is assumed in the model. A last explanation for the poorer fit in observed than simulated data lies in the cubic spline itself that guarantees continuity and smoothness at the knots at the expense of closeness to data points.

Number and location of knots were estimated from dataset 2: Concentration of somatic cells started to increased 14 days before diagnosis up to the 12 days after diagnosis and returned to values pre-infection values 27 days after diagnosis (Fig. 3). This is characteristic of acute infections with short peaks in SCS, as observed in clinical cases associated with *E. coli* under non-experimental conditions (e. g., [24]). This was also described in quarters experimentally infected with *E. coli*: SCS returned to pre-infection values after a period of 21 to 28 days [25, 26]. An additional argument is that highest SCS were between 6.5 and 7.5 (Fig. 3). Indeed, SCS are regularly higher than 6.4 in infections by major pathogens (as reviewed by [27]).

Even though no information was found in the literature, estimated rates in the absence and presence of bacterial infection (ν and β, respectively) were realistic. The credibility of ν can be discussed in relation to s_0 that represents SCS in the absence of infection. It was estimated here at 3.84 which is close to the value of 3.91 observed by [28] in cows that were repeatedly and consistently cultured negative. It was slightly below values reported by [29] for bacteriologically negative quarters (between 4.22 and 5.23). The rate of extra-recruitment of cells during infection is represented by β. Its estimate was significantly different from null which is necessary for the resolution of mammary infections [30]. The value of β can be discussed in relation to chemotactic indexes (CI) obtained in in vitro experiments. Indeed, a CI is the number of neutrophils that migrated towards a chemo-attractant to the number of neutrophils that migrated towards a control medium. Similarly, the ratio $(\beta x_i + \nu)/\nu$ represents SCS that migrated towards mammary gland infected with x_i bacteria to SCS that migrated towards uninfected mammary gland. Its value was estimated at 1.3 for $x_i = 4$. It is close to the CI value found by [31] who observed CI of neutrophils from mammary glands inoculated with $\sim 10^4$ CFU/ml of *E. coli* (i. e., $x_i = 4$ on the log scale) was 1.2 times the pre-infection CI value. Similarly, [32] observed the CI of neutrophils from glands infected with *S. aureus* was 1.2 times the CI of non-mastitic ($<7.5\ 10^5$ SCC/ml) mammary secretions. In Fig. 2, bacterial concentration increased as values of β decreased. Correspondingly, [33] observed a delayed chemotactic response in cows with high vs moderate bacterial concentrations during the first 120 h after experimental infection with the same amount of *E.coli*.

Standard errors for υ and β were high and this suggests recruitment rates varied among cows. If confirmed, such finding suggests that recruitment rates could be considered in breeding programs to improve the level of resistance of the population because individual variability is a prerequisite to such programs. Of course, it remains to determine whether this variability is of genetic origin.

As shown in model [1], estimates of direct and indirect resistance levels are ω and $\omega\ \beta$, respectively. Estimates of direct and indirect tolerance levels could also be estimated by adding a third equation to model [1]: $dm_i/dt = \delta\ (m_0 - m_i) - (\eta\ x_i + \varepsilon\ y_i)$.

Where m_i is the milk quantity produced by mammary secretory cells at a particular point in time i. The first term includes the natural rate (δ) at which secretory cells proliferate and die as a result of apoptosis [34]. Parameter η is an indicator of the ability of the cow to tolerate negative effects on milk-secreting tissues (and other components of the mammary gland) of bacterial multiplication and production of toxins, i.e., the ability of the cow to directly tolerate the infection. Parameter ε is an indicator of the ability of the cow to tolerate negative effects of the immune response triggered by the infection and more particularly, milk loss mediated by the increase in the concentration of phagocytic cells, i.e., the ability of the cow to indirectly tolerate the infection. If $\eta = \varepsilon = 0$, the animal is completely tolerant and produces at the level observed during health. If not, milk drops due to the infection. In this equation, all other effects, such as resource intake, management, month in milk or age, are assumed fixed. It is also assumed that each secretory cell produces the same quality of milk so that m_i are directly related to the concentration of secretory cells.

Conclusions

Results suggest PDA is valuable to estimate, at the individual level and in field studies, rates of neutrophilic recruitment and killing, both of which are components of innate resistance to infectious pathogens. Given the economic and health implications of infectious diseases, a more frequent evaluation of these components in commercial populations could lead to more efficient strategies of disease control and treatments and a better description of host–pathogen interactions.

Abbreviations

ODE: Ordinary differential eqs.; SCC: somatic cell count; SCS: somatic cell score

Acknowledgements

The author thanks the "Association Wallone de l'élevage" and the OSaM Team for sharing data.

Funding

Not applicable.

Authors' contributions

Not applicable.

Competing interests

The author declares that she has no competing interests.

Consent for publication

Not applicable.

Reference

1. Thompson-Crispi K, Atalla H, Miglior E, Mallard BA. Bovine mastitis: frontiers in immunogenetics. Frontiers Immunol. 2014;5:493–503.
2. Hillerton JE, Berry EA. Treating mastitis in the cow–a tradition or an archaism. J Appl Microbiol. 2005;98:1250–5.
3. Bradley AJ, Breen JE, Payne B, White V, Green MJ. An investigation of the efficacy of a polyvalent mastitis vaccine using different vaccination regimens under field conditions in the United Kingdom. J Dairy Sci. 2015;98: 1706–20.
4. Råberg L, Sim D, Read A. Disentangling genetic variation for resistance and tolerance to infectious diseases in animals. Science. 2007;318:812–4.
5. Brenau P, Lefèvre L, Rau A, Laloë D, Pisoni G, Moroni P, et al. Contribution of mammary epithelial cells to the immune response during early stages of a bacterial infection to *Staphylococcus aureus*. Vet res. 2014;45:16–36.
6. Kolaczkowska E, Kubes P. Neutrophil recruitment and function in health and inflammation. Nature rev Immunol. 2013;13:159–75.
7. Paape M, Mehrzad J, Zhao X, Detilleux J, Burvenich C. Defense of the bovine mammary gland by polymorphonuclear neutrophil leukocytes. J Mammary Gland Biol Neoplasia. 2002;7:109–21.
8. Barlow JW, White LJ, Zadoks RN, Schukken YH. A mathematical model demonstrating indirect and overall effects of lactation therapy targeting subclinical mastitis in dairy herds. Prev vet med. 2009;90:31–42.
9. Detilleux JC. A mathematical model to study resistance and tolerance to infection at the animal and population levels: application to *E. coli* mastitis. Front Genet. 2012;3:146–55.
10. Kumar R, Clermont G, Vodovotz Y, Chow CC. The dynamics of acute inflammation. J Theor Biol. 2004;230:145–55.
11. Vodovotz Y, Clermont G, Chow C, An G. Mathematical models of the acute inflammatory response. Curr Opin Crit Care. 2004;10:383–90.
12. Brewer D, Barenco M, Callard R, Hubank M, Stark J. Fitting ordinary differential equations to short time course data. Phil Trans R soc a. 2008;366:519–44.
13. Poyton AA, Varziri MS, McAuley KB, MvLellan PJ, Ramsay JO. Parameter estimation in continuous-time dynamic models using principal differential analysis. Comp Chemical Engin. 2006;30:698–708.
14. Lekstrom-Himes JA, Gallin JI. Immunodeficiency diseases caused by defects in phagocytes. N Engl J med. 2000;343:1703–14.
15. Detilleux JC, Koehler KJ, Freeman AE, Kehrli ME, Kelly DH. Immunological parameters of periparturient Holstein cattle: genetic variation. J Dairy Sci. 1994;77:2640–50.
16. Kelm SC, Detilleux JC, Freeman AE, Kehrli ME Jr, Dietz AB, Fox LK, et al. Genetic association between parameters of inmate immunity and measures of mastitis in periparturient Holstein cattle. J Dairy Sci. 1997;80:1767–75.
17. Alizon Z, van Baalen M. Acute or chronic? Within-host models with immune dynamics, infection outcome, and parasite evolution. Am Nat. 2008;172: E244–56.
18. Munz P, Hudea I, Imad J, Smith RJ. When zombie attack: mathematical modelling of an outbreak of zombie infection. In: Tchuenche JM, Chiyaka C, editors. Infectious disease modelling research progress. Hauppage NY: Nova Science Publishers; 2011. p. 133–50.
19. Reding E, Theron L, Detilleux J, Bertozzi C, Hanzen C. LAECEA: un outil fédérateur d'aide à la décision pour le suivi de la santé mammaire dans les élevages bovins laitiers wallons. In: Proc 18èmes rencontres autour de la recherche sur les ruminant. INRA - Institut national de la recherche agronomique: Paris; 2011.
20. Hagnestam-Nielsen C, Emanuelson U, Berglund B, Strandberg E. Relationship between somatic cell count and milk yield in different stages of lactation. J Dairy Sci. 2009;92:3124–33.
21. White IMS, Thompson R, Brotherstone S. Genetic and environmental smoothing of lactation curves with cubic splines. J Dairy Sci. 1999;82:632–8.
22. Hertl JA, Schukken YH, Welcome FL, Tauer LW, Gröhn YT. Pathogen-specific effects on milk yield in repeated clinical mastitis episodes in Holstein dairy cows. J Dairy Sci. 2014;97:1465–80.
23. Elazar S, Gonen E, Livneh-Kol A, Rosenshine I, Shpigel NY. Neutrophil recruitment in endotoxin-induced murine mastitis is strictly dependent on mammary alveolar macrophages. Vet res. 2010;41:10–24.
24. de Haas Y, Barkema HW, Veerkamp RF. The effect of pathogen-specific clinical mastitis on the lactation curve for somatic cell count. J Dairy Sci. 2002;85:1314–23.
25. Erskine RJ, Wilson RC, Riddell MG Jr, Tyler JW, Spears HJ, Davis BS. Intramammary administration of gentamicin as treatment for experimentally induced *Escherichia coli* mastitis in cows. Am J vet res. 2012;53:375–81.

26. Pyörälä S, Kaartinen L, Käck H, Rainio V. Efficacy of two therapy regimens for treatment of experimentally induced *Escherichia coli* mastitis in cows. J Dairy Sci. 1994;77:453–61.
27. Ruegg PL, Pantoja JCF. Understanding and using somatic cell counts to improve milk quality. Irish J Agric Food res. 2013;52:101–17.
28. Laevens H, Deluker H, Schukken YH, de Meulemeester L, Vandermeersch R, de Muelenaere E, et al. Influence of parity and stage of lactation on the somatic cell count in bacteriologically negative dairy cows. J Dairy Sci. 1997; 80:3219–26.
29. Djabri B, Bareille N, Beaudeau F, Seegers H. Quarter milk somatic cell count in infected dairy cows: a meta-analysis. Vet res. 2002;33:335–57.
30. Rambeaud M, Pighetti GM. Impaired neutrophil migration associated with specific bovine CXCR2 genotypes. Infect Immun. 2005;73:4955–9.
31. Shuster DE, Kehrli M, Rainard P, Paape M. Complement fragment C5a and inflammatory cytokines in neutrophil recruitment during intramammary infection with *Escherichia coli*. Infect Immun. 1997;65:3286–92.
32. Barber MR, Yang TJ. Chemotactic activities in nonmastitic and mastitic mammary secretions: presence of interleukin-8 in mastitic but not nonmastitic secretions. Clin Diagn lab Immunol. 1998;5:82–6.
33. Kremer WDJ, Noordhuizen-Stassen EN, Grommers FJ, Daemen AJJM, Brand A. Blood polymorphonuclear leukocyte chemotaxis during experimental *Escherichia coli* bovine mastitis. J Dairy Sci. 1993;76:2613–8.
34. Cappio-Borlino A, NPP M, Pulina G. Mathematical modelling of milk production in dairy sheep. In: Pulina G, Bencini R, editors. Dairy sheep nutrition. Italy: Cabi Publishing, Sassari; 2004. p. 13–30.

Rapid detection of infectious bovine Rhinotracheitis virus using recombinase polymerase amplification assays

Peili Hou, Hongmei Wang*, Guimin Zhao, Chengqiang He and Hongbin He*

Abstract

Background: Infectious bovine rhinotracheitis virus (IBRV) is a major pathogen in cattle and has led to significant economic losses to the dairy industry worldwide, and therefore a more optimal method for the rapid diagnosis of IBRV infection is highly needed. In this study, we described the development of a lateral flow dipstrip (LFD) of isothermal recombinase polymerase amplification (RPA) method for rapid detection of IBRV.

Methods: Distinct regions were selected as a candidate target for designing the LFD-RPA primers and probes. The analytical sensitivity of the RPA assay was determined using ten-fold serially diluted IBRV DNA. The specificity of the assay was assessed with other viral pathogens of cattle with similar clinic and other herpesviruses. The clinical performance was evaluated by testing 106 acute-phase high fever clinical specimens.

Results: RPA primers and probe were designed to target the specific conserved UL52 region fragment of IBRV. The detection could be completed at a constant temperature of 38 °C for 25 min, and the amplification products were easily visualized on a simple LFD. The detection limit of this assay was 5 copies per reaction of IBRV DNA and there was no cross-reactivity with other viruses causing bovine gastrointestinal and respiratory infections or other herpesviruses. The assay performance on acute-phase high fever clinical samples collected from cattle with no vaccine against IBRV, which were suspected to be infected with IBRV, was validated by detecting 24 fecal, 36 blood, 38 nasal swab and 8 tissue specimens, and compared with SYBR Green I based real-time PCR. The coincidence between IBRV LFD-RPA and real-time PCR was 100%.

Conclusion: IBRV LFD-RPA was fast and much easier to serve as an alternative to the common measures used for IBRV diagnosis, as there is reduction in the use of instruments for identification of the infected animals. In addition, this assay may be the potential candidate to be used as point-of-care diagnostics in the field.

Keywords: Infectious bovine rhinotracheitis virus (IBRV), Recombinase polymerase amplification (RPA), Lateral-flow dipstrip (LFD), Rapid detection

Background

Infectious bovine rhinotracheitis virus (IBRV), often referred to as bovine herpesvirus 1 (BoHV-1), is responsible for infectious bovine rhinotracheitis (IBR). IBR is highly contagious, and can cause a diverse range of clinical manifestations from upper respiratory disease, rhinitis, vulvovaginitis, traeheitis, enteritis, conjunctivitis, abortion and encephalitis, to fatal systemic infection in neonatal calves [1]. IBRV can also induce immune suppression that contributes to the severity of disease manifestation. In addition, IBRV is one of the bovine respiratory disease complex pathogens, which is the leading cause of cattle death around the world [2–4]. Taken together, it is a major disease of cattle leading to significant economic losses to the dairy industry worldwide [5, 6]. Several developed countries such as Germany, have adopted immunization and eradication of pathogen-positive animals for IBR control [7]. Therefore, early identification of IBRV positive animals is critical for disease control and elimination programs to diminish its burden on the dairy industry.

* Correspondence: hongmeiwang@sdnu.edu.cn; hongbinhe@sdnu.edu.cn
Key Laboratory of Animal Resistant Biology of Shandong, Ruminant Diseases Research Center, College of Life Sciences, Shandong Normal University, No. 88 East Wenhua Road, Jinan City, Shandong Province, China

At present, IBRV can be routinely detected using cell culture, polymerase chain reaction (PCR), immune-histopathology, and enzyme-linked immunosorbent assay (ELISA) as well as the virus neutralization test [8–10]. However, currently available diagnostic tests remain laboratory-based and require sophisticated instruments operated by specially trained personnel. Although isothermal amplification techniques such as the loop-mediated isothermal amplification (LAMP) have been offered as a simple, rapid and alternative molecular pathogen diagnostic tool for point-of-care testing in the field [11, 12], the LAMP assay needs four to six primers, leading to longer amplicons and possibly more difficult to design in the case of highly variable viruses.

Recombinase polymerase amplification (RPA), is a novel isothermal alternative to PCR, which targets and amplifies DNA from clinical samples with high sensitivity and specificity [13]. The technology takes advantage of three major proteins, including recombinase proteins, single-strand binding proteins (SSB), and polymerases, and relies on two specific oligonucleotide primers and a probe, and can specifically amplify nucleic acid sequences ranging from trace levels to detectable amounts of product in an isothermal format in less than 30 min. RPA products can be detected by gel electrophoresis, probe-based fluorescence monitoring or lateral flow dipsticks depending on the specific primers and/or probe configuration. Although RPA technology has been widely used for detection of various pathogens since its initial development [14–19], to date, there is no RPA assay developed for IBRV detection.

In this study, RPA primer and probe combinations were designed, and screened to permit LFD-RPA detection of IBRV. The development of a combination of LFD-RPA detection for IBRV was described. Finally, the performance of the RPA assay on acute phase fever clinical samples was evaluated and the results compared with SYBR Green I real time PCR.

Methods

Viruses, cell and clinical specimens

IBRV/BoHV-1.1/BarthaNu/67 strain, bovine herpesvirus 5 (BoHV-5)/N569 strain, bovine viral diarrhea virus (BVDV)/NADL strain, bovine parainfluenza virus type 3 (BPIV-3)/BN-1 strain were preserved in our laboratory, and the viruses were cultured in the Madin-Darby Bovine Kidney (MDBK) cell using the Dulbecco's Modified Eagle Medium (DMEM, HyClone, USA), containing antibiotics (1000 UI/L penicillin, 100 mg/L streptomycin) with 8% horse serum. Other bovine virus strains for cross reactivity testing used in this study were provided by full-length cloned cDNA: entire genome sequence of bovine respiratory syncytial virus (BRSV)/A51908strain, bovine ephemeral fever virus (BEFV)/(Gene Bank No: NC_002526.1), bovine enterovirus (BEV)/VG-5-27strain, bovine coronavirus (BcoV)/ENT strain (Gene Bank No:NC_003045.1), respectively. A total of 106 acute-phase high fever clinical specimens (24 fecal, 36 blood, 38 nasal swab and 8 tissue specimens) were collected from cattle farms suspected to be infected with IBRV in Shandong Province, China.

Isolation of DNA/RNA, cDNA synthesis

IBRV and other herpesviruses DNA were extracted from 200 μL of infected cell culture supernatant using the UNIQ-10 viral DNA extraction kit (Sangon Biotech Co., Ltd., Shanghai, China). RNA from BVDV, BPIV-3 was prepared from 200 μL of infected cell culture supernatant using the QIAamp viral RNA minikit according to manufacturer's instructions (Qiagen, Germany), respectively. The DNA/RNA was eluted in 50 μL of nuclease-free water. The extracted RNA was used as template for cDNA synthesis using the RevertAid™ First Strand cDNA Synthesis Kit (Fermentas, Canada). All templates were stored at −70 °C until further needed.

Generation of DNA standard

The IBRV UL52 region fragment (300 bp) were synthesized by Jierui Biotech (Shanghai, China) and cloned into pEASY-T3 vector, designated as UL-T3-RPA. The UL-T3-RPA standard DNA was extracted with Plasmiad Mini kit (Tiangen, Beijing) and measured using a Nanodrop ND-1000 spectrophotometer (Thermo Scientific, Dreieich, Germany). The DNA copy number was calculated by the equation: DNA cope number = $(M \times 6.02 \times 10^{23} \times 10^{-9})/(n \times 660)^{28}$, M: molecular weight, n: plasmid concentration measured at 260 nm. DNA standard was stored at −20 °C until further used.

Design of RPA primers and specific LF probe for IBRV

The highly conserved region of IBRV was screened and selected in GenBank database (GenBank: AJ004801.1, E01200.1, NC_001847.1, JX898220.1, KM258880.1). Eight forward primers and reverse primers, and nine LF probes (Table 1) were designed according to RPA instruction manual from TwistDx (TwistDx, Ltd., Cambridge, United Kingdom). In summary, the length of 30 bp to 35 bp for RPA Primers is recommended. TwistAmp™ LF Probe oligonucleotide backbone includes a 5′-antigenic label FAM group, an internal abasic nucleotide analogue 'dSpacer' and a 3′-polymerase extension blocking group C3-spacer. One amplification primer opposing TwistAmp™ LF Probe is labeled with Biotin at its 5′ end, thus dual-labeled amplicon can be detected simultaneously. Oligonucleotide RPA primers and LF probes used in the study were synthesized by Sangon Biotech (Shanghai, China).

Table 1 The sequences of primers and probes designed in this study

Primers	Oligonucleotide sequences (5'to3')	Product sizes (bp)	Location
1F:	5′-GGCAAGCGCCGCGAAGGAAACCAAGTCG-3′	236	4013–7237
1R:	【Biotin】 5′-GGCTTTACTCCAACAGCGGTGCGACTCCCTTC-3′		
1LF:	5′-【FAM】 GCGAAGGAAACCAAGTCGGGGAAGGCGAGTC[dSpacer]CGAGGGGTTAGGCG【C3-spacer】-3′		
2F	5′- GGGGACGGCCACGTACACTTGCTCGTCGTAGAGG –3′	187	19,597–20,823
2R:	【Biotin】5′- TCTGTCCGACGGCGGCAACGGCAACCCAATC –3′		
2-1LF1:	AAAGGCGTTTCGCAGCGAGGCGCCAAAGGG[dSpacer]CTCAGCAGGGCGGAGAC-3′		
2-2LF2:	5′-【FAM】 AGGCGTTTCGCAGCGAGGCGCCAAAGGGG[dSpacer]TCAGCAGGGCGGAGACGT【C3-spacer】-3′		
3F:	5′- ACACGAGGTCGCCGCCCGTGAAGACGCCGTTGTT –3′	142	23,526–25,889
3R	【Biotin】5′- CCAATGGACGGAAAGGTGCCCGCCTCCCAGAT –3′		
3LF:	5′-【FAM】 CCGTTGTTGGTGGCCTTGCGGATCTTGCAG[dSpacer]AGTAGAGCCCCGTCTTA【C3-spacer】-3′		
4-1F:	5′- TTGACAAAGACCGAGTCCGTGTCGCCGTAAACCA –3′	274	45,238–48,978
4-1R:	【Biotin】5′- TCGATAAGCAGCAGGCCGCCATCAAGGTCGTGT –3′		
4-1LF:	5′-【FAM】 TGTGGCCCAGCGCTCGTGTATGTACCGCCG[dSpacer]GTCTCGAGCAGCATGTC【C3-spacer】-3′		
4-2F	5′-GCTTTCCGACCAGCGCCGAATCTTGGATGCAGT –3′	250	47,151–47,397
4-2R:	【Biotin】5′- GGCCAAAACCGCTTTCAGAAGCAGAGCAAGGTGA –3′		
4-2LF:	5′-【FAM】 CCGCAAAGTGCCGAGGGATGTCCTTGTAGT[dSpacer]CAGGTCCACCTTCCGCT【C3-spacer】-3′		
4-3F:	5′- GCCACCGCCGACAGCTCCAGGTGGGGCAAGTAC –3′	295	47,151–47,397
4-3R:	【Biotin】5′- CGGGCCAAAACCGCTTTCAGAAGCAGAGCAAGGT –3′		
4-3LF:	5′-【FAM】 CACCTTCCGCTCCCGCAGGGCCTCCTCGGC[dSpacer]ACGGCGTTGAGCTTGTA【C3-spacer】-3′		
4-4F	:5′- CTTTCCGACCAGCGCCGAATCTTGGATGCAGTA –3′	154	47,151–47,397
4-4R:	【Biotin】5′- CAGCTACAAGCTCAACGCCGTGGCCGAGGAGGC –3′		
4-4LF:	5′-【FAM】 CCGCAAAGTGCCGAGGGATGTCCTTGTAGT[dSpacer]CAGGTCCACCTTCCGCTC【C3-spacer】-3′		
gB-F:	5′- ACACGGACCGCGTGCCCGTGGGCATGGGCGAGATCA –3′	257	55,015–58,579
gB-R:	【Biotin】5′- GCAGTTCACAGAGGTGCCCGTGCGGTAGAGCC –3′		
gB-LF:	5′-【FAM】 AGCGGGCGCAAGGTGGTGGCCTTTGACCGC[dSpacer]ACGACGACCCCTGGGAG【C3-spacer】-3′		

Note: *F*: Forward primer; *R*: Reverse primer; *LF* Probe; *FAM* Carboxyfluorescein; *dSpacer* A tetrahydrofuran residue; C3-spacer: 3′-block

Laboratory based RPA assays

TwistAmp™ nfo kits were supplied as dry enzyme pellets in eight strips within vacuum-sealed pouches (TwistDx, Ltd., Cambridge, United Kingdom). The IBRV RPA was performed in a 50 μL final reaction volume according to the instructions outlined in the Twist Amp nfo kit manual. The rehydration solution contained an optimized blend of DNA template and primers and a LF probe. Each reconstituted reaction mixture contained 2 μL DNA template, 2.1 μL (10 μM) Primer, 0.6 μL (10 μM) TwistAmp™ LF Probe, 29.5 μL Rehydration Buffer. Resuspend the reaction pellet with 47.5 μL of the rehydration solution, and then the reaction was initiated by adding 2.5 μL of Magnesium Acetate (280 mM). The tubes were then incubated at 38 °C in an incubator block for 4 min. As recommended, the samples were blended up and down 6–8 times after 4 min' incubation, and an additional incubation was continued for 21 min. In addition, in each run, a positive template control supplied with the Twist Amp nfo kit (primers/probe and template) and a negative template control (nuclease-free) water were included.

The amplicon of TwistAmp™ LF Probe system was visualised using a simple 'sandwich' LFD assay. Milenia's Genline Hybridetect-1 or Hybridetect-2 lateral flow strips duplexes labeled with anti-FAM gold conjugates and anti-Biotin antibodies from Milenia GmbH (Germany) were used in this study for detection of LFD-RPA amplified nucleic acids. 2 μL of hybridization products were mixed with 98 μL of PBST (1 × Phosphate Buffered Saline with 0.1% Tween-20) running buffer. The LFD were then placed into the PBST dilution in a 96-well plate. The positive amplification product might be indicated by both test line and control line on the strip visualized simultaneously after 5 min, the negative control (no template) should generate a separate control line found further up test line on the strip. The absence of a control line on the LFD indicates the strip could not work correctly.

The outcome of TwistAmp™ LF Probe systems were also analyzed by agarose gel-electrophoresis (AGE). In brief, the amplification product was purified by commercial PCR purification kits. The comparable size of required amount of the amplification products were visualized by electrophoresis on a 2% agarose-gel.

Determination of sensitivity and specificity of the assay

To determine the limit of IBRV genomic DNA copies, ten-fold serial dilutions of the standard UL-T3-RPA plasmid ranging from 5×10^8 to 5×10^{-1} DNA copies per reaction were detected within the same sample run. The operation steps were performed according to section of laboratory based RPA assays. The assay sensitivity assessment was also carried out by PCR assay, and the IBRV DNA amplification condition were previously described [20]. Briefly, the nucleotide sequences of the primers were as follows: BF: 5′-AGACCCCAGTTGTGATGAATGC-3′ and BR: 5′-ACACGTCCAGCACGAACACC-3′. The amplification conditions consisted of a preliminary denaturation step of 95 °C for 4 min, 35 cycles of denaturation at 95 °C for 1 min, primer annealing at 58 °C for 45 s, and extension at 72 °C for 45 s and a final cycle of 72 °C for 5 min, and the size of amplification product is 183 bp. Two methods were operated with the same amount of template.

The specificity of the assay was assessed among other viral pathogens of cattle with similar clinical signs or other herpesviruses. DNA and RNA extracts were prepared from cell culture supernatant of BoHV-5, BVDV, BPIV-3, respectively, and cDNA of BVDV, BPIV-3 were prepared as mentioned above. Clone of full-length genome of BRSV, BEFV, BEV and BcoV were supplied as templates in the LFD-RPA reaction. Additionally, DNA extracted from 5×10^5 DNA copies per reaction of IBRV and IBRV-free samples were used as a positive control and a negative control respectively.

Clinical specimen preparation

A total of 106 acute-phase high fever clinical specimens including 24 fecal, 36 blood specimens, 38 nasal swabs and 8 tissue specimens were collected from in non-vaccinated herds suspected to be infected with IBRV in Shandong Province, China. Tissue specimens were homogenized in 10 mM phosphate buffered saline (PBS) with a dilution of 1:10 (*W*/*V*), centrifuged at 10,000×g at 4 °C for 15 min, sample suspension was collected until used. Fecal and swabs were placed immediately in 1 mL PBS and mixed by pulse-vortexing for 20 s after collection. 200 μL sample suspension was separated for DNA extraction using magnetic beads (Dynabeads®SILANE viral NA kit, Life Technologies, Darmstadt, Germany) according to the manufacturer's instructions. In summary, 200 μL of sample suspension was incubated with 50 μL (20 $mgmL^{-1}$) of proteinase K and 300 μL of lysis/binding buffer (viral NA) for 5 min at room temperature, and then 150 μL of isopropanol and 50 μL (2 mg) of Dynabeads were added and incubated at room temperature for 10 min followed by two washing steps. Viral DNA bound to the Dynabeads was left to dry at room temperature for 5 min before eluting in 50 μL of elution buffer. A volume of 2 μL of DNA extracted from each swab specimen was used as a template in the RPA reactions. The minute was how long before a test line was observed on the LFD.

SYBR green I real-time PCR for amplification of IBRV

The primer pairs for SYBR Green I real-time PCR used for amplification of IBRV were IBRV-F: 5′- ACGGACG ACGAGCTGGGACT-3′, IBRV-R: 5′-CGGCAGCGAAA CCATGAAAT-3′. Real-time PCR was performed on a LightCycler480 Real-time PCR System using SYBR® Premix Ex Taq™ II (TliRNaseH Plus) reagents (Takara BioInc, Japan) according to the Manufacturer's instructions. The reaction was carried out in a 20 μL volume containing 10 μL 2 × SYBR Premix Ex Taq II, 0.5 μL of forward and reverse primers (20 μM), respectively, 2 μL of DNA and 7 μL DNase-free water. The real-time PCR was performed as follows 1 cycle of 95 °C for 5 min, followed by 45 cycles of 95 °C for 30 s and 63 °C for 30 s. Fluorescent signal was collected during the elongation step. In diagnostic real-time PCR assay, it was customary to regard results between C_T 35 and 40 as equivocal and above C_T 40 as negative.

Results

Design and optimization of RPA primers and probe

Based on alignment analysis of infections bovine rhinotracheltis virus (GenBank: AJ004801.1, E01200.1, NC_001847.1, JX898220.1, KM258880.1), six distinct regions were selected as a candidate target for designing the LFD-RPA primers and probes. Eight forward primers and eight reverse primers labeled at the 5′ end with biotin for the detection of IBRV were designed to screen candidate primer pairs and probe (Table 1). Then nine LF probe combinations with primers were employed for further validation in this study. The candidate primers/probe for the LFD-RPA assay were screened by performing with TwistAmp™ nfo reactions and preliminarily analyzed on 2% agarose gel with labeled amplicons. The initial agarose gel result showed that Primer set 4-2F/4-2R/4-2LF yielded specific amplification efficiency for the RPA assay, and produced the expected size of the product was 250 base-pairs (Fig. 1a), while the primers/probe targeting glycoprotein gB of the IBRV genome in this study could not be used to amplify effectively in the initial screen (data not show). In order to determine the best pairs of primers/probe for maximum effective amplification, a series of staggered primers with 1–5 base intervals upstream and downstream

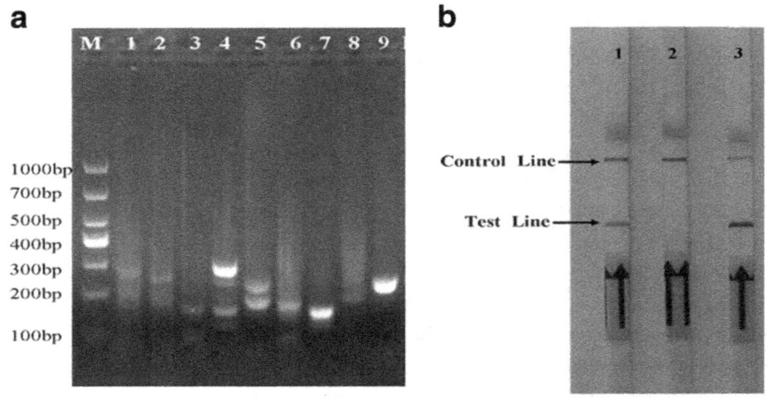

Fig. 1 Validating the designed primers/probe of IBRV LFD-RPA assay. **a** Agarose gel electrophoresis of RPA products generated using designed primers/probes. Lane M: molecular weight standard (DNA Marker1000). Lane 1 to 9: designed primer and probe sets. Especially, Lane 5 was primers/probe set 4-2F/4-2R/4-2LF, and the expected size of the product was 247 bp. **b** Lateral-flow strip end-point analysis of RPA products generated using optimal designed primers/probes set 4F/4R/4LF. Lane 1: positive control (supplied by Twist Ampnfo kit); Lane 2: negative control (DNase-free water); Lane 3: IBRV amplicons performed with RPA primer pair 4F/4R/4LF. Samples were tested in triplicate with one reaction displayed in figure for each triplicate

of the original 4-2F/4-2R/4-2LF sequences were designed to obtain optimal primers for IBRV RPA, LFD-RPA results indicated that Primer set 4F/4R/4LF presented the most efficient amplification with expected size of 247 bp (Table 2), showing a test line within 5 min on the LFD (Fig. 1b).

Sensitivity and specificity of the RPA reaction

The analytical sensitivity of the RPA assay was determined using the IBRV DNA extracted from ten-fold serially diluted IBRV DNA ranging from 5×10^{-1} to 5×10^{8} copies per reaction, and the minimum virus detection limits of RPA were as low as 5 copies per reaction (Fig. 2a). The amplified products in the IBRV LFD RPA reaction were also detected by subsequent agarose gel electrophoresis (Fig. 2b). To detect the stability of the RPA method, the stability of the assay using DNA extracted from 5×10^{0} DNA copies per reaction of IBRV and negative controls were also evaluated in 3 replicates, respectively. The detection limits of the method showed the same result (Fig. 2c). As compared, all these ten-fold serially diluted templates were detected by conventional PCR, the sensitivity of the gold standard conventional PCR was 5×10^{2} DNA copies per reaction. Therefore, the sensitivity of our RPA-LFD assay was at least 100 times higher than that of the routine PCR assay (Fig. 2d).

Table 2 RPA primers and probe used for the rapid detection of IBRV

Name	Sequence (5'to 3')
4F	5'-TTCCGACCAGCGCCGAATCTTGGATGCAGTACT-3'
4R	5'-【Biotin】GGCCAAAACCGCTTTCAGAAGCAGAGCAAGGTGA-3'
4LF	5'-【FAM】CCGCAAAGTGCCGAGGGATGTCCTTGTAGT【dSpacer】CAGGTCCACCTTCCGCT【C3-spacer】-3'

Note: *F* Forward primer; *R* Reverse primer; *LF* probe; *FAM* Carboxyfluorescein; *dSpacer* A tetrahydrofuran residue; C3-spacer: 3'-block

The specificity of the assay was assessed with other viral pathogens of cattle with similar clinic and other herpesviruses such as bovine herpesvirus5 (BoHV-5).As shown in Fig. 3a, no cross-reactions of the BVDV, BPIV-3, BRSV, BEFV, BEV, BcoV, and BoHV-5 were observed and the amplicons in these viruses examined by the IBRV RPA-LFD assay were also tested with agarose gel electrophoresis Fig. 3b.

RPA performances using clinical specimens

One hundred six clinical specimens were collected from suspected cases, and viral DNA extracted using magnetic beads were used as templates for detection. In all cases, clinical specimens were subjected to conventional PCR, RPA, and compared with the real-time PCR assay. The results of those assays showed that a total of 76 clinical specimens were tested positive by conventional PCR, while the same performance that 84 specimens were detected positive by IBRV RPA nucleic acid amplification assays on LFD within 5 min, and with the Cycle threshold (C_T) values below 35 using the SYBR Green I real-time PCR assay. This particular RPA therefore was highly sensitive compared with the real-time PCR, and there was very good correlation between the results from RPA and SYBR Green I real-time PCR of the same sample (Table 3). In addition, the results show that IBRV RPA-LFD may be an ideal method to detect the IBRV genome in low resource settings.

Discussion

Rapid and reliable nucleic acid tests are the gold-standard for the detection of a wide variety of infectious pathogens. Recent studies have shown that isothermal amplification techniques such as RPA and LAMP could be developed to amplify nucleic acids, which require neither high precision

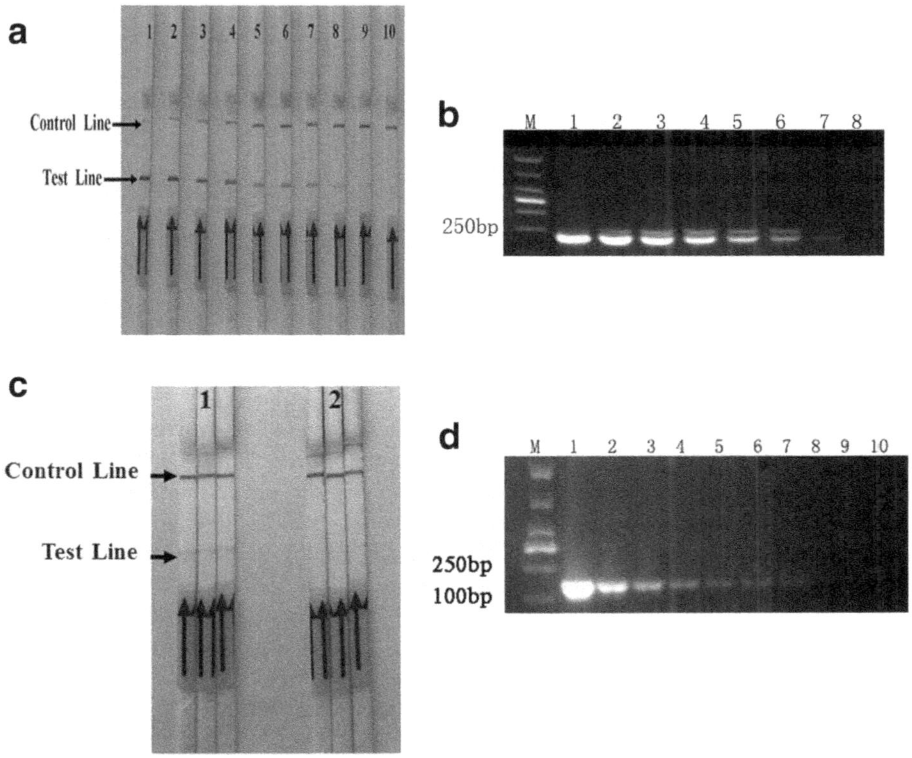

Fig. 2 Sensitivity of the LFD-RPA assay. **a** Molecular sensitivity of RPA using total DNA extracted from 10-fold serially diluted IBRV-infected cell as template. IBRV templates of lane 1 to 10 in these reactions extracted from ten-fold serially diluted virus range from 5×10^8 to 5×10^{-1} DNA copies per reaction. Samples were tested in triplicate with one reaction displayed in figure for each triplicate. **b** IBRV RPA reaction products (247 bp) could be detected on a 2% agarose gel. Lane 1 to 9 were represented IBRV RPA reactions extracted from ten-fold serially diluted IBRV templates range from 5×10^6 to 5×10^{-1} DNA copies per reaction. **c** Repeatability of limits detection. The sensitivity of the assay using IBRV DNA extracted from 5 copies per reaction of IBRV DNA and negative control (DNase-free water) were also evaluated in 3 replicates, respectively. **d** Sensitivity of conventional PCR. Molecular sensitivity of conventional PCR uses the same template amount as the IBRV LFD-RPA assay. Templates of lane 1 to 10 in these reactions extracted from ten-fold serially diluted virus genome DNA range from 5×10^8 to 5×10^{-1} copies per reaction. Samples were tested in triplicate with one reaction displayed in figure for each triplicate

instrument for amplification nor elaborate methods for detection of the amplified products [21]. Among those isothermal amplification assays, RPA is a powerful, innovative nucleic acid test, which could be useful for low resource settings [22, 23]. RPA outperforms over LAMP currently developed for IBRV diagnosis. One advantage is that RPA reaction only utilizes two primers and one probe and three binding sites, in contrast, the LAMP assay needs at least four primers and six binding sites. In addition, RPA reagents provided in a lyophilized pellet are stable

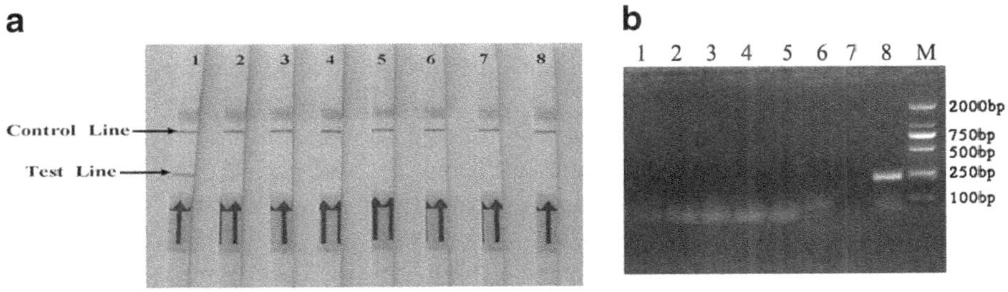

Fig. 3 Specificity of the LFD-RPA assay. **a** The specificity of the IBRV RPA-LFD assay was assessed for other viral pathogens genome cDNA of cattle that present similarly in the clinic other herpesviruses such as bovine herpesvirus5 (BoHV-5). Lanes 1: positive control. Lanes 2 to 8: BVDV, BPIV-3, BRSV, BEFV, BEV, BcoV and BoHV-5, respectively. Samples were tested in triplicate with one reaction displayed in figure for each triplicate. **b** The specificity of the IBRV RPA-LFD products could be displayed on a 2% agarose gel. Lanes 1 to 7: BVDV, BPIV-3, BRSV, BEFV, BEV, BcoV and BoHV-5, respectively, Lane 8: positive control. Lane M: molecular weight standard (DNA Marker 2000)

Table 3 Comparative performance of LFD-RPA, PCR and SYBR Green I real time qPCR assays for detection of IBRV suspected clinical specimens

Samples name	PCR		LFD-RPA		Real-time qPCR		LFD-RPA/Real-time qPCR		LFD-RPA/ PCR/ Real-time qPCR	
	P	N	P	N	P	N	P	N	P	N
fecal	18	6	20	4	20	4	20	4	18	4
blood	30	6	32	4	32	4	32	4	30	4
nasal swab	20	18	24	14	24	14	24	14	20	14
lymph node	3	0	3	0	3	0	3	0	3	0
spleen	3	0	3	0	3	0	3	0	3	0
lung	2	0	2	0	2	0	2	0	2	0
Total	76	30	84	22	84	22	84	22	76	22

Note: *P* Positive; *N* Negative

even when stored for 3 weeks at 45 °C, which allow independence from the cooling chain [24, 25].

The most important step of RPA is to identify the appropriate primers and probes. However, there is no ideal design support software available for RPA. In this study, different conserved genomic regions were selected for olignucleotide design (Table 1). Several primer and probe combinations were initially evaluated for target sequences and two products generated by RPA primer pair and probe were distinct in size on an agarose gel to exclude non-specific amplification (Fig. 1a). It is worth mentioning that, unlike PCR-based DNA amplification assays, it should be noted that the primer and probe set of RPA is much more stringent as it requires longer primers (30–35 bases) and probes (46–52 bases) leading to the potential of formation of secondary structures. Moreover, after several optimization screening, one optimal set of the primers and probe limited to the UL52 regions functioning DNA replication can be successfully used to amplify an exact sequence-matched template (Fig. 1b) since replacement, increase, decrease or mismatch of single base will have a significant impact on the result of amplification [26]. Furthermore, we also found that IBRV molecular detection with RPA assay poses unique challenges because the genome of IBRV was rich in GC content. In retrospect, given recently published data describing glycoprotein-based IBRV detection assay, loop-mediated isothermal amplification (LAMP) or PCR-based assays have been reported to detect IBRV in biological samples [27, 28]. In the present study, none of the primers targeting glycoprotein gB within the same region of the genome of LAMP and PCR could be used to amplify effectively in the initial screen (Table 1), this may be due to the long probe formed folded secondary structures and had an impact upon hybridization to target, or perhaps there are different regions for primer design between RPA and LAMP/PCR.

With regard to analytical sensitivity, the RPA developed in this study showed a performance limit of detection of 5 copies per reaction of IBRV DNA (Fig. 2a and b) equaled to Real Time PCR, which was at least 100 times higher than that of the routine PCR assay (Fig. 2d). The study of specificity showed that no cross-detection between IBRV and other bovine infectious virus or bovine herpesvirus 5 (Fig. 3a and b). It should be noted that the high sensitivity and specificity of this assay gave the credit to good use of gold-labeled anti-FAM and anti-Biotin antibodies to capture RPA product simultaneously. The clinical performance of PCR, LFD-RPA and SYBR Green I based PCR assays were detected using 106 suspected clinical specimens, the clinical sensitivity of both LFD-RPA and SYBR Green I real-time assays was 100%, while PCR showing the lower detection might be due to some clinical samples containing low viral titers. Although LFD-RPA is not appropriate for the quantitative analysis of nucleic acid, an important feature of the method is the LFD-RPA assay under normal circumstances outperforms other isothermal amplification assays in terms of simplicity and sensitivity, because it only requires a simple heat block to run and the results can also be visualized by LFD with naked eyes inspection.

This methodology of LFD-RPA might be uniquely appropriate for application of visual field testing due wholly to the RPA enzymes can be short-term storage and transport at ambient temperatures in a lyophilized pellet, and conducted without a precise incubation temperature (body temperature) [29]. Moreover, some samples only require simple preparation and processing before RPA. It has also been shown that RPA tolerates multiple known PCR inhibitors, including hemoglobin (50 gL^{-1}), heparin (0.5 U), undiluted serum, and ethanol (4%v/v) [17]. However, some components of nucleic acids extracted from clinical sample have an influence on RPA reaction such as the concentrations of background DNA in whole blood [30]. To fulfill the full potential of developed IBRV LFD-RPA at the point of care in field conditions, we evaluated several simple methods for clinical sample extraction including direct sample lysis with heat lysis, alkaline lysis (0.2 M KOH or 0.5% SDS) and Dynabeads® magnetic separation. We found that Dynabeads® magnetic separation worked well. Similar sensitivities were obtained from viral genome extraction kit. Heat and alkaline lysis did not result insufficient recovery of positive DNA (data not shown). Although Dynabeads® magnetic separation technology is easily adapted to automated liquid handling platforms, other methodology platform to perform sample preparation will be further required to optimize.

Conclusion

This workpackage has developed a rapid, robust, cost-effective and highly sensitive LFD-RPA assay for the detection of IBRV. In addition, the rapid LFD-RPA for IBRV may save much time in epidemiological surveillance and aid in identification of latent IBRV infected individuals in beef and dairy farms. Furthermore, it may be serves as a model platform for detecting other bovine pathogens.

Abbreviations

BcoV: Bovine coronavirus; BEFV: Bovine ephemeral fever virus; BEV: Bovine enterovirus; BoHV-1: Bovine herpesvirus 1; BPIV-3: Bovine parainfluenza virus type 3; BRSV: Bovine respiratory syncytial virus; BVDV: Bovine viral diarrhea virus; DMEM: Dulbecco's modified eagle medium; ELISA: Enzyme-linked immunosorbent assay; IBRV: Infectious bovine rhinotracheitis virus; LAMP: Loop-mediated isothermal amplification; LFD: Lateral flow dipstrip; MDBK: Madin-darby bovine kidney; PBS: Phosphate buffered saline; PCR: Polymerase chain reaction; RPA: Recombinase polymerase amplification; SSB: Single-strand binding proteins

Acknowledgments

Not applicable.

Funding

This work was partially supported by grants from National Natural Science Fund of China (31,502,064, 31,672,556), Taishan Scholar and Distinguished Experts (H. H.), Shandong Major Agricultural Application Technology Innovation Project (H.W), Primary Research & Developement Plan of Shandong Province(2015GNC113006, 2016GNC113006).

Authors' contributions

H.HB designed and instructed the experiments. H.PL and W.HM performed the experiments and drafted the manuscript. H.CQ and Z.GM collected and provided clinical specimens. All the authors have read and approved the final manuscript.

Consent for publication

Not applicable.

Competing interests

The authors declared no potential conflicts of interest with respect to the research, authorship, and/or publication of this article.

References

1. Straub OC. Advances in BHV1 (IBR) research. Dtsch Tierarztl Wochenschr. 2001;108(10):419–22.
2. Kirchhoff J, Uhlenbruck S, Goris K, Keil GM, Herrler G. Three viruses of the bovine respiratory disease complex apply different strategies to initiate infection. Vet Res. 2014;45:20.
3. Muylkens B, Thiry J, Kirten P, Schynts F, Thiry E. Bovine herpesvirus 1 infection and infectious bovine rhinotracheitis. Vet Res. 2007;38(2):181–209.
4. Nandi S, Kumar M, Manohar M, Chauhan RS. Bovine herpes virus infections in cattle. Anim Health Res Rev. 2009;10(1):85–98.
5. Raaperi K, Orro T, Viltrop A. Epidemiology and control of bovine herpesvirus 1 infection in Europe. Vet J. 2014;201(3):249–56.
6. Newcomer BW, Givens D. Diagnosis and control of viral diseases of reproductive importance: infectious bovine Rhinotracheitis and bovine viral diarrhea. Vet Clin North Am Food Anim Pract. 2016;32(2):425–41.
7. Nardelli S, Farina G, Lucchini R, Valorz C, Moresco A, Dal Zotto R, Costanzi C. Dynamics of infection and immunity in a dairy cattle population undergoing an eradication programme for infectious bovine Rhinotracheitis (IBR). Prev Vet Med. 2008;85(1–2):68–80.
8. Biswas S, Bandyopadhyay S, Dimri U, Patra PH. Bovine herpesvirus-1 (BHV-1) – a re-emerging concern in livestock: a revisit to its biology, epidemiology, diagnosis, and prophylaxis. Vet Q. 2013;33(2):68–81.
9. Graham DA, Mawhinney KA, McShane J, Connor TJ, Adair BM, Merza M. Standardization of enzyme-linked immunosorbent assays (ELISAs) for quantitative estimation of antibodies specific for infectious bovine rhinotracheitis virus, respiratory syncytial virus, parainfluenza-3 virus, and bovine viral diarrhea virus. J Vet Diagn Invest. 1997;9(1):24–31.
10. Yang SH, Wang CF, Gao YD, Liu WH, Yan-Qin LI, Zhong JF. Fast Diagnosis of IBRV by Nested-PCR Method. Acta Ecologiae Animalis Domastici. 2007;28(4): 81–3.
11. Fu S, Qu G, Guo S, Ma L, Zhang N, Zhang S, Gao S, Shen Z. Applications of loop-mediated isothermal DNA amplification. Appl Biochem Biotechnol. 2011;163(7):845–50.
12. Suwancharoen D, Sittiwicheanwong B, Wiratsudakul A. Evaluation of loop-mediated isothermal amplification method (LAMP) for pathogenic Leptospira spp. detection with leptospires isolation and real-time PCR. J Vet Med Sci. 2016;78(8):1299–302.
13. Piepenburg O, Williams CH, Stemple DL, Armes NA. DNA detection using recombination proteins. PLoS Biol. 2006;4(7):e204.
14. Boyle DS, Lehman DA, Lillis L, Peterson D, Singhal M, Armes N, Parker M, Piepenburg O, Overbaugh J. Rapid detection of HIV-1 Proviral DNA for early infant diagnosis using recombinase polymerase amplification. MBio. 2013;4(2):49–52.
15. Euler M, Wang Y, Nentwich O, Piepenburg O, Hufert FT, Weidmann M. Recombinase polymerase amplification assay for rapid detection of Rift Valley fever virus. J Clin Virol. 2012;54(4):308–12.
16. Euler M, Wang Y, Heidenreich D, Patel P, Strohmeier O, Hakenberg S, Niedrig M, Hufert FT, Weidmann M. Development of a panel of recombinase polymerase amplification assays for detection of biothreat agents. J Clin Microbiol. 2013;51(4):1110–7.
17. Kersting S, Rausch V, Bier FF, Nickisch-Rosenegk v. M: rapid detection of plasmodium falciparum with isothermal recombinase polymerase amplification and lateral flow analysis. Malar J. 2014;13:99.
18. Murinda SE, Ibekwe AM, Zulkaffly S, Cruz A, Park S, Razak N, Paudzai FM, Ab Samad L, Baquir K, Muthaiyah K, et al. Real-time isothermal detection of Shiga toxin-producing Escherichia Coli using recombinase polymerase amplification. Foodborne Pathog Dis. 2014;11(7):529–36.
19. Xia X, Yu Y, Hu L, Weidmann M, Pan Y, Yan S, Wang Y. Rapid detection of infectious hypodermal and hematopoietic necrosis virus (IHHNV) by real-time, isothermal recombinase polymerase amplification assay. Arch Virol. 2015;160(4):987–94.
20. Yason CV, Harris LM, Mckenna PK, Wadowska D, Kibenge FS. Establishment of conditions for the detection of bovine herpesvirus-1 by polymerase chain reaction using primers in the thymidine kinase region. Can J Vet Res. 1995;59(2):94.
21. Niemz A, Ferguson TM, Boyle DS. Point-of-care nucleic acid testing for infectious diseases. Trends Biotechnol. 2011;29(5):240–50.
22. Zaghloul H, El-Shahat M. Recombinase polymerase amplification as a promising tool in hepatitis C virus diagnosis. World J Hepatol. 2014;6(12):916–22.
23. James A, Macdonald J. Recombinase polymerase amplification: emergence as a critical molecular technology for rapid, low-resource diagnostics. Expert Rev Mol Diagn. 2015;15(11):1475–89.
24. Notomi T, Okayama H, Masubuchi H, Yonekawa T, Watanabe K, Amino N, Hase T. Loop-mediated isothermal amplification of DNA. Nucleic Acids Res. 2000;28(12) E63.

25. Lillis L, Siverson J, Lee A, Cantera J, Parker M, Piepenburg O, Lehman DA, Boyle DS. Factors influencing recombinase polymerase amplification (RPA) assay outcomes at point of care. Mol Cell Probes. 2016;30(2):74–8.
26. Daher RK, Stewart G, Boissinot M, Boudreau DK, Bergeron MG. Influence of sequence mismatches on the specificity of recombinase polymerase amplification technology. Mol Cell Probes. 2015;29(2):116–21.
27. El-Kholy AA, Abdelrahman K, Soliman H. Rapid detection of BoHV-1 genomic DNA by loop-mediated isothermal amplification assay. J Virol Methods. 2014;204:81–5.
28. Pawar SS, Meshram CD, Singh NK, Sonwane AA, Saini M, Rautmare SS, Muglikar DM, Mishra BP, Gupta PK. Rapid detection of bovine herpesvirus 1 in bovine semen by loop-mediated isothermal amplification (LAMP) assay. Arch Virol. 2014;159(4):641–8.
29. Crannell ZA, Rohrman B, Richards-Kortum R. Equipment-free incubation of recombinase polymerase amplification reactions using body heat. PLoS One. 2014;9(11):e112146.
30. Rohrman B, Richards-Kortum R. Inhibition of recombinase polymerase amplification by background DNA: a lateral flow-based method for enriching target DNA. Anal Chem. 2015;87(3):1963–7.

5

Bovine tuberculosis visible lesions in cattle culled during herd breakdowns: the effects of individual characteristics, trade movement and co-infection

Andrew W. Byrne[1,2*], Jordon Graham[1], Craig Brown[1], Aoibheann Donaghy[1], Maria Guelbenzu-Gonzalo[1], Jim McNair[1], Robin Skuce[1], Adrian Allen[1] and Stanley McDowell[1]

Abstract

Background: Bovine tuberculosis (bTB), caused by *Mycobacterium bovis*, remains a significant problem for livestock industries in many countries worldwide including Northern Ireland, where a test and slaughter regime has utilised the Single Intradermal Comparative Cervical Tuberculin (SICCT) test since 1959.

We investigated the variation in post-mortem confirmation based on bTB visible lesion (VL) presence during herd breakdowns using two model suites. We investigated animal-level characteristics, while controlling for herd-level factors and clustering. We were interested in potential impacts of concurrent infection, and therefore we assessed whether animals with evidence of liver fluke infection (*Fasciola hepatica*; post-mortem inspection), *M. avium* reactors (animals with negative *M. bovis-avium* (*b-a*) tuberculin reactions) or Bovine Viral Diarrhoea Virus (BVDV; RT-PCR tested) were associated with bTB confirmation.

Results: The dataset included 6242 animals removed during the 14 month study period (2013–2015). bTB-VL presence was significantly increased in animals with greater *b-a* reaction size at the disclosing SICCT test (e.g. $b\text{-}a = 5$-9 mm vs. $b\text{-}a = 0$ mm, adjusted Odds ratio (aOR): 14.57; $p < 0.001$). *M. avium* reactor animals ($b\text{-}a < 0$) were also significantly more likely to disclose VL than non-reactor animals ($b\text{-}a = 0$; aOR: 2.29; $p = 0.023$). Animals had a greater probability of exhibiting lesions with the increasing number of herds it had resided within (movement; log-herds: aOR: 2.27–2.42; $p < 0.001$), if it had an inconclusive penultimate test result (aOR: 2.84–3.89; $p < 0.001$), and with increasing time between tests (log-time; aOR: 1.23; $p = 0.003$). Animals were less likely to have VL if they were a dairy breed (aOR: 0.79; $p = 0.015$) or in an older age-class (e.g. age-quartile 2 vs. 4; aOR: 0.65; $p < 0.001$). Liver fluke or BVDV variables were not retained in either multivariable model as they were non-significantly associated with bTB-VL status ($p > 0.1$).

Conclusions: Our results suggest that neither co-infection of liver fluke nor BVDV had a significant effect on the presence of VLs in this high-risk cohort. *M. avium* tuberculin reactors had a significantly increased risk of disclosing with a bTB lesion, which could be related to the impact of co-infection with *M. avium* subsp. *paratuberculosis* (MAP) affecting the performance of the SICCT however further research in this area is required. Movements, test history, breed and age were important factors influencing confirmation in high-risk animals.

Keywords: Bovine TB, *Mycobacterium bovis*, BVDV, Liver fluke, Paratuberculosis, Co-infection, Johne's disease, MAP, Fascioliasis, Gamma interferon, Skin tests, Cattle

* Correspondence: andrew.byrne@afbini.gov.uk
[1]Agri-food and Biosciences Institute, Veterinary Science Division, Stormont, Belfast, Northern Ireland BT43SD, UK
[2]School of Biological Sciences, Queen's University Belfast, Belfast, Northern Ireland, UK

Background

Despite decades of research into bovine tuberculosis (bTB), caused by *Mycobacterium bovis*, there still remains limitations in our ability to explain the variation in bTB detectability and confirmation infection within cattle [1–4]. Furthermore, animal-level analyses relating to pathological findings from surveillance have not been as frequently investigated, in comparison with epidemiological studies concentrating on herd-level factors [5, 6].

Bovine TB in Northern Ireland remains a significant chronic problem, with continual maintenance of the disease in the national herd despite a coordinated compulsory statutory scheme in place since the 1950s [7, 8]. This national scheme has been predicated on an ante-mortem test and cull regime, and supplemented with additional continual slaughter house surveillance systems [7]. The Single Intradermal Comparative Cervical Tuberculin (SICCT) test is the statutory ante-mortem test, and as dictated by legislation, all animals deemed to be standard reactors are compulsorily culled. Additional animals may be culled if 'severe' interpretation of the test is implemented during herd breakdowns, or through the ancillary use of the Interferon-γ test or serological tests, in an attempt to remove exposed animals [9–11]. However, all of these tests have limitations in terms of sensitivity (especially SICCT and serological tests) and specificity (especially the interferon-γ test), meaning some infected animals can be missed from breakdown herds or some non-infected animals needlessly culled [9, 12–14].

Recently, co-infection of other pathogens has been highlighted as a potential factor affecting the efficacy of the current systems to identify and remove infected animals from endemic bTB countries like the UK and Ireland [15–22]. Bovine Viral Diarrhoea Virus (BVDV) [15], liver fluke (*Fasciola hepatica*; [19]) and Johne's disease (caused by *Mycobacterium avium* subsp. *paratuberculosis* [21, 23]) have all been suggested to be implicated in the epidemiology of bovine TB either by actively exacerbating infection, potentially leading to increase *M. bovis* transmission, increasing host susceptibility, or by affecting the performance of tests used to detect bTB infection.

Here we investigate the variation in post-mortem confirmation (presence of bTB visible lesions; VL) of at-risk animals culled in Northern Ireland during 2013–2015. All animals removed were ante-mortem positive for bTB, or negative at-risk animals in direct contact with infected animals. Building on the previous work by O'Hagan et al. [4] in Northern Ireland, we hypothesised that confirmation would be significantly associated with variations in the SICCT test reaction size, the animal's test history, movement history (trade), and herd-level characteristics where the animal resided before slaughter [1, 3, 4]. Controlling for such risk factors, we then also utilised these data to explore the hypotheses that co-infection (exposure to BVDV, liver fluke or non-bTB *Mycobacterium*) may be significantly associated (either in positively or negatively) with the probability of bTB confirmation.

Methods

The study design was a retrospective observational case-control study. The study population was animals slaughtered as part of bTB herd breakdowns (where bTB has been detected in the herd via one or more positive statutory tests) in Northern Ireland. Cases were exposed animals with bTB visible lesions (VL), a metric of post-mortem confirmation, as used elsewhere (e.g. [1–4, 24–27]). Controls were animals without VL detected at slaughter. 97% of animals with lesions were laboratory confirmed (histopathology and/or culture) and a previous risk factor study of bovine reactors from Northern Ireland suggested that little difference in parameter estimates occurred when comparing VL with bacteriologically confirmed samples [4]. Extensive details of the TB program in Northern Ireland are presented in [7], and specific details of the processing of reactors and the determination of cases is presented in [4]. Briefly, reactor animals are sent to slaughter where post-mortem examination (PME) within the abattoir for evidence of infection through the presence of VLs is undertaken [4]. During the study period, 99% of samples were processed in one specific slaughterhouse, which would reduce the inter-abattoir variability in detection of lesions [1, 2]. The routine PME includes palpation of the lungs, liver and tongue, and incision of the lungs, heart, and liver. In reactor animals, examination of the lymph nodes of the head, chest and mesenterium, lungs, pleura, peritoneum, and the prescapular, popliteal, iliac, precrural lymph nodes was undertaken [4].

The dataset contained records from animals that were culled from the 27th of November 2013 to the 27th of January 2015. All animals were culled as they were deemed reactors to the Single Intradermal Comparative Cervical Tuberculin (SICCT) test (either standard interpretation or severe interpretation), gamma interferon test positive or animals in-contact with test positive animals.

Metrics of co-infection

The primary goal of this study was to investigate potential interactions between endemic diseases and *M. bovis* confirmation (VL). We investigated whether there was any evidence of interaction between BVDV positivity or exposure, liver fluke post-mortem status, and *Mycobacterium avium* complex exposure. All culled animals in the dataset had a tissue sample (ear-tag notch) available, which was stored at −70°c. These samples were used to prospectively test for BVDV virus using a commercial real time RT-PCR test (Virotype BVDV RT-PCR, Qiagen) as described before [22, 28]. All samples were first batch screened by RT-PCR, and individual samples within positive batches were then tested using antigen-capture ELISA test (Herd Check BVDV antigen/serum plus, IDEXX Laboratories) to detect viraemic animals. BVDV-bTB interaction was then assessed using two variables: (i) a direct BVDV RT-PCR positive test assigned to the animal, indicating the animal has active infection with BVDV (ii) indirect herd-level exposure, with all animals within a herd with a positive BVDV animal being considered exposed. Liver fluke status was also assessed with three metrics of infection using surveillance data [29]: (i) *Fascioliasis* recorded at slaughter, indicating that active infection (the presence of *Fasciola hepatica* in the liver) was occurring at time of death (1 = active infection; 0 = non-active infection) (ii) Liver fluke damage recorded at slaughter, indicating that the animal had been infected in the past, with resulting scar tissue in the liver, however the animal was not currently infected (1 = historic infection; 0 = non-historic infection) (iii) the animal was either found to have *Fascioliasis* or liver fluke damage at slaughter (1 = active infection or historic infection; 0 = non-active and non-historic infection). Please note, that category three is related to the other categories and so could not be entered into the same model.

Potential exposure to non-bTB *Mycobacterium* was assessed using the relative reaction size to the bovine and *M. avium* Purified Protein Derivative (PPD) tuberculin used during the disclosing test [30–33]. The comparative skin test (SICTT) used in Northern Ireland assigns test status to animals based on the bovine tuberculin reaction size subtracted by the avian reaction size (*b-a*), with positive bias values indicating a reaction to the bovine tuberculin greater than to the avian tuberculin (i.e. net bias), and negative reaction sizes indicating a reaction to avian tuberculin greater than to the bovine tuberculin. A bTB "standard reactor", one deemed positive to the statutory test and required to be culled by law, is one whereby the $b\text{-}a > 4$ mm. The relationship between PPD reaction size and VL presence was non-linear (Additional file 1; and see Additional file 2) – and was modelled by categorising the values into one of six types, three non-standard reactors (1. Avium reactor ($b\text{-}a < 0$ mm), 2. Non-reactor ($b\text{-}a = 0$ mm); 3. Inconclusive bovine reactor ($b\text{-}a > 0$ & $< =4$ mm)) and three standard reactor categories (4. "Small bovine reactors" ($b\text{-}a > 4$ & $b\text{-}a < 10$ mm); 5. "Large bovine reactors" ($b\text{-}a > =10$ & $b\text{-}a < 20$ mm); 6. "Hyper bovine reactors" ($b\text{-}a > =20$ mm)). We considered *M. avium* reactors as potentially indicative of exposure to non-bTB *Mycobacterium*, including *Mycobacterium avium* subsp. *paratuberculosis* the agent of Johne's disease in cattle [30, 32, 33], a notifiable pathogen in Northern Ireland. To further explore the impact of *M. avium* reactors on lesion presence, the effect of the individual bovine PPD reaction was assessed using descriptive statistics and univariable models. For this, a single intradermal tuberculin (SIT) test results was established as positive if the net bovine PPD reaction was >4 mm.

Other co-factors

We concentrated on animal-level variables in this study, while controlling for herd-level clustering. Factors investigated in our models are presented Table 1. These variables were chosen as we hypothesised that they could be influential in the ante-mortem test variability, confirmation, or pathology or because previous research suggested that they may be important (e.g. [3–5, 16, 25]).

Response variable and modelling approach

We developed models where the outcome was binary - bTB VL presence or absence [1–4]. The primary source of data for these analyses was the Northern Ireland Animal and Public Health Information System (APHIS; [34]). The presence of a lesion at slaughter was modelled using a multivariable binary logit random effects model, with the random effect capturing the potential non-independence of animals coming from the same herds [35]. The significance of this clustering was measured using a likelihood ratio test, compared with a regular logit regression model. Unlike previous studies [4], we did not include slaughter house as a random effect, as 99% of all animals within the dataset were processed at the same abattoir.

Throughout we used a two-step model building strategy – univariable model screening and multivariable model building. The functional form was assessed using LOWESS graphing, with suitable transforms of predictors implemented to improve model fit (e.g. natural logarithm transform; Additional file 1; Additional file 3; and see Additional file 2). We fitted separate univariable models for each independent variable of interest, and all variables that were significant at $p < 0.15$ were candidates for a multivariable model building process. The variables tested during the model building for the logistic regression model are presented in Table 1 below. Correlations amongst independent variables were assessed, and where necessary, variables were dropped if highly correlated (i.e. to reduce the possibility of multi-collinearity; [35, 36]). The decision to include a variable amongst a correlated pair was based on which variable improved the model fit more, as assessed by Akaike's Information Criteria (AIC). Backwards elimination was then used to establish parsimonious models [35], with final competing models compared using AIC and Bayesian Information Criteria (BIC) values [37, 38]. Models with lower Information Criteria (IC) values were considered preferred models. It should be noted, that ICs could not be used to compare models of differing number of observations [37]. In that case (for example, model with or without the *b-a* variable), were

Table 1 Variables assessed for association with post-mortem presence of bTB visible lesions

Variable	Description
Reason for removal	Categorical; 1. Negative in contact; 2. IFN-γ; 3. SICCT
Bovine reaction size	Reaction to bovine tuberculin injection (in mm) during skin testing for bTB
Avian reaction size	Reaction to avian tuberculin injection (in mm) during skin testing for bTB
b-a reaction difference	Bovine reaction minus avian reaction to tuberculin injection during skin testing for bTB (in mm)
BVD test result	Binary; RT-PCR test result for ear-tag samples
Inconclusive BVDV result	Binary; inconclusive RT-PCR test result for ear-tag samples
Indirect BVDV test result	Binary; if one animal in a herd tests + for BVDV then all animals from that herd gets assigned an indirect +; otherwise -
Fascioliasis	Binary; Presence of active infection of *F. hepatica* = 1; absence of active infection = 0
Fluke damage	Binary; Presence of fluke damage = 1; absence of fluke damage = 0
Fluke general	Binary; Presence of either Fascioliasis or fluke damage = 1; absence of Fascioliasis and absence of fluke damage = 0
VL	Binary; presence of a bTB like visible lesion (VL)
Age-quartiles	Animal age in years at death; categorised into quartiles.
Breed	Breed of animal (breeds associated with dairy or non-dairy)
Sex	Male or female
Associated herds	Number of herds from birth to death
Number of lifetime moves	Number of movements from birth to death, including market moves
Time since last test	Time from penultimate to ultimate test
bTB Herd history (4 years)	Binary, whether the last herd the animal resided in had a history of bTB over the preceding 4 years
Penultimate SICCT reading	Whether the animal was a severe interpretation reaction at penultimate test (binary)
Total reactors at disclosure	Total number of reactors disclosed during the breakdown where the animal was SICCT positive (Breakdown size). Note, that the breakdown was defined as the total period over which the herd was restricted, with the total number animals removed over that period.
Herd size	Total animals within the herd at time of testing; categorised into quartiles
Number of purchased animals	Number of bought-in animals during the last 3 years; categorised into quartiles
Region	Location based on three categories (North, South-west, South-east)

considered simply as separate competing models, and duly reported. First order interaction terms were fitted for variables retained after backwards model building, and only retained if they improved the fit of the model and were significant at an $p < 0.05$. Covariate patterns were assessed using visual plots. The discriminatory ability of the final models were assessed by estimating the Area Under the ROC Curve (AUC). Models with an AUC > 0.7 were considered "adequate" [39]. All modelling was undertaken with Stata SE 14 (Stata Corp., 2015).

Results

Descriptive results of the dataset

The dataset included a total of 6242 animals with an ante-mortem and post-mortem record, from 1335 herds; however not all variables in the dataset were complete. Overall, 5198 animals were recorded in the dataset as "positive" skin reactors (5198/6242; 83%). A further 458 animals (458/6242; 7.3%) were designated as gamma positive, with 586 (586/6242; 9.4%) being designated as negative in contacts (NIC). Of these 6242 animals with an associated post-mortem result, 40% (2504) had visible lesions disclosed at slaughter. Of the 5198 standard reactor animals within the dataset, 2444 (47%) disclosed with visible lesions at slaughter.

Overall, there were 5698 animals with a *b-a* value recorded at the disclosing SICCT test (Table 2). Descriptive statistics relating to the breakdown and VL percentage are presented in Table 2. Not all animals were tested for gamma interferon, as this test was a supplementary test to the SICCT tests. There were 355 of these animals with gamma interferon as their disclosing test (355/5698; 6.2%), 20 of which were VL positive (5.6%). There were 20 animals from 5698 that were negative to all ante-mortem tests (20/5698; 0.35%); 2 were VL positive (10%). Five hundred ninety-six animals were inconclusive reactors to both standard and severe interpretation SICCT tests (596/5698; 10%), 142 of which were VL positive (24%). There were 259 animals that were inconclusive to severe interpretation but negative to both gamma and standard (259/5698; 4.6%; Table 2), 19 of which were VL positive (7.3%).

Factors associated with lesion presence - *Univariable models*

We present the univariable associations in Table 3, however a thorough description of the univariable model findings is presented in Additional file 2.

Multivariable random effect logit model – Lesion presence

After univariable model fitting, there were 14 independent variables offered to the full model ($p < 0.15$ in univariable models). Correlation analysis amongst independent variables found that the lifetime number of market movements and the number of herds (log(no. associated herds)) the animal resided in during its lifetime were strongly correlated ($r = 0.83$; $p < 0.001$). We retained only log(no. associated herds) variable to avoid collinearity in our model, and because this was a far superior predictor of lesion presence in the univariable model (ΔAIC: 208). Purchase also

Table 2 Tabulation of bTB test results by standard interpretation (positive, negative or inconclusive) SICCT, severe (sev.) interpretation SICCT, and Interferon-γ, and the percentage (%) which disclosed bTB visible lesions (VL) at slaughter

	Gamma negative/untested (% VL+)			Gamma positive (% VL+)			Row totals
Standard interpretation	Sev. Neg.	Sev. Pos.	Sev. Incon.	Sev. Neg.	Sev. Pos.	Sev. Incon.	
Neg.	2/20 (10%)	0	19/259 (7%)	3/20 (15%)	0	16/320 (5%)	40/619 (6%)
Pos.	0	2224/4235 (53%)	0	0	0	0	2224/4235 (53%)
Inconclusive	0	69/248 (28%)	138/581 (24%)	0	0	4/15 (27%)	211/844 (21%)
Column totals	2/20 (10%)	2293/4483 (51%)	157/840 (19%)	3/20 (15%)	0	20/335 (6%)	

The gamma results only relate to animals designated for removal due to the gamma test result only; these data only relate to the cohort of animals where a *b-a* reading was recorded ($n = 5698$)

significantly correlated with log(no. associated herds) ($r = 0.46$; $p < 0.001$), but was not significantly associated with the outcome at univariable level ($p = 0.114$) and so was also dropped from the model building process.

Two competing models were run before model building with either the *b-a* reaction size included or the test result (skin test positive, gamma positive, or NIC animals). This was due to the number of animals without a *b-a* value ($n = 544$ missing values); 81% (440/544) of these animals were NIC animals.

The final model (Table 4) including *b-a* as a predictor significantly explained variation in the dataset (Wald χ^2 (df: 9) = 772.86; $p < 0.001$), and displayed significant variation in animal risk across herds (σ: 1.13; ρ: 0.28; LR test of $\rho = 0$: $p < 0.001$). The model exhibited adequate discriminatory ability with an AUC of 0.75 (95%CI: 0.74–0.77). The model was based on 5698 observations, with an average of 4.3 animals per herd. The probability of an animal disclosing a lesion at slaughter varied significantly by *b-a* reaction size, the number of herds the animal resided in during its lifetime, breed and penultimate test result. Animals with net positive bovine increase ($b\text{-}a > 0$) had a significantly higher risk of having a lesion at slaughter ($P < 0.001$), than non-reactors. Furthermore, this pattern increased with increasing *b-a* size; for example, in comparison with non-reactors ($b\text{-}a = 0$), animals with reaction sizes of 1-4 mm were 6.31 times more likely to have a lesion ($p < 0.001$), whereas animals with reaction sizes 5-9 mm were 14.57 times more likely to have a lesion ($p < 0.001$). Animals who were *M. avium* tuberculin reactors ($b\text{-}a < 0$; $n = 151$) were also significantly more likely to disclose with a lesion relative to non-reactor animals (OR: 2.29; $p = 0.023$).

There was significant positive relationship between the log-number of herds an animal resided within and lesion risk (log-herds: OR: 2.27; $p < 0.001$). Dairy breed animals had significantly lower odds of having a lesion at slaughter relative to non-dairy animals (OR: 0.79; $P = 0.015$). Animals that were positive reactors on their penultimate skin test under severe interpretation were 3.98 times more likely to have a lesion at slaughter than negative animals. There was no significant difference between animals without a penultimate test result and those who tested negative ($p = 0.201$).

The second model significantly explained variation in the dataset (Wald χ^2 (df: 9) = 448.18; $p < 0.001$; Table 5), and revealed significant variation in the probability of lesion disclosure across herds (significant herd random effect; LR test of $\rho = 0$: $p < 0.001$). The model exhibited fair to adequate discriminatory ability with an AUC of 0.69 (95%CI: 0.67–0.70). The final model contained 5823 animals, from 1286 herds, with an average of 4.5 animals per herd. Animals were significantly more likely to disclose with lesions if they were removed due to being SICCT test reactors (OR: 14.62; $p < 0.001$) in comparison with negative in-contact animals. There was no significant difference in the probability of VL presence between negative in-contacts and animals removed due to gamma interferon results ($p = 0.738$). Animals with a positive penultimate severe interpretation result were significantly more likely to have a lesion than (severe interpretation) test negative animals (OR = 2.84; $p < 0.001$). There was no difference between animals without a penultimate test result and test negative animals ($p = 0.135$). There was significant variation in the probability of a lesion across age quartiles; the highest risk was associated with quartiles 1 and 2. Animals in age quartile 3 (OR: 0.63) and quartile 4 (OR: 0.65) were of significantly lower odds of having a lesion relative to quartile 2 ($P < 0.001$), respectively. There was no significant difference between age quartile 1 and 2 ($p = 0.446$). There was a significant higher odds of lesion detection with the increasing (log) number of herds an animal resided within during their life (OR per unit increase: 2.42; $p < 0.001$). Finally, there was a significant positive relationship between lesion presence and time since last (penultimate) test (OR per log unit increase in days: 1.23; $p = 0.003$).

Additional analysis of non-reactors and net *M. avium* PPD reactors

There were 151 animals with net increases in *M. avium* PPD reactions ($b\text{-}a < 0$), 37 of which would have been SIT reactors (24.5%). 11.92% (18/151) of these animals had VLs. 7/37 SIT positive animals had VLs (18.9%); 11/103 non-SIT animals had VLs (9.7%). This difference in the probability of lesion disclosure was non-

Table 3 Univariable random effects logit models predicting the probability of an animal disclosing with a visible lesion at slaughter

Variable (outcome = VL) Risk factors at animal level	N-positive (% positive)		N	OR (95%CI)	*P*-value
b-a PPD reaction size			5698		<0.001
	18 (11.92%)	<0 mm		2.39 (1.19–4.82)	
	22 (4.7%)	0 mm		Ref.	
	211 (25%)	1-4 mm		7.16 (4.32–11.87)	
	691 (36.64%)	5-9 mm		15.97 (9.8–26.01)	
	884 (59.81%)	10-19 mm		45.47 (27.8–74.37)	
	649 (74.51%)	>20 mm		109.53 (65.52–183.10)	
Reason for removal			6242		<0.001
	30 (5.12%)	Negative in contact		Ref.	
	30 (6.55%)	Removed due to IFN-γ result		1.32 (0.72–2.38)	
	2444 (47.02%)	Removed due to SICCT result		20.83 (13.58–31.95)	
BVD			6242		0.106
	2500 (99.84%)	BVD Negative		Ref.	
	4 (0.16%)	BVD positive		0.33 (0.08–1.26)	
BVD (indirect)			6242		0.165
	2407 (40.41%)	BVD Negative		Ref.	
	97 (33.92%)	BVD positive		0.60 (0.29–1.23)	
Fascioliasis			6242		0.292
	2372 (40.33%)	Fascioliasis Negative		Ref.	
	132 (36.57%)	Fascioliasis Positive		0.86 (0.65–1.13)	
Liver fluke damage			6242		0.997
	2161 (40.27%)	Liver damage Negative		Ref.	
	343 (39.16%)	Liver damage Positive		1.00 (0.83–1.2)	
Liver fluke exposure			6242		0.55
	2029 (40.53%)	Facioliasis and damage Negative		Ref.	
	475 (38.43%)	Facioliasis or damage Positive Mean		0.95 (0.81–1.11)	
Age-quartiles			6231		<0.001
	612 (39.74%)	≤ 1.53 years		0.77 (0.64–0.92)	
	704 (45.48%)	1.53–2.86 years		Ref.	
	580 (36.64%)	2.86–5.58 years		0.69 (0.58–0.83)	
	607 (38.91%)	≥5.58 years		0.76 (0.63–0.91)	
Breed			6242		<0.001
	1517 (44.29%)	Non-dairy		Ref.	
	987 (35.04%)	Dairy		0.73 (0.61–0.86)	
Sex			6242		0.406
	517 (39.26%)	Male		Ref.	
	1987 (40.35%)	Female		1.07 (0.90–1.26)	
Associated herds			6242		<0.001
		Log(No. associated herds)		2.84 (2.45–3.30)	
No. Market moves			6242		0.028
		Market moves		1.04 (1–1.08)	
Time since last test			5831		<0.001

Table 3 Univariable random effects logit models predicting the probability of an animal disclosing with a visible lesion at slaughter *(Continued)*

Variable (outcome = VL) Risk factors at animal level	N-positive (% positive)		N	OR (95%CI)	*P*-value
		Log(Time in days between tests)		1.59 (1.40–1.80)	
Herd bTB history			6242		<0.001
	1188 (35.83%)	No bTB		Ref.	
	1316 (44.98%)	bTB		2.13 (1.76–2.57)	
Penultimate herd bTB history			6242		0.044
		No bTB		Ref.	
		bTB		2.02 (1.02–4.00)	
Penultimate test results			6242		<0.001
	2246 (39.94%)	Severe interpretation negative on penultimate test		Ref.	
	84 (59.15%)	Severe interpretation positive on penultimate test		2.42 (1.57–3.72)	
	174 (36.48%)	No previous test result		0.84 (0.64–1.09)	
Breakdown size			6242		0.001
		per additional reactor		0.99 (0.98–0.99)	
Herd size			6237		0.044
(quartiles)	716 (45.99%)	≤71		Ref.	
	637 (41.26%)	72–158		0.86 (0.66–1.1)	
	491 (33.22%)	159–279		0.71 (0.54–0.93)	
	658 (39.69%)	≥280		0.72 (0.54–0.94)	
Purchases			6017		0.114
(quartiles)	593 (41.61%)	≤7			Ref.
	683 (43.98%)	8–31		1.12 (0.86–1.46)	
	542 (35.38%)	32–100		1.22 (0.91–1.64)	
	582 (38.62%)	≥101		1.44 (1.06–1.94)	
Region			6242		0.171
	629 (46.35%)	1. North (Derry, Larne, Ballymena and Coleraine)		Ref.	
	863 (38.2%)	2. South-West (Omagh, Enniskillen and Dungannon)		0.91 (0.7–1.18)	
	1012 (38.54%)	3. South-east (Newtownards, Newry and Armagh)		0.78 (0.61–1.01)	

significant (OR: 2.18; $p = 0.136$). The mean *M. avium* PPD reaction size for avium reactors with lesions was 5.82 mm ($n = 11$; SD: 3.12; Range: 2-12 mm), while the mean *M. avium* PPD reaction size for avium reactors without lesions was 4.01 mm ($n = 103$; SD: 2.05; Range: 1–12 mm), a significant difference (linear regression: $p = 0.010$).

For non-reactors ($b\text{-}a = 0$), 22/468 (4.7%) of animals had VLs. There was a significantly greater proportion of VL positive animals with positive SIT test results (16.0% (4/25)) than SIT negative animals (4.1%; 18/443; OR: 4.50; $p = 0.011$). For animals with a $b\text{-}a = 0$ test reading, the mean *M. avium* PPD reaction size was non-significantly larger in animals with a VL (0.83 mm; range 0-4 mm) than animals without a VL (0.49 mm; range 0-4 mm) at slaughter (linear regression: $p = 0.242$).

Discussion

Overall, this study has shown that there is significant variation in the probability of cattle exhibiting a VL at slaughter that were culled as part of herd breakdowns in Northern Ireland. This variation can be attributed to animal-level characteristics, exposure during life histories, and potentially to exposure to other *Mycobacteria*.

Table 4 Random effect multivariable logit model assessing the variation in the presence of bTB visible lesions. Test result modelled as categories of the bovine-avian Purified Protein Derivative (PPD) tuberculin reaction size ($n = 5698$)

Predictor	Categories	OR	Std. Err.	z	*P*	Lower 95% CI	Upper 95% CI
b-a PPD reaction size							
	<0 mm	2.29	0.83	2.28	0.023	1.12	4.65
	0 mm	Ref.					
	1-4 mm	6.31	1.64	7.07	<0.001	3.79	10.51
	5-9 mm	14.57	3.66	10.66	<0.001	8.90	23.85
	10-19 mm	42.59	10.79	14.81	<0.001	25.92	69.98
	>20 mm	103.03	27.29	17.50	<0.001	61.31	173.15
Log(No. associated herds)		2.27	0.19	9.76	<0.001	1.92	2.67
Breed	Non-dairy	Ref.					
	Dairy	0.79	0.08	−2.43	0.015	0.65	0.96
Penultimate test results	Negative	Ref.					
	Severe interpretation positive	3.98	0.93	5.93	<0.001	2.52	6.28
	No previous test result	1.08	0.17	0.48	0.629	0.79	1.48
Constant		0.02	0.01	−14.95	<0.001	0.01	0.03
RE	ρ^a	0.28	0.03			0.23	0.33

[a]Intra-class correlation

Co-infection

Co-infections have been highlighted as a significant modulator of immune responses to the challenge of bacterial infections, including tuberculosis [40–44]. Recent studies suggest that bovine TB could be affected, either through mechanisms of increased pathology, increased transmission, susceptibility or decreased detection, by pathogens such as BVDV [15, 22, 45], liver fluke (*F. hepatica*; 18, 19, 44], and Johne's Disease (JD; [20, 42, 46]; but see [47]).

During the present study BVDV exposure was assessed in two ways – a positive BVDV RT-PCR test result, or an indirect exposure metric based on the presence of a test positive animal disclosed within the animal's final herd. The first metric represent Persistently Infected (PI) animals, which were rare in the dataset (0.27%), with the second metric representing potentially 'exposed' cattle. We did not find any significant (at $P < 0.05$) animal-level associations between these BVDV statuses and the probability of an animal having a lesion at slaughter. This

Table 5 Random effect multivariable logit model assessing the variation in the presence of bTB visible lesions. Bovine TB test result modelled as categories (reasons) leading to animal removal ($n = 5823$)

Predictor	Categories	OR	Std. Err.	z	*P*	Lower 95% CI	Upper 95% CI
Reason for removal	Negative in contact	Ref.					
	Removed due to IFN-γ result	1.11	0.34	0.33	0.738	0.61	2.03
	Removed due to SICCT result	14.62	3.32	11.80	<0.001	9.36	22.83
Penultimate test results	Negative	Ref.					
	Severe interpretation positive	2.84	0.65	4.54	<0.001	1.81	4.46
	No previous test result	0.62	0.20	−1.49	0.135	0.33	1.16
Age-class	≤ 1.53 years	1.08	0.11	0.76	0.446	0.88	1.33
	1.53–2.86 years	Ref.					
	2.86–5.58 years	0.63	0.06	−4.77	<0.001	0.53	0.76
	≥5.58 years	0.65	0.06	−4.37	<0.001	0.54	0.79
Log(No. associated herds)		2.42	0.19	11.26	<0.001	2.07	2.82
Log(Time in days between tests)		1.23	0.09	2.95	0.003	1.07	1.41
Constant		0.01	0.00	−11.15	<0.001	0.01	0.02
RE	ρ^a	0.26	0.02			0.21	0.31

[a]Intra-class correlation

could be partially due to the small number of test positive animals found within the cohort, reducing the power to detect an effect. Other research from this cohort suggested that the apparent indirect exposure of animals in herds where BVDV positive cattle were found was negatively associated with the minimum lesion counts found in animals – a finding which would not be generally consistent with the proposed mechanisms by which BVDV might impact bTB epidemiology [15, 22, 45, 48, 49]. Some have suggested that acute BVDV infection could lead to the rapid progression of bTB in co-infected animals [50]. However, experimental studies failed to show significant differences in *M. bovis* shedding patterns between co-infected (BVDV and *M. bovis*) and infected (*M. bovis* only) animals [15]. Previous research suggested that acute BVDV infection could temporarily compromise *ante-mortem* tests for bTB, by suppressing the immunological response to tuberculin PPDs [45]. Herd-level research from Northern Ireland suggested that, when controlling for confounders (especially herd-size which is a herd-level risk factor for both bTB and BVDV), there was no significant relationship between bTB and BVDV herd risk based on 2827 herds [22]. Results from populations outside Northern Ireland suggest that acute BVDV cases may in some cases exacerbate infection [50] or impact on *ante-mortem* tests ability to detect *M. bovis* in truly infected animals [45], but that these affects are not readily demonstrated with herd- and animal-level epidemiological population-level datasets in Northern Ireland [22]. However, as pointed out previously [22], biosecurity practices implemented in the management of BVDV could potentially have benefits for bTB management (but see [51]).

Liver fluke (*F. hepatica*) infection has been suggested to negatively impact the control of *M. bovis* in Britain and Ireland [18, 19, 44, 52]. Experimental work has found that a proportion of co-infected animals with Bacille Calmette Guerin (BCG) can be misdiagnosed using IFN-γ or SICCT tests [52]. Claridge et al. [19] presented both experimental and epidemiological evidence to suggest that co-infection with liver fluke was associated with reduced SICCT tests disclosure (underascertainment of 27–38%) in England and Wales. Experimental data presented in that paper suggested that co-infected animals exhibited significantly lower *b-a* reactions to the skin test at 10 and 21 weeks post-innoculation [19]. However, at both time points all co-infected animals would still have been deemed standard reactors (i.e. $b\text{-}a > 4$ mm). Despite these experimental and epidemiological data, during the present study, three metrics of liver fluke infection (Fascioliasis, fluke damage, and either Fascioliasis/fluke damage) were tested and none were significantly associated with the probability of an animal having a visible lesion at slaughter. However, other research from this population has suggested a negative relationship between maximum visible lesion size and liver fluke presence has been found [53]. This appears perhaps contrary to the hypothesis to an immunological suppression hypothesis [54–56], but reflects other recent data suggesting the potential for the induction of latency [57]. Further research is on-going into this latter hypothesis (Byrne et al. In prep.).

There was evidence from the present study that reaction to *M. avium* Purified Protein Derivative (PPD) tuberculin (negative *b-a* values), was significantly associated with visible lesion presence at slaughter. These animals would not have been classed as standard reactors to bovine tuberculosis, suggesting that animals with bTB visible lesions that strongly react to *M. avium* tuberculin will have increased risk of going undetected. The *M. avium* PPD comparator was introduced to increase specificity in areas where non-specific reactions could occur [13], however at a potential loss of sensitivity relative to the SIT test. For non-reactor animals and *M. avium* PPD reactors, a proportion of animals strongly reacted to the bovine PPD, and would have been classed as SIT reactors. It is possible that such *M. avium* reactors have been exposed to non-*bovis* mycobacteria, including *Mycobacterium avium* subsp. *paratuberculosis* (MAP) the etiological agent of Johne's disease (JD; [30, 32, 33, 58]). Previous research has suggested that the comparative skin test can be used as a preliminary diagnostic for JD in cattle [32]. Gilardoni et al. [32] suggests animals with JD react positively to both bovine and avian tuberculins, but generally greater intensity to avian PPD. However, because of the non-specific nature of the avium tuberculin reaction, it is not possible to disaggregate exposure to MAP or other members of the *M. avium* complex. Recently in Ireland, Kennedy et al. [33] found a significant association between the reactions sizes (most markedly in animals reacting to both avian and bovine PPD) during a SICCT test and an ELISA test for MAP. Increases in tuberculin sizes at day 10 and day 16 post-inoculation was associated with increases in sample/positive ratio for the JD ELISA blood test. However, this study failed to elucidate whether tuberculin reaction sizes can be indicative of exposure to MAP, or if their results were due to cross reactivity. Our findings need to be further investigated with a larger dataset, and from cohorts that include non-breakdown herds, to verify whether this is a general pattern. Further research investigating specifically JD and bTB is on-going in Northern Ireland (Lahuerta-Marin, Byrne et al., personal communication). It should be noted that previous research has found significant effects of JD on bTB in cattle herds ([32, 42, 46, 59, 60], and vice-versa: [61]), and so co-management should be considered if managing both infections when present in the same herd, and careful attention to the interpretation of comparative tests where co-infection is suspected.

Individual characteristics, herd-level factors, and life histories

Animals classed as of a dairy breed exhibited significant differences to beef breed types in post-mortem confirmation of bTB VL. Dairy breeds were dominated by Friesian and Holstein breeds (91% of total); in comparison, beef breeds were made up of a number of dominant breed types (Limousin, Charolais, Aberdeen Angus, Simmental, and Belgian Blue (86% of total)). We found in this high risk cohort that dairy breed animals tended to be significantly less likely to disclose with a VL, suggesting diagnostics for bTB may be behaving differently amongst herd types [25]. Recent research suggests that some tests may have differing characteristics depending on breed type [14], with data from chronic herds in Northern Ireland suggesting that the SICCT test may not perform as well in dairy herds as it does in beef herds [12]. Genetic susceptibility may also be a factor [62], with evidence from an Irish cattle population to suggest that Holstein cattle are the least susceptible breed examined, with Simmental and Charolais beef breeds being most susceptible [63]. In the current study dataset, for breeds with >300 animals represented, the highest proportion of animals confirmed were Charolais (46.08% confirmed bacteriologically) and Simmental (45.05% confirmed), while the least likely breeds to confirm were Friesian (32.22% confirmed) and Holstein (37.97% confirmed) at *post-mortem* (Additional file 4; also see [64]). It is currently difficult to ascertain whether the effect is due to increased resistance, non-specific skin test reactions or a reduced pathogenesis and lesion formation in dairy cattle [25]. However, there is evidence to suggest that confirmed breakdown recurrence is more frequent in dairy relative to non-dairy herds in Britain and Northern Ireland [65, 66]. Dairy herds tend to have an older age profile, which also affects risk (see below), however in this cohort there was little difference in the mean age of dairy breed animals (4.0 years) and non-dairy animals (3.8 years).

Age-class was another significant variable affecting the probability of an animal being confirmed (with VL; similar to [4]). The results of the present study suggested an increased risk for animals within the first and second quartiles, relative to other age-classes. Brooks-Pollock et al. [67] working in GB found that bTB risk increased with age up to the highest risk age group at 12 and 36 months old before risk declining. Potentially this pattern emerged due to the detection and removal of infected animals, with surviving cohorts of animals could have lower rates of infection. The same authors presented data on VL confirmation which suggested that confirmation risk declined with age. Anergy due to repeated testing could be a factor affecting the immunological response to the tuberculin tests with age [68, 69]. Interestingly, Clegg et al. [70] when undertaking a case-control study of non-reactor bTB confirmed animals in Ireland found that cases tended to be older than the national average age at slaughter, mirroring previous results [1] that suggested confirmation risk increased with age in non-reactors.

We found that the movement history of animals was a significant factor associated with increased probability of an animal being confirmed to have lesions found at abattoir. This suggests that movement through multiple premises may increase an animal's risk significantly, or increase the pathological response if exposed during their lifetime. Lifetime moves were not previously associated with animal-level risk in Northern Ireland [4] in a study assessing the *post-mortem* confirmation risk of reactors. However, movement has been highlighted as a bTB risk factor in other studies (e.g. [71, 72]). In the present study, there was a significant positive relationship between increasing age and movement ($p < 0.001$), and with beef animals relative to dairy breed animals ($p < 0.001$). Therefore, the compounding effects of potential increased exposure (across multiple premises and animals), older animals, and being more likely a beef animal may have contributed to this finding. Stress due to movement may also be a significant driver of this pattern, as stress is known to negatively affect the immunocompetency of cattle [73, 74]. Lifetime number of herds an animal resided within significantly correlated with lifetime market moves and the number of animal purchases (i.e. buying in) the disclosing herds made in the 3 years before the disclosing test. Therefore, animals which resided in many herds, also made many market moves, and markets are known to be highly connected nodes within cattle trade networks in Northern Ireland [75] and elsewhere (e.g. GB, Denmark and Italy; [76–78]), which potentially increases exposure to infectious hosts and contributes to disease spread [70, 71]. Herds that purchased many animals also tended to buy-in animals with greater market-move histories (e.g. animals in herds in the fourth quartile of purchasing had on average 2.2 more market moves than animals in the first purchasing quartile; linear regression; $p < 0.001$). Finally, there was also an association between movement history and the time between the penultimate and disclosing tests – for example, for each additional market move, the time between tests increased by 5.5 days (linear regression; $p < 0.001$). While animals should be tested on average once per year in Northern Ireland (as part of an Annual Herd Test (AHT) or other follow-up tests), this may not always be the case with animals that move frequently across herds which undertake testing at different times of the year. While the average time between penultimate and disclosing test in this high-risk cohort was approximately 6 months (mean: 156 days), the longest time period between tests was almost 2 years (665 days). This pattern could be a factor in the time to detection of infection.

Finally, we provide evidence that the penultimate SICCT test result was significantly associated with *post-mortem* presence of a lesion at slaughter. Severe interpretation reactors were significantly more likely to confirm with a lesion at death. Similar results with a significantly increased risk of *post-mortem* confirmation in reactors has been demonstrated in other studies in Northern Ireland [4] and Ireland [70]. This could indicate that such animals in high-risk herds represent exposed animals in the early stages of infection that may have been missed by the SICCT test and so could pose a future risk [79, 80]. Indeed, Clegg et al. [79, 80] found that inconclusive reactors (animals which had reaction sizes of >2 mm on the bovine tuberculin injection site and between 1 and 4 mm > the avian response) had significantly increased future risk of bTB relative to non-reactor animals within the same herds or in comparison with animals in the national herds in Ireland. Furthermore, Lahuerta-Marin et al. [81] also showed how SICCT negative, but INF-γ test positive animals left on farm constituted to farms a significant future breakdown risk. In herds with significant recurrent problems, indicators of future risk could be considered when managing herd breakdown risk.

Limitations and future direction

There were some limitations with regards this study. Firstly, post-mortem diagnostics for bovine TB has limitations in terms of variable sensitivity (e.g. see [12, 13]), though the slaughter house surveillance does exhibit high specificity (>99%). Similarly, abattoir carcass assessment for liver fluke infection can exhibit limited sensitivity and specificity at the animal level (e.g. 68%SE, 88% SP in Scotland; [82]), though there is no assessments of Northern Irish abattoir performance yet nor how transferrable the results are from other countries [29]. Part of the issue relates to inter-abattoir variation in surveillance effectiveness [1, 2], however, we largely controlled for this by having 99% of samples being processed through a single experienced slaughter house. While the sensitivity and specificity of the RT-PCR BVDV test is very high [>99%; 28], the animal level prevalence was very low (lower than expected given routine surveillance data), which may have diminished the power to detect an effect, if present. We did however, endeavour to overcome this, by assessing indirect effects of exposure, as BVDV is highly contagious within herds with actively excreting animals [28]. Future studies will directly assess the impact of MAP on bTB test diagnostics in Northern Ireland, to help refine and assess the validity of the present findings. Liver fluke exposure will be assessed systematically in Northern Ireland using a prospective study design assessing bulk milk antigens using high performance ELISA tests at herd levels, to assess the herd level nexus between liver fluke and bTB risk.

Conclusion

There is significant animal-level variation in the *post-mortem* presence of VL from animals removed as part of bTB breakdowns in Northern Ireland. In this dataset, we found limited robust evidence of BVDV impacts on metrics of *post-mortem* confirmation, concurring with previous herd-level analyses. We did not find evidence to support liver fluke infection impacting on VL presence during this study. Exposure to *Mycobacteria* other than *M. bovis* may also have an impact on the SICCT test performance, with *M. avium* PPD reactors exhibiting higher probability of confirmation than non-reactor animals. We hypothesize that this effect could be partially due to exposure to *Mycobacterium bovis* subsp. *paratuberculosis* (MAP) the etiological agent of Johne's disease, but this needs further confirmatory research. There was a strong significant relationship between visible lesion presence and increasing positive bovine tuberculin bias over the avian tuberculin reaction. Visible lesion presence in this high risk cohort was related to breed (decreased in dairy breeds relative to non-dairy), age (older animals are less likely to have lesions), movement history (increased risk with how many herds an animal resided in) and whether the animal was inconclusive to the SICCT at its penultimate test (previous test results can be a predictor of future risk).

Additional files

Additional file 1: Figure S1. Graphical exploratory assessment of the relationship between the probability of bovine TB visible lesion (VL) presence and the bovine minus avian tuberculin (*b-a*) reaction sizes (mm) at the disclosing test for cattle culled in Northern Ireland during bTB breakdowns ($n = 5698$). The LOWESS curve (grey solid line) is a locally weighted regression line (bandwidth: 0.5); orange line represent *b-a* as a log-transformed predictor. Note, that the log-transformed predictor fails to address the increasing risk at negative *b-a* values, due to this the *b-a* variable was modelled as a categorical variable.

Additional file 2: Supplementary material 1. Detailed description of univariable associations between candidate predictors of TB-visible lesion presence.

Additional file 3: Figure S2. Relationship between the probability of an animal having a bTB visible lesion at slaughter and the time between the penultimate and disclosing skin tests in cattle in Northern Ireland. Orange line represents a locally weighted regression line (non-linear regression fit; LOWESS); Grey line represents the predicted fit from the log-transformed predictor variable (log(time in days)).

Additional file 4: Figure S3. The point estimated linear predictions from a random effects logit regression model for the presence of bTB visible lesions (VL) at slaughter amongst recorded cattle breeds for *Mycobacterium bovis* exposed cattle slaughtered in Northern Ireland. The grey dots represent point estimates; dots farther from zero line represent animals with higher or lower risk of disclosing with a lesion at slaughter relative to the population average. Orange circles represent weighted sample sizes. Outliers include (grey arrows): BGA = Belted Galloway highest risk of VL; SHB = Short horn beef cattle lowest risk of VL. Highly represented breeds are highlighted.

Abbreviations
AUC: Area under the ROC curve; bTB: Bovine tuberculosis; BVDV: Bovine Viral Diarrhoea Virus; JD: Johne's Disease; MAP: *Mycobacterium avium* subsp. *paratuberculosis*; VL: bTB visible lesion

Acknowledgements
We would like to acknowledge the work of TB teams within the veterinary service of Northern Ireland, and helpful discussions with Dr. Angela Lahuerta-Marin at AFBI.

Funding
This work was funded as part of a broader study of concurrent infections and their role in bTB epidemiology in Northern Ireland (48005 (122035): 15/3/10 – bTB Endemic Diseases; PI: Dr. Andrew Byrne) funded under the Evidence and Innovation (E&I) Scheme by the Department of Agriculture and Rural Development (DAERA; www.daera-ni.gov.uk).

Authors' contributions
Study design/planning: AWB, JG, AA, MGG, SM; Database construction and data interpretation: JG; Analysis: AWB; Interpretation of results: AWB, AA, RS; Laboratory work (prospective BVDV testing of all samples for this study), generated data and interpretation of data: MGG, CB, AD; Initial draft of the manuscript: AWB; Drafting and critical revision of the manuscript: AWB, AA, JM, RS, SM, MGG. All authors read and approved the final manuscript.

Competing interests
The authors declare that they have no competing interests.

Consent for publication
NA

References
1. Frankena K, White PW, O'Keeffe J, Costello E, Martin SW, van Grevenhof EM, More SJ. Quantification of the relative efficiency of factory surveillance in the disclosure of tuberculosis lesions in attested Irish cattle. Vet Rec. 2007;161:679–84.
2. Olea-Popelka F, Freeman Z, White P, Costello E, O'Keeffe J, Frankena K, Martin W, More S. Relative effectiveness of Irish factories in the surveillance of slaughtered cattle for visible lesions of tuberculosis, 2005-2007. Irish Vet J. 2012;65:2.
3. Shittu A, Clifton-Hadley RS, Ely ER, Upton PU, Downs SH. Factors associated with bovine tuberculosis confirmation rates in suspect lesions found in cattle at routine slaughter in great Britain, 2003–2008. Prev Vet Med. 2013;110(3):395–404.
4. O'Hagan MJ, Courcier EA, Drewe JA, Gordon AW, McNair J, Abernethy DA. Risk factors for visible lesions or positive laboratory tests in bovine tuberculosis reactor cattle in Northern Ireland. Prev Vet Med. 2015 Jul 1;120(3):283–90.
5. Humblet MF, Boschiroli ML, Saegerman C. Classification of worldwide bovine tuberculosis risk factors in cattle: a stratified approach. Vet Res. 2009;40(5):1–24.
6. Skuce RA, Allen AR, McDowell SW. Herd-level risk factors for bovine tuberculosis: a literature review. Vet Med Int. 2012 Jun;28:2012.
7. Abernethy DA, Denny GO, Menzies FD, McGuckian P, Honhold N, Roberts AR. The Northern Ireland programme for the control and eradication of *Mycobacterium bovis*. Vet Microbiol. 2006;112(2):231–7.
8. Robinson PA. Farmers and bovine tuberculosis: Contextualising statutory disease control within everyday farming lives. J. Rural. Stud. 2017;55:168–80.
9. Lahuerta-Marin A, McNair J, Skuce R, McBride S, Allen M, Strain SA, Menzies FD, McDowell SJ, Byrne AW. Risk factors for failure to detect bovine tuberculosis in cattle from infected herds across Northern Ireland (2004–2010). Res Vet Sci. 2016 Aug 31;107:233–9.
10. McCallan L, Brooks C, Couzens C, Young F, McNair J, Byrne AW. Assessment of serological tests for diagnosis of bovine tuberculosis. Vet Rec. 2017 Apr 5: vetrec-2016. doi:10.1136/vr.104272
11. McCallan L, Brooks C, Couzens C, Young F, McNair J, Byrne AW. Performance of serological tests for bovine tuberculosis in cattle herds in Northern Ireland. BioRxiv. 235184. https://doi.org/10.1101/235184.
12. Lahuerta-Marin, A., Milne, M.G., McNair, J., Skuce, R., McBride, S., Menzies, F., McDowell, S.J.W., Byrne, A.W., Handel, I.G., Bronsvoort, M.B.C. 2017. Bayesian latent class estimation of sensitivity and specificity parameters of diagnostic tests for bovine tuberculosis in chronic herds-Northern Ireland. Vet J, In review.
13. De la Rua-Domenech R, Goodchild AT, Vordermeier HM, Hewinson RG, Christiansen KH, Clifton-Hadley RS. Ante mortem diagnosis of tuberculosis in cattle: a review of the tuberculin tests, γ-interferon assay and other ancillary diagnostic techniques. Res Vet Sci. 2006;81(2):190–210.
14. Nuñez-Garcia J, Downs SH, Parry JE, Abernethy DA, Broughan JM, Cameron AR, Cook AJ, de la Rua-Domenech R, Goodchild AV, Gunn J, More SJ. Meta-analyses of the sensitivity and specificity of ante-mortem and post-mortem diagnostic tests for bovine tuberculosis in the UK and Ireland. Prev Vet Med. 2017. doi:10.1016/j.prevetmed.2017.02.017
15. Kao RR, Gravenor MB, Charleston B, Hope JC, Martin M, Howard CJ. *Mycobacterium bovis* shedding patterns from experimentally infected calves and the effect of concurrent infection with bovine viral diarrhoea virus. J R Soc Interface. 2007;4(14):545–51.
16. Broughan JM, Judge J, Ely E, Delahay RJ, Wilson G, Clifton-Hadley RS, Goodchild AV, Bishop H, Parry JE, Downs SH. A review of risk factors for bovine tuberculosis infection in cattle in the UK and Ireland. Epidemiol. Infect. 2016;144:2899–926.
17. Godfray HC, Donnelly CA, Kao RR, Macdonald DW, McDonald RA, Petrokofsky G, Wood JL, Woodroffe R, Young DB, McLean AR. A restatement of the natural science evidence base relevant to the control of bovine tuberculosis in great Britain. Proc R Soc B Biol Sci. 2013 Oct 7;280(1768):20131634.
18. Flynn RJ, Mulcahy G, Welsh M, Cassidy JP, Corbett D, Milligan C, Andersen P, Strain S, McNair J. Co-infection of cattle with *Fasciola hepatica* and *Mycobacterium bovis*–immunological consequences. Transbound Emerg Dis. 2009;56(6–7):269–74.
19. Claridge J, Diggle P, McCann CM, Mulcahy G, Flynn R, McNair J, Strain S, Welsh M, Baylis M, Williams DJ. *Fasciola hepatica* is associated with failure to detect bovine tuberculosis in dairy cattle. Nat Commun. 2012;3:853.
20. Álvarez J, De Juan L, Bezos J, Romero B, Sáez JL, Gordejo FR, Briones V, Moreno MÁ, Mateos A, Domínguez L, Aranaz A. Interference of paratuberculosis with the diagnosis of tuberculosis in a goat flock with a natural mixed infection. Vet Microbiol. 2008;128(1):72–80.
21. Álvarez J, De Juan L, Bezos J, Romero B, Sáez JL, Marqués S, Domínguez C, Mínguez O, Fernández-Mardomingo B, Mateos A, Domínguez L. Effect of paratuberculosis on the diagnosis of bovine tuberculosis in a cattle herd with a mixed infection using interferon-gamma detection assay. Vet Microbiol. 2009;135:389–93.
22. Byrne AW, Guelbenzu-Gonzalo M, Strain SA, McBride S, Graham J, Lahuerta-Marin A, Harwood R, Graham DA, McDowell S. Assessment of concurrent infection with bovine viral diarrhoea virus (BVDV) and *Mycobacterium bovis*: a herd-level risk factor analysis from Northern Ireland. Prev Vet Med. 2017;141:38–47.
23. Aagaard C, Govaerts M, Meikle V, Gutiérrez-Pabello JA, McNair J, Andersen P, Suárez-Güemes F, Pollock J, Espitia C, Cataldi A. Detection of bovine tuberculosis in herds with different disease prevalence and influence of paratuberculosis infection on PPDB and ESAT-6/CFP10 specificity. Prev Vet Med. 2010;96(3):161–9.
24. Vicente J, Höfle U, Garrido JM, Acevedo P, Juste R, Barral M, Gortazar C. Risk factors associated with the prevalence of tuberculosis-like lesions in fenced wild boar and red deer in south central Spain. Vet Res. 2007;38(3):451–64.
25. Downs SH, Broughan JM, Goodchild AV, Upton PA, Durr PA. Responses to diagnostic tests for bovine tuberculosis in dairy and non-dairy cattle naturally exposed to Mycobacterium Bovis in great Britain. Vet J. 2016 Oct 31;216:8–17.
26. Nalapa DP, Muwonge A, Kankya C, Olea-Popelka F. Prevalence of tuberculous lesion in cattle slaughtered in Mubende district, Uganda. BMC Vet Res. 2017 Mar 21;13(1):73.
27. Gallagher MJ, Higgins IM, Clegg TA, Williams DH, More SJ. Comparison of bovine tuberculosis recurrence in Irish herds between 1998 and 2008. Prev. Vet. Med. 2013 Sep 1;111(3):237–44.
28. Guelbenzu-Gonzalo MP. Benchmarking and control of bovine viral diarrhoea in Northern Ireland dairy and suckler herds. Thesis, Queens University Belfast. 2015.
29. Byrne AW, McBride S, Lahuerta-Marin A, Guelbenzu M, McNair J, Skuce RA, McDowell SW. Liver fluke (Fasciola Hepatica) infection in cattle in Northern Ireland: a large-scale epidemiological investigation utilising surveillance data. Parasit Vectors. 2016;9(1):209.

30. Ameni G, Aseffa A, Engers H, Young D, Gordon S, Hewinson G, Vordermeier M. High prevalence and increased severity of pathology of bovine tuberculosis in Holsteins compared to zebu breeds under field cattle husbandry in central Ethiopia. Clin Vaccine Immunol. 2007;14(10):1356–61.
31. Bermingham ML, More SJ, Good M, Cromie AR, Higgins IM, Brotherstone S, Berry DP. Genetics of tuberculosis in Irish Holstein-Friesian dairy herds. J Dairy Sci. 2009;92(7):3447–56.
32. Gilardoni LR, Paolicchi FA, Mundo SL. Bovine paratuberculosis: a review of the advantages and disadvantages of different diagnostic tests. Rev Argent Microbiol. 2012;44(3):201–15.
33. Kennedy AE, Byrne N, O'Mahony J, Sayers RG. Investigations and implications of associations between mycobacterial purified protein derivative hypersensitivity and MAP-antibody ELISA in Irish dairy cows. Res. Vet. Sci. 2017;115:13–6.
34. Houston R. A computerised database system for bovine traceability. Rev Sci Tech. 2001;20(2):652.
35. Dohoo I, Martin W, Stryhn H. Veterinary epidemiologic research. Canada: University of Prince Edward Island; 2009.
36. Belsley DA, Kuh E, Welsch RE. Regression diagnostics: identifying influential data and sources of collinearity (Vol. 571). New York: Wiley; 2005.
37. Burnham KP, Anderson DR. Model selection and multimodel inference a practical information-theoretic approach. New York: Springer; 2002.
38. Schwarz G. Estimating the dimension of a model. Ann Stat. 1978;6(2):461–4.
39. Hosmer, D.W., Lemeshow, S. 2000. Applied logistic regression. 2. New York, NY: John Wiley & Sons, USA.
40. Kamal SM, El Sayed Khalifa K. Immune modulation by helminthic infections: worms and viral infections. Parasite Immunol. 2006 Oct 1;28(10):483–96.
41. Resende Co T, Hirsch CS, Toossi Z, Dietze R, Ribeiro-Rodrigues R. Intestinal helminth co-infection has a negative impact on both anti-mycobacterium tuberculosis immunity and clinical response to tuberculosis therapy. Clin. Exp. Immunol. 2007;147(1):45–52.
42. Bezos J, de Juan L, Romero B, Álvarez J, Mazzucchelli F, Mateos A, Domínguez L, Aranaz A. Experimental infection with Mycobacterium Caprae in goats and evaluation of immunological status in tuberculosis and paratuberculosis co-infected animals. Vet Immunol Immunopathol. 2010 Feb 15;133(2):269–75.
43. Salgame P, Yap GS, Gause WC. Effect of helminth-induced immunity on infections with microbial pathogens. Nat Immunol. 2013;14(11):1118–26.
44. Lucena AN, Cuartero LG, Mulcahy G, Zintl A. The immunoregulatory effects of co-infection with *Fasciola hepatica*: From bovine tuberculosis to Johne's disease. Vet J. 2017;222;9–16.
45. Charleston B, Hope JC, Carr BV, Howard CJ. Masking of two in vitro immunological assays for Mycobacterium Bovis (BCG) in calves acutely infected with non-cytopathic bovine viral diarrhoea virus. Vet Rec. 2001; 149(16):481–4.
46. Aranaz A, Bezos J, Álvarez J, Romero B, Lozano F, Paramio JL, López-Sánchez J, Mateos A, Domínguez L. Assessment of diagnostic tools for eradication of bovine tuberculosis in cattle co-infected with Mycobacterium Bovis and M. Avium subsp. paratuberculosis. Vet Res. 2006;37(4):593–606.
47. Dunn JR, Kaneene JB, Grooms DL, Bolin SR, Bolin CA, Bruning-Fann CS. Effects of positive results for Mycobacterium Avium subsp paratuberculosis as determined by microbial culture of feces or antibody ELISA on results of caudal fold tuberculin test and interferon-γ assay for tuberculosis in cattle. J Am Vet Med Assoc. 2005;226:429–35.
48. Menzies FD, Neill SD. Cattle-to-cattle transmission of bovine tuberculosis. Vet J. 2000;160:92–106.
49. Pollock JM, Neill SD. *Mycobacterium bovis* infection and tuberculosis in cattle. Vet J. 2002;163:115–27.
50. Monies RJ, Head JC. Bovine tuberculosis in housed calves. Vet Rec. 1998; 145(25):743.
51. Cardwell JM, Van Winden S, Beauvais W, Mastin A, De Glanville WA, Hardstaff J, Booth RE, Fishwick J, Pfeiffer DU. Assessing the impact of tailored biosecurity advice on farmer behaviour and pathogen presence in beef herds in England and Wales. Prev Vet Med. 2016;135:9–16.
52. Flynn RJ, Mannion C, Golden O, Hacariz O, Mulcahy G. Experimental *Fasciola hepatica* infection alters responses to tests used for diagnosis of bovine tuberculosis. Infect Immun. 2007;75:1373–81.
53. Byrne AW, Graham J, Brown C, Donaghy A, Guelbenzu-Gonzalo M, McNair J, Skuce R, Allen A, McDowell S. Modelling the variation in skin-test tuberculin reactions, post-mortem lesion frequency and pathology in cattle culled during bovine tuberculosis herd breakdowns. Transbound Emerg Dis. 2018. In press.
54. Ezenwa VO, Etienne RS, Luikart G, Beja-Pereira A, Jolles AE. Hidden consequences of living in a wormy world: nematode-induced immune suppression facilitates tuberculosis invasion in African buffalo. Am Nat. 2010;176:613–24.
55. Jolles AE, Ezenwa VO, Etienne RS, Turner WC, Olff H. Interactions between macroparasites and microparasites drive infection patterns in free-ranging African buffalo. Ecology. 2008;89:2239–50.
56. O'Leary S, O'sullivan MP, Keane J. IL-10 blocks phagosome maturation in mycobacterium tuberculosis–infected human macrophages. Am J Respir Cell Mol Biol. 2011;45(1):172–80.
57. Garza-Cuartero L, O'sullivan J, Blanco A, McNair J, Welsh M, Flynn RJ, Williams D, Diggle P, Cassidy J, Mulcahy G. Fasciola Hepatica infection reduces Mycobacterium Bovis burden and mycobacterial uptake and suppresses the pro-inflammatory response. Parasite Immunol. 2016 Jul 1; 38(7):387–402.
58. Kalis CH, Collins MT, Hesselink JW, Barkema HW. Specificity of two tests for the early diagnosis of bovine paratuberculosis based on cell-mediated immunity: the Johnin skin test and the gamma interferon assay. Vet. Microbiol. 2003;97(1):73–86.
59. Walravens K, Marché S, Rosseels V, Wellemans V, Boelaert F, Huygen K, Godfroid J. IFN-γ diagnostic tests in the context of bovine mycobacterial infections in Belgium. Vet Immunol Immunopathol. 2002 Sep 10;87(3):401–6.
60. Seva J, Sanes JM, Ramis G, Mas A, Quereda JJ, Villarreal-Ramos B, Villar D, Pallares FJ. Evaluation of the single cervical skin test and interferon gamma responses to detect Mycobacterium Bovis infected cattle in a herd co-infected with Mycobacterium Avium subsp paratuberculosis. Vet Microbiol. 2014;171(1):139–46.
61. Lilenbaum W, Ferreira R, Marassi CD, Ristow P, Oelemann WMR, Fonseca LDS. Interference of tuberculosis on the performance of ELISAs used in the diagnosis of paratuberculosis in cattle. Braz J Microbiol. 2007;38(3):472–7.
62. Allen AR, Minozzi G, Glass EJ, Skuce RA, McDowell SWJ, Woolliams JA, Bishop, SC. Bovine tuberculosis: the genetic basis of host susceptibility. Proc R Soc B. 2010. p.rspb20100830.
63. Richardson IW, Bradley DG, Higgins IM, More SJ, McClure J, Berry DP. Variance components for susceptibility to *Mycobacterium bovis* infection in dairy and beef cattle. Genet. Sel. Evol. 2014;46(1):77.
64. Wright DM, Allen AR, Mallon TR, McDowell SW, Bishop SC, Glass EJ, Bermingham ML, Woolliams JA, Skuce RA. Field-isolated genotypes of *Mycobacterium bovis* vary in virulence and influence case pathology but do not affect outbreak size. PloS One. 2013;8(9):e74503.
65. Doyle LP, Gordon AW, Abernethy DA, Stevens K. Bovine tuberculosis in Northern Ireland: risk factors associated with time from post-outbreak test to subsequent herd breakdown. Prev Vet Med. 2014;116(1):47–55.
66. Karolemeas, K., McKinley, T.J., Clifton-Hadley, R.S., Goodchild, A.V., Mitchell, A., Johnston,W.T., Conlan, A.J., Donnelly, C.A.,Wood, J.L., 2011. Recurrence of bovine tuberculosis breakdowns in great Britain: risk factors and prediction. Prev Vet Med. 102, 22–29.
67. Brooks-Pollock E, Conlan AJ, Mitchell AP, Blackwell R, McKinley TJ, Wood JL. Age-dependent patterns of bovine tuberculosis in cattle. Vet Res. 2013; 44(1):97.
68. Radunz BL, Lepper AWD. Suppression of skin reactivity to bovine tuberculin in repeat tests. Australian Vet J. 1985;62(6):191–4.
69. Coad M, Clifford D, Rhodes SG, Hewinson RG, Vordermeier HM, Whelan AO. Repeat tuberculin skin testing leads to desensitisation in naturally infected tuberculous cattle which is associated with elevated interleukin-10 and decreased interleukin-1 beta responses. Vet Res. 2010;41(2):1–12.
70. Clegg TA, Good M, More SJ. Risk factors for cattle presenting with a confirmed bTB lesion at slaughter, from herds with no evidence of within-herd transmission. Prev Vet Med. 2016;126:111–20.
71. Gilbert M, Mitchell A, Bourn D, Mawdsley J. Cattle movements and bovine tuberculosis in great Britain. Nature. 2005;435:491.
72. Ramirez-Villaescusa AM, Medley GF, Mason S, Green LE. Herd and individual animal risks associated with bovine tuberculosis skin test positivity in cattle in herds in south west England. Prev Vet Med. 2009;92:188–98.
73. Carroll JA, Forsberg NE. Influence of stress and nutrition on cattle immunity. Vet Clin N Am Food Anim Pract. 2007;23:105–49.
74. Ryan TJ, Livingstone PG, Ramsey DS, De Lisle GW, Nugent G, Collins DM, Buddle BM. Advances in understanding disease epidemiology and implications for control and eradication of tuberculosis in livestock: the experience from New Zealand. Vet Microbiol. 2006;112:211–9.
75. Brown E, Marshall AH, Mitchell H, Byrne AW. Analysing cattle movements in Northern Ireland using social network analysis. In: Brennan M, Lindberg A, editors. Society for Veterinary Epidemiology and Preventive Medicine – Proceedings. Tallinn, Estonia. 21–23 March. 2018.

76. Robinson SE, Christley RM. Exploring the role of auction markets in cattle movements within great Britain. Prev Vet Med. 2007;81:21–37.
77. Bigras-Poulin M, Thompson RA, Chriél M, Mortensen S, Greiner M. Network analysis of Danish cattle industry trade patterns as an evaluation of risk potential for disease spread. Prev Vet Med. 2006;76:11–39.
78. Natale F, Giovannini A, Savini L, Palma D, Possenti L, Fiore G, Calistri P. Network analysis of Italian cattle trade patterns and evaluation of risks for potential disease spread. Prev Vet Med. 2009;92:341–50.
79. Clegg TA, Good M, Duignan A, Doyle R, More SJ. Shorter-term risk of *Mycobacterium bovis* in Irish cattle following an inconclusive diagnosis to the single intradermal comparative tuberculin test. Prev Vet Med. 2011;102: 255–64.
80. Clegg TA, Good M, Duignan A, Doyle R, Blake M, More SJ. Longer-term risk of *Mycobacterium bovis* in Irish cattle following an inconclusive diagnosis to the single intradermal comparative tuberculin test. Prev Vet Med. 2011; 100(3):147–54.
81. Lahuerta-Marin A, Gallagher M, McBride S, Skuce R, Menzies F, McNair J, McDowell SW, Byrne AW. Should they stay, or should they go? Relative future risk of bovine tuberculosis for interferon-gamma test-positive cattle left on farms. Vet Res. 2015;46(1):90.
82. Mazeri S, Sargison N, Kelly RF, Barend M, Handel I. Evaluation of the performance of five diagnostic tests for *Fasciola hepatica* infection in naturally infected cattle using a Bayesian no gold standard approach. PLoS One. 2016;11(8):e0161621.

6

Multicentric lymphoma in buffaloes in the Amazon region, Brazil

Cairo H S De Oliveira[1,2†], José D Barbosa[3†], Karine A Damasceno[4], Geovanni D Cassali[4], Carlos MC Oliveira[3], Rômulo C Leite[1,3] and Jenner K P Reis[1*]

Abstract

Background: The presence of lymphoma in buffaloes was first reported in India in the 1960s. The disease is similar to Enzootic Bovine Leucosis (EBL) caused by *Bovine leukemia virus* (BLV) in cattle; however, according to our results and those of other studies, the etiology of these lymphomas in buffalo do not appear to be associated with BLV. The objectives of this study are to describe four cases of the disease in buffaloes belonging to the same herd in the Amazon region of Brazil and to perform a clinical-anatomopathological, immunohistochemical, and etiological study of the lymphomas.

Results: Over a period of ten years, four buffaloes were observed presenting progressive weight loss, swelling of peripheral lymph nodes, and nodules in the subcutaneous tissue. Upon necropsy, whitish-colored tumor masses were observed in the form of nodules in the subcutaneous tissue, along with miliary nodules on the serosal surfaces of abdominal and thoracic organs and tumors in lymph nodes and other organs. Neoplastic lymphocyte proliferation was observed through histopathology. An immunohistochemical study revealed that the neoplasias were formed by proliferation of predominantly B lymphocytes. The presence of BLV genome was not detected in the lymphomas when using the real-time PCR technique, nor was it detected through immunohistochemical staining using monoclonal antibodies against two viral proteins. *Bovine herpesvirus 6* was not detected in the tumors. However, *Bovine immunodeficiency virus* (BIV) was detected in samples of lymphoma and in the lymph nodes and kidneys of one of the animals.

Conclusions: The occurrence of lymphoma in buffaloes is reported for the first time in Brazil and is characterized by B-cell multicentric lymphoma. The etiology of the disease does not appear to be associated with BLV; however, the detection of BIV in samples of lymphoma from one sick animal deserves further study, considering the oncogenic potential of this virus.

Keywords: Lymphoma, Buffalo, BIV, BLV, BoHV-6, Brazil

Background

In Brazil, the buffalo population is estimated at roughly 1.3 million heads, with 66 % of these animals raised in the northern region of the country, mainly in the state of Pará [1]. The main breeds raised in Brazil are Murrah, Mediterranean, Jafarabadi and Carabao, which are intended for beef production, mainly extensive, but are also used for milk production in a semi-intensive system.

The buffaloes are commonly raised in the same manner as cattle because their appearance is phenotypically similar to this species. Many owners and veterinarians employ the same management tools used in cattle when raising buffaloes and forget the particularities of each species. Similarly, researchers transfer studies performed in cattle to the buffalo species without first conducting more detailed investigations.

For 10 years, our research group has observed the occurrence of a lymphoproliferative disease in buffaloes in the Amazon region, state of Pará, Brazil. Lymphoma is a malignant neoplasm of the immune system characterized

* Correspondence: jenner@ufmg.br
†Equal contributors
[1]Laboratório de Retroviroses, Departamento de Medicina Veterinária Preventiva, Escola de Veterinária, Universidade Federal de Minas Gerais, Avenida Antônio Carlos 6627, Belo Horizonte, Minas Gerais, Brazil
Full list of author information is available at the end of the article

by neoplastic proliferation of lymphocytes, which causes the formation of tumor masses in various organs. In buffaloes, the occurrence of lymphoma has been reported since 1967 in India [2].

The lesions are characterized by floccules (miliary nodules), nodules, and papillae of continuous growth and velvety appearance on the parietal and visceral surfaces of the serosal membranes of organs. The involvement of lymph nodes occurs through mild tumefaction with varying degrees of swelling [3, 4].

The etiology of this illness in buffaloes is still unclear, and due to the multicentric character of the tumors, some authors suggest the involvement of a viral agent [5]. In cattle, the emergence of lymphomas are associated with infection by *Bovine leukemia virus* (BLV), which causes Enzootic Bovine Leucosis (EBL), in which one to five percent of infected animals develop lymphoma, 20 to 30 % develop persistent lymphocytosis, and the majority remain asymptomatic for long periods [6, 7].

More recent studies have described the occurrence of lymphoma in buffaloes in Venezuela [8] and India [9]. In these studies, the authors discussed the conditions as being cases of EBL but failed to demonstrate the presence of this virus in the sick animals.

Our group has detected the presence of some viruses infections in buffaloes in Brazil including *Bovine herpesvirus 6* (BoHV-6) but no causal link to any diseases has so far been established [10]. *Bovine immunodeficiency virus* (BIV) was studied in 607 samples of DNA taken from the whole blood of buffaloes in Brazil and was detected in 4.4 % of cases using molecular biology techniques [11]. In cattle, BIV has been associated with the occurrence of lymphoma and lymphadenopathy in experimentally inoculated animals [12], but in buffaloes their role is unknown.

A closer study of the etiology of lymphomas in buffalo has not been undertaken, and few reports of this disease can be found in the world literature. In Brazil, the occurrence of lymphoma in buffaloes has never been reported. The objectives of this study were to describe four cases of lymphoma in buffaloes from one herd in the Amazon region and to conduct a clinical-anatomopathological, immunohistochemical, and etiological study of this disease.

Methods

Animals

Four buffaloes manifesting clinical symptoms indicative of lymphoma (clinical cases 01, 02, 03 and 04), belonging to a property in the Amazon region (property A-PA), were studied. The property was located in the city of Castanhal, state of Pará, Brazil (1°18'12.4"S 47°56'30.8"W), and breeding of cattle and buffaloes was used for reproduction.

Epidemiological data, such as breed, age, sex and breeding system, were obtained through technical evaluations and informal consultations with handlers and the owner. The owner allowed the study and has signed a consent term.

All procedures and animal handling followed the ethical principles in animal experimentation, adopted by the Ethics Committee in Animal Experimentation of UFMG/CEUA, under Protocol n° 133/2012.

Clinical and anatomopathological study

The animals were clinically evaluated for the presence and location of tumor nodules, enlargement of peripheral lymph nodes, appetite, and body condition.

The four animals were subjected to an anatomopathological exam in which fragments of tumor tissue were collected and fixed in 10 % formalin and sent to the Animal Pathology Department of the Animal Health Project in the Amazon of the Federal Rural University of Rio de Janeiro (Universidade Federal Rural do Rio de Janeiro), where they were processed routinely for histology and embedded in paraffin. The fragments were sectioned at 5 μm, stained with hematoxylin and eosin (HE) and evaluated through optical microscopy. In clinical case 04, fragments of the kidneys, lymph nodes, salivary gland, testis, liver, and spleen were also collected.

Immunohistochemical study

An immunohistochemical examination was performed on the tumor and organ fragments of animal 04 to characterize the type of lymphocytes present in the lymphomas.

For the immunohistochemical study, 4-μm sections were placed on gelatinized slides, and the antigenic sites were recovered with the solution Dako Cytomation Target Retrieval Solution, Citrate pH 6.0 (Dako, Carpinteria, CA, USA), before overnight incubation with anti-CD79a antibodies (marker for B lymphocytes – clone HM47/A9, DBS, Pleasanton, CA, USA), at a dilution of 1:500, and anti-CD3 (marker for T lymphocytes – clone CD3-12, University of California, Davis, CA, USA), at a dilution of 1:200. Subsequently, the commercial secondary antibody Dako Advance HRP (Horseradish Peroxidase) Link (Dako, Carpinteria, CA, USA) was added, along with the enzyme Dako Advance HRP Enzyme, the reaction with DAB (3,3'-Diaminobenzidine, Dako Liquid DAB + Substrate Chromogen System) was revealed, and counter staining with Mayer's Hematoxylin was performed.

To evaluate the presence of BLV viral proteins, immunohistochemical analysis was performed with monoclonal antibodies against the gp51 glycoproteins of the viral envelope (VMRD, Pullman, WA, USA), at a dilution of 1:100 and against the p24 protein of the viral capsid

(VMRD, Pullman, WA, USA), at a dilution of 1:500. For the positive control of the reactions, FLK (fetal lamb kidney) cells continuously infected with BLV were grown on glass slides for 48 hours, fixed with acetone for 30 minutes, and processed together with the tumor fragments using a method similar to the one described above.

The slides were observed under an optical microscope for qualitative assessment of the presence or absence of staining by specific antibodies.

Etiologic study

Three agents, BLV, BoHV-6 and BIV, were studied using PCR in fragments of lymphoma and organs from animal 04.

The tissue samples embedded in paraffin were sectioned at 5 µm and subjected to DNA extraction using a QIAamp DNA Mini Kit (Qiagen, Germany) according to the manufacturer's recommendations for formalin-fixed, paraffin-embedded (FFPE) samples.

Frozen samples of tumor fragments from animal 04 were also subjected to DNA extraction with the above mentioned kit according to the manufacturer's recommendations for fresh tissue samples.

The DNA samples were subjected to seminested PCR for BIV to detect the *pol* gene – the region that encodes the DNA polymerase enzyme – amplifying a 385-bp fragment in the outer reaction and a 154-bp fragment in the internal reaction, according to previously standardized methodology [13]. Real-time PCR was performed (qPCR) for BLV to detect the LTR gene, amplifying a 120-bp fragment according to a previous study [14]. Lastly, BoHV-6 was investigated by means of seminested PCR for the *pol* gene [10].

A positive sample for the BIV seminested PCR was cloned from the external reaction in pGEM®-T Easy Vector System II (Promega, EUA) according to the manufacturer's recommendations, transformed and multiplied in DH5alpha bacteria. Two plasmid clones were extracted using a miniprep kit (Wizard Plus SV Minipreps DNA Purification Systems, Promega, USA). The region of the insertion (385 bp) in the plasmid was subjected to nucleotide sequencing using the seminested PCR external reaction primers in an ABI 3130 sequencing machine using Big Dye chemistry and POP7 polymer (Applied Biosystems, USA).

The sequence obtained (isolated Castanhal04) was evaluated for quality and edited for contig assembly on the web at http://www.biomol.unb.br/phph/. The sequence was blasted to evaluate the degree of similarity with the reference sequence for BIV in GenBank (GenBank database, National Center for Biotechnology Information), access code M32690.1 (isolated R-29), along with the isolates OK (GenBank: U34389.1), FL112 (GenBank: L06524.1) and FL491 (GenBank: L06525.1), which were aligned using the ClustalW method in the Mega5.2 program.

Results

In 2004, two buffaloes were observed presenting progressive weight loss, enlarged lymph nodes ranging from 2 to 20 times their normal size, and nodules of varying sizes in the subcutaneous tissue. The first case was observed in a female buffalo of the Murrah breed (01), and the second in an animal of the Mediterranean breed (02) (Fig. 1a and b).

In 2010, one Murrah female buffalo (03) was observed presenting the following main clinical signs: swelling of the abdominal region and progressive weight loss (Fig. 1c). In 2013, a male animal, of the Mediterranean breed (04), was observed presenting weight loss and great difficulty urinating and defecating (tenesmus and strangury), and upon rectal palpation, a tumor mass was noted at the entrance of the pelvic cavity on the right side (Fig. 1d).

All cases occurred on a single property where the buffaloes are raised together with cattle in a semi-intensive system. The farm maintains a buffalo herd of approximately 20 animals and a cattle herd of 30 animals, and over a 10-year period, four lymphoma cases in buffaloes were observed, including an animal that was introduced to this herd two years ago (animal 04). This history raised the hypothesis that the disease could have been transmitted horizontally. It was not possible to obtain information on the degree of kinship of the animals. Table 1 presents all evaluated cases and information on breed, sex, age and location of lymphoma lesions observed during necropsy.

After identification of the disease, the animals quickly progressed to a state of great debility, with anorexia, cachexia, collapse and evolution of the nodules observed in the subcutaneous tissue and peripheral lymph nodes.

At the necropsy of animals 01 and 02, whitish nodules were observed, with sizes varying from 3 to 10 cm in diameter, diffuse along subcutaneous tissue (Fig. 2a). These nodules were soft in consistency when cut and were multilobular. The lymph nodes lost their normal morphology, and the surface appeared smooth and shiny with nodular areas of a whitish color (Fig. 2a and b).

In animal 03, the presence of tumor masses was observed in the serosa of the rumen, omasum, abomasum, intestines, liver, gallbladder, peritoneum, omentum, spleen, heart and pericardial sac. These masses appeared in the form of miliary nodules of continuous growth with a velvety or cauliflower appearance on the parietal and visceral surfaces of organs (Fig. 2d and e).

In animal 04, the presence of a large tumor mass was observed, measuring 35 × 20 cm, located at the entrance to the pelvic cavity (Fig. 2f and g). This mass was compressing the rectum and urethra, making defecation and urination difficult for the animal, and the mass

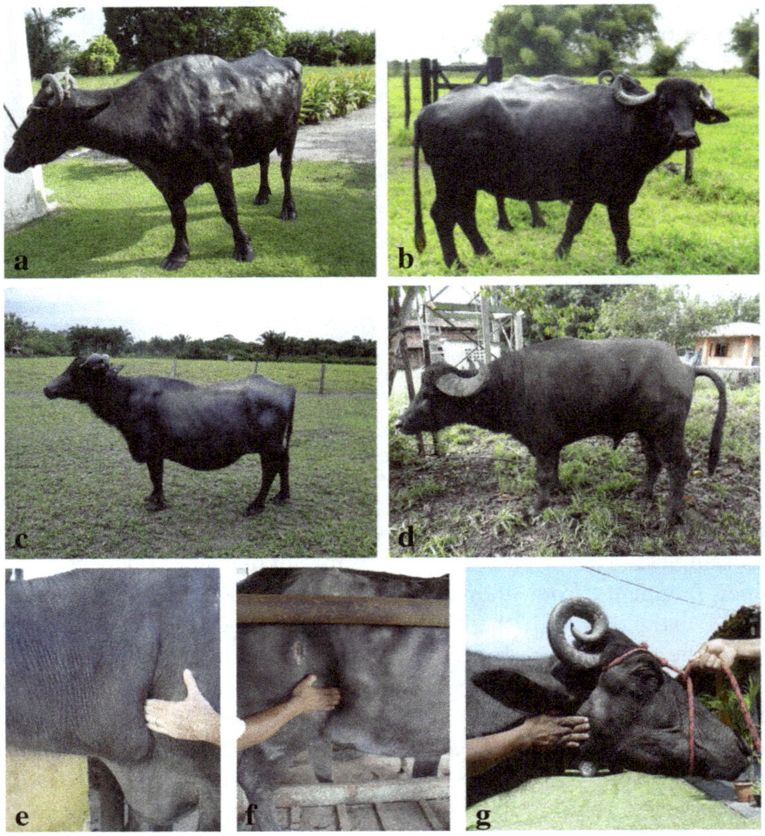

Fig. 1 Lymphoma in buffaloes. **a** Animal 01 presenting subcutaneous nodules and weight loss. **b** Animal 02. **c** Animal 03 with swelling in the abdominal region. **d** Animal 04 with tenesmus and stranguria. Lymphadenopathy: **e** superficial cervical lymph node (pre-scapular) - animal 02, **f** subiliac lymph node (pre-crural) and **g** parotid lymph node - animal 01

infiltrated into the pelvic musculature in a small area. The consistency of the mass was friable, and the cut surface was multilobulated, with a whitish to beige color and the appearance of fat (Fig. 2g).

Lymphadenopathy was observed in all of the cases in peripheral (Fig. 1e, f and g) or internal lymph nodes. Tumor masses were observed in various organs, especially the abomasum (Fig. 2c), intestines and heart (Table 1).

Histopathological analysis of the nodules and lymph nodes revealed the presence of tumor masses, characterized by the proliferation of round, discretely pleomorphic cells with little cytoplasm, large nuclei, and ovoid rounded basophilic shape, sometimes with loose chromatin and prominent nucleoli, compatible with lymphocytes. The presence of delicate fibrovascular tissue interweaving with the neoplastic process was observed. Eosinophilic areas were observed with cells in karyorrhexis and karyolysis, characterizing coagulative necrosis. The normal architecture of the lymph nodes was completely or partially replaced by neoplastic masses. Vascular invasion by neoplastic cells was also observed in the tumor masses (Fig. 3a and b).

When observed microscopically, whitish areas in the parenchyma of the liver and kidneys of animals 01 and 02 corresponded to areas of neoplastic tissue infiltration, which replaced the normal organ architecture.

An additional movie file shows the clinical signs, gross pathology and histopathology in more detail [see Additional file 1].

In the immunohistochemical analysis of pieces of tumor tissue from animal 04, the neoplastic cells showed immunoreactivity with the anti-CD79 antibody in the plasma membrane, characterizing the cells as B lymphocytes. Few cells expressed CD3, indicating the lack of T lymphocytes (Fig. 3c and d).

For BLV infection by immunohistochemistry analyses, FLK cells persistently infected with BLV were used. In these cells were observed production of viral p24 and gp51 proteins demonstrated by anti-p24 and anti-gp51 antibodies respectively (Fig. 3e). No staining was observed in neoplastic lymphocytes in lymph nodes and tumor fragments from animal 04 when the same antibodies were used (Fig. 3f). The DNA samples extracted from the frozen tumor fragments and the paraffin-embedded tissues

Table 1 Epidemiological and pathological data of four clinical cases of lymphoma in buffaloes from one property (A-PA) located in the state of Pará, Amazon region, Brazil

Clinical cases	01	02	03	04
Sex	Female	Female	Female	Male
Breed	Murrah	Mediterranean	Murrah	Mediterranean
Age	Over 10 years	Over 10 years	Over 10 years	Over 10 years
Date of necropsy	11/07/2004	12/15/2004	11/12/2010	02/08/2013
Areas with the presence of neoplasia				
Subcutaneous	+++	+++		
Digestive system				
Serosa of the rumen			+++	++
Serosa of the omasum			+++	
Mucosa of the abomasum	+	+	+	
Serosa of the intestine			+++	
Liver	+	++	+++	
Gallbladder			+++	
Peritoneum		++	+++	
Omentum		+	+++	
Lymphatic system				
Parotid lymph node	+++	++		
Submandibular lymph node	+++			
Pre-scapular lymph node	+++			
Pre-crural lymph node	+++	++		
Iliofemoral lymph node	+++			++
Mediastinal lymph node	+	+		
Cardiorespiratory System				
Heart		+++		+++
Pericardial sac				++
Lung		+	+	
Parietal pleura			++	
Spleen	+		++	
Other findings			Presence of a large amount of yellowish fluid in the abdominal and thoracic cavity	Tumor masses located at the entrance of the pelvic cavity measuring 35 × 20 cm compressing the rectum and urethra, causing tenesmus and stranguria. Thickening of the bladder wall

(+) Barely affected, (++) moderately affected and (+++) very affected

of the liver, kidneys, salivary gland, lymph node, testis and tumor fragments tested negative for BLV through the qPCR technique and for BoHV-6 through seminested PCR. However, the samples of frozen and paraffin-embedded tumor fragments of the lymph nodes and kidneys tested positive for BIV through seminested PCR.

The nucleotide sequence obtained from the amplification of a 385-bp fragment of the *pol* gene of BIV from the frozen tumor sample of animal 04 (Castanhal04 isolate) was deposited in GenBank under access number KP202180. This sample showed 99 % similarity with the R-29 isolate of BIV in cellular culture, originally obtained from cattle with persistent lymphocytosis in 1972, 92 % with the OK isolate, 92 % with the FL112 isolate, and 91 % with the FL491 isolate. The alignment of nucleotides between the Castanhal04 isolate and the R-29 reference isolate showed only one transition point mutation at position 390, with the exchange of a G (guanine) for an A (adenine) (Fig. 4).

Discussion

The occurrence of lymphoma has been reported in buffaloes only in India [2–5, 15, 16] and Venezuela [8]. This is the first report of the disease in buffaloes in Brazil.

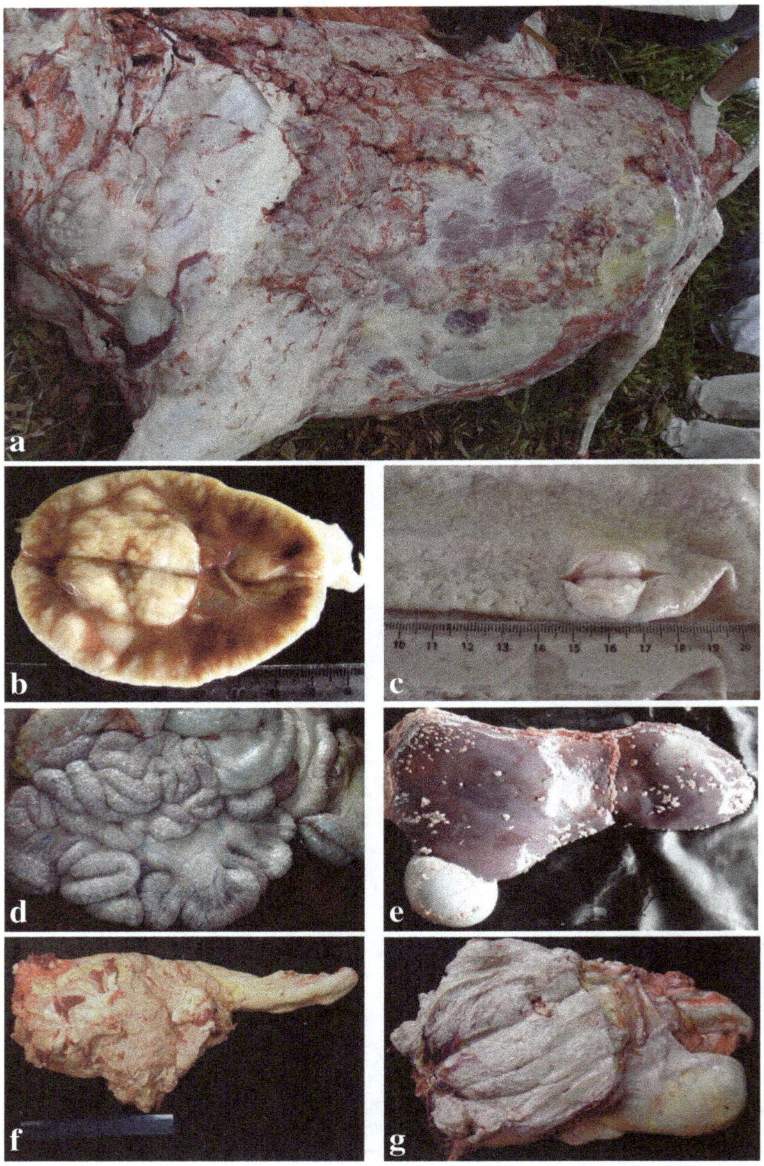

Fig. 2 Macroscopic lesions in buffaloes with multicentric lymphoma. **a** Subcutaneous tissue with whitish nodules of different sizes and swelling of pre-scapular lymph node. **b** Surface of a lymph node with the presence of a tumor mass. **c** Tumor nodule in the abomasum. **d** Miliary nodules in the serosa of the intestines and mesentery. **e** Miliary nodules on the serosa of the liver and gallbladder. **f** Tumor mass measuring 35 x 20 cm located at the entrance of the pelvic cavity of a buffalo. **g** Surface of the tumor mass seen in **f**, characterized by a whitish coloration and fatty appearance. **a-c** from animal 01, **d-e** from animal 03 and **f-g** from animal 04

The involvement of various organs and systems of the sick animals revealed the multicentric character of the disease, a fact also mentioned by other authors [8, 16]. In our study, only older animals were affected, suggesting that lymphoma in buffaloes is a chronic illness. In India, 17.8 % of adult animals were observed to have lymphoma lesions during slaughter; the rate was 1.23 % in animals up to two years old [3].

The pathological and histological lesions were similar to those observed by other authors [16]. Some authors reported the presence of large quantities of lymphoblasts and/or lymphocytes [5] and numerous mitotic figures in the histopathology of the tumor nodules. In this study, large quantities of lymphocytes and few cells in mitosis were observed. In the immunohistochemical analysis, the staining of most of the cells by the anti-CD79 antibody indicates that the tumors were characterized by the proliferation of B lymphocytes, a finding which has not yet been investigated in other studies.

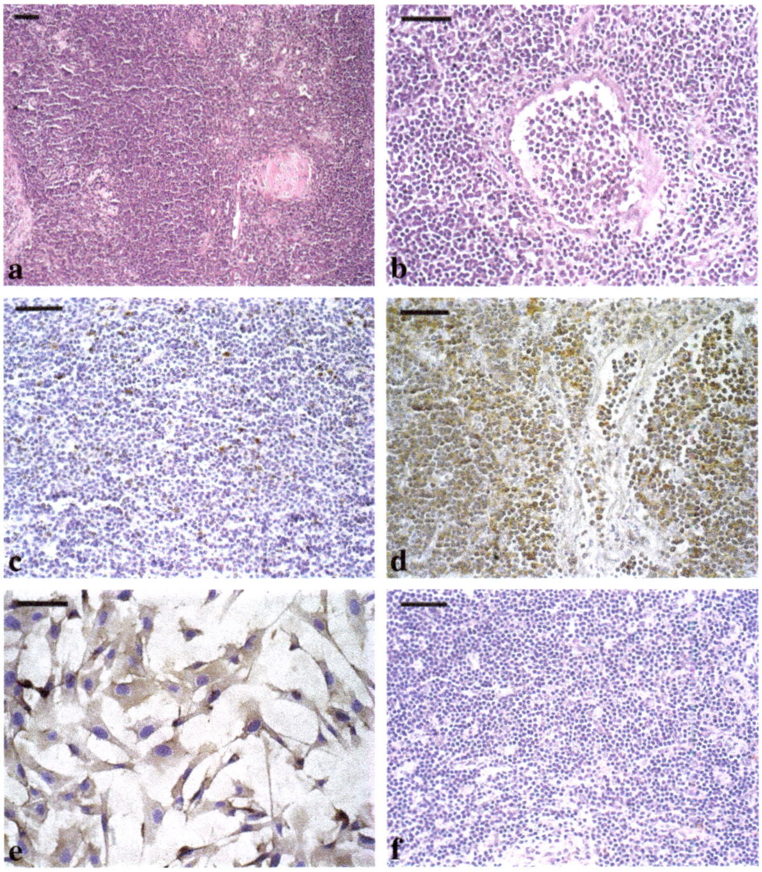

Fig. 3 Histology and immunohistochemistry of clinical case 04. **a** Histological section of lymph node showing neoplastic lymphocytes, with loss of organ architecture. HE. **b** Tumor mass from pelvic cavity showing vascular invasion area for neoplastic cells. HE. **c** Membrane marking with anti-CD3 antibody. Immunohistochemical reaction with Mayer's Hematoxylin counterstaining. **d** Labeling of membranes with anti-CD79 antibody. Immunohistochemical reaction with Mayer's Hematoxylin counterstaining. **e** FLK cells with cytoplasmic staining using an anti-p24 antibody for BLV. Immunohistochemical reaction with Mayer's Hematoxylin counterstaining. **f** Tumor mass from pelvic cavity with absence of staining using an anti-p24 antibody for BLV. Immunohistochemical reaction with Mayer's Hematoxylin counterstaining. Bars = 50 μm

In cattle with lymphoma caused by BLV, the macroscopic evaluation and histopathology of the tumors are similar to those observed in buffaloes in this study. In cattle, the tumors can occur in a multicentric form in various organs of the body, including the liver, lymph nodes, spleen, eyeballs, abomasum, rumen, and nervous system, among others. The histopathology is characterized by the proliferation of medium to large cells, lymphocytic and lymphoblastic in origin and with low mitotic indices. These cells have the phenotype of B lymphocytes, and necrotic areas are observed in the tumor masses [17, 18].

The etiology of this disease in buffaloes is still unclear. We suspect the involvement of a transmissible etiologic agent, as animal 04 presented the lymphoproliferative disease two years after its introduction into the herd of property A-PA, where the disease has been observed since the year 2004. Lymphoma in domestic animals can occur in spontaneous form associated with genetic and relatedness, although the degree of relationship of the sick buffaloes could not be accessed, the animals were obtained from different herds and does not seems to have any kinship. Additionally, lymphoma caused by genetic or undefined causes generally occur in younger animals, like sporadic leucosis in cattle not associated with BLV infection [19], unlike the cases in buffaloes that affected only older animals.

Due to the anatomopathological characteristics of the lymphomas in the buffaloes, some authors have diagnosed the disease as EBL [8, 9], but the involvement of BLV is unproven. Another important observation is that all of the animals in our study exhibited leukocytosis by lymphocytosis, like the other apparently healthy buffalo in the herd (data not shown), very similar to that observed in cattle infected with BLV [6, 7]. However, tumor and organ samples of a buffalo with lymphoma tested

```
                    1       10        20        30        40        50        60        70        80
                    |--------+---------+---------+---------+---------+---------+---------+---------|
     R29_M32690.1   CCTCCAGGAATTAAGGAATGTGAACACTTAACTGCAATAGATATAAAAGATGCCTACTTTACTATCCCTTTACATGAGGA
Castanhal04_KP202180 ................................................................................
      OK_U34389.1   ...................................TT...............................CC.G.....A..
    FL112_L06524.1  .......................G............T................................C.G........
    FL491_L06525.1  .......................G............T................................C.G........

                    81      90       100       110       120       130       140       150       160
                    |--------+---------+---------+---------+---------+---------+---------+---------|
     R29_M32690.1   CTTTAGACCCTTTACAGCCTTCTCTGTAGTCCCTGTAAATCGAGAAGGACCTATAGAGAGGTTCCAGTGGAATGTTCTAC
Castanhal04_KP202180 ................................................................................
      OK_U34389.1   ............C............A..................................A...................
    FL112_L06524.1  ...........AC.............................G.................A.A.................
    FL491_L06525.1  ...........AC............T......................G...........A.AT................

                    161    170       180       190       200       210       220       230       240
                    |--------+---------+---------+---------+---------+---------+---------+---------|
     R29_M32690.1   CACAAGGATGGGTATGTAGCCCTGCCATTTATCAGACTACCACCCAGAAGATTATAGAAAACATTAAAAAGAGTCACCCA
Castanhal04_KP202180 ................................................................................
      OK_U34389.1   ..................................A........T.................A..C.GG.GA..C......
    FL112_L06524.1  ...................T........C.....A........T.G.G..........T.G...A....G.G..T.....
    FL491_L06525.1  .......G...........T........C.....A........T.G.G................A....G.G..T.....

                    241    250       260       270       280       290       300       310       320
                    |--------+---------+---------+---------+---------+---------+---------+---------|
     R29_M32690.1   GATGTCATGTTGTATCAATATATGGATGATTTGTTGATTGGGTCTAATAGGGATGATCATAAGCAAATAGTGCAGGAAAT
Castanhal04_KP202180 ................................................................................
      OK_U34389.1   ..CA.......A.......................A..C........C..A.......................A..G..
    FL112_L06524.1  ...........A....................A..............C..A..........................T..
    FL491_L06525.1  ...........A....................A..............C..AA.............G.....A.....T..

                    321    330       340       350       360       370       380  385
                    |--------+---------+---------+---------+---------+---------+----|
     R29_M32690.1   CAGGGATAAGTTAGGATCATATGGTTTCAAGACTCCAGATGAAAAGGTCCAGGAAGAGAGAGTGA
Castanhal04_KP202180 ...........................................................A.....
      OK_U34389.1   T......G.........................C.........................A.....
    FL112_L06524.1  T......G.......G...........T.....C.......................A..G....
    FL491_L06525.1  T......G..........C........T.....C..........................G....
```

Fig. 4 ClustalW alignment of the nucleotide sequence from part of the *pol* gene of BIV. Comparison of the isolated sequence of the sample of lymphoma of a buffalo from the state of Pará, Brazil, Castanhal04 isolate (GenBank: KP202180), with the reference sample for R-29 (GenBank: M32690.1), and the isolates for OK (GenBank: U34389.1), FL112 (GenBank: L06524.1) and FL491 (GenBank: L06525.1). Castanhal04 and R-29 showed 99 % similarity, with only one transition point mutation at position 380 of the alignment. The positions of the nucleotides are shown in accordance with the R-29 isolate (.), indicating the identity of the nucleotides

negative for BLV by qPCR and immunohistochemical analysis, which reinforces the hypothesis that this virus is not involved in the etiology of lymphoma in buffaloes. In a previous study, we used serological and molecular tests to evaluate 315 samples from buffaloes in Brazil, and the presence of BLV was not detected in any of the animals [20].

Gammaherpesviruses are known to have oncogenic potential [21, 22]. In humans, *Epstein-Barr virus* (EBV) is associated with the occurrence of Hodgkin lymphoma, Burkitt's lymphoma, and diffuse lymphoma of large B cells, among others [23]. BoHV-6, a gammaherpesvirus initially detected in samples of bovine lymphomas caused by BLV [24], was not detected in samples of lymphoma from buffaloes evaluated in our study, despite its previous detection in the peripheral blood of other buffaloes from the same herd [10].

In contrast, samples of tumor fragments, kidneys and lymph nodes were positive for BIV, a retrovirus of the genus *Lentivirus*. This is the first detection of BIV in samples of lymphoma from buffaloes, and the sequence of nucleotides of Castanhal04 isolate had high similarity with the R-29 reference sequence. During a study of BIV pathogenesis, four calves, negative for BLV, were inoculated with the R-29 strain of BIV. One animal developed lymphadenopathy and monocytosis 160 days after inoculation. The calf died 203 days after inoculation, diagnosed with multicentric T cells lymphoma [12].

In cats, animals infected with the lentivirus *Feline immunodeficiency virus* (FIV) are five times more likely to develop B cell lymphoma [25]. The virus acts indirectly in the induction of tumors [26, 27], reducing the immune system's surveillance mechanisms due to immunodeficiency, and may be involved in the polyclonal expansion of B cells, which predisposes the animal to mutations leading to oncogenesis [25]. Therefore, the importance of the detection of BIV in the buffalo species should be considered.

In slaughterhouses in the Amazon region, buffalo carcasses are being condemned as cases of tuberculosis or EBL due to the presence of neoplasia in various organs. Thus, the occurrence of lymphoma in buffalo seems to be larger than we actually realize.

Conclusions

Buffaloes in the Amazon region have displayed a neoplastic disease characterized by multicentric B-cell lymphoma, but its pathogenesis is still unclear. The disease is observed in older animals, and the main clinical signs are progressive weight loss, lymphadenopathy, and the presence of nodules in the subcutaneous tissue. BIV was detected in the tumor samples, lymph nodes and kidneys of one sick animal. Thus the oncogenic role of this virus should be considered and investigated in future studies.

Abbreviations

BIV: Bovine immunodeficiency virus; BLV: Bovine leukemia virus; BoHV-6: Bovine herpesvirus 6; bp: base pair; CEUA: Ethics Committee in Animal Experimentation; DNA: Deoxyribonucleic acid; EBL: Enzootic Bovine Leucosis; FFPE: Formalin-fixed, paraffin-embedded; FIV: Feline immunodeficiency virus; FLK: Fetal lamb kidney; HE: Hematoxylin and eosin; LTR: Long repeated terminal; PCR: Polymerase chain reaction; qPCR: Real time PCR; UFMG: Universidade Federal de Minas Gerais; μm: Micrometers

Acknowledgements

The authors thanks the Pós-graduação in Animal Science from Universidade Federal do Pará (UFPA) for the financial support for English proofreading. The authors also thank all colleagues from the Laboratório de Retroviroses (EV-UFMG), Hospital de Grandes Animais - UFPA, and the Laboratório de Patologia Comparada (ICB-UFMG) for their technical support.

Funding

Financial support for this study was provided by the Instituto Nacional de Ciência e Tecnologia - Pecuária (INCT-Pecuária), the Conselho Nacional de Desenvolvimento Científico e Tecnológico (CNPq), the Coordenação de Aperfeiçoamento de Pessoal de Nível Superior (CAPES) and Fundação de Amparo à Pesquisa do Estado de Minas Gerais (FAPEMIG). JKPR, RCL and JDB received fellowships from CNPq.

Authors' contributions

CHSO: experimental design and article preparation; this work is part of the author's doctoral thesis. JDB: attendance of clinical cases and macroscopic analysis. KAD and GDC: immunohistochemical analyses. CMCO: performance of necropsies. RCL and JKPR: coordinators of the study and contributed to the writing of the manuscript. All authors read and approved the final manuscript.

Competing interests

The authors declare that they have no competing interests.

Consent for publication

Not applicable.

Author details

[1]Laboratório de Retroviroses, Departamento de Medicina Veterinária Preventiva, Escola de Veterinária, Universidade Federal de Minas Gerais, Avenida Antônio Carlos 6627, Belo Horizonte, Minas Gerais, Brazil. [2]Setor de Medicina Veterinária Preventiva, Escola de Veterinária e Zootecnia, Universidade Federal de Goiás, Goiânia, Goiás, Brazil. [3]Hospital Veterinário de Grandes Animais, Instituto de Medicina Veterinária, Universidade Federal do Pará, Castanhal, Pará, Brazil. [4]Laboratório de Patologia Comparada, Instituto de Ciências Biológicas, Universidade Federal de Minas Gerais, Belo Horizonte, Minas Gerais, Brazil.

References

1. Produção da Pecuária Municipal. Instituto Brasileiro de Geografia e Estatística. v.41. Brasil: Produção da Pecuária Municipal; 2013.
2. Bhattacharya P. Lymphosarcoma in Indian buffaloes. Bull Off Int Epizoot. 1967;68(1):149–50.
3. Singh CM. Lymphosarcoma in Indian buffaloes. B bl Haematol. 1968;30:237–43.
4. Singh B, Singh KP, Parihar NS, et al. Lymphosarcomatous involvement of reproductive and endocrine organs in Indian buffalo. Zentralbl Veterinarmed A. 1980;27(7):583–92.
5. Singh CM, Singh B, Parihar NS. Pulmonary involvement in lymphosarcoma of Indian buffaloes. Bibl Haematol. 1973;39:220–7.
6. Ghysdael J, Bruck C, Kettmann R, et al. Bovine leukemia virus. Curr Top Microbiol Immunol. 1984;112:1–19.
7. Bartlett PC, Norby B, Byrem TM, et al. Bovine leukemia virus and cow longevity in Michigan dairy herds. J Dairy Sci. 2013;96(3):1591–7.
8. Vale-Echeto OE, Montiel-Urdaneta N, Simoes D, et al. Linfoma multicéntrico o linfosarcoma multicéntrico en Búfalo de agua (Bubalus buballs): Estudio Anatomopatológico. Reporte de un caso Revista Científica. 2009;19:257–63.
9. Chand N, Deshmukh S, Banga HS, et al. Bovine ymphosarcoma in a buffalo (Bubalus bubalis). Vet Pract. 2012;13(1):114.
10. De Oliveira CH, de Oliveira FG, Gasparini MR, et al. Bovine herpesvirus 6 in buffaloes (Bubalus bulalis) from the Amazon region. Brazil Trop Anim Health Prod. 2015;47(2):465–8.
11. Albernaz TT, Leite RC, Reis JKP, et al. Molecular detection of bovine immunodeficiency virus in water buffaloes (Bubalus bubalis) from the Amazon retion. Brazil Trop Anim Health Prod. 2015. doi:10.1007/s11250-015-0884-6.
12. Rovid AH, Carpenter S, Miller LD, et al. An atypical T-cell lymphosarcoma in a calf with bovine immunodeficiency-like virus infection. Vet Pathol. 1996; 33(4):457–9.
13. Rodrigues AS. Detecção molecular do vírus da immunodeficiência bovina (BIV) em bovinos do estado de Minas Gerais. In: 59f. Dissertação (Mestrado em Ciência Animal) - Escola de Veterinária. Belo Horizonte: Universidade Federal de Minas Gerais; 2014.
14. Jimba M, Takeshima SN, Murakami H, et al. BLV-CoCoMo-qPCR: a useful tool for evaluating bovine leukemia virus infection status. BMC Vet Res. 2012;8:167.
15. Gupta PP, Singh B, Gill BS. Some uncommon neoplasms of Indian water buffaloes (Bubalus bubalis). Zentralbl Veterinarmed A. 1977;24(6):511–9.
16. Singh B, Singh KP, Parihar NS, et al. Clinicopathological studies on lymphosarcoma in Indian buffaloes (Bubalus bubalis). Zentralbl Veterinarmed A. 1979;26(6):468–81.
17. Chiba T, Hiraga M, Aida Y, et al. Immunohistologic studies on subpopulations of lymphocytes in cattle with enzootic bovine leukosis. Vet Pathol. 1995;32(5):513–20.
18. Malatestinic A. Bilateral exophthalmos in a Holstein cow with lymphosarcoma. Can Vet J. 2003;44(8):664–6.
19. Grünberg W, Eisenberg SW. Atypical form of sporadic bovine leukosis (SBL) in the Netherlands. Vet Rec. 2013 173(16):398.
20. De Oliveira, C. H. S., Resende, C. F., Oliveira, C. M. C., Barbosa, J. D., Fonseca Junior, A. A., Leite, R. C., Reis, J. K. P. (2016). Absence of Bovine leukemia virus (BLV) infection in buffaloes from Amazon and southeast region in Brazil. Prev Vet Med. http://dx.doi.org/10.1016/j.prevetmed.2016.05.002
21. Ackermann M. Pathogenesis of gammaherpesvirus infections. Vet Microbiol. 2006;113(3-4):211–22.
22. Cesarman E. Gammaherpesviruses and lymphoproliferative disorders. Annu Rev Pathol. 2014;9:349–72.
23. Thorley-Lawson DA, Hawkins JB, Tracy SI, et al. The pathogenesis of Epstein-Barr virus persistent infection. Curr Opin Virol. 2013;3(3):227–32.

24. Rovnak J, Quackenbush SL, Reyes RA, et al. Detection of a novel bovine lymphotropic herpesvirus. J Virol. 1998;72(5):4237–42.
25. Beatty J. Viral causes of feline lymphoma: retroviruses and beyond. Vet J. 2014;201(2):174–80.
26. Beatty JA, Lawrence CE, Callanan JJ, et al. Feline immunodeficiency virus (FIV)-associated lymphoma: a potential role for immune dysfunction in tumourigenesis. Vet Immunol Immunopathol. 1998;65(2-4):309–22.
27. Schmiedt CW, Grimes JA, Holzman G, et al. Incidence and risk factors for development of malignant neoplasia after feline renal transplantation and cyclosporine-based immunosuppression. Vet Comp Oncol. 2009;7(1):45–53.

7

Virulence gene profiles: alpha-hemolysin and clonal diversity in *Staphylococcus aureus* isolates from bovine clinical mastitis in China

Limei Zhang[1], Jian Gao[1], Herman W. Barkema[2], Tariq Ali[1], Gang Liu[1], Youtian Deng[1], Sohail Naushad[2], John P. Kastelic[2] and Bo Han[1*]

Abstract

Background: *Staphylococcus aureus*, a common cause of bovine mastitis, is known for its ability to acquire to antimicrobial resistance and to secrete numerous virulence factors that can exacerbate inflammation. In addition, alpha-hemolysin has an important role in *S. aureus* infections, diversity of the *hla* gene (that produces alpha-hmolysin) in *S. aureus* isolated from bovine mastitis has not been well characterized. The objective was, therefore, to determine diversity of virulence genes, *hla* gene sequences, and clonal profiles of *S. aureus* from bovine mastitis in Chinese dairy herds, and to evaluate inter-relationships.

Results: The antimicrobials resistance varies from as low as 1.9% (2/103) for CTX to as high as 76.7% (79/103) for penicilin in the 103 isolates and 46 (44.7%) *S. aureus* were determined as multi-resistant isolates with diverse resistance patterns. Thirty-eight virulence gene patterns (with variable frequencies) were identified in the 103 isolates and correlated with MLST types, indicating a great diversity. Although the *hla* gene also had great diversity (14 genotypes), Hla peptides were relatively more conserved. With 7 clonal complexes identified from 24 *spa* types and 7 MLST types. Regarding the letter, ST 97 was the dominant type in *S. aureus* from bovine mastitis in China. Furthermore, based on phylogenetic analysis, there was a distinct evolutionary relationship between the *hla* gene and MLST.

Conclusion: Multi-resistant *S. aureus* occurred in bovine mastitis with diverse resistance patterns. The diversity of virulence gene profiles, especially the *hla* gene and, their relationship with molecular types were reported for the first time in *S. aureus* from bovine mastitis, which will be useful for future studies on immunogenicity and vaccine development. In addition, based on the distinct evolutionary relationship between the *hla* gene and MLST types, we inferred that the *hla* gene has potential role for molecular typing of *S. aureus*.

Keywords: *Staphylococcus aureus*, Virulence gene, *Hla*, MLST, *spa*, Bovine mastitis

Background

Bovine mastitis causes huge economic losses in the global dairy industry by decreasing the quality and quantity of milk produced, as well as compromising dairy cow health and welfare. *Staphylococcus aureus*, one of the most prevalent etiologic agents, has an important role in clinical and subclinical mastitis, characterized by persistent and recurrent infections with low cure rates in response to antimicrobial therapy [1–3].

Staphylococcus aureus is known for the ability to develop resistance to antimicrobial agents (e.g. methicillin-resistant *S. aureus*, vancomycin-intermediate *S. aureus*, and vancomycin-resistant *S. aureus*) and to secrete numerous virulence factors to exacerbate inflammation. As an alternative to antimicrobials, anti-virulence therapies interfere with bacterial toxins or virulence factors and/or pathways that regulate their production [4]. Allen et al. [5] proposed that a combination of anti-virulence compounds

* Correspondence: hanbo@cau.edu.cn
[1]College of Veterinary Medicine, China Agricultural University, Yuan Ming Yuan West Road No. 2, Haidian District, Beijing 100193, People's Republic of China
Full list of author information is available at the end of the article

targeting various virulence factors would be a more effective solution than conventional treatments. Therefore, characterization of virulence gene profiles and clonal diversity among *S. aureus* populations are very important in development of anti-virulence therapies [6–9].

Alpha-hemolysin (Hla) toxin is the most emphasized and characterized virulence factor [10] in *S. aureus*. Changes in key amino acid residues may affect Hla activity. For example, a H35L substitution had no hemolytic or lethal activity, whereas a C259T substitution resulted in a premature stop codon and a significant reduction in Hla production [11–13]. Additionally, promising results have been obtained using Hla as a candidate for developing a vaccine to prevent *S. aureus* infections [14–16]. However, variation in Hla peptide sequences could affect vaccine efficacy. It is therefore important to characterize genetic polymorphism of the *hla* gene.

To date, several studies on diversity of *hla* gene of *S. aureus* originating from humans have been reported [13, 17, 18]; however, there is paucity of research regarding sequence variability of this gene in *S. aureus* isolates from bovine mastitis. The objective was to determine virulence gene patterns and *hla* gene diversity in *S. aureus* from bovine mastitis and link them with potential molecular clones, as determined by multilocus sequence type (MLST) and *spa* typing.

Methods

A total of 103 *S. aureus* isolates from 1021 clinical mastitis samples collected from 2013 to 2016 on 19 dairy farms in 9 provinces of China were used in this study (Table 1). Isolates were identified as *S. aureus* according to conventional methods, including Gram staining, colony morphology, hemolysis, catalase and tube coagulase test, as well as 16S rRNA, *coa* and *nuc* gene sequence analysis, as described [6, 10].

Table 1 Distribution of the 103 *Staphylococcus aureus* clinical mastitis isolates according to region and herd

Region	Herd	No. of milk samples	No. of isolates	Total isolates of region
Beijing	a	407	41	48
	b	53	5	
	c	28	2	
Ningxia	d	46	5	16
	e	31	4	
	f	29	3	
	g	28	3	
	h	28	1	
Heilongjiang	i	56	11	11
Hebei	j	38	6	11
	k	23	4	
	l	22	1	
Inner Mongolia	m	25	3	5
	n	22	2	
Liaoning	o	15	2	4
	p	15	2	
Guangdong	q	98	3	3
Shandong	r	40	3	3
Henan	s	17	2	2
Total	19	1021	103	103

Extraction of genomic DNA

Genomic DNA of all 103 isolates was extracted using Bacteria Genomic DNA Kit (CW, Beijing, China) according to the manufacturer's instructions and stored at − 20 °C. In addition, quantity and quality of DNA were assessed using a Nanodrop ND-1000 spectrophotometer (Thermoscientific, Wilmington, DE).

Antimicrobial susceptibility testing

To analyze the antibiotic susceptibility profiles of the 103 isolates, minimum inhibitory concentrations (MICs) of a panel of 11 different antibiotics were determined using the broth microdilution method and resistance breakpoints for ampicillin (AMP, 0.5 mg/L), augmentin (AMX/CA, 32 mg/L), cefotaxime (CTX, 8 mg/L), ceftriaxone (CRO, 8 mg/L), ciprofloxacin (CIP, 4 mg/L), clindamicin (CL, 8 mg/L), erythromycin (E, 8 mg/L), gentamicin (GM, 16 mg/L), oxacillin (OX, 0.5 mg/L), penicillin (P, 0.25 mg/L), tetracycline (TE, 16 mg/L) as described in CLSI (2013) [19]. *S. aurues* ATCC 29213 was used as uality control in this study.

Antimicrobial agents above were selected either according to their availability in commercial products or working as representative of an antibiotic family. And those which were found to be resistant to at least three or more of antimicrobial agents were defined as multidrug resistant isolates.

Detection of virulence genes

All *S. aureus* isolates were screened by polymerase chain reaction (PCR) for the following virulence genes: fibronectin binding proteins A and B (*fnbA* and *fnbB*), clumping factors A and B (*clfA* and *clfB*), α-, β-, γ-, and δ-hemolysin (*hla, hlb, hlc* and *hld*), intracellular adhesion A and D (*icaA* and *icaD*), toxic shock syndrome toxin (*tsst*), and enterotoxins (*sea, seb, sec, see, seg* and *sei*). Primer sequences and PCR methods have been described [8, 20, 21]. Products amplified by PCR were sequenced by Beijing Sunbiotech Co. (Beijing, China). Virulence gene profiles were analyzed as binary data using the Maximum Parsimony tree by MEGA6 [22, 23]. Evolutionary distances were computed using the p-distances method and were in units of the number of base differences per site [24].

Genotyping of *hla* gene and phylogenetic analysis

Primers used for amplification of the complete 960 bp *hla* gene were: *hla*F1 (5′- TTAGCCGAAAAACATCATTTC -3′) and *hla*R1 (5′- TTATTCCCGACGAAATTCCAA -3′), as described Mocca et al. (2014) [15]. The PCR was performed with initial denaturation at 95 °C for 5 min, followed by 33 cycles of 94 °C for 1 min, 55 °C for 1 min, 72 °C for 1 min, and a final extension at 72 °C for 10 min. Products were sent to Beijing Sunbiotech Co. (Beijing, China) for bidirectional sequencing using both primers: *hla*F2 (5′- GAAGTTATCGGCTAAAGTTATAA -3′) and *hla*R2 (5′- CATAATTAATACCCTTTTTCTC -3′ [15]. All PCR-amplified products were sequenced twice.

Staphylococcus aureus strain WOOD46 (GenBank accession no. X01645) was selected as the reference strain, as reported [13, 16, 25–27], and *hla* gene sequences were aligned using BioEdit v7.0.9 (Micro Focus, Newbury, UK) to designate genotypes. Corresponding peptide sequences were deduced and aligned to determine the presence of amino acid substitutions. NetPhosBac 1.0 Server (http://www.cbs.dtu.dk/services/NetPhosBac-1.0) was used to predict serine and threonine phosphorylation sites in Hla peptide sequences, which were identified with non-synonymous amino acid substitutions [28]. In addition, phylogenetic trees of the *hla* gene and 7 MLST alleles in the collection were generated by MEGA6 (http://www.megasoftware.net/) using the neighbor-joining method by the Kimura 2-parameter model with 1000 bootstrap replicates [22].

Molecular typing

Staphylococcus aureus isolates that harbored the *hla* gene were genotyped by staphylococcal protein A (*spa*) typing (http://spa.ridom.de/index.shtml) using SPATypeMapper software (download at http://www.clondiag.com/filead min/Media/Downloads/SPATypeMapper_0_6.zip) and multilocus sequence typing (MLST; http://saureus.mlst.net/) [9, 29]. In addition, the goeBURST algorithm (http://goeBURST.phyloviz.net) was used to infer evolutionary associations of MLST types (STs).

Statistical analyses

Associations between virulence gene profiles, Hla peptide types and clonal background were analyzed using a Chi-square or Fisher's exact test, as appropriate, on contingency tables (virulence types or Hla peptide types vs clonal backgrounds or geography; virulence types vs Hla peptide types) using SPSS 23.0 (SPSS Inc., Chicago, IL). Statistical significance was defined as $P < 0.05$.

Results

Antimicrobial resistance patterns

Overall, there were only 5 *S. aureus* isolates susceptible to all tested antimicrobial compounds, as shown in Table 2. And a total of 46 (44.7%) *S. aureus* were determined as multi-resistant isolates with diverse resistance patterns. In addition, the antimicrobials resistance varies from as low as 1.9% (2/103) for CTX to as high as 76.7% (79/103) for penicillin.

Table 2 Antimicrobial resistance patterns of *S. aureus* strains isolated from clinical mastitis in cows

Number of types of resistance	Patterns of resistance	*S. aurues* (*n* = 103)
0 (5)		5
1 (8)	CL	2
	CRO	1
	E	3
	AMP	2
2 (45)	P, AMP	39
	CIP, AMP	1
	OX, E	1
	E, P	1
	CIP, P	1
	OX, AMP	1
	OX, CIP	1
3 (28)	OX, P, AMP	2
	CIP, AMP, P	4
	P, AMP, CL	3
	E, P, AMP	14
	P, AMP, CRO	1
	AMX/CA, P, AMP	1
	OX, E, CL	1
	TE, AMP, P	2
4 (13)	OX, E, CIP, CL	1
	OX, AMX/CA, P, AMP	1
	E, AMX/CA, P, AMP	1
	OX, E, AMP, CL	1
	OX, TE, E, AMP	1
	OX, CIP, P, AMP	1
	E, CIP, AMP, CL	3
	TE, E, P, AMP	1
	OX, E, P, AMP	1
	E, P, AMP, CL	2
≥5 (5)	OX, E, P, CTX, AMP	1
	GM, E, P, AMP, CL	1
	GM, E, CIP, AMP, CL	1
	OX, E, CIP, P, AMP, CL	1
	OX, TE, GM, E, CIP, P, CTX, AMP, CL, CRO	1

AMP ampicillin, *AMX/CA* augmentin, *CFX/K* cephalexin/kanamycin, *CIP* ciprofloxacin, *CL* clindamycin, *CRO* ceftriaxone, *CTX* cefotaxime, *E* erythromycin, *GM* gentamicin, *OX* oxacillin, *P* penicillin, *TE* tetracycline

Virulence gene profiles

The PCR amplification results of 17 virulence genes are shown in Additional file 1: Figure S1, Additional file 2: Figure S2, Additional file 3: Figure S3 and Additional file 4: Figure S4, and their relative frequency in 103 clinical mastitis *S. aureus* are shown (Fig. 1). Among them, *clfB* and *icaA* genes were detected in 100% of isolates, followed by *clfA* ($n = 99$; 96%), *hld* ($n = 98$; 95%), *fnbA* ($n = 97$; 94%), *hla* ($n = 93$; 90%), *hlc* ($n = 91$; 88%), *fnbB* ($n = 88$; 85%) and *hlb* ($n = 82$; 80%), *tsst* ($n = 31$; 30%), *icaD* ($n = 26$; 25%), *sec* ($n = 22$; 21%), *sei* ($n = 5$; 5%), *seg* (n = 3; 3%), *seb* and *see* (n = 2; 2%). None of the 103 *S. aureus* isolates had the *sea* gene.

The 103 *S. aureus* isolates comprised 38 virulence gene profiles, which were then categorized into 5 clusters (A to E; Fig. 1). Geographic distribution of these clusters are shown (Table 3). Prevalence of virulence clusters differed among herds from different provinces. Different virulence cluster combinations appeared in herds from different provinces with only 2 exceptions (Herds m and q and Herds s and l; Table 3). Isolates from herds in same province usually had similar cluster combinations. Predominant clusters therefore differed among provinces ($P < 0.01$): Cluster A was the most frequently detected in Beijing herds, Cluster D in herds from Ningxia, and Cluster C in herds from Hebei and Heilongjiang.

Genotyping based on *hla* gene

Using *S. aureus* strain WOOD 46 as a reference sequence, 22 single nucleotide mutations were detected, 4 in the signal peptide encoding portion (nucleotide positions − 42, − 22, − 6 and − 5) and 18 on the mature *hla* encoding sequence (nucleotide positions 47, 144, 214, 237, 255, 262, 399, 438, 453, 498, 499, 519, 606, 686, 765, 797, 824, 833) (Table 4). As a result 14 *hla*

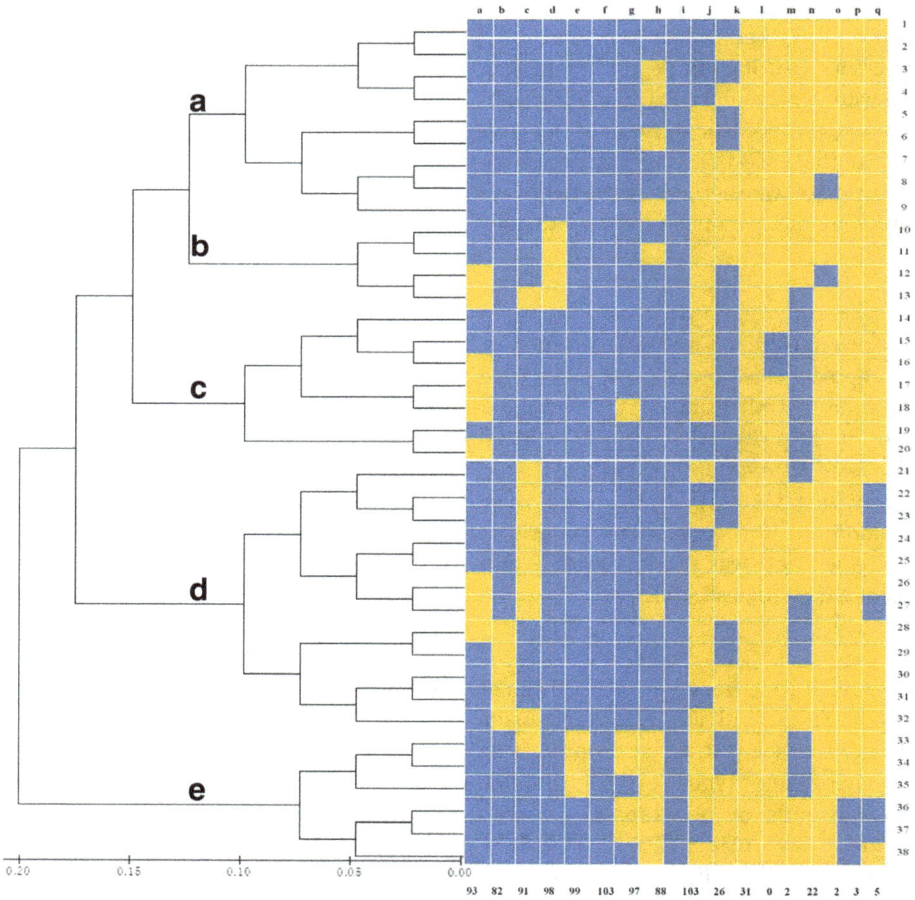

Fig. 1 Analysis of virulence gene profiles of 103 Chinese *Staphylococcus aureus* isolates from bovine clinical mastitis. This dendrogram was generated based on the presence/absence of virulence genes with the sum of branch length = 0.91629109. The tree is drawn to scale, with branch lengths in the same units as those of the evolutionary distances used to infer the phylogenetic tree. (**a-e**) refer to different virulence gene clusters. Blue boxes indicate the presence and yellow boxes the absence of the corresponding virulence genes, and the number on the right refer to the virulence profile patterns, whereas the number under the box refer to the corresponding number of positive isolates in each virulence gene. (a-q), refers to the virulence genes in order: *hla, hlb, hlc, hld, clfA, clfB, fnbA, fnbB, icaA, icaD, tsst, sea, seb, sec, see, seg, sei*

Table 3 Distribution of virulence gene clusters and Hla peptide sequence types in *Staphylococcus aureus* from 103 cases of clinical mastitis

Province	Herd	Virulence cluster					Hla peptide type									
		A	B	C	D	E	I	II	III	IV	V	VI	VII	VIII	IX	X
Beijing	a	36	2	–	3	–	35	–	3	–	–	–	–	1	1	1
	b	4	–	–	–	1	3	–	–	2	–	–	–	–	–	–
	c	1	1	–	–	–	2	–	–	–	–	–	–	–	–	–
Ningxia	d	–	–	–	5	–	5	–	–	–	–	–	–	–	–	–
	e	–	–	–	4	–	4	–	–	–	–	–	–	–	–	–
	f	–	–	–	3	–	3	–	–	–	–	–	–	–	–	–
	g	–	–	–	3	–	3	–	–	–	–	–	–	–	–	–
	h	–	–	–	1	–	1	–	–	–	–	–	–	–	–	–
Heilongjiang	i	3	–	4	4	–	7	–	–	–	–	1	–	–	–	–
Hebei	j	1	1	1	3	–	4	–	–	–	–	–	–	–	–	–
	k	–	–	4	–	–	2	–	–	–	–	–	–	–	–	–
	l	1	–	–	–	–	1	–	–	–	–	–	–	–	–	–
Inner Mongolia	m	–	–	–	–	3	–	2	–	–	–	–	1	–	–	–
	n	–	–	1	1	–	2	–	–	–	–	–	–	–	–	–
Liaoning	o	1	–	–	1	–	2	–	–	–	–	–	–	–	–	–
	p	1	–	–	1	–	1	–	–	–	–	–	–	–	–	–
Guangdong	q	–	–	–	–	3	1	2	–	–	–	–	–	–	–	–
Shandong	r	1	1	1	–	–	1	–	–	–	–	–	–	–	–	–
Henan	s	2	–	–	–	–	–	–	–	–	2	–	–	–	–	–

- No isolates

genotypes were identified based on nucleotide sequence analysis and 10 peptide sequence types (I to X) among 93 isolates with the *hla* gene (Tables 4 and 5). Amongst the 14 *hla* genotypes, Genotype 1 contained 65 (70%) isolates (Table 4).

Hla peptide type I, composed of *hla* genotypes 1, 2, 4, 6 and 11, was present in 18 herds, peptide sequence type II was in 2 herds, whereas others were identified in only 1 herd with 1 or 2 isolates, indicating that Hla peptide were conserved among herds (Table 3).

Three results were obtained from the prediction of serine and threonine phosphorylation sites among the 92 complete peptide sequences (Fig. 2). Figure 2a presents the prediction results of peptide sequence type I, II, V, VII and IX, which were same as the reference strain. Conversely, there were variations at position 300 in Fig. 2b (results of peptide sequence types III, IV and VIII) and position 100 in Fig. 2c (result of peptide sequence type VI) when comparing with that of the reference strain. Type A was the most dominant in the 93 isolates ($n = 86$, 93%), indicating that the Hla peptide sequence was conserved to an extent (Table 5)

Molecular typing

The analysis of 103 *S. aureus* isolates by *spa* typing revealed 24 *spa* types, of which 19 were known types (t189, t127, t2699, t359, t237, t4682, t521, t730, t224, t6297, t2756, t131, t1234, t267, t034, t529, t518 and t528), 3 others were reported for the first time (t16314, t16315, and t17095), and 2 were unassigned types with repeats r07r23r12r21r17r34r34r33r34r13 (UK-1) and r07r16r34r33r13r26 (UK-2) (Table 6).

In addition, 7 MLST types were obtained, which clustered into 7 clonal complexes. Of them, ST97, composed of 82 isolates, was detected in 12 herds from 7 provinces and shared by 15 *spa* types, whereas other MLST types were present in isolates from only 1 or 2 provinces (Table 6). In addition, there was great diversity among isolates within or between herds. Nine of the 19 herds contained > 1 *spa* type (Table 6).

Phylogenetic tree of *hla* gene

According to nucleotide diversity, the 93 *hla* sequences branched into 3 distinct major clusters (Fig. 3a). Furthermore, the corresponding ST types were also grouped into various clusters: ST97 and ST1 were in Cluster A, ST118 was in Cluster B, whereas ST 50, ST705 and ST479 were grouped into Cluster C (Fig. 3a). The position of STs in the tree constructed by the concatenated sequences of the 7 housekeeping genes used in MLST was almost the same as that of *hla* tree, with only ST705 as an exception (Fig. 3b).

Table 4 Nucleotide mutations and corresponding amino acid substitutions of *Staphylococcus aureus* from cases of clinical mastitis

Geno type	No.	Nucleotide mutation position/corresponding amino acid substitution[a]																			
		−42	−22	−6 &-5	47	144	214	237	255	262	399	438	453	498	499	519	606	686	765	797	824	833
		C	G	GG	G	C	G	C	G	T	C	G	T	C	T	T	T	C	T	A	C	T
1	65	–[b]	A	AA	–	–	–	–	–	–	–	–	–	–	–	–	–	–	–	–	–	–
			S[b]	G(−2)N																		
2	5	–	A	AA	–	–	–	–	–	C	T	C	G	–	–	–	C	–	C	–	–	–
			S	G(−2)N						S	S	S	S				S		S			
3	4	T	A	AA	–	–	–	–	–	–	T	C	G	–	–	–	C	–	C	–	–	–
		S	S	G(− 2)N							S	S	S				S		S			
4	4	–	A	AA	–	–	–	–	–	–	–	–	–	T	–	–	–	–	–	–	–	–
			S	G(−2)N										S								
5	3	–	A	AA	–	–	–	–	–	–	–	–	–	–	–	–	–	–	–	–	–	A
			S	G(−2)N																		S278Y
6	2	–	A	AA	–	–	–	–	A	–	–	–	–	–	–	–	–	–	–	–	–	–
			S	G(−2)N					S													
7	2	–	A	AA	–	–	–	–	–	–	–	–	–	–	–	–	–	–	–	–	–	T
			S	G(−2)N																		S278F
8	2	–	A	AA	–	T	–	–	–	–	–	–	–	–	–	–	C	–	C	C	T	–
			S	G(−2)N		S											S		S	S	T275I	
9	1	–	A	AA	–	–	A	–	A	–	–	–	–	–	–	–	–	–	–	–	–	–
			S	G(−2)N			Q72S		S													
10	1	–	A	AA	T	–	–	–	–	–	T	C	G	–	–	–	C	–	C	–	–	–
			S	G(−2)N	S16I						S	S	S				S		S			
11	1	–	A	AA	–	–	–	A	–	–	–	–	–	–	–	–	–	–	–	–	–	–
			S	G(−2)N				S														
12	1	–	A	AA	–	–	–	–	–	–	–	–	–	–	–	–	–	G	–	–	–	A
			S	G(−2)N														A229G				S278Y
13	1	–	A	AA	–	–	–	–	–	–	–	–	–	–	–	A	–	–	–	–	–	–
			S	G(−2)N												N173 K						
14	1	–	A	AA	–	–	–	–	–	–	–	–	–	–	D[b]	–	–	–	–	–	–	–
			S	G(−2)N											W167G[c]							

[a]Nucleotide/peptide positions were designated relative to the first nucleotide/amino acid of the mature -hemolysin (*S. aureus* WOOD46)
[b]*S* synonymous mutation, *D* deletion mutation, – = no mutation;
[c]The deletion at nucleotide position 499 of Genotype 14 resulted in peptide termination at residue position 169

Relationships among virulence gene profiles, *hla* genotypes and clonal typing

Isolates in *hla* type 1/peptide I were present in 5 virulence gene clusters in various proportions, revealing great diversity of virulence genes, whereas isolates in other *hla* genotypes and peptide types demonstrated simplex virulence gene profile (Table 5). Nevertheless, there was no association between *hla* gene genotypes and virulence gene profiles ($P = 0.12$), and no association between Hla peptide types and virulence gene profiles ($P = 0.80$).

Isolates belonging to the same ST may comprise same virulence gene profile. Isolates from ST705 were grouped into Cluster E, whereas ST50 isolates were included in Cluster D. With the exception ST97 and ST1, in which isolates were sprinkled in more than 3 clusters (Table 7). Hence, there was a correlation between virulence gene profiles and molecular clones ($P < 0.01$).

Each Hla peptide sequence type was only present in 1 ST type, except for peptide I, which had isolates in ST97, ST705, ST50, and ST1 (Table 7). Similarly, isolates belonging to the same ST harbored same peptide type, except for ST97, in which isolates were clustered into 7 peptide sequence types (I, V, VI, VII, VIII, IX and X) (Table 5). Therefore, Hla peptide types and ST types were correlated ($P < 0.01$).

Table 5 Association between *hla* peptide types and virulence gene profiles of 93 *Staphylococcus aureus* isolated from clinical mastitis

Prediction of phosphorylation sites (n)	Peptide type	*hla*	Virulence gene profile cluster				
			A	B	C	D	E
A (85)	I (77)	1	37	3	6	18	1
		2	0	0	0	5	0
		4	3	0	0	1	0
		6	0	0	1	0	1
		11	1	0	0	0	0
	II (4)	3	4	0	0	0	0
	V (2)	8	2	0	0	0	0
	VII (1)	10	0	0	0	0	1
	IX (1)	13	1	0	0	0	0
B (6)	III (3)	5	2	0	0	1	0
	IV (2)	7	2	0	0	0	0
	VIII (1)	12	1	0	0	0	0
C (1)	VI (1)	9	1	0	0	0	0
	X (1)	14	1	0	0	0	0

Discussion

It is important to monitor antimicrobial resistance in veterinary medicine. As a frequent and major contagious pathogen in bovine mastitis, *S. aureus* readily becomes resistant to antimicrobials and causes persistent noncurable intramammary infection. Recent investigations on antimicrobial resistance of *S. aureus* are available [30–33]. However, lacking of a common clinical breakpoint for antibiotics which are frequently used to treat mastitis make it difficult to comparing with other data. Overall, the percentage of antimicrobial resistant *S. aureus* in this study is much higher (76.7% vs 25%) in resistant to penicillin according to the work of de Jong et al. [31].

In the present study, the 17 virulence genes were distributed with varying frequencies among *S. aureus* isolates. Consistent with previous research, none of the 103 isolates contained the *pvl* gene [34, 35], whereas adhesin genes (*clfA*, *clfB*, *fnbA* and *fnbB*) were the most prevalent. In contrast, Gogoi-Tiwari et al. (2015) reported that *fnbB* was only present in 1.3% of *S. aureus* isolates, which was much lower than in our study (85%) [36]. Thompson et al. (2014) reported a lower occurrence of

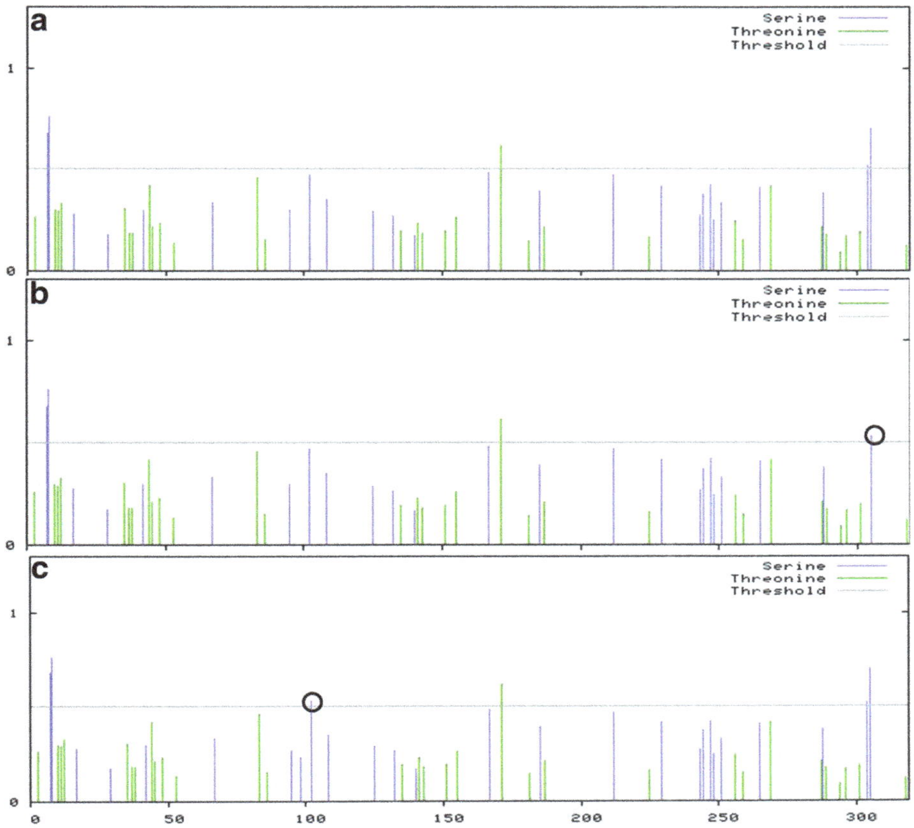

Fig. 2 Phosphorylation sites prediction of Hla peptide types with non-synonymous substitutions. The score for each serine or threonine residue is plotted against the sequence position of that residue. When the score is > 0.5, the residue is a predicted phosphorylation site. Variations from the reference sequence are indicated by black circles. **a**) Phosphorylation sites prediction of reference strain WOOD46 and Hla peptide I, II, V, VII, IX; **b**) Phosphorylation sites prediction of Hla peptide type III, IV and VIII; **c**) Phosphorylation sites prediction of Hla peptide type VI and X

Table 6 Distribution of *spa* typing and MLST types of 103 *Staphylococcus aureus* isolated from clinical mastitis in China

Clonal complex (CC)	MLST type	Spa type	[a]BJ			NX					HJ	HB			IM		LN		GD	SD	HN
			a	b	c	d	e	f	g	h	i	j	k	l	m	n	o	p	q	r	s
CC1 (90)	ST188	t189	0	0	0	0	0	0	0	0	0	0	0	0	0	0	0	0	0	0	2
	ST1	t127	0	0	0	0	0	0	0	0	0	0	0	0	0	0	0	0	0	2	0
		t2699	0	0	0	0	0	0	0	0	0	0	0	0	0	0	0	1	0	0	0
		t17095	0	0	0	0	0	0	0	0	0	0	0	0	0	0	1	0	0	0	0
		UK02	0	0	0	0	0	0	0	0	0	0	0	1	0	0	1	0	0	0	0
	ST97	t359	25	1	1	0	0	0	0	0	0	0	0	0	0	0	0	0	0	0	0
		t4570	12	0	0	0	0	0	0	0	0	0	0	0	0	0	0	0	0	0	0
		t237	0	0	0	0	0	0	0	0	6	0	0	0	0	0	0	0	0	0	0
		t4682	0	1	0	0	0	0	0	0	2	0	0	0	0	0	0	0	0	0	0
		t521	0	0	0	0	4	0	0	0	1	0	0	0	0	0	0	0	0	0	0
		t730	0	0	0	0	0	0	0	0	1	3	4	0	0	1	0	0	0	1	0
		t16314	0	2	0	0	0	0	0	0	0	0	0	0	0	0	0	0	0	0	0
		t16315	3	1	0	0	0	0	0	0	0	0	0	0	0	0	0	0	0	0	0
		t224	0	0	0	5	0	0	0	0	0	0	0	0	0	0	0	0	0	0	0
		t6297	0	0	0	0	0	0	3	0	0	0	0	0	0	0	0	0	0	0	0
		t2756	0	0	0	0	0	0	0	1	0	0	0	0	0	0	0	0	0	0	0
		t131	1	0	0	0	0	0	0	0	0	0	0	0	0	0	0	0	0	0	0
		t1234	0	0	1	0	0	0	0	0	0	0	0	0	0	0	0	0	0	0	0
		t267	0	0	0	0	0	0	0	0	1	0	0	0	0	0	0	0	0	0	0
		UK01	0	0	0	0	0	0	0	0	0	1	0	0	0	0	0	0	0	0	0
CC7(1)	ST398	T034	0	0	0	0	0	0	0	0	0	0	0	0	0	0	1	0	0	0	0
CC12(5)	ST705	t529	0	0	0	0	0	0	0	0	0	0	0	0	2	0	0	0	3	0	0
CC22(6)	ST50	t518	0	0	0	0	0	3	0	0	0	2	0	0	0	1	0	0	0	0	0
CC30(1)	ST479	t528	0	0	0	0	0	0	0	0	0	0	0	0	1	0	0	0	0	0	0

[a]*BJ* Beijing, *NX* Ningxia, *HJ* Heilongjiang, *HB* Hebei, *IM* Inner Mongolia, *GD* Guangdong, *SD* Shandong, *HN* Henan, *LN* Liaoning

sec gene in MSSA than the current study (14 vs 21%, respectively) [37]. In the present study, 30% clinical isolates of *S. aureus* contained the *tsst* gene, whereas in another study [35], none of 47 *S. aureus* mastitis isolates were positive for this gene. In agreement with a previous study, none of the isolates harbored the *sea* gene; this was the gene most frequently encountered from food poisoning in humans and subclinical mastitis cases in cattle [6, 38]. Li et al. (2017) reported that no enterotoxin gene was present in ST97, ST188 or ST398 isolates, which was different from the current study, where some ST97 isolates had *seb*, *sec* and *see* genes [38]. Overall, virulence gene patterns of *S. aureus* isolates had variable distributions among herds from different regions.

There were many reports regarding contribution of α-hemolysin to the pathogenesis of *S. aureus* infection, including cell signaling pathways that govern cell proliferation, cytokine secretion, inflammatory responses and cell-cell interactions [39–42]. Although polymorphisms in the *hla* promoter region have been described [43], the range of genetic diversity and evolution of this toxin was only assessed in human [43–45], with no report of a large representative collection of *S. aureus* from dairy cows. Among the 22 single nucleotide mutations, 14 (64%) mutations were the same as those isolates from humans [13], Among the 22 single nucleotide mutations, 14 (64%) were the same as reported earlier from human isolates, indicating that transmission of *S. aureus* might occur between cows and humans, which would be of great relevance to public health security. The high degree of *hla* gene diversity was in accordance with other reports [17, 23]. However, with the analysis of Hla peptide sequences in this study, we predicted that most (n = 86) isolates carried the same phosphorylation site as in our reference strain; therefore, we inferred that Hla peptide sequences were conserved. Although influence of the different phosphorylation sites was uncertain with regards to their influence on the 3-dimensional structure stability of the protein [23], Burnside et al. (2015) reported that a serine/threonine kinase and phosphatase regulated expression of hemolysin in *S. aureus* [46]. Therefore, the exact influence of disparate phosphorylation sites here

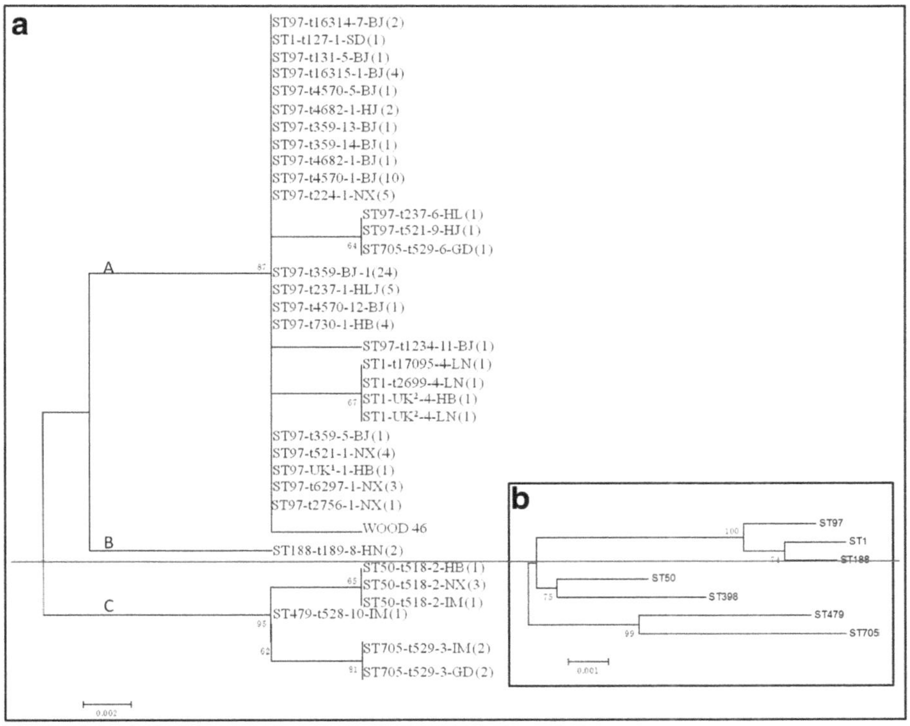

Fig. 3 Phylogenetic trees of *hla* gene (**a**) and concatenated sequences of MLST alleles (**b**) in *Staphylococcus aureus* isolates. The percentage of the trees in which the associated *hla* sequence clustered together is shown next to the branches. The tree is drawn to scale, with branch lengths measured in number of substitutions per site. Evolutionary analyses were conducted in MEGA6. Note: BJ = Beijing; NX = Ningxia; SD = Shandong; HB = Hebei; LN = Liaoning; HN = Henan; GD = Guangdong; IM = Inner Mongolia; HJ = Heilongjiang. The number after regions refers to the corresponding *hla* type

remains to be studied. Sharma-Kuink et al. (2015) co-related peptide polymorphism to random mutations in nature and selective pressure from the immune system, due to generation of antibodies that bind to alpha-toxins [17]. In this study, the correlation between *hla* gene genotype/ peptides types and geography partly supported the above conclusion. In addition, variations in peptide sequences may influence Hla functionality and may change antigenic epitopes and potentially cause vaccine failure, as reported [15, 16].

Analysis of *hla*-based phylogenetic tree revealed 3 clusters with distinct nucleotide diversity and the ST types of isolates in Cluster A were ST97 and ST1, Cluster B were ST118 and Cluster C were ST 50, ST705 and ST479. Therefore, we inferred that the *hla* gene in *S. aureus* is evolving at varying rates in various genetic backgrounds. This was very similar to a previous study [23]. Interestingly, the tree based on MLST sequences was almost as same as the *hla* tree, revealing that the *hla* gene evolved with MLST background.

Table 7 Association between virulence gene clusters and Hla peptide types, and MLST types and *spa* types

MLST type	*Spa* type	Virulence gene cluster					Hla peptide sequence type									
		A	B	C	D	E	I	II	III	IV	V	VI	VII	VIII	IX	X
ST97	t359, t237, t4682, t521, t730, t16314, t16315, t224, t6297, t2756, t131, t1234, t267, UK-1	45	5	11	20	1	66	0	0	0	1	3	2	1	1	1
ST705	t529	0	0	0	0	5	1	4	0	0	0	0	0	0	0	0
ST50	t518	0	0	0	6	0	5	0	0	0	0	0	0	0	0	0
ST1	t127, t2699, t17095, UK-2	4	0	1	1	0	5	0	0	0	0	0	0	0	0	0
ST479	t528	0	0	0	0	1	0	0	0	[illegible]	0	0	0	0	0	0
ST188	t189	2	0	0	0	0	0	0	2	0	0	0	0	0	0	0
ST398	t034	0	0	0	1	0	0	0	0	0	0	0	0	0	0	0

Based on analysis of clonal diversity, the 103 *S. aureus* isolates had 24 *spa* types and 7 MLST types, with t359, t730 and ST97 present in most isolates, consistent with previously reports in which ST97 was also the dominant ST type in *S. aureus* from bovine mastitis from China [38, 47]. Conversely, ST239 was reported to be the dominant ST type among 608 hospital-acquired *S. aureus* isolates recovered from human respiratory specimens, sterile body fluids, *S. aureus* bacteremia and non-*S. aureus* bacteremia patients in China [47, 48]. Importantly, 5 new *spa* types (t16314 from Beijing, t16315 from Beijing, t17095 from Liaoning, UK-1 from Hebei and UK-2 from Liaoning and Hebei) were reported for the first time in this study, indicating evolutionary occurrence of unique clones in the region. Most herds harbored at least 3 *spa* types, indicating diversity of the clonal background. When comparing *spa*/ ST types with distribution of isolates, there was a correlation, despite the presence of disparate molecular types.

Notably, there was no correlation between *hla* gene/ peptide types and virulence gene clusters. Both virulence gene profile and *hla* gene/peptide types were associated with the molecular clone background, consistent with previous studies in which there was a strong correlation between *hla* gene/ peptide types and clonal background of isolates from human [13]. In addition, there were also differences in virulence genes of various molecular types of strains [38]. Therefore, clone background should be taken into consideration when using Hla as a candidate for vaccines.

The distribution on peptide types, virulence gene profile and molecular clone according to geographical location was not determined, due to the large variation in numbers of *S. aureus* isolates in herds and provinces. However, based on the difference of virulence cluster and *spa* types among herds, we inferred that geography might be an important factor when developing effective treatment strategies for bovine mastitis.

Conclusions

Multi-resistant *S. aureus* occurred in bovine mastitis with diverse resistance patterns. A great diversity of virulence gene patterns and *spa* typing was determined; *hla* gene evolved with MLST types; ST97 was the dominant types in *S. aureus* from bovine mastitis in China and virulence gene patterns were correlated with MLST types. All of these finding will be useful for future studies on anti-virulence therapies, immunogenicity and vaccine development. In addition, the similarity in diversity of *hla* gene from both humans and bovines make great significance in public health security.

Additional files

Additional file 1: Figure S1. Original picture of PCR result-1: *hla*; 2: *hlb*; 3: *hlc*; 4: *icaD*; 5: *sec*; 6: *sei*; 7: *seg*; 8: *icaA*; 9: *tsst*; 10: *coa*; 11: *nuc*; 12: *clfA*; 13: *clfB*; 14: *fnbA*; 15: *fnbB*.

Additional file 2: Figure S2. Original picture of PCR result of *hld* gene.

Additional file 3: Figure S3. Original picture of PCR result of *seb* gene.

Additional file 4: Figure S4. Original picture of PCR result of *see* gene.

Abbreviations

AMP: Ampicillin; AMX/CA: augmentin; CIP: Ciprofloxacin; CL: Clindamicin; *clfA*: clumping factors A; *clfB*: clumping factors B; CRO: Ceftriaxone; CTX: Cefotaxime; E: Erythromycin; *fnbA*: fibronectin binding proteins A; *fnbB*: fibronectin binding proteins B; GM: Gentamicin; Hla: Alpha-hemolysin; *hla*: α- hemolysin; *hlb*: β-hemolysin; *hlc*: γ-hemolysin; *hld*: δ-hemolysin; *icaA*: intracellular adhesion A; *icaD*: intracellular adhesion D; MICs: Minimum inhibitory concentrations; MLST: Multilocus sequence type; OX: Oxacillin; P: penicillin; PCR: Polymerase chain reaction; *S. aureus*: *Staphylococcus aureus*; *sea*: *Staphylococcus aureus* enterotoxin a; *sec*: *Staphylococcus aureus* enterotoxin c; *see*: *Staphylococcus aureus* enterotoxin e; *seg*: *Staphylococcus aureus* enterotoxin g; *sei*: *Staphylococcus aureus* enterotoxin i; *spa*: staphylococcal protein A; STs: MLST types; TE: tetracycline; *tsst*: toxic shock syndrome toxin

Acknowledgments

The authors thank all the milking technicians, farm veterinarians and the commercial farms supporting the samples collection.

Funding

This research was financially supported by the National Natural Science Foundation of China (No. 31772813, 31572587 and No. 31550110200) and the National Key R&D Project (No. 2016YFD0501203), which beared the expenses, and High-end Foreign Experts Recruitment Program (No. GDT20171100013), with which we got the English native speakers revise the manuscript.

Authors' contributions

BH conceived and designed the experiment. LZ performed the research and wrote the manuscript, GL and YD collected the *S. aureus* isolates from milk samples, JG assisted in the result analysis. HWB, TA, SN and JPK revised the manuscript. All authors read and approved the final manuscript.

Ethics approval and consent to participate

The current work was carried out according to the ethical guide lines of China Agricultural University (CAU), Beijing. Prior to the initiation of this study, proper approval was obtained from the ethics committee of College of Veterinary Medicine, China Agricultural University, Beijing. Furthermore, sampling was performed in accordance to the standard protocols of National Mastitis Council (NMC). There are no vulnerable populations involved, and no endangered species was used in the experiments. Farm managers provided verbal consent to collect the milk samples.

Consent for publication

Not applicable.

Competing interests

The authors declare that they have no competing interests

Author details
[1]College of Veterinary Medicine, China Agricultural University, Yuan Ming Yuan West Road No. 2, Haidian District, Beijing 100193, People's Republic of China. [2]Department of Production Animal Health, Faculty of Veterinary Medicine, University of Calgary, Calgary, AB T2N 4N1, Canada.

References

1. Barkema HW, Schukken YH, Zadoks RN. Invited review: the role of cow, pathogen, and treatment regimen in the therapeutic success of bovine *Staphylococcus aureus* mastitis. J Dairy Sci. 2006;89:1877–95.
2. Schukken YH, Günther J, Fitzpatrick J, Fontaine MC, Goetze L, Holst O, Leigh J, Petzl W, Schuberth HJ, Sipka A, Smith DGE, Quesnell R, Watts J, Yancey R, Zerbe H, Gurjar A, Zadoks RN, Seyfert HM. Host-response patterns of intramammary infections in dairy cows. Vet Immun Immunopathol. 2011; 144:270–89.
3. Gao J, Barkema HW, Zhang L, Liu G, Deng Z, Cai L, Shan R, Zhang S, Zou J, Kastelic JP, Han B. Incidence of clinical mastitis and distribution of pathogens on large Chinese dairy farms. J Dairy Sci. 2017;100:4797–806.
4. Kong C, Neoh HM, Nathan S. Targeting *Staphylococcus aureus* toxins: a potential form of anti-virulence therapy. Toxins. 2016;8:72.
5. Allen RC, Popat R, Diggle SP, Brown SP. Targeting virulence: can we make evolution-proof drugs? Nat Rev Microbiol. 2014;12:300–8.
6. Yang FL, Li XS, Liang XW, Zhang XF, Qin GS, Yang BZ. Detection of virulence-associated genes in *Staphylococcus aureus* isolated from bovine clinical mastitis milk samples in Guangxi. Trop Anim Health Prod. 2012;44: 1821–6.
7. Mitra SD, Velu D, Bhuvana M, Krithiga N, Banerjee A, Shome R, Rahman H, Ghosh SK, Shome BR. *Staphylococcus aureus* spa type t267, clonal ancestor of bovine subclinical mastitis in India. J Appl Microbiol. 2013;114:1604–15.
8. Martins KB, Faccioli-Martins PY, Riboli DF, Pereira VC, Fernandes S, Oliveira AA, Dantas A, Zafalon LF, da Cunha Mde L. Clonal profile, virulence and resistance of *Staphylococcus aureus* isolated from sheep milk. Braz J Microbiol. 2015;46:535–43.
9. Roetzer A, Haller G, Beyerly J, Geier CB, Wolf HM, Gruener CS, Model N, Eibl MM. Genotypic and phenotypic analysis of clinical isolates of *Staphylococcus aureus* revealed production patterns and hemolytic potentials unlinked to gene profiles and source. BMC Microbiol. 2016;16:13.
10. Wang D, Zhang L, Zhou X, He Y, Yong C, Shen M, Szenci O, Han B. Antimicrobial susceptibility, virulence genes, and randomly amplified polymorphic DNA analysis of *Staphylococcus aureus* recovered from bovine mastitis in Ningxia, China. J Dairy Sci. 2016;99:9560–9.
11. Menzies BE, Kernodle DS. Site-directed mutagenesis of the alpha-toxin gene of *Staphylococcus aureus*: role of histidines in toxin activity in vitro and in a murine model. Infect Immun. 1994;62:1843–7.
12. McGavin MJ, Arsic B, Nickerson NN. Evolutionary blueprint for host- and niche-adaptation in *Staphylococcus aureus* clonal complex CC30. Front Cell Infect Microbiol. 2012;2:48.
13. Xiao M, Zhao R, Zhang Q, Fan X, O'Sullivan MV, Li DF. Genotypic diversity of *Staphylococcus aureus*α-hemolysin gene (*hla*) and its association with clonal background: implications for vaccine development. PLoS One. 2016;11: e0149112.
14. Adhikari RP, Thompson CD, Aman MJ, Lee JC. Protective efficacy of a novel alpha hemolysin subunit vaccine (AT62) against *Staphylococcus aureus* skin and soft tissue infections. Vaccine. 2016;34:6402–7.
15. Mocca CP, Brady RA, Burns DL. Role of antibodies in protection elicited by active vaccination with genetically inactivated alpha hemolysin in a mouse model of *Staphylococcus aureus* skin and soft tissue infections. Clin Vaccine Immunol. 2014;21:622–7.
16. Oscherwitz J, Cease KB. Identification and validation of a linear protective neutralizing epitope in the β-pore domain of alpha toxin. PLoS One. 2015; 10:e0116882.
17. Sharma-Kuinkel BK, Wu Y, Tabor DE, Mok H, Sellman BR, Jenkins A, Yu L, Jafri HS, Rude TH, Ruffin F, Schell WA, Park LP, Yan Q, Thaden JT, Messina JA, Fowler VG Jr, Esser MT. Characterization of alpha-toxin hla gene variants, alpha-toxin expression levels, and levels of antibody to alpha-toxin in hemodialysis and postsurgical patients with Staphylococcus Aureus bacteremia. J Clin Microbiol. 2015;53:227–36.
18. Tabor DE, Yu L, Mok H, Tkaczyk C, Sellman BR, Wu Y, Oganesyan V, Slidel T, Jafri H, McCarthy M, Bradford P, Esser MT. *Staphylococcus aureus* Alpha-toxin is conserved among diverse hospital respiratory isolates collected from a global surveillance study and is neutralized by monoclonal antibody MEDI4893. Antimicrob Agents Chemother. 2016;60:5312–21.
19. Clinical and Laboratory Standards Institute. Performance standards for antimicrobial disk and dilution susceptibility tests for bacteria isolated from animals. Approved standard-fourth edition. 2013; CLSI document VET01-A4, Wayne, PA.
20. Lin Y, Barker E, Kislow J, Kaldhone P, Stemper ME, Pantrangi M, Moore FM, Hall M, Fritsche TR, Novicki T, Foley SL, Shukla SK. Evidence of multiple virulence subtypes in nosocomial and community-associated MRSA genotypes in companion animals from the upper midwestern and northeastern United States. Clin Med Res. 2011;9:7–16.
21. Kot B, Szweda P, Frankowska-Maciejewska A, Piechota M, Wolska K. Virulence gene profiles in *Staphylococcus aureus* isolated from cows with subclinical mastitis in eastern Poland. J Dairy Res. 2016;83:228–35.
22. Tamura K, Stecher G, Peterson D, Filipski A, Kumar S. MEGA6: molecular evolutionary genetics analysis version 6.0. Mol Biol Evol. 2013;30:2725–9.
23. Tavares A, Nielsen JB, Boye K, Rohde S, Paulo AC, Westh H, Schonning K, de Lencastre H, Miragaia M. Insights into alpha-hemolysin (Hla) evolution and expression among *Staphylococcus aureus* clones with hospital and community origin. PLoS One. 2014;(7):e98634.
24. Li YL, Han GM, He SE, Zhang ZJA. New strategy for construction of phylogenetic tree based on DNA molecular marker data. China J Bioinformatics. 2007;4:168–70.
25. Gray GS, Kehoe M. Primary sequence of the alpha-toxin gene from *Staphylococcus aureus* wood 46. Infect Immun. 1984;46:615–8.
26. Koziel J, Chmiest D, Bryzek D, Kmiecik K, Mizgalska D, Maciag-Gudowska A, Shaw LN, Potempa J. The Janus face of alpha-toxin: a potent mediator of cytoprotection in staphylococci-infected macrophages. J. Innate Immunity. 2015;7:187–98.
27. Rauch S, Gough P, Kim HK, Schneewind O, Missiakas D. Vaccine protection of leukopenic mice against *Staphylococcus aureus* bloodstream infection. Infect Immun. 2014;82:4889–98.
28. Miller ML, Soufi B, Jers C, Blom N, Macek B, Mijakovic I. NetPhosBac – a predictor for Ser/Thr phosphorylation sites in bacterial proteins. Proteomics. 2009;9:116–25.
29. Jamrozy DM, Fielder MD, Butaye P, Coldham NG. Comparative genotypic and phenotypic characterisation of methicillin-resistant *Staphylococcus aureus* ST398 isolated from animals and humans. PLoS One. 2012;7:e40458.
30. Abdi RD, Gillespie BE, Vaughn J, Merrill C, Headrick SI, Ensermu DB, D'Souza DH, Agga GE, Almeida RA, Oliver SP, Kerro Dego O. Antimicrobial resistance of *Staphylococcus aureus* isolates from dairy cows and genetic diversity of resistant isolates. Foodborne Pathog Dis. 2018; https://doi.org/10.1089/fpd.2017.2362.
31. de Jong A, Garch FE, Simjee S, Moyaert H, Rose M, Youala M, Siegwart E, VetPath Study Group. Monitoring of antimicrobial susceptibility of udder pathogens recovered from cases of clinical mastitis in dairy cows across Europe: VetPath results. Vet Microbiol. 2018;213:73–81.
32. Kulangara V, Nair N, Sivasailam A, Sasidharan S, Kollannur JD, Syam R. Genotypic and phenotypic β-lactam resistance and presence of PVL gene in staphylococci fromdry bovine udder. PLoS One. 2017;12:e0187277.
33. Haubert L, Kroning IS, Iglesias MA, da Silva WP. First report of the Staphylococcus Aureus isolate from subclinical bovine mastitis in the south of Brazil harboring resistance gene dfrG and transposon family Tn916-1545. Microb Pathog. 2017;113:242–7.
34. Prashanth K, Rao KR, Reddy PV, Saranathan R, Makki AR. Genotypic characterization of *Staphylococcus aureus* obtained from humans and bovine mastitis samples in India. J Global Infect Dis. 2011;3:115–22.
35. Feltrin F, Alba P, Kraushaar B, Ianzano A, Argudín MA, Di Matteo P, Porrero MC, Aarestrup FM, Butaye P, Franco A, Battisti A. A livestock-associated, multidrug-resistant, methicillin-resistant *Staphylococcus aureus* clonal complex 97 lineage spreading in dairy cattle and pigs in Italy. Appl Environ Microbiol. 2016;82:816–21.
36. Gogoi-Tiwari J, Waryah CB, Eto KY, Tau M, Wells K, Costantino P, Tiwari HK, Isloor S, Hegde N, Mukkur T. Relative distribution of virulence-associated factors among Australian bovine *Staphylococcus aureus* isolates: potential relevance to development of an effective bovine mastitis vaccine. Virulence. 2015;6:419–23.
37. Thompson T, Brown PD. Comparison of antibiotic resistance, virulence gene profiles, and pathogenicity of methicillin-resistant and methicillin-

susceptible *Staphylococcus aureus* using a caenorhabditis elegans infection model. Pathog Glob Health. 2014;108:283–91.

38. Li T, Lu H, Wang X, Gao Q, Dai Y, Shang J, Li M. Molecular characteristics of *Staphylococcus aureus* causing bovine mastitis between 2014 and 2015. Front Cell Infect Microbiol. 2017;7:127.
39. Mairpady Shambat S, Haggar A, Vandenesch F, Lina G, van Wamel WJB, Arakere G, Svensson M, Norrby-Teglund A. Levels of alpha-toxin correlate with distinct phenotypic response profiles of blood mononuclear cells and with agr background of community-associated *Staphylococcus aureus* isolates. PLoS One. 2014;9:e106107.
40. Maurer K, Reyes-Robles T, Alonzo F 3rd, Durbin J, Torres VJ, Cadwell K. Autophagy mediates tolerance to *Staphylococcus aureus* Alpha-toxin. Cell Host Microbe. 2015;17:429–40.
41. Popov LM, Marceau CD, Starkl PM, Lumb JH, Shah J, Guerrera D, Cooper RL, Merakou C, Bouley DM, Meng W, Kiyonari H, Takeichi M, Galli SJ, Bagnoli F, Citi S, Carette JE, Amieva MR. The adherens junctions control susceptibility to *Staphylococcus aureus* Alpha-toxin. PNAS. 2015;112:14337–42.
42. Tkaczyk C, Kasturirangan S, Minola A, Jones-Nelson O, Gunter V, Shi YY, Rosenthal K, Aleti V, Semenova E, Warrener P, Tabor D, Stover CK, Corti D, Rainey G, Sellman BR. Multimechanistic monoclonal antibodies (MAbs) targeting *Staphylococcus aureus* Alpha-toxin and clumping factor a: activity and efficacy comparisons of a MAb combination and an engineered bispecific antibody approach. Antimicrob Agents Chemother. 2017;61: e00629-17.
43. Liang X, Hall JW, Yang J, Yan M, Doll K, Bey R, Ji Y. Identification of single nucleotide polymorphisms associated with hyperproduction of alpha-toxin in *Staphylococcus aureus*. PLoS One. 2011;6:e18428.
44. DeLeo FR, Kennedy AD, Chen L, Wardenburg JB, Kobayashi SD, Mathema B, Braughton KR, Whitney AR, Villaruz AE, Martens CA, Porcella SF, McGavin MJ, Otto M, Musser JM, Kreiswirth BN. Molecular differentiation of historic phage-type 80/81 and contemporary epidemic *Staphylococcus aureus*. PNAS. 2011;108:18091–6.
45. Burnside K, Lembo A. De los Reyes M, Iliuk a, BinhTran NT, Connelly JE. Regulation of hemolysin expression and virulence of *Staphylococcus aureus* by a serine/threonine kinase and phosphatase. PLoS One. 2015;5:e11071.
46. Wang D, Wang Z, Yan Z, Wu, J, Ali T, Li J, Han B. Bovine mastitis *Staphylococcus aureus*: antibiotic susceptibility profile, resistance genes and molecular typing of methicillin-resistant and methicillin-sensitive strains in China. Infect. Genet. Evol. 2015; 31: 9–16.
47. Li T, Song Y, Zhu Y, Du X, Li M. Current status of *Staphylococcus aureus* infection in a central teaching hospital in shanghai, China. BMC Micorob. 2013;13:153.
48. Jiang B, Yin S, You B, Huang G, Yang Z, Zhang Y, Chen Y, Chen J, Yuan Z, Rao X, Hu X, Gong Y, Peng Y. A 5-year survey reveals increased susceptibility to glycopeptides for methicillin-resistant *Staphylococcus aureus* isolates from *Staphylococcus aureus* bacteremia patients in a Chinese burn center. Front Microbiol. 2017;8:2531.

Genetic diversity assessment of Tunisian *Mycobacterium bovis* population isolated from cattle

Saif Eddine Djemal[1*], Mariam Siala[1,2], Salma Smaoui[3,4,5], Sana Kammoun[3,4,5], Chema Marouane[3,4,5], Javier Bezos[6,7], Feriele Messadi-Akrout[3,4,5], Beatriz Romero[7] and Radhouane Gdoura[1]

Abstract

Background: The genetic diversity of *M. bovis* in Tunisia is still underestimated despite the implementation of an eradication program. The lack of data about spatial distribution of the *M. bovis* population hinders the control of bovine tuberculosis (bTB) progress. This study represents the largest molecular analysis of *M. bovis* isolates in Tunisia. It is aimed to upgrade the understanding of bTB epidemiology and the geographical distribution of the infection. Tuberculosis research was performed in cattle ($n = 149$) with TB-compatible lesions collected over 5 months from a slaughterhouse located in Sfax, Tunisia.

Results: Ninety-four animals were found to be infected by *M. bovis* and two others by *M. caprae*. Spoligotyping revealed twenty-five patterns, SB0120, SB0134, and SB0121 being the most prevalent profiles (36.4%, 11.4%, and 7.2%, respectively). Three new spoligotypes were detected: SB2345, SB2344 and SB2343. MIRU-VNTR analysis classified the isolates in seventy-three profiles and showed a large genotypic variety observed within the main spoligotype which was split into several MIRU-VNTR types: 29 in SB0120 ($h = 0.983$), 10 in SB0134 ($h = 0.981$) and 7 in SB0121 ($h = 1$). Genotyping revealed a common pattern in different geographic regions. It also showed that Sfax, located in southern-Tunisia, represents a high-risk area with an elevated genetic diversity.

Conclusions: Spatial analysis may provide insights into disease transmission, which affects the effectiveness of eradication campaigns in cattle.

Keywords: *Mycobacterium Bovis*, Genetic diversity, Spoligotyping, MIRU-VNTR typing

Background

Bovine tuberculosis (bTB) is one of the seven endemic zoonoses neglected worldwide, especially in developing countries [1]. It is mainly caused by *M. bovis*, a member of the *Mycobacterium tuberculosis* complex (MTBC). *M. bovis* has a wide host range and can affect various target species, including domesticanimals, mainly cattle. *M. bovis* can be transmitted from animals to humans in close contact including aerosols, consuming unpasteurized milk or dairy products and less often by skin contact.

* Correspondence: saifjemal@hotmail.fr
[1]Department of Life Sciences, Research Laboratory of Environmental Toxicology-Microbiology and Health (LR17ES06), Faculty of Sciences, University of Sfax-Tunisia, Sfax, Tunisia
Full list of author information is available at the end of the article

A national bTB control program has been implemented in Tunisia since 1984 based essentially on the intra-dermal tuberculin skin testing and routine slaughterhouse meat inspections of dairy cattle [2].

In fact, there are two livestock sectors characterized as follows:

- The organized intensive livestock belonging to the state and subjected to the bTB eradication program.
- The private sector is the so-called unorganized Tunisian livestock, which consists of 60 to 70% of the whole bovine livestock and extensive or semi-extensive cattle herds belonging to private owners [3]. Nevertheless, the bTB is still prevalent mainly in the private sector where disease control is based on a scarce veterinary activity limited to visual

inspection of carcasses in slaughterhouses without routine intra-dermal tuberculin skin testing. From January to August 2013, 499 cows showed TB-compatible lesions during the meat inspection among 37,060 slaughtered animals [4]. Moreover, the majority of Tunisian cattle are not registered and cattle movement control schemes are unknown. Most of the bTB cases in Tunisia are discovered during meat inspection of cattle slaughtered at regular slaughterhouses when gross visible lesions typical of the disease are detected. However, in two recent Tunisian studies, *M. bovis* was isolated from milk and in 35% of the cattle exhibiting lesions [3, 5]. This suggests that bTB caused by *M. bovis* still persists in animals and thus could affect ecosystems and cause human extra-pulmonary tuberculosis (EPTB). In fact, in Tunisia, the prevalence of *M. bovis* as a causative agent of EPTB is high and divergent from studies in African countries [6]. Recently, Ghariani et al. and Siala et al. have shown that *M. bovis*, the agent of bovine TB, is a major cause of lymphadenitis TB with a frequency of 57% in north and 76% in south Tunisia, respectively [7, 8]. Consumption of not well-cooked meat and drinking raw milk from infected animals are common practices and could be the main causes of human EPTB [7, 8].

Spacer oligonucleotide typing (spoligotyping) and Variable Number of Tandem Repeat (VNTR) typing have been shown to be efficient tools to discriminate between *M. bovis* isolates [9, 10].

The ability to compare *M. bovis* isolates in the same country and among countries could help understand the distribution of *M. bovis* strains. In Tunisia, a large-scale study has not yet been possible since the two existing studies have analysed a low size of samples. In addition, based on the strong historical commercial links between Tunisia and France (the main cattle supplier of Tunisia), a thorough description of the genetic discrimination power of VNTR on French strains of the same spoligotyping group previously published by Hauer et al. [11] could clarify whether the French input to the Tunisian *M. bovis* population could exist?

Therefore, the main goal of the present work was to study the genetic diversity of a large *M. bovis* population using spoligotyping and VNTR typing and to identify a potential exchange of strains between Tunisia and France.

Methods

Samples

Lung, liver, and lymph nodes (retropharyngeal/mandibular, mediastinal/bronchial, portal and mesenteric) were collected from 149 dairy cattle (Frisonne-Holstein breed) with TB-compatible lesions during the veterinary inspection of carcasses. The samples were only taken from the private unorganized livestock sector slaughtered in the largest slaughterhouse in the south of Tunisia from November 2014 to April 2015. Animals belonged to ten geographic regions of Tunisia: Sfax ($n = 63$), Ariana ($n = 1$), Gabes ($n = 3$), Mahdia ($n = 13$), Sidi bouzid ($n = 6$), Kairouan ($n = 1$), Beja ($n = 1$), Jendouba ($n = 1$), Manouba ($n = 4$) and Monastir ($n = 3$). Cattle were 48 male less than 18 month old calves and 101 cull dairy cows aged more than 5 years. Data about municipality and city of origin were obtained from the Ministry of Agriculture according to a registration number given to each cattle.

Bacterial isolation

Five to ten grams of lymph nodes or lung without fat were cut into small pieces (approx. 50–100 mg) and macerated in 20 mL sterile distilled water in a Stomacher (BagMixer) until an even suspension was obtained. Tissues from each animal were processed separately. An equal volume of 4% (*w*/*v*) NaOH was added to the aliquot of tissue suspension to give a final concentration of 2%. After the addition of NaOH, the suspension was vigorously shaken and then incubated at 37 °C for 30 min, after which time the suspension was neutralized with 10% H_2SO_4. The treated tissue suspensions were centrifuged at 3000 g for 20 min and then the supernatant was discarded. Culture media Colestos (Bio-Rad, France) and Lowenstein–Jensen (Bio-Rad, France) were inoculated with the sediment using a cotton swab. The applicator was recharged with sediment before each medium slope was inoculated. The inoculated medium was incubated at 37 °C for 12–15 weeks and examined weekly for the presence of colonies [4].

Identification of MTBC by IS*6110*-PCR

A loopful of each isolate was harvested into 200 ul TE buffer (10 mM Tris-HCl, pH 8 ± 0; 1 mM EDTA) in screw-cap 1.5 ml microcentrifuge tubes and boiled for 20 min. After centrifugation in 9000 g for 20 min, the supernatant was transferred to fresh tubes. All DNA extracts were used as template for the identification of MTBC by amplifying the insertion sequence IS*6110*.

A conventional PCR for the detection of the MTBC was performed to test the DNA samples extracted as well as positive and negative controls, following a previously described protocol [12]. DNA was amplified using 1.25 units of Takara Ex Taq DNA polymerase (Takara *Ex taq*, Otsu, Shiga, Japan) and 1 µl of DNA extract. PCR was carried out in a Gene-Amp PCR System 9700 (Applied Biosystems, Foster City, CA, USA). PCR amplification products were visualized using ethidium bromide staining after agarose gel electrophoresis.

Spoligotyping and MIRU-VNTR typing

The MTBC strains were spoligotyped as described by Kamerbeek et al. [13] using the spoligotyping membrane made by the VISAVET Health Surveillance Centre (Madrid, Spain). The spoligotyping patterns were assigned according to the Mbovis.org website [14].

MIRU-VNTR analysis was carried out as described by Roring et al. [15] amplifying the loci ETR-A and ETR-B [9], MIRU 4, MIRU 31, MIRU 26 [16, 17], and QUB 3232, QUB 11a, QUB 11b and QUB 26 [15, 18]. The amplification program consisted of 15 min at 95 °C, followed by 40 cycles of 30 s at 95 °C, 60 s at 60 °C, and 120 s at 72 °C. Amplicon sizes were estimated by electrophoresis on a 2.5% agarose gel at 45 V during 5 h, using 100-bp ladder (Biotools B&M Labs, Madrid, Spain) and the number of repeats was calculated. The VNTR profiles were named by a P followed by a correlated number (i.e. P1, P2, P3, etc.).

Data analysis

A dendogram was built with the unweighted pair group method with arithmetic average (UPGMA) and NJ (Neighbour Joining) clustering methods using the MIRU-VNTR data using Tree graph 2 software. A group of two or more isolates sharing the same MIRU-VNTR pattern was defined as a cluster. The discriminative power of each typing method was calculated using the Hunter–Gaston diversity index (HGDI) [19] using the website application http://insilico.ehu.es/.

Results

Among the 149 cattle samples with suspicious TB lesions collected between November 2014 and April 2015, live mycobacteria were detected by culture in 99 animals (66.4%), 96 isolates belonged to *M. tuberculosis* complex and three to atypical mycobacteria. No coinfection with other strains was found in any sample.

Three profiles were typical of *M. bovis*, and two were classified as *M. caprae* (SB2024 and SB0418 patterns) (Figs. 1 and 2). The discriminatory power of spoligotyping was $h = 0.842$.

The most predominant spoligotypes were the SB0120 ($n = 35$, 36.4%), SB0134 ($n = 11$, 11.4%), and SB0121 ($n = 7$, 7.2%). Three new spoligotyping profiles were described (SB2345, SB2344, and SB2343). The geographic distribution of the different spoligotypes is shown in Fig. 1. The region of Sfax showed a very high level of genetic diversity with 20 out of the 25 detected spoligotypes.

The frequency of the three most detected spoligotypes in our strains (SB0120, SB0121, SB0134) was quite similar to those presented in Tunisia by Lamine-Khemiri et al. [3] and are also the three most frequent types observed in France by Hauer et al. [11] (Additional file 1).

All the 96 MTBC isolates were genotyped using nine MIRU-VNTR loci. Seventy-three different VNTR profiles were found (Fig. 2) and two of them were associated to the *M. caprae* isolates (P62 and P68). The discriminatory power for the MIRU-VNTR technique was high ($h = 0.992$). The discriminatory power of the nine individual loci ranged from 0.158 to 0.727. The

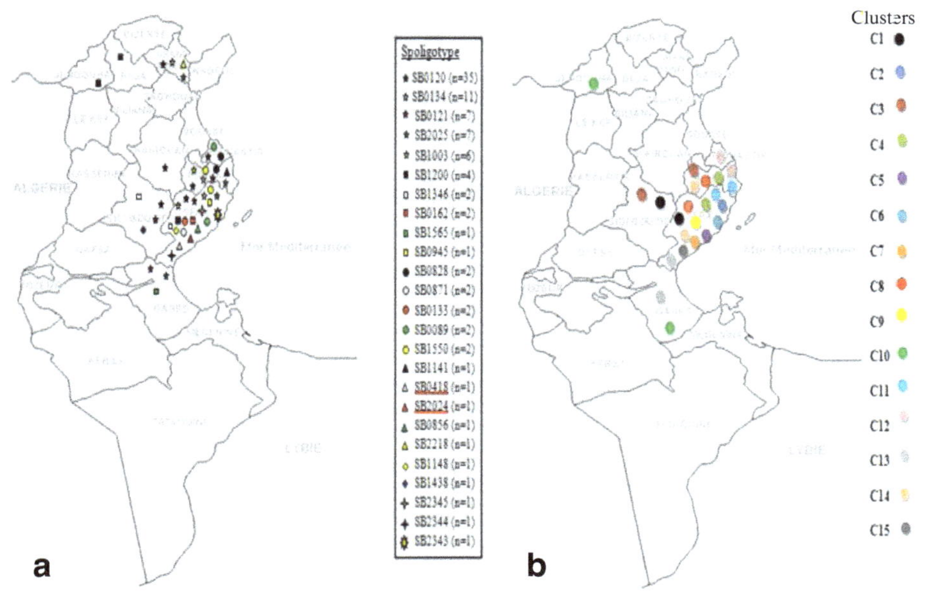

Fig. 1 Geographical distribution of clusters and spoligotypes. **a** Distribution of twenty five spoligotypes distributed on ten Tunisian regions. The two *M.caprae* spoligotypes are underlined with red color. **b** Distribution of fifteen clusters identified using the UPGMA algorithm

1

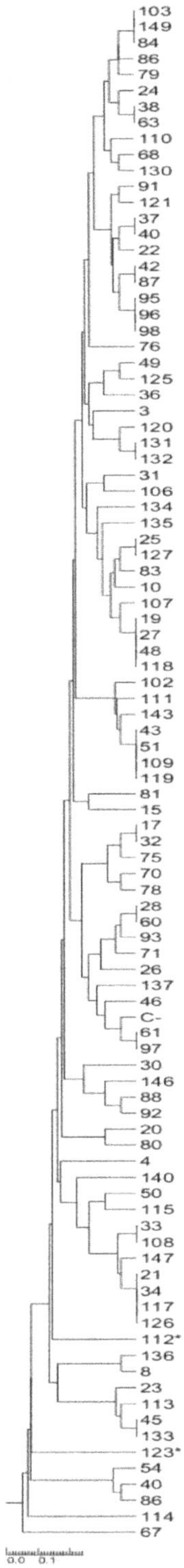

Isolates	Binary code	ST	ETR-A	ETR-B	QUB11a	QUB3232	QUB26	QUB11b	MIRU26	MIRU31	MIRU4	VNTR profile	Region	Clusters
103	1100111101111110111111111110011111111100000	SB2345	5	5	11	6	5	2	5	3	3	P1	Sfax	C1
149	1101111101111110111111111100000111111100000	SB1438	5	5	11	6	5	2	5	3	3	P1	Sidibouzid	C1
84	1101111101111110111111111111111111111100000	SB0120	5	5	11	6	5	2	5	3	3	P1	Sfax	C1
86	1101111101111110111111111111111111111100000	SB0120	5	5	11	6	5	1	5	3	3	P2	Mahdia	
79	1101111101111110111111111111111111111100000	SB0120	5	5	11	6	5	5	5	3	3	P3	Sfax	
24	1101111101111110111111111111111111111100000	SB0120	5	5	11	7	5	3	5	3	3	P4	Mahdia	
38	1101111101111110111111111111111111111100000	SB0120	5	5	11	7	5	2	5	3	3	P5	Sfax	C2
63	1101111101111110111111111111111111111100000	SB0120	5	5	11	7	5	2	5	3	3	P5	Sfax	C2
110	1101111101111110111111111111111111111100000	SB0120	5	5	11	6	5	4	5	3	2	P6	Kairouan	
68	1100011101111110111111111111111111111100000	SB0134	5	5	11	6	5	4	5	3	3	P7	Ariana	
130	1101111101111010111111111111111111111100000	SB2218	5	5	11	4	5	4	5	3	3	P8	Manouba	
91	1101111101111110111111111111111111111100000	SB0120	4	3	11	6	5	3	5	3	3	P9	Sfax	
121	1101111101111110111111111111111111111100000	SB0120	5	3	11	6	5	3	5	3	3	P10	Sfax	
37	1101111101111110111111111111111111111100000	SB0120	4	2	11	6	5	3	5	3	3	P11	Mahdia	C3
40	1101111101111110111111111111111111111100000	SB0120	4	2	11	6	5	3	5	3	3	P11	Sidi bouzid	C3
22	1101111101111110111111111111111111111100000	SB0120	4	7	11	6	5	3	5	3	3	P12	Sfax	
42	1101111001111110111111111111111111111100000	SB1550	5	5	11	6	5	3	5	3	3	P13	Mahdia	C4
87	1101111001111110111111111111111111111100000	SB1550	5	5	11	6	5	3	5	3	3	P13	Sfax	C4
95	1101111101111110111111111111111111111100000	SB0120	4	5	11	6	5	3	5	3	3	P14	Sfax	C5
96	1101111101111110111111111111111111111100000	SB0120	4	5	11	6	5	3	5	3	3	P14	Sfax	C5
98	1101111101111110111111111111111111111100000	SB0120	4	5	11	6	5	3	5	3	3	P14	Sfax	C5
76	1101111101111110111111111111111111111100000	SB0120	4	5	11	5	5	5	5	3	3	P15	Sfax	
49	1101111101111110111111111111111111111100000	SB0120	5	3	11	6	5	2	5	3	3	P16	Mahdia	
125	1101111101111100111111111111111111111100000	SB0856	3	3	11	6	5	2	5	3	3	P17	Sfax	
36	1101111101111110111011111111111111111100000	SB0121	2	3	8	6	5	2	5	3	3	P18	Gabes	
3	1101111101111110111111111110011111111100000	SB1200	5	6	10	7	5	2	5	3	3	P19	Jendouba	
120	1101111101111110111111111110011111111100000	SB1200	5	6	11	6	5	2	5	3	3	P20	Beja	
131	1101111101111110111111111110011111111100000	SB1200	5	6	11	6	5	2	4	3	3	P21	Sfax	C6
132	1101111101111110111111111110011111111100000	SB1200	5	6	11	6	5	2	4	3	3	P21	Sfax	C6
31	1101111101111110111111111111111111111100000	SB0120	5	5	11	4	4	4	5	3	3	P22	Sidi bouzid	
106	1101111101111110111111111111111111111100000	SB0120	5	5	11	5	4	3	5	3	3	P23	Sfax	
134	1101110101111110111111111110111111111100000	SB1003	5	4	11	6	3	1	5	3	3	P24	Sfax	
135	1100000101111110111111111111111111111100000	SB0133	5	3	11	6	2	4	5	3	3	P25	Sfax	
25	0000000000000000000000111111111111111100000	SB0162	5	4	11	6	5	4	5	3	3	P26	Sfax	C7
127	0000000000000000000000111111111111111100000	SB0162	5	4	11	6	5	4	5	3	3	P26	Sfax	C7
83	1101111101111110111111111111111111111100000	SB0120	5	4	11	8	5	4	5	3	3	P27	Manouba	
10	1101111101111110111111111111111111111100000	SB0120	5	6	11	6	5	4	5	3	3	P28	Sfax	
107	1101110101111110111111111110111111111100000	SB1003	5	6	11	6	4	4	5	3	3	P29	Sfax	
19	1101110101111110111111111110111111111100000	SB1003	5	4	11	6	4	4	5	3	3	P30	Sfax	C8
27	1101110101111110111111111110111111111100000	SB1003	5	4	11	6	4	4	5	3	3	P30	Sfax	C8
48	1101110101111110111111111110111111111100000	SB1003	5	4	11	6	4	4	5	3	3	P30	Mahdia	C8
118	1101110101111110111111111110111111111100000	SB1003	5	4	11	6	4	4	5	3	3	P30	Sfax	C8
102	1101111101111110111111111111111111111100000	SB0120	3	5	9	6	2	3	5	3	3	P31	Monastir	
111	1101111101111110111111111111111111111100000	SB0120	3	5	11	6	2	3	6	3	3	P32	Sfax	
143	1101111101111110111111111111111111111100000	SB0120	3	5	11	6	2	2	5	3	3	P33	Sfax	
43	1101111101111110111111111111111111111100000	SB0120	3	5	11	6	2	3	5	3	3	P34	Sfax	C9
51	1101111101111110111111111111111111111100000	SB0120	3	5	11	6	2	3	5	3	3	P34	Sfax	C9
109	1101111101111110111111111111111111111100000	SB0120	3	5	11	6	2	3	5	3	3	P34	Sfax	C9
119	1101111101111110111111111111111111111100000	SB0120	3	5	11	6	2	3	5	3	3	P34	Sfax	C9
81	1101111101111110111111111111111111111100000	SB0120	4	5	11	6	1	4	5	3	3	P35	Sfax	
15	1101111101111110111111111111111111111100000	SB0120	4	5	11	6	5	4	4	3	4	P36	Sfax	
17	1101111101111110111111111111111111111100000	SB0120	5	5	10	6	2	4	5	4	3	P37	Manouba	C10
32	1101111101111110111111111101111111111100000	SB1565	5	5	10	6	2	4	5	4	3	P37	Gabes	C10
75	1101111101111110111111111111111111111100000	SB0120	5	7	10	6	2	4	5	4	3	P38	Sfax	
70	1100000101111110111111111111111111111100000	SB0133	5	5	11	6	2	4	5	4	3	P39	Sfax	
78	1101111101111110111111111111111111111100000	SB0120	5	5	11	6	4	4	5	4	3	P40	Sidi bouzid	
28	1100011101111110111111111111111111111100000	SB0134	5	4	11	3	5	4	5	4	3	P41	Sfax	C11
60	1100011101111110111111111111111111111100000	SB0134	5	4	11	3	5	4	5	4	3	P41	Mahdia	C11
93	1100011101111110111111111100000111111100000	SB2344	5	4	11	5	5	4	5	4	3	P42	Sfax	
71	1100011101111110111111111111111111111100000	SB0134	5	2	11	3	5	4	5	4	3	P43	Sfax	
26	1100011101111110111111111111111111111100000	SB0134	5	4	11	6	5	4	5	4	3	P44	Mahdia	
137	1101111101111110111111111100011111111100000	SB1148	5	5	11	7	5	6	5	4	3	P45	Sfax	
46	1100011101111110111110111111111111111100000	SB0134	5	3	11	6	5	1	5	4	3	P46	Sfax	
C-	1100011101111110111111111111111111111100000	SB0134	5	4	11	6	5	2	5	4	3	P47	Sfax	
61	1101111101111110111111111111111111011100000	SB0828	5	5	11	6	5	2	5	4	3	P48	Mahdia	C12
97	1101111101111110111111111111111111011100000	SB0828	5	5	11	6	5	2	5	4	3	P48	Monastir	C12
30	1001111101111110111011111111111000111100000	SB2343	5	4	10	5	5	2	3	3	3	P49	Sfax	
146	1100011101111110111111111111111111111100000	SB0134	5	2	7	5	5	2	5	3	3	P50	Sfax	
88	1100011101111110111111111111111111111100000	SB0134	5	5	7	5	5	4	5	3	3	P51	Sfax	
92	1100011101111110111111111111111111111100000	SB0134	5	4	7	5	5	4	5	3	3	P52	Mahdia	
20	1101111101111110111111111111111111111100000	SB0120	4	5	11	9	5	3	5	4	3	P53	Sfax	
80	1101111101111110111111111111111111111100000	SB0120	7	6	11	9	5	3	5	4	3	P54	Sfax	
4	1100011101111100111111111111111111111100000	SB0945	6	4	8	4	3	3	5	3	3	P55	Sfax	
140	1101111100111110111111111111111111111100000	SB0871	6	5	11	4	4	2	2	3	3	P56	Sfax	
50	1101111101111110111011111111111111111100000	SB0121	6	4	10	7	5	2	5	3	3	P57	Sfax	
115	1101111101111110111011111111111111111100000	SB0121	6	4	10	7	4	4	5	3	3	P58	Sidi bouzid	
33	1100011101111110111110111110111111111100000	SB2025	6	6	10	6	4	2	5	3	3	P59	Gabes	C13
108	1100011101111110111110111110111111111100000	SB2025	6	6	10	6	4	2	5	3	3	P59	Sfax	C13
147	1100011101111110111110111110111111111100000	SB2025	6	5	10	6	4	4	5	3	3	P60	Manouba	
21	1100011101111110111110111110111111111100000	SB2025	6	5	10	6	4	2	5	3	3	P61	Mahdia	C14
34	1100011101111110111110111110111111111100000	SB2025	6	5	10	6	4	2	5	3	3	P61	Sfax	C14
117	1100011101111110111110111110111111111100000	SB2025	6	5	10	6	4	2	5	3	3	P61	Sfax	C14
126	1100011101111110111110111110111111111100000	SB2025	6	5	10	6	4	2	5	3	3	P61	Sfax	C14
112*	0100000000000000111111111101111111111100000	SB0418	5	1	11	10	3	4	5	2	3	P62	Sfax	
136	1100011101111110111101111111111111111100000	SB0089	3	3	11	8	5	6	4	3	3	P63	Monastir	
8	1100011101111110111101111111111111111100000	SB0089	3	3	11	8	5	4	4	3	3	P64	Sfax	
23	1101111101111110111011111111111110111100000	SB1346	2	3	11	7	5	2	5	3	2	P65	Sidi bouzid	
113	1101111101111110111011111111111111111100000	SB0121	4	3	11	7	5	2	3	3	2	P66	Sfax	
45	1101111101111110111011111111111111111100000	SB0121	4	3	11	7	5	2	5	3	2	P67	Sfax	C15
133	1101111101111110111011111111111110111100000	SB1346	4	3	11	7	5	2	5	3	2	P67	Sfax	C15
123*	0100000000000000111111110101000011111100000	SB2024	5	3	6	9	2	4	5	4	9	P68	Sfax	
54	1101111101111110111011111111111111111100000	SB0121	8	4	9	7	2	1	2	3	3	P69	Sfax	
40	1101111101111110111111111111111111111100000	SB0120	4	2	11	6	5	3	5	3	3	P70	Sidi bouzid	
86	1101111101111110111011011111111111111100000	SB1141	9	4	10	7	2	1	2	3	3	P71	Mahdia	
114	1100011101111110111111111111111111111100000	SB0134	3	2	7	5	5	4	5	2	4	P72	Sfax	
67	1101111100111110111111111111111111111100000	SB0871	6	2	6	3	4	3	2	4	3	P73	Sfax	

Fig. 2 (See legend on next page.)

(See figure on previous page.)
Fig. 2 Dendogram of cluster analysis. Dendrogram generated with the UPGMA (unweighted pair group method with arithmetic average) and Neighbour Joining (NJ) clustering methods using the MIRU-VNTR data using Tree graph 2 software showing the genetic relationships of the 96 *Mycobacterium bovis* isolates. A group of two or more isolates sharing the same MIRU-VNTR pattern is defined as a cluster. ST: Spoligotype as defined in the *M. bovis* Spoligotype Database website (http://www.mbovis.org). * Isolate corresponding to *M. caprae*

loci with higher diversity were QUB-11b, ETR-B, ETR-A, QUB-3232, QUB26 and QUB-11a with a discriminatory power *h* corresponding to 0.727, 0.724, 0.650, 0.583, 0.577, and 0.445, respectively. The MIRU 31, MIRU26 and MIRU 4 loci displayed a very little allelic diversity (0.370, 0.249, and 0.158, respectively).

Our results showed a large genotypic variety observed within the main spoligotypes which was split into several MIRU-VNTR types as previously shown in Tunisia and in France [3, 11]. MIRU-VNTR typing results for 6 common loci (ETR A, ETR B, MIRU4 (ETRD), QUB11a, QUB11b and QUB3232) were available for strains from Tunisia and France showing shared genotypes (Additional file 1).

MIRU-VNTR analysis showed a large genotypic variety observed within the main spoligotype that was split into several MIRU-VNTR types: 29 in SB0120 ($h = 0.983$), 10 in SB0134 ($h = 0.981$) and 7 in SB0121 ($h = 1$). Genotyping revealed a pattern common for different geographic regions (P11, P13, P30, P41, P48, P59 and P61) (Fig. 1, Fig. 2). Our results showed that Sfax, located in southern Tunisia, represents a high-risk area with a high level of genetic diversity with 20 and 63 out of the 25 and the 73 detected spoligotypes and genotypes, respectively.

Fifteen clusters including 36 isolates (37.5%) were identified using the UPGMA algorithm and the largest three clusters (C1, C10 and C15) had four isolates; while most clusters had only two (Fig. 2). The most common VNTR profiles P30, P34 and P61 were found in four isolates each. Moreover, most clusters showed the same spoligotyping pattern for all isolates. Isolates with the spoligotyping patterns SB1438, SB2345, and SB0120 presented a similar MIRU-VNTR profile (P1: 5.5.11.6.5.2.5.3.3). It also occurred in the case of isolates with spoligotypes SB0120 and SB1565 where MIRU-VNTR profiles were P37: 5.5.10.6.2.4.5.4.3, and in isolates with spoligotypes SB1346 and SB0121 (MIRU-VNTR profile P67: 4.3.11.7.5.2.5.3.2) (Fig. 2). When both typing techniques were combined, the level of discrimination was 0.993 and 78 different spoligo–MIRU–VNTR types were observed.

For SB0120, the main MIRU-VNTR pattern (MV16), 5.5.3.11.4.6 identified in our study was detected in the Central East of France in the Côte d'Or region. Additionally, pattern MV6 (5.5.3.11.4.4) was identified for strains with SB0120 from France and Tunisia. Interestingly, four genotypes (MV21, MV10, MV53 and MV63) detected in our strains with an SB0120 spoligotype pattern from Sfax were previously described by Lamine-Khmiri et al. in the same region [3] but not detected in strains from France [11] (Table 1, Additional file 1). Moreover, MIRU-VNTR genotype MV53 (6.5.3.10.2.6) was detected according to our study in strains corresponding to the spoligotype SB2025; which highlights matching results only with the study conducted by Lamine-Khmiri et al. [3] (Table 1, Additional file 1). Interestingly, the pattern MV36 (5.4.3.11.4.6) was obtained in strains with spoligotype pattern SB0134 from Tunisia and France.

Discussion

Our study represented a large analysis including 96 characterized *M. bovis* out of 149 slaughtered cattle from ten Tunisian regions showing TB compatible lesions in the lymph nodes after routine inspection. However, two Tunisian studies have previously reported data about bTB in Tunisia analyzing only 35 and 6 *M. bovis* isolates out of 100 cattle and 306 milk samples, respectively [3, 5]. The allelic diversity of spoligotype patterns among the *M. bovis* strains isolated in our study ($h = 0.842$) were relatively more than the ones previously found by Lamine-Khemiri et al. and Kahla et al. (0.733 and 0.753, respectively) in Tunisia [3, 5]. This fact could be mainly due to the differences in the number of isolates.

Of the 25 detected *M. bovis* spoligotype patterns, 8 patterns, accounting for 75% of all the isolated strains, have previously been detected in strains isolated from

Table 1 Shared MIRU-VNTR genotypes of strains with spoligotype pattern SB0120 from Tunisia and France

	Tunisia		France
VNTR type	This study	Lamine-Khemiri et al. [3]	Hauer et al. [11]
MV6	5.5.3.11.4.4£	5.5.3.11.4.4£	5.5.3.11.4.4£
MV16	5.5.3.11.4.6€		5.5.3.11.4.6€
MV21	5.5.3.11.2.6¥	5.5.3.11.2.6¥	
MV10	3.5.3.11.3.6¥	3.5.3.11.3.6¥	
MV53	6.5.3.10.2.6¥	6.5.3.10.2.6¥	
MV63	5.6.3.11.2.6¥	5.6.3.11.2.6¥	

Results from Tunisia and France have previously been published. [3, 11] Additional file 1 shows more details concerning the comparison of our results to those of two previous studies. £Matching patterns of strains from the two Tunisian studies and France. € Matching patterns of strains from our study and France. ¥ Matching patterns of strains from our study and Lamine-Khemiri et al. MV53 genotype was also detected in strains with SB2025 genotype in our study and in Tunisia previously published by Lamine-Khemiri et al

Tunisia [3]. The frequency of three common spoligotypes most detected in our strains (SB0120, SB0121, SB0134) are quite similar to those detected in Tunisia by Lamine-Khemiri et al. [3], in Algeria by Sahraoui et al. [20] are also in France by Hauer et al. [11]. They were also found in other European countries as Italy, Spain and Portugal [10, 21, 22]. Our present results corroborate previous studies showing a more frequent occurrence of *M. bovis* strains of spoligotype pattern SB0120 causing bTB in Tunisia (36–37%), in Algeria (39%) [20] and in France since 1978 accounting for 26% as mentioned by Hauer et al. [11]. Interestingly, the spoligotype SB0134 was identified as the second predominant type in Tunisia, the second most frequently isolated type in France [11] and was highly prevalent in cattle from neighbouring Algeria [20]. SB0121,the third most abundant spoligotype in our study (7.2%), is also present in France (6%) [11], and more frequently found in Algeria (21%) [20].

The comparative study of the Tunisian and French spoligotypes and MIRU-VNTR profiles could further support the French input to the Tunisian *M. bovis* population considering the striking similarity. There have been very strong historical commercial links between Tunisia and France starting during the French colonial period. The importation of French cattle could explain the majority of our genotypic results and the similarity with the *M. bovis* French population genotypes is concerned. The Food and Agriculture Organization in Tunisia, states documentation concerning the imported breeds in Tunisia originated from North America and Europe only from 1986 to 1989 [23]. Therefore the increased effort to control bTB in Europe or North America had already allowed almost eradication of the disease [24]. Thus, introduction of *M. bovis* from Europe into African countries has previously been suggested [10, 25]. In addition, Sahraoui et al. [20] mentioned that some strains of *M. bovis* found in Algeria may have been independently introduced from France (or more generally continental Europe). In fact, in Tunisia, the introduction of cattle from neighboring countries such Algeria and Lybia via non controlled routes is continuing up to date; which is considered one of the main sources of the maintenance of the infection in Tunisian cattle due to the absence of control and eradication campaigns. In addition, there are exclusive Tunisian spoligotypes clearly derived from strains SB0120, SB0134 or SB0121; some of which have already been described [11, 20], suggesting that the imported strains mutated in Tunisia. On the other hand, *M. bovis* mutates rather slowly; it is then highly possible that these mutated strains have long existed in the territory and that possibly spillback to the breed animals was introduced in the country.

The origin farms of the animals could not be traced since samples were taken only from cattle belonged to the private unorganized livestock characterized by a multiple selling of the animals prior to slaughter. However, the majority of animals could be dairy cattle; thus it is very improbable that animals had come from the same herds. Thus, our study demonstrates the importance of the elaboration of a tracing system which could be a useful tool for bTB monitoring.

Our findings emphasize previous claims that cattle could be infected by *M. caprae* spoligotypes (SB0418, SB2024) [3, 6]. Interestingly, the SB2024 profile has recently been described in Tunisia [3] whereas the spoligotype SB0418 has been mentioned in Central and Eastern European countries [10, 26, 27] as the most frequent spoligotype found in human and animal isolates [3, 27]. The current study raises the issue of a cross contamination in and between cattle and goats during their breeding or importation. In Tunisia, the herd of goats was estimated at 1.5 million head. In the North, goats are reared in extensive mixed farming systems with sheep and cows. Meanwhile, almost 60% of the goats are located in the Center and South of Tunisia, reared in semi-intensive oasis systems, in small herds [28]. However, to our knowledge, no data is available about the importation of small ruminants in the country although the introduction of *M. caprae* infected cattle and/or goats from other countries could be possible.

The spatial distribution of the *M. bovis* strains reveals the existence of isolates with shared spoligotypes and MIRU-VNTR profiles between different geographic Tunisian regions: Sfax and Gabes (P59), Sfax and Mahdia (P13, P30, P4 and P61), Mahdia and Monastir (P48), and Mahdia and Sidi Bouzid (P11), which revealed the movement of animals between them. This exchange event is probably related to economic facts like the trade of infected animals and the geographical distribution in the area. In fact, Sfax, Gabes, Mahdia, Sidi bouzid, and Monastir regions are contiguous states which may facilitate the movement of cattle among them.

Isolates corresponding to the cluster C1 (SB0120, SB1438 and SB2345 spoligotypes), showed the same MIRU-VNTR allelic profile, and SB1438 and SB2345 could be probably derived from a SB0120 isolate. In a similar way, isolates corresponding to clusters C10 and C15 have identical MIRU-VNTR allelic profiles, and the loss of a single spacer could be compatible with a one-step evolution (SB0120 → SB1565; SB0121 → SB1346, respectively) asmentioned by Romero et al. [29]. It has also been hypothesized that the appearance of new strains diverged from pre-existing clones which have lost spacers [29–32]. However, the molecular techniques used in our study cannot determine the oldest strains. Thus, further analysis by whole genome sequencing would be interesting for this purpose.

Conclusions

The molecular data obtained until now would greatly support and provide hints to improve the national eradication campaign since it helps to determine the origin of outbreaks and better understand the link in-between btB transmission. Further laboratory testing, periodic sampling from different slaughterhouses and additional herd epidemiological studies should be conducted to determine the exact bTB prevalence and to further understand the mode of transmission.

Acknowledgments

This work is part of a doctoral thesis by Saif Eddine Djemal.
This work was supported by the research program of the Ministry of Higher Education and Scientific Research, Tunisia.
We would like to acknowledge Wissem Gdoura for his assistance with laboratory testing of specimens and also Mohamed Ghariani and Lilia Chaker for coordinating this study at the Regional Hygiene Care Mycobacteriology Laboratory, Hedi-Chaker University Hospital, Sfax, Tunisia. We thank the VISAVET Centre in Spain for the training course in molecular techniques, specially J. Gimeno and F. Lozano.
This work was supported by the Programa de Tecnologías Avanzadas en Vigilancia Sanitaria (TAVS) from the Comunidad de Madrid (ref. S2013/ABI-2747).
The authors are eventually grateful to Kamel MAALOUL, translator and English professor for having proofread the manuscript.

Funding

No specific funding for this work.

Authors' contributions

SD conception and design of the study, sampling of animals, culturing of Mycobacteria, molecular typing, VNTR typing, writing of the manuscript. MS conception and design of the study, writing and review of the manuscript. SS conception and design of the study, participated in the manipulation for the isolation of strains of Mycobacterium and for molecular gene characterization, interpreted the results and revised critically the manuscript. SK and CM Data curation. JB contribution in paper writing and review. FM-A Participated in the study design, interpretation of results and revised critically the manuscript. BR principal supervision and support for molecular typing, VNTR typing at Centro de Vigilancia Sanitaria Veterinaria (VISAVET), Madrid, Spain writing of the manuscript. RG Supervised the experimental work, interpretation of results and revised critically the manuscript. All authors read and approved the final manuscript.

Consent for publication

Not applicable

Competing interests

The authors declare that they have no competing interests.

Author details

[1]Department of Life Sciences, Research Laboratory of Environmental Toxicology-Microbiology and Health (LR17ES06), Faculty of Sciences, University of Sfax-Tunisia, Sfax, Tunisia. [2]Department of Biology, Preparatory Institute for Engineering Studies, University of Sfax-Tunisia, Sfax, Tunisia. [3]Department of Microbiology, Regional Hygiene Care Mycobacteriology Laboratory, Hedi-Chaker University Hospital, Sfax, Tunisia. [4]Department of Biology, Faculty of Pharmacy, University of Monastir-Tunisia, Monastir, Tunisia. [5]Department of Microbiology, National Reference Laboratory of Mycobacteria, Research Unit (UR12SP18), A, Mami University Hospital of Pneumology, Ariana, Tunisia. [6]MAEVA SERVET SL. C/ de la Fragua 3, 28749, Alameda del Valle, Madrid, Spain. [7]Centro de Vigilancia Sanitaria Veterinaria (VISAVET), Universidad Complutense, Avda. Puerta de Hierro s/n, 28040 Madrid, Spain.

References

1. Olea-Popelka F, Muwonge A, Perera A, Dean AS, Mumford E, Erlacher-Vindel E, et al. Zoonotic tuberculosis in human beings caused by Mycobacterium Bovis—a call for action. Lancet Infect Dis. 2017;17:e21–5.
2. Cosivi O, Grange JM, Daborn CJ, Raviglione MC, Fujikura T, Cousins D, et al. Zoonotic tuberculosis due to Mycobacterium Bovis in developing countries. Emerg Infect Dis. 1998;4:59–70.
3. Lamine-Khemiri H, Martínez R, García-Jiménez WL, Benítez-Medina JM, Cortés M, Hurtado I, et al. Genotypic characterization by spoligotyping and VNTR typing of Mycobacterium Bovis and Mycobacterium Caprae isolates from cattle of Tunisia. Trop Anim Health Prod. 2014;46:305–11.
4. Corner LA, Gormley E, Pfeiffer DU. Primary isolation of Mycobacterium Bovis from bovine tissues: conditions for maximising the number of positive cultures. Vet Microbiol. 2012;156:162–71.
5. Kahla IB, Boschiroli ML, Souissi F, Cherif N, Benzarti M, Boukadida J, et al. Isolation and molecular characterisation of Mycobacterium Bovis from raw milk in Tunisia. Afr Health Sci. 2011;11:2–5.
6. Müller B, Steiner B, Bonfoh B, Fané A, Smith NH, Zinsstag J. Molecular characterisation of Mycobacterium Bovis isolated from cattle slaughtered at the Bamako abattoir in Mali. BMC Vet Res. 2008;4:26.
7. Ghariani A, Jaouadi T, Smaoui S, Mehiri E, Marouane C, Kammoun S, et al. Diagnosis of lymph node tuberculosis using the GeneXpert MTB/RIF in Tunisia. Int J Mycobacteriology. 2015;4:270–5.
8. Siala M, Smaoui S, Taktak W, Hachicha S, Ghorbel A, Marouane C, et al. First-time detection and identification of the mycobacterium tuberculosis complex members in extrapulmonary tuberculosis clinical samples in south Tunisia by a single tube tetraplex real-time PCR assay. Pluschke G, editor. PLoS Negl Trop Dis. 2017;11:e0005572.
9. Frothingham R, Meeker-O'Connell WA. Genetic diversity in the mycobacterium tuberculosis complex based on variable numbers of tandem DNA repeats. Microbiology. 1998;144:1189–96.
10. Haddad N, Ostyn A, Karoui C, Masselot M, Thorel MF, Hughes SL, et al. Spoligotype diversity of Mycobacterium Bovis strains isolated in France from 1979 to 2000. J Clin Microbiol. 2001;39:3623–32.
11. Hauer A, De Cruz K, Cochard T, Godreuil S, Karoui C, Henault S, et al. Genetic evolution of Mycobacterium Bovis causing tuberculosis in livestock and wildlife in France since 1978. PLoS One. 2015;10:e0117103.
12. Eisenach KD, Cave MD, Bates JH, Crawford JT. Polymerase chain reaction amplification of a repetitive DNA sequence specific for mycobacterium tuberculosis. J Infect Dis. 1990;161:977–81.
13. Kamerbeek J, Schouls LEO, Kolk A, Van Agterveld M, Van Soolingen D, Kuijper S, et al. Simultaneous detection and strain differentiation of mycobacterium tuberculosis for diagnosis and epidemiology. J Clin Microbiol. 1997;35:907–14.
14. Smith NH, Upton P. Naming spoligotype patterns for the RD9-deleted lineage of the mycobacterium tuberculosis complex; www.Mbovis.org. Infect Genet Evol J Mol Epidemiol Evol Genet Infect Dis. 2012;12:873–6.
15. Roring S, Scott A, Brittain D, Walker I, Hewinson G, Neill S, et al. Development of variable-number tandem repeat typing of Mycobacterium Bovis: comparison of results with those obtained by using existing exact tandem repeats and Spoligotyping. J Clin Microbiol. 2002;40:2126–33.
16. Supply P, Mazars E, Lesjean S, Vincent V, Gicquel B, Locht C. Variable human minisatellite-like regions in the mycobacterium tuberculosis genome. Mol Microbiol. 2000;36:762–71.
17. Allix C, Walravens K, Saegerman C, Godfroid J, Supply P, Fauville-Dufaux M. Evaluation of the epidemiological relevance of variable-number tandem-repeat genotyping of Mycobacterium Bovis and comparison of the method with IS6110 restriction fragment length polymorphism analysis and Spoligotyping. J Clin Microbiol. 2006;44:1951–62.
18. Skuce RA, McCorry TP, McCarroll JF, Roring SM, Scott AN, Brittain D, et al. Discrimination of mycobacterium tuberculosis complex bacteria using novel VNTR-PCR targets. Microbiology. 2002;148:519–28.

19. Hunter PR, Gaston MA. Numerical index of the discriminatory ability of typing systems: an application of Simpson's index of diversity. J Clin Microbiol. 1988;26:2465–6.
20. Sahraoui N, Müller B, Guetarni D, Boulahbal F, Yala D, Ouzrout R, et al. Molecular characterization of Mycobacterium Bovis strains isolated from cattle slaughtered at two abattoirs in Algeria. BMC Vet Res. 2009;5:4.
21. Duarte EL, Domingos M, Amado A, Botelho A. Spoligotype diversity of Mycobacterium Bovis and Mycobacterium Caprae animal isolates. Vet Microbiol. 2008;130:415–21.
22. Rodríguez S, Romero B, Bezos J, de Juan L, Alvarez J, Castellanos E, et al. High spoligotype diversity within a Mycobacterium Bovis population: clues to understanding the demography of the pathogen in Europe. Vet Microbiol. 2010;141:89–95.
23. FAO. Tunisie : Rapport National sur les Ressources Génétiques animales [Internet]. 2001 [cited 2017 May 16]. Available from: http://ftp.fao.org/docrep/fao/010/a1250e/annexes/CountryReports/Tunisia.pdf
24. Caffrey JP. Status of bovine tuberculosis eradication programmes in Europe. Vet Microbiol. 1994;40:1–4.
25. Njanpop-Lafourcade BM, Inwald J, Ostyn A, Durand B, Hughes S, Thorel M-F, et al. Molecular typing of Mycobacterium Bovis isolates from Cameroon. J Clin Microbiol. 2001;39:222–7.
26. Prodinger WM, Eigentler A, Allerberger F, Schönbauer M, Glawischnig W. Infection of red deer, cattle, and humans with Mycobacterium Bovis subsp. caprae in western Austria. J Clin Microbiol. 2002;40:2270–2.
27. Erler W, Martin G, Sachse K, Naumann L, Kahlau D, Beer J, et al. Molecular fingerprinting of Mycobacterium Bovis subsp. caprae isolates from central Europe. J Clin Microbiol. 2004;42:2234–8.
28. Ammar H, Boda R, Ben Younes M, López S. Goat breeding systems in the South of Tunisia (Tataouine). Options Méditerranéennes Econ. Soc. Environ. Sustain. Sheep Goat Prod Syst A. 2011. p. 283–88.
29. Romero B, Aranaz A, Sandoval Á, Álvarez J, de Juan L, Bezos J, et al. Persistence and molecular evolution of Mycobacterium Bovis population from cattle and wildlife in Doñana National Park revealed by genotype variation. Vet Microbiol. 2008;132:87–95.
30. Van Embden JDA, Van Gorkom T, Kremer K, Jansen R, Van der Zeijst BAM, Schouls LM. Genetic variation and evolutionary origin of the direct repeat locus of mycobacterium tuberculosis complex bacteria. J Bacteriol. 2000;182:2393–401.
31. Smith NH, Dale J, Inwald J, Palmer S, Gordon SV, Hewinson RG, et al. The population structure of Mycobacterium Bovis in great Britain: clonal expansion. Proc Natl Acad Sci U S A. 2003;100:15271–5.
32. Aranaz A, Romero B, Montero N, Álvarez J, Bezos J, de Juan L, et al. Spoligotyping profile change caused by deletion of a direct variable repeat in a mycobacterium tuberculosis Isogenic laboratory strain. J Clin Microbiol. 2004;42:5388–91.

9

Spatial analysis for bovine viral diarrhea virus and bovine herpesvirus type 1 infections in the state of Paraíba, northeastern Brazil

Leíse Gomes Fernandes[1], Edviges Maristela Pituco[2], Adriana Hellmeister de Campos Nogueira Romaldini[2], Eliana De Stefano[2], Inácio José Clementino[3], Amanda Rafaela Alves Maia[1], Carolina de Sousa Américo Batista Santos[1], Clebert José Alves[1] and Sérgio Santos de Azevedo[1*]

Abstract

Background: Bovine Viral Diarrhea Virus (BVDV) and Bovine Herpesvirus type 1 (BoHV-1) cause reproductive problems in cattle and restrictions on international trade in animals worldwide. Both infections were detected in cattle herds in the Paraíba state, Northeastern Brazil, however, the spatial distribution and geographic identification of positive herds for these viruses has never been examined. Therefore, the aim of this study was to describe the spatial pattern of apparent prevalence estimate and to identify spatial clustering of positive herds of BVDV and BoHV-1 infections in cattle herds from the state of Paraíba, Northeastern Brazil.

Results: The herd-level prevalence for BVDV and BoHV-1 infections in Paraíba were, respectively, 65.5% (95% CI: 61.1–69.7) and 87.8% (95% CI: 84.5–90.5). The average apparent within-herd prevalence of BVDV was 31.8% and of BoHV-1 was 62.4%. The predicted prevalence was highest (0.42–0.75) for BVDV in the west, north and eastern part of Sertão and in the central and eastern part of Agreste/Zona da Mata. For BoHV-1, the highest predicted prevalence (0.74–0.97) was in some local areas across Sertão and throughout the eastern part of Agreste/Zona da Mata. Six significant clusters were detected for BVDV, a primary cluster covering the eastern Sertão region, with 11 herds, radius of 24.10 km and risk relative (RR) of 2.21 ($P < 0.001$) and five smaller significant clusters, involving one or two herds in Agreste/Zona da Mata region with a high RR. A significant clustering of BoHV-1 positive herds ($P < 0.001$) was detected in Agreste/Zona da Mata region with a radius of 77.17 km and a RR of 1.27, with 103 cases. Consistency was found between kriging and SatScan results for identification of risk areas for BVDV and BoHV-1 infections.

Conclusions: The clusters detected contemplated different areas of the state, with BVDV cluster located in the Sertão and BoHV-1 in Agreste/Zona da Mata stratum. Through the risk mapping, it was possible to identify the areas in which the risk is significantly elevated, coincided with areas where there are borders with other states and in which there is a high movement of animals.

Keywords: Cattle, Epidemiology, Cluster analysis, BVDV, BoHV-1, Kriging estimate

* Correspondence: sergio@vps.fmvz.usp.br
[1]Laboratory of Transmissible Diseases, Academic Unit of Veterinary Medicine, Center of Rural Technology and Health, Federal University of Campina Grande, Patos, PB 58700-970, Brazil
Full list of author information is available at the end of the article

Background

The reproductive infectious diseases are those that cause more damage in productivity in cattle herds, assuming importance viral agents, especially Bovine Viral Diarrhea Virus (BVDV) and Bovine Herpesvirus type 1 (BoHV-1), which cause reproductive problems in both beef and milk cattle, and restrictions on international trade for animals and animal products [1–3].

BVDV is a member of the genus *Pestivirus,* which belongs to the *Flaviviridae* family, and although capable of manifesting in different clinical presentations and acute, sub acute or chronic character, the reproductive consequences of this virus and its persistent infection have greater economic and epidemiological importance [4, 5]. The transmission may occur by a wide range of body fluids (nasal discharge, urine, milk, semen, saliva and fetal fluids), indirect contacts (airborne transmissions, contaminated material or iatrogenic) and via the placenta to the fetus, resulting in the birth of an immunotolerant and persistently infected (PI) calf [6]. The PI animals result from uterine exposure to noncytopathic strains of BVDV before development of fetal immunocompetence (generally before 125 days of gestation) [7]. PI calves are often weak at birth or die before one year of age, but others may not show clinical signs, being epidemiologically important due to shed large amounts of virus, acting as constant sources of infection for susceptible animals [8]. The detection and removal of PI animals and vaccination of susceptible animals are key strategies for the control of herds from BVDV [9, 10].

The BoHV-1 is a alphaherpesvirus belonging to the genus *Varicellovirus*, which infects cattle and presents clinical manifestations such as pustular vulvovaginitis or balanoposthitis, abortion, rhinotracheitis and meningoencephalitis, and causes great economic losses to the livestock industry [11, 12]. This virus may be transmitted by respiratory and genital secretions of infected individuals through direct and indirect contact, such as contaminated materials, contaminated semen or airbone transmission [13]. BoHV-1 has the ability to cause latent infections, and periodically, BoHV-1 may be reactivated, and then shed and transmitted, which guarantees its perpetuation and spread in herds, thus being the main obstacle to the establishment of control measures [14].

The seroprevalence of BVDV and BoHV-1 have numerous references available all over the world, with variable values, but generally higher, depending on the control measures practiced [15]. In Brazil, regional data obtained from serological surveys reveal significant spread of the virus in beef and dairy herds [16–18]. In the state of Paraíba, Thompson et al. [19] found anti-BVDV antibodies in 22.2% of animals and 88.9% of herds and anti-BoHV-1 antibodies in 46.6% of animals and 100% of herds. These authors concluded that the within-herd spread of BVDV and BoHV-1 were relatively slow and its ubiquitous nature makes it difficult to generalize the rate of among-herds spread.

BVDV and BoHV-1 infections occur in cattle herds in the state of Paraíba, however, the spatial distribution and geographic identification of positive herds for these viruses has never been examined. According to Carpenter [20], whether it is an outbreak investigation or epidemiological research, more emphasis should be placed on the spatial and temporal components of health events in order to identify unusual occurrences of events that happen close together in either time and/or space.

Spatial analysis of infectious diseases allows for the detection of disease clusters, which can occur due to common risk factors among herds or the transmission between neighbors herds, being a useful tool in epidemiological surveillance providing better visualization and hypothesis survey for the occurrence of clusters, facilitating the elaboration of control strategies [21]. Hence, the present study aimed to describe the spatial pattern of apparent prevalence estimate of BVDV and BoHV-1 infections in cattle herds from the state of Paraíba, Northeastern Brazil, including identification of areas with increased risk of occurrence of these viruses.

Methods

Characterization of the study area

The state of Paraíba, located in the Northeastern region of Brazil, is characterized by warm weather throughout the year. The state is geographically subdivided into the following four regions, based mostly on vegetation type and rainfall: (i) Zona da Mata (Atlantic forest), (ii) Agreste, (iii) Borborema, and (iv) Sertão. The Zona da Mata and Agreste have relatively higher rainfall regimes [22]. Borborema and Sertão (semi-arid region) are typically within the Caatinga biome, a xeric forest and a forest of thorns composed by cacti, thick plants, spiny brush and adapted arid grasses [23]. The climate is characterized by a warm and semi-arid climate, with average temperatures of 27 °C, and the average annual rainfall is typically ≈500 mm. There are typically two seasons: a rainy season from February to May, and a long drought period from June to January. However, occurrences of droughts lasting more than one year are also characteristic of the region [24].

The animal husbandry has an increasingly important in the Agreste, Borborema and Sertão regions, where small cattle-raising farms and family farms are widespread. The cattle are usually reared extensively on native Caatinga in most of the Borborema and Sertão farms. Following the Brazilian scenario of milk production, in the state of Paraíba around 69% of milk was produced in small cattle-raising farms [25].

Data source

The data used in this study were obtained from a survey of bovine brucellosis in the state of Paraíba made by the National Program for Control and Eradication of Brucellosis and Tuberculosis, in which samples were collected from September 2012 to January 2013. In total, 2443 cows aged ≥24 months were sampled from 478 herds.

Study design

The state of Paraíba was divided into three sampling groups: sampling stratum 1 (mesoregion of Sertão), sampling stratum 2 (mesoregion of Borborema), and sampling stratum 3 (mesoregions of Zona da Mata and Agreste) (Fig. 1). When this stratification scheme was proposed, the operational capacity of the Agricultural and Livestock Defense Service of the State of Paraíba (SEDAP) was considered based on the areas of action of its regional units in order to ensure that the veterinarians and agricultural and livestock technicians from the SEDAP could conduct the fieldwork. For each sampling stratum, a pre-established number of herds with reproductive activity (primary sampling units) were randomly selected and then, a pre-established number of unvaccinated cows aged ≥24 months were randomly and systematic selected (secondary sampling units), using the following criteria: 10 animals were sampled in herds with up to 99 cows aged over 24 months; 15 animals were sampled in herds with 100 or more cows aged over 24 months; and all animals were sampled in those with up to 10 cows aged over 24 months.

The field activities included blood collection and sending the samples to the laboratory. The coordinates in each herd were identified using a global positioning system device (GPS).

BoHV-1 and BVDV serological diagnosis

For the serological diagnosis of BVDV and BoHV-1 infections the virus-neutralization test was used [26, 27]. The cytopathic viral strains BVDV-1 (NADL) and BoHV-1 supplied by the Virology Institute of the Veterinary Medicine College of Hanover, Germany were used. The technique was performed in two stages, screening and titration, and a sample was considered positive when it presented a titer ≥10 for BVDV and ≥2 for BoHV-1. The neutralizing antibodies titers were considered the reciprocal of the higher serum dilutions capable of inhibiting the viral replication and the consequent production of cytopathic effect of BVDV and BoHV-1. The infectious titer ($TCID_{50:}$ infective doses for 50% of cell cultures) used was $10^{5.61}TCID_{50}/50$ μL for BVDV and $10^{6.25}$ $TCID_{50}/50$ μL for BoHV-1, determined by the Reed and Müench method [28].

Herd-level case definition

The herd-level case definition was based on the size of the population (cows aged ≥24 months), number of females sampled, an intra-herd apparent prevalence of 50%, and the sensitivity and specificity of the virus-neutralization test of 95 and 99.5% for BVDV [29] and 94.4% and 93.2% for BoHV-1 [30], respectively, with the goal of obtaining a herd sensitivity and specificity of ≥90%. After simulations using Herdacc software, a herd was deemed positive for BVDV when at least one positive animal was detected, and for BoHV-1 infection, a herd was considered positive if it included at least one

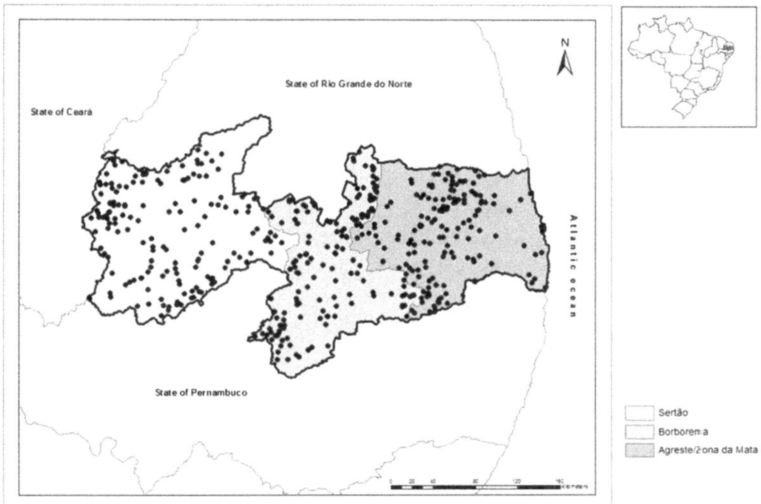

Fig. 1 Spatial localization of cattle herds in the State of Paraíba, Northeastern Brazil, according to sampling stratum. Detail shows Paraíba state within Brazil

positive animal in herds of up to seven females; two positive animals in herds of 8–99 females; and three positive animals in herds with more than 99 females.

Apparent prevalence calculations

EpiInfo 6.04 software was used to calculate the apparent prevalences and respective confidence intervals [31]. Stratified random sampling was used to calculate the herd-level prevalence in the state of Paraíba [32]. The required parameters were as follows: (a) condition of the herd (positive or negative), (b) sampling stratum to which the herd belonged, and (c) statistical weight. The statistical weight was determined by applying the following formula [31]:

$$Weight = \frac{\text{number of herds in the stratum}}{\text{number of herds sampled in the stratum}}$$

The calculation of the herd-prevalence per sampling stratum employed the sampling design of a simple random sample by using the following parameters: (a) number of positive herds and (b) number of herds sampled in the stratum.

Spatial analysis

Identification of the herd, geographical coordinates and results of serological tests were included in a database for spatial analysis. Firstly, the Cuzick–Edwards' k-nearest neighbor method [33] was used to detect the possibility of spatial clustering at herd level using the ClusterSeer 2.5.1 software (BioMedware, Ann Arbor, MI, United States). Existence of potential spatial clustering was analyzed at each of the first 10 neighborhood levels, and the overall p-value was adjusted for multiple comparisons with the Simes approach. In a second step, scan statistics by the SatScan software version 9.0 [34] was used to identify local clusters of positive herds. A Bernoulli model was applied, the scanning window was circular, and the spatial size of scan window was limited to 25% of the total population. Because of the high herd-level prevalences for BVDV and BoHV-1, analysis was not run on herd-level, and then considering within-herd prevalence. The statistical significance level was set as 0.05 and the maps were constructed with the ArcGIS software.

The kriging method was used to estimate the spatial pattern of apparent within-herd prevalence of BoHV-1 and BVDV. By this method, it is possible to produce a smooth surface of predicted prevalence and a map of prediction variance [35]. Kriging is based on the spatial correlation between measurements which is modelled by the semivariogram, and work well on stationary and non-stationary rates [36]. Directional semivariograms in four directions (north, north-east, east, south-east) were fitted to test for anisotropy. It was used an exponential model described below and fitted to the sample semivariogram [35]:

$$\gamma(d) = C_o + C\left(1- \exp\left(-\frac{d}{a}\right)\right)$$

where the parameters were nugget (c_o), partial sill (c), and range (a).

Results

Figure 1 shows the spatial location of the herds in the state of Paraíba. The herd-level prevalence for BVDV and BoHV-1 infections in Paraíba were, respectively, 65.5% (95% CI: 61.1–69.7) and 87.8% (95% CI: 84.5–90.5) (Table 1). Two proprieties were excluded because they showed errors in their geographic coordinates, totaling 476 herds used in the spatial analysis. Figure 2 shows the spatial localization of positive and negative herds for BVDV (Fig. 2a) and BoHV-1 (Fig. 2b). The average apparent within-herd prevalence of BVDV was 31.8%, ranging from 0% to 100%, and for BoHV-1 it was 62.4% ranging from 0% to 100%. Figures 3 and 4 show the kriging estimate of the apparent within-herd prevalences for BVDV and BoHV-1, respectively.

Sample semivariograms with fitted exponential model are shown in Fig. 5. For BVDV, parameters were: nugget = 0.02, partial sill = 0.10, and range = 13.9 km; and for BoHV-1, parameters were: nugget = 0.01, partial sill = 0.10, and range = 13.0 km. The predicted prevalence was highest (0.42–0.75) for BVDV (Fig. 3a) in the west, north and eastern part of Sertão and in the central and eastern part of Agreste/Zona da Mata. For BoHV-1 (Fig. 4a), the

Table 1 Census data of the cattle population in the State of Paraíba, Northeastern Brazil, according to sampling stratum, and herd-level prevalence for BVDV and BoHV-1

Sampling stratum	No. of herds	Tested	BVDV			BoHV-1		
			Positive	Prevalence	95% CI	Positive	Prevalence	95% CI
Sertão	24,356	159	118	74.2	[66.8–80.4]	145	91.2	[85.6–94.7]
Borborema	11,603	160	79	49.4	[41.7–57.1]	130	81.3	[74.4–86.6]
Agreste/Zona da Mata	18,398	159	102	64.2	[56.4–71.3]	139	87.4	[81.3–91.8]
Stateof Paraíba	54,357	478	299	65.5	[61.1–69.7]	414	87.8	[84.5–90.5]

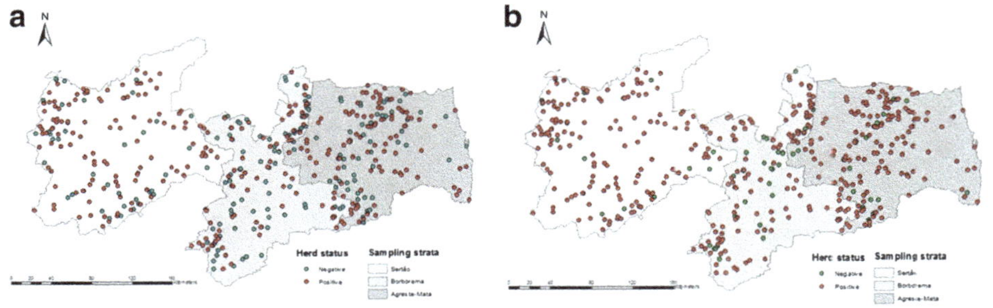

Fig. 2 Spatial localization of positive and negative herds in the State of Paraíba, Northeastern Brazil: **a** Herd status of BVDV **b** Herd status of BoHV-1

highest predicted prevalence (0.74–0.97) was in some local areas across Sertão and thoughout the eastern part of Agreste/Zona da Mata. The prediction variance reflects the location of tested herds: low values in the western part of Sertão and north, central and southern part of Agreste/ Zona da Mata for BVDV (Fig. 3b) and north and central part of Agreste/Zona da Mata for BoHV-1 (Fig. 4b), where herd density was high.

The Cuzick–Edwards' test identified statistically significant ($P < 0.05$) spatial clustering of BVDV and BoHV-1 cases at $k = 18$ and $k = 7$ neighborhood levels, respectively. Using Bernoulli model, six significant clusters were detected for BVDV and one significant cluster for BoHV-1 (Table 2, Fig. 6). There was no spatial overlap among clusters. For BVDV, a primary cluster covered the eastern Sertão region, with 11 herds, radius of 24.10 km and the risk for infection was 2.21 (relative risk (RR) = 2.21; $P < 0.001$) times higher in herds located inside cluster than in those located elsewhere. The others significant BVDV clusters were smaller, involving one or two herds in Agreste/Zona da Mata region, near the border of the Borborema mesoregion, however, with a high relative risk. The BoHV-1 cluster covered the Agreste/Zona da Mata region with a radius of 77.17 km and a relative risk of 1.27 ($P < 0.001$), with 103 cases.

Discussion

In Brazil, prevalence rates of BVDV range from 22.2% to 85.4% [18, 37, 38], and seropositivity frequencies of BoHV-1 between 18% and 90% were frequently observed in non-vaccinated herds throughout the different geographical areas of Brazil [39–41]. In the Northeastern Brazil, seroprevalences for BVDV infection of 72.6% [42] and 51.1% in family farms [43] in Pernambuco state, and for BoHV-1 infection of 79.5% [44] also in Pernambuco state, 62.67% [45] in Sertão of Paraíba and 63.23% [46] in Maranhão state have been reported. The herd-level seroprevalences for BVDV (65.5%) and BoHV-1 (87.8%) estimated for Paraíba state in this survey indicate that these viruses are present in most herds of the state.

In this work, six significant clusters were detected for BVDV infection and one significant cluster for BoHV-1. Similar results were found by kriging and SatScan for identification of risk areas (location of areas with high apparent within-herd prevalence) for BVDV and BoHV-1 infections: the western part of Sertão for BVDV and the western part of Agreste/ Zona da Mata for BoHV-1.

The primary cluster for BVDV was detected in the Sertão region, with a radius of 24.10 km, and covering its eastern region. The Sertão was the stratum of higher prevalence for BVDV and is bordered on the north by Rio Grande do Norte state, west by Ceará

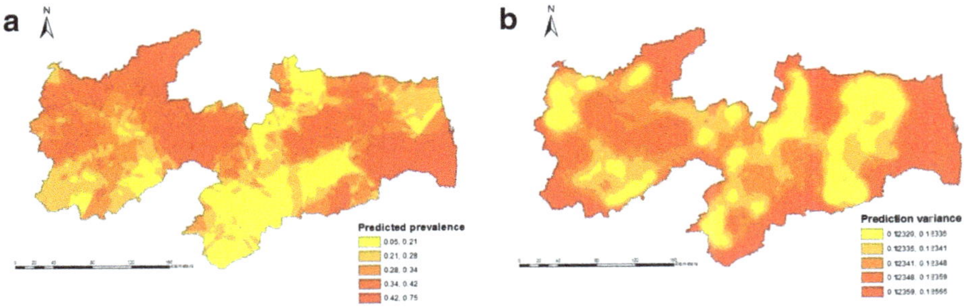

Fig. 3 Apparent within-herd prevalences for BVDV in the State of Paraíba, Northeastern Brazil: **a**) Kriging surface of predicted apparent prevalence and (**b**) the variance of kriging estimates of predicted apparent prevalence

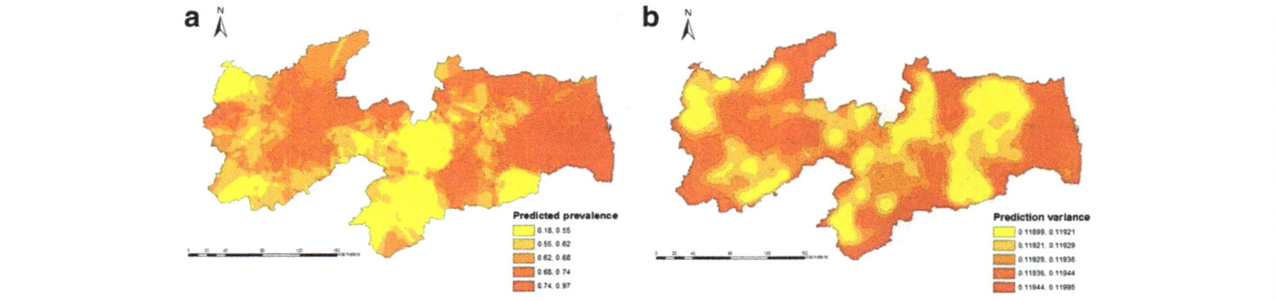

Fig. 4 Apparent within-herd prevalences for BoHV-1 in the State of Paraíba, Northeastern Brazil: **a** Kriging surface of predicted apparent prevalence and (**b**) the variance of kriging estimates of predicted apparent prevalence

state, and south by Pernambuco state. Border regions are always associated as risk factors, since in these regions there are large circulations of animals due to intense trade and often without knowledge of the health status of animals [47–49]. This circumstance corroborates what happens in the Sertão, where most of the properties are familiar or subsistence, predominating the mixed exploration, semi-confined farming, low technification and no veterinary assistance [50], increasing the risk in the herds of these properties.

Furthermore, recently BVDV was isolated in a herd in Pombal, a municipality of the Sertão mesoregion [51]. Knowing that PI animals are the main sources of infection of BVDV, and animal purching and pasture rental were identified as risk factors associated with herd-level seroprevalence for BVDV infection in the State of Paraíba [52], it is important to consider that the cluster for BVDV may have PI herds. Ersbøll et al. [53] in a study on the dynamics of BVDV infection among neighboring herds in Denmark found that the presence of PI-herds increased the risk of a herd becoming infected (PI-herd), showing *odds ratios* (OR) of 1.37, 1.40 and 1.70 for 1, 2, and ≥3 PI-herds in the neighborhood, respectively, as well as the risk of becoming a PI-herd was negatively associated with the mean distance from the neighboring herds (OR = 0.7 for an increase of 1 km), concluding that the occurrence of PI-herd in a certain area has influence on the risk of a neighbor herd becoming infected.

In Brazil, Hein et al. [54] found two BVDV clusters of dairy herds in the Arroio do Meio region, Rio Grande do Sul state, a primary (P = 0.391) and a secondary (P = 0.773) by scanning analysis, but both without statistical significance. According to the author, the occurrence of no association may have been due to the scan test limitation or because transmission of the virus via aerosols or other vehicles is not an effective way to disseminate. Kirchgessner et al. [55] in an exploratory cluster analysis identified clusters in different locations for domestic livestock and white-tailed deer in New York state, United States, suggesting that BVDV is maintained independently in domestic livestock herds in the western part of the state and in the white-tailed deer population in the northwestern part. According to the authors, the spatial point pattern analyses provide information

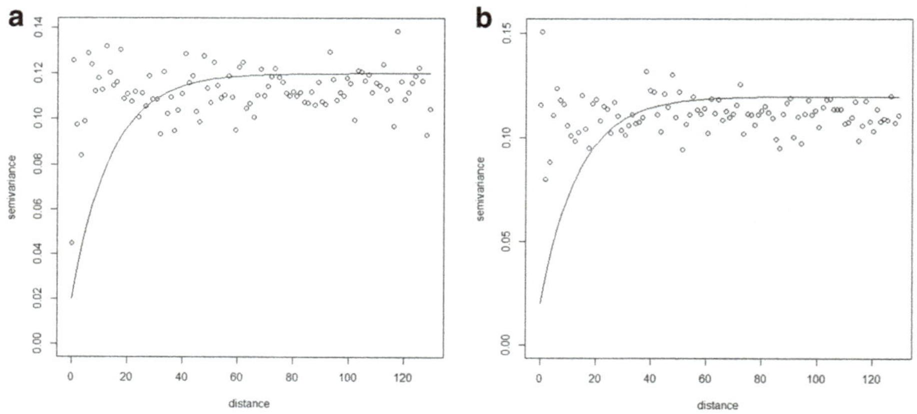

Fig. 5 Sample semivariograms with fitted model (solid line) used to generate kriging surface of predicted within-herd prevalence of BVDV (**a**) and BoHV-1 (**b**)

Table 2 Statistically significant clusters of herds with a high within-herd prevalence of BVDV and BoHV-1 in the state of Paraíba, Northeastern Brazil

Radius (km)	No. of herds in cluster	No. of cases in cluster		RR[a]	*p*-value
		Observed	Expected		
BVDV					
24.10[b]	11	55	25.87	2.21	< 0.001
2.11	2	8	2.59	3.11	0.045
0	1	13	4.53	2.90	0.004
0	1	10	3.23	3.12	0.005
0	1	10	3.23	3.12	0.005
0	1	10	3.23	3.12	0.005
BoHV-1					
77.17	103	359	297.39	1.27	< 0.001

[a]Relative risk
[b]Primary cluster

necessary for the epidemiological risk assessment that should precede the development of any regional BVDV management plan.

The significant BoHV-1 cluster ($P < 0.001$) showed a radius of 77.17 km with 103 herds whose 359 animals were positive when it was expected 297 positive animals, and involved a large part of the Agreste/Zona da Mata stratum, which has a high herd-level prevalence (87.4%). Despite the seroprevalence is high throughout the state, the presence of a significant BoHV-1 cluster requires epidemiological interpretation of its spatial distribution and, consequently, the decisions based on that evidence [56]. The mesoregions of Agreste and Zona da Mata had the highest rainfall in the state and a bovine livestock characterized by dairy farms and predominant confined rearing [50]. Miranda et al. [57] detected BoHV-1 clusters in southeastern Brazil and observed that disease clusters may occur either because herds share common risk factors or via transmission between herds through the movement of infected animals. The high prevalence of BoHV-1 in the Agreste/Zona da Mata stratum and the presence of cluster suggest that the relationship between the cases and the spread of the virus is due to the proximity of the animals in the herd [20]. BoHV-1 clusters were detected in the state of Rio Grande do Sul, in which the most significant ($P = 0.00027$) had a radius of 122.33 km, with 173 properties, 109 positive animals, and RR of 1.31, showing a moderate presence of BoHV-1 infection in the southern herds [20].

In addition to the presence of PI animals for BVDV infection and purchasing untested cattle, other environmental or management factors may be influencing the intra and inter herd transmission for both infections in the state of Paraíba, mainly in high-risk areas. Such factors could be the lack of biosafety procedures in herds, extensive breeding, mixing cattle of different ages and from multiple sources, communal grazing and absence of vaccination.

In the risk mapping described in this study, there is a significant relation between the spatial effect and the development of the diseases, indicating that there are some important predisposing factors in the occurrence of infections studied. The herds of Paraíba and neighbor's

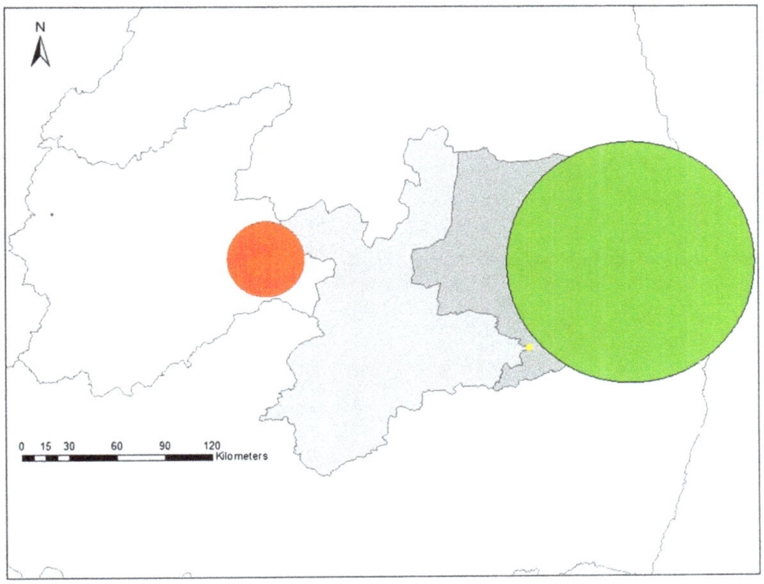

Fig. 6 Significant clusters of herds with a high apparent within-herd prevalence of BVDV (primary cluster: red, secondary clusters: yellow) and BoHV-1 (green)

states might be sharing common risk factors or transmission routes among herds through the movement of infected animals, animal purchasing without the knowledge of the health status of animals, pasture rental, or absence of permanent veterinary assistance.

There may be other variables not considered in this work that can determine the spatial distribution pattern for both BVDV and BoHV-1 infections in a particular area. These variables may be potential risk factors that influence a higher risk of disease in areas of greater spatial effect, therefore, further works should be considered.

Conclusions

The spatial analysis enabled the identification of spatial clustering of risk for BVDV and BoHV-1 in the state of Paraíba. The clusters detected contemplated different areas of the state, with BVDV cluster located in the Sertão stratum and BoHV-1 in Agreste/Zona da Mata stratum. Through the risk mapping, it was possible to identify the areas in which the risk is significantly elevated, coinciding with areas where there are borders with other states and in which there is a high movement of animals. Clusters detection analysis enabled a better view of the occurrence of the BoHV-1 and BVDV and its result indicates the highest risk areas in the state of Paraíba, facilitating control strategies for specific actions and directed to those areas.

Abbreviations

BoHV-1: Bovine Herpesvirus type 1; BVDV: Bovine Viral Diarrhea Virus; GPS: global positioning system; OR: odds ratio; PI: persistently infected; RR: Risk Relative; SEDAP: Agricultural and Livestock Defense Service of the State of Paraíba; $TCID_{50}$: 50% Tissue culture Infective Dose

Acknowledgements

The authors would like to thank the SEDAP for help during the sample collection.

Funding

This study was funded by the Conselho Nacional de Desenvolvimento Científico e Tecnológico (CNPq), under the codes 471571/2011-3, 302131/2012-4, and 476596/2013-0.

Authors' contributions

LF conducted the serological diagnosis tests and drafted the manuscript. EP, AR and ES conducted the serological diagnosis tests. IC, AM, CS and CA conducted the field activities and study design, and were involved in the preparation of the methods. SA conceived the study, participated in its design and coordination of the study and performed the spatial analysis. All authors read and approved the final manuscript.

Consent for publication

Not applicable.

Competing interests

The authors declare that they have no competing interests.

Author details

[1]Laboratory of Transmissible Diseases, Academic Unit of Veterinary Medicine, Center of Rural Technology and Health, Federal University of Campina Grande, Patos, PB 58700-970, Brazil. [2]Laboratory of Bovidae Viruses, Biological Institute, São Paulo, SP 04014-900, Brazil. [3]Department of Veterinary Medicine, Federal University of Paraíba, Areia, PB 58397-000, Brazil.

References

1. Del Fava C, Pituco EM, D'Angelo JL. Herpesvírus bovino tipo 1 (HVB-1): revisão e situação atual no Brasil. Rev Educ Cont Vet Med Zootec2002;5:300–312.
2. Del Fava C, Arcaro JRP, Pozzi CR, Júnior IA, Fagundes H. Manejo sanitário para o controle de doenças da reprodução em um sistema leiteiro de produção semi-intensivo. Arq Inst Biol. 2003;70:25–33.
3. Junqueira JRC, Freitas JC, Alfieri AF, Alfieri AA. Reproductive performance evaluation of a beef cattle herd naturally infected with the BoHV-1, BVDV and *Leptospira hardjo*. Semin: Cien Agrar. 2006;27:471–80.
4. Rodning SP, Givens MD, Marley MSD, Zhang Y, Riddell KP. Reproductive and economic impact following controlled introduction of cattle persistently infected with bovine viral diarrhea virus into a naive group of heifers. Theriogenology 2012; https://doi.org/10.1016/j.theriogenology.2012.05.031.
5. Newcomer BW, Givens D. Diagnosis and control of viral diseases of reproductive importance: Infectious Bovine Rhinotracheitis and Bovine Viral Diarrhea Vet Clin North Am - Food Anim Pract 2016; https://doi.org/10.1016/j.cvfa.2016.01.011.
6. Lanyon SR, Hill FI, Reichel MP, Brownlie J. Bovine viral diarrhoea: pathogenesis and diagnosis. Vet J. 2014; https://doi.org/10.1016/j.tvjl.2013.07.024.
7. McClurkin AW, Littledike ET, Cutlip RC, Frank GH, Coria MF, Bolin SR. Production of cattle immunotolerant to bovine viral diarrhea virus. Can J Comp Med. 1984;48:156–61.
8. Rüfenacht J, Schaller P, Audigé L, Knutti B, Küpfer U, Peterhans E. The effect of infection with bovine viral diarrhea virus on the fertility of Swiss dairy cattle. Theriogenology. 2001;56:199–210.
9. Presi P, Heim D. BVD eradication in Switzerland — a new approach. Vet Microbiol 2010; https://doi.org/10.1016/j.vetmic.2009.09.054.
10. Hay KE, Ambrose RCK, Morton JM, Horwood PF, Gravel JL, Waldron S, et al. Effects of exposure to bovine viral diarrhoea virus 1 on risk of bovine respiratory disease in Australian feedlot cattle. Prev Vet Med. 2016; https://doi.org/10.1016/j.prevetmed.2016.01.025.
11. Nandi S, Kumar M, Manohar M, Chauhan RS. Bovine herpes virus infections in cattle. Anim Health Res Rev. 2009;10:85–98.
12. Biswas S, Bandyopadhyay S, Dimri U, Patra PH. Bovine herpesvirus-1 (BHV-1) – a re-emerging concern in livestock : a revisit to its biology, epidemiology, diagnosis, and prophylaxis.Vet Q 2013; https://doi.org/10.1080/016e52176.2013.799301.
13. Raaperi K, Nurmoja I, Orro T, Viltrop A. Seroepidemiology of bovine herpesvirus 1 (BHV1) infection among Estonian dairy herds and risk factors for the spread within herds. Prev Vet Med. 2010; https://doi.org/10.1016/j.prevetmed.2010.06.001.
14. Raaperi K, Orro T, Viltrop A. Epidemiology and control of bovine herpesvirus 1 infection in Europe. Vet J 2014; https://doi.org/10.1016/j.tvjl.2014.05.040.
15. Lucchese L, Benkirane A, Hakimi I, Idrissi A El. Seroprevalence study of the main causes of abortion in dairy cattle in Morocco. Vet Ital 2016; https://doi.org/10.12834/VetIt.388.1813.1
16. Affonso IB, Amoril JG, Alexandrino B, Buzinar, MG, Medeiros ASR, Samara SI, Anticorpos contra o Herpesvírus Bovino Tipo 1 (BoHV-1) nas dez regiões de planejamento do estado de Goiás, Brasil. Ci Anim Bras 2010; https://doi.org/10.5216/cab.v11i4.6318.
17. Fino TCM, De Melo CB, Ramos AF, Leite RC. Diarréia bovina a vírus (BVD) - uma breve revisão. Rev Bras Med Vet. 2012;34:131–40.
18. Flores EF, Weiblen R, Cargnelutti JF, Bauermann V, Spilki FR, Mori E, et al. Emerging animal viruses: real threats or simple bystanders? Pesq Vet Bras. 2013;33:1161–73.
19. Thompson JA, Leite RMH, Gonçalves VSP, Leite RC, Bandeira DA, Herrmann GP, et al. Spatial and hierarchical variances and age covariances for seroprevalence to *Leptospira interrogans* serovar hardjo, BoHV-1 and BVDV

for cattle in state of Paraíba, Brazil. Prev Vet Med. 2006; https://doi.org/10.1016/j.prevetmed.2006.05.010.
20. Carpenter TE. Methods to investigate spatial and temporal clustering in veterinary epidemiology. Prev Vet Med. 2001; https://doi.org/10.1016/S0167-5877(00)00199-9.
21. Silva GS, Machado G, Santiago Neto W, Hein HE, Santos DV, Medeiros AAR, et al. Estudo de prevalência e análise espacial de varredura do herpesvírus bovino no estado do Rio Grande do Sul (BoHV-1). In: 2° Encontro Nacional de Epidemiologia Veterinária. Biológico. 2015;77(Suppl 1):11–64. http://www.biologico.sp.gov.br/uploads/docs/bio/suplementos/v77_supl_1/54.pdf. Accessed 07 Feb 2017
22. Cabrera AL, Willink A. Biogeografía de America Latina. Organización de los Estados Americanos: Washington; 1973.
23. Andrade-Lima D. The Caatinga dominium. Rev Bras Bot. 1981;4:149–53.
24. Batista JS, Riet-Correa F, Teixeira MMG, Madruga CR, Simões SDV, Maia TF. Trypanosomiasis by Trypanosomavivax in cattle in the Brazilian semiarid: description of an outbreak and lesions in the nervous system. Vet Parasitol. 2007;143:174–81.
25. IBGE. Instituto Brasileiro de Geografia e Estatística (IBGE). Censo agropecuário 2006. http://www.ibge.gov.br/estadosat/temas.php?sigla=pb&tema=censoagro. (2006). Accessed 07 Feb 2017.
26. OIE, World Organization for Animal Health. Bovine Viral Diarrhea. In: Manual of Diagnostic Tests and Vaccines for Terrestrial Animals. http://www.oie.int/fileadmin/Home/eng/Health_standards/tahm/2.04.07_BVD.pdf (2015) Accessed 07 Feb 2017.
27. OIE, World Organization for Animal Health. Infectious Bovine Rhinotracheitis/ Infectious Pustular Vulvovaginitis. In: Manual of Diagnostic Tests and Vaccines for Terrestrial Animals, http://www.oie.int/fileadmin/Home/eng/Health_standards/tahm/2.04.12_IBR_IPV.pdf (2010). Accessed 07 Feb 2017.
28. Reed LJ, Muench HA. Simple method of estimating fifty percent endpoints. Am J Hyg. 1938;27:493–7.
29. Corbett EM, Grooms DL, Bolin SR, Bartlett B, Grotelueschen DM, Corbett EM, et al. Use of sentinel serology in a bovine viral diarrhea virus eradication program. J Vet Diagn Investig 2011; https://doi.org/10.1177/1040638711403412.
30. Cárdenas AB, Arango CJJ, Maya JJM, Hirose JAM, Bernal AO. Comparison between three diagnostic tests to detect abortion caused by infectious bovine rhinotracheitis in dairy herds. Vet Méx. 2006;2:151–63.
31. Dean AG, Dean JA, Coulombier D, Brendel KA, Smith DC, Burton AH, et al. Epi info, version 6: a word processing, database, and statistics program for public health on IBM compatible microcomputers. Atlanta: Center for Diseases Control and Prevention; 1996. file:///C:/Users/Sergio%20Santos/Downloads/cdc_23189_DS1.pdf.
32. Thrusfield M. Veterinary epidemiology. 3rd ed. Oxford: Blackwell Science; 2007.
33. Cuzick J, Edwards R. Spatial clustering for inhomogeneous populations. J R Statist Soc B. 1990;52:73–104.
34. Kulldorff M, Nagarwalla N. Spatial disease clusters: detection and inference. Stat Med. 1995;14:799–810.
35. Bihrmann K, Nielsen SS, Toft N, Ersbøll AK. Spatial differences in occurrence of paratuberculosis in Danish dairy herds and in control programme participation. Prev Vet Med. 2012;103:112–9.
36. Gotway CA, Wolfinger RD. Spatial prediction of counts and rates. Stat Med. 2003;22:1415–32.
37. Quincozes CG, Fischer G, Hübner SDO, Vargas GDA, Vidor T, Brod CS. Prevalence and factors associated with bovine viral diarrhea virus infection in south of Rio Grande do Sul. Semina: Ciên Agrár. 2007;2:269–76.
38. Almeida LL, Miranda ICS, Hein HE, Neto WS, Costa EF, Marks FS, et al. Herd-level risk factors for bovine viral diarrhea virus infection in dairy herds from southern Brazil. Res Vet Sci 2013; https://doi.org/10.1016/j.rvsc.2013.08.009.
39. Lovato LT, Weiblen R, Tobias FL, Moraes MP. Herpesvírus bovino tipo 1: inquérito soro-epidemiológico no rebanho leiteiro do Estado do Rio Grande do Sul. Brasil Ciênc Rural. 1995;25:425–30.
40. Takiuchi E, Alfieri AF, Alfieri AA. Bovine herpervirus type 1: infection and diagnosis methods. Semina: Ciên Agrár. 2001;1:203–9.
41. Dias JA, Alfieri AA, Gonc VSP. Seroprevalence and Risk factors of bovine herpesvirus 1 infection in cattle herds in the state of Parana. Transbound Emerg Dis 2013; https://doi.org/10.1111/j.1865-1682.2012.01316.x
42. Castro RS, Melo LEH, Abreu SRA, Muniz AMM, Albuquerque APS. Anticorpos neutralizantes contra pestivírus em soros bovinos do Estado de Pernambuco. Pesq Agropec Bras. 1993;28:1327–31.
43. Rêgo JMP, Batista Filho AFB, Oliveira PRF, Borges JM, França CAB, Ribeiro CP, et al. Epidemiological analysis of infection by the bovine viral diarrhea virus on family farms in Brazil. Semina: Ciên Agrár 2016; https://doi.org/10.5433/1679-0359.2016v37n6p4119.
44. Silva FS, Oliveira JMB, Batista Filho AFB, Ribeiro CP, Pituco EM, Pinheiro Junior JW. Seroepidemiological survey of infection bovine herpesvirus type 1 (BoHV-1) in cattle in the state of Pernambuco. Acta Sci Vet. 2015;55:1–11.
45. Melo CB, Azevedo EO, Alfaro AEP, Lobato ZIP, Lobato FCF, Leite RC. Anticorpos neutralizantes contra herpesvirus bovino 1 (HVB 1) em bovinos do sertão da Paraíba. Ciênc Vet Tróp. 1999;2:43–4.
46. Freitas EJP, Lopes CER, Moura Filho JM, Sá JS Santos HP, Pereira HM. Frequency of antibodies against bovine herpesvirus type 1 (BoHV-1) in beef cattle not vaccinated. Semina: Ciên Agrár. 2014; https://doi.org/10.5433/1679-0359.2014v35n3p1301.
47. Alban L, Stryhn H, Kjeldsen AM, Ersboll AK, Skjoth F, Christensen J, et al. Estimating transfer of bovine virus-diarrhoea virus in Danish cattle by use of register data. Prev Vet Med. 2001;52:133–46.
48. Gates MC, Woolhouse MEJ, Gunn GJ, Humphry RW. Relative associations of cattle movements, local spread, and biosecurity with bovine viral diarrhoea virus (BVDV) seropositivity in beef and dairy herds. Prev Vet Med. 2013; https://doi.org/10.1016/j.prevetmed.2013.07.017.
49. Gates MC, Humphry RW, Gunn GJ, Woolhouse MEJ. Not all cows are epidemiologically equal : quantifying the risks of bovine viral diarrhoea virus (BVDV) transmission through cattle movements. Vet Res 2014; https://doi.org/10.1186/s13567-014-0110-y.
50. Clementino IJ, Pimenta CLRM, Fernandes LG, Bezerra CDS, Alves CJ, Dias RA, et al. Characterization of cattle raising in Paraíba state, northeastern Brazil. Semina: Ciên Agrár. 2015; https://doi.org/10.5433/1679-0359.2015v36n1p557.
51. Weber MN, Silveira S, Machado G, Groff FHS, Mósena ACS, Budaszewski RF, et al. High frequency of bovine viral diarrhea virus type 2 in southern Brazil. Virus Res 2014; https://doi.org/10.1016/j.virusres.2014.07.035.
52. Fernandes LG, De Campos Nogueira AH, De Stefano E, Pituco EM, Ribeiro CP, et al. Herd-level prevalence and risk factors for bovine viral diarrhea virus infection in cattle in the state of Paraíba, northeastern Brazil. Trop Anim Health Prod 2015; https://doi.org/10.1007/s11250-015-0937-x.
53. Ersbøll AK, Ersbøll BK, Houe H, Alban L, Kjeldsen AM. Spatial modelling of the between-herd infection dynamics of bovine virus diarrhoea virus (BVDV) in dairy herds in Denmark. Preev Vet Mec 2010; https://doi.org/10.1016/j.eprevetmed.2010.08.004.
54. Hein HE, Payão C, Costa EDF, Almeida LL, Gustavo L. Análise espacial de Diarréia Viral Bovina (BVD) em propriedades leiteiras na região de Arroio do Meio (RS). 2008. http://www.lume.ufrgs.br/handle/10183/45529. Accessed 07 Feb 2017.
55. Kirchgessner MS, Dubovi EJ, Whipps CM. Spatial point pattern analyses of bovine viral diarrhea virus infection in domestic livestock herds and concomitant seroprevalence in wild white-tailed deer (*Odocoileus virginianus*) in New York state, USA. J Vet Diagn Investig 2013; https://doi.org/10.1177/1040638713479121.
56. Ávila LN, Perez AM, Neto JSF, Ferreira F, Telles EO, Dias RA, et al. Análise de detecção de cluster na caracterização espaço- temporal da tuberculose bovina no Estado da Bahia. Pesq Vet Bras. 2013;33:1313–8.
57. Miranda ICS, Hein HE, Costa EF, Machado G, Neto WS, Marks FS, et al. Prevalence survey and spatial analysis of bovine herpesvirus. In: International Symposia on veterinary epidemiology and economics (ISVEE). 2012. http://www.sciquest.org.nz/node/81153. Accessed 07 Feb 2017.

10

In silico and phylogenetic analyses of partial *BbRAP-1*, *BbCP2*, *BbSBP-4* and *BbβTUB* gene sequences of *Babesia bovis* isolates from cattle in South Africa

Phillip Senzo Mtshali[1] and Moses Sibusiso Mtshali[1,2*]

Abstract

Background: Bovine babesiosis is one of the most economically important tick-borne diseases threatening the livestock industry globally including South Africa. This disease is induced by members of *Babesia bovis* species. Antigenic variations among geographical strains of *B. bovis*, and these heterogeneities are cited as the mechanism by which parasites evade from host immune system and they hamper the successful development of a single vaccine that could confer absolute protection. Given the economic importance of livestock industry in South Africa, the extent of genetic diversity among field isolates of *B. bovis* merits extensive investigation.

In this study, we genetically characterized partial genes of *B. bovis* and studied the phylogenetic relationship among *B. bovis* isolates of South African origin. The genes, which were PCR-amplified from bovine samples collected from different locations across South Africa, coded for rhoptry-associated protein 1 (*BbRAP-1*), cysteine peptidase 2 (*BbCP2*), spherical body protein 4 (*BbSBP-4*) and β-tubulin (*BbβTUB*). Phylogenies were inferred from newly determined sequences using the neighbour-joining approach.

Results: Nested PCR assays with gene-specific primers indicated that, of the 54 bovine samples tested, 59.3% (32/54; 95% CI = 46.0–71.3%), 27.8% (15/54; 95% CI = 17.6–40.9%), 37.0% (20/54; 95% CI = 25.4–50.4%) and 29.6% (16/54; 95% CI = 19.1–42.8%) possessed *BbRAP-1*, *BbCP2*, *BbSBP-4* and *BbβTUB* fragments, respectively. Sequencing of PCR-generated fragments revealed that nucleotide sequences of each of the four genes were highly conserved among the *B. bovis* isolates examined. Phylogenetic analyses of *BbCP2*, *BbSBP-4* and *BbβTUB* sequences indicated a close phylogenetic relatedness among South African-derived sequences and those of global *B. bovis* strains.

Conclusion: The data reported in this study indicated that there is a high conservation among the genes of *B. bovis* isolates from cattle in South Africa. These findings give an indication that immunologically important proteins encoded by these genes could potentially be considered for exploitation as viable candidates for inclusion in recombinant subunit vaccines.

Keywords: *Babesia bovis*, Cattle, South Africa, Nested PCR assays, Phylogenies

* Correspondence: sibusiso.mtshali@nrf.ac.za
[1]Veterinary Parasitology Programme, Research and Scientific Services Department, National Zoological Gardens of South Africa, Pretoria 0001, South Africa
[2]Parasitology Research Programme, Department of Zoology and Entomology, University of the Free State, QwaQwa Campus, Phuthaditjhaba 9866, South Africa

Background

Babesia bovis is an intraerythrocytic protozoan parasite and an important aetiological agent of bovine babesiosis. This tick-borne disease is considered an economically important constraint to livestock production in tropical and subtropical regions of the world [1]. While *B. bigemina* (another agent of babesiosis) can be transmitted by both *Rhipicephalus microplus* and *R. decoloratus*, the confirmed tick vector of *B. bovis* in southern Africa is *R. microplus* [2].

Cattle infected by *B. bovis* are characterized by high fever, ataxia, anorexia and sometimes nervous signs [3]. Further, *B. bovis* remains the most pathogenic microorganism compared to other *Babesia* species and induces a more severe disease due to the sequestration of infected red blood cells in cerebral capillaries, thus resulting in parasitaemia levels of less than 1% in the circulating blood [4, 5]. On the other hand, the disease caused by *B. bigemina* is milder and is characterized by anaemia, fever and haemoglobinuria. Infections by *B. bigemina* do not involve sequestration of infected red blood cells and the levels of parasitaemia in blood often exceed 10% [3]. Therefore, it remains pivotal that effective control measures are implemented in an endeavour to curtail cattle mortalities resulting from *Babesia* infections.

In South Africa, vaccination against *B. bovis* is a method that is widely exploited to immunize cattle against babesiosis. This follows that the cattle which recover from primary acute infection remain persistently infected and serve as reservoirs for parasite transmission to other animals [4]. Nevertheless, it is worth noting that the available vaccines are based on bovine blood infected with live attenuated strains of the parasite [6, 7]. Although these vaccines confer protective immunity, the major limitation associated with the use of attenuated vaccines relate to the possible transmission of other blood-borne pathogens [6]. In addition, the production of live vaccines requires artificial infection of cattle in order to attain high parasitaemia levels in the blood, and this often constitutes important ethical implications [8].

According to Torina et al. [9], the success in the development of vaccines against babesial infections is impeded by the presence of heterogeneities in some parasite proteins. In particular, studies are focused on surface proteins that can confer high level of protection and better safety in comparison to currently used vaccines [10]. Many of these proteins might play a crucial role in erythrocyte invasion and are therefore the targets for vaccine development [9]. Several genes encoding these *B. bovis* proteins with immunogenic potential are known, and thanks to the complete genome sequencing of an American *B. bovis* T2Bo strain that these surface proteins were identified [11]. However, it must be acknowledged that there is still a dearth of information regarding the conservation of genes encoding potential immunogenic proteins in South African isolates of *B. bovis*.

In this context, the present study was borne out of the need to characterize the genes encoding rhoptry-associated protein 1 (*BbRAP-1*), cysteine peptidase 2 (*BbCP2*), spherical body protein 4 (*BbSBP-4*) and β-tubulin (*BbβTUB*) in *B. bovis* isolates from South African field bovine samples.

Methods

Blood samples

Field bovine samples ($n = 54$) were randomly selected to validate the nested PCR assays developed in this study. These samples form part of the sample collection of the Veterinary Parasitology Programme (National Zoological Gardens of South Africa: NZG, South Africa), and the collection of these samples was approved by the NZG Research Ethics and Scientific Committee. Animal owners gave verbal informed consent for the collection of the samples for the epidemiological survey, and animals were not involved in any clinical trials or treatments. All blood samples were maintained at −20°C prior to DNA extraction.

DNA extraction

Genomic DNA was extracted using ZR Genomic DNA™-Tissue MiniPrep kit (Zymo Research Corporation, Irvine, CA, USA) according to the manufacturer's instructions. DNA quantification was performed using a NanoDrop® ND-1000 (NanoDrop Technologies Inc., Wilmington, USA).

Primer design

Nested PCR primers used for amplifying *B. bovis*-specific *BbRAP-1* genes from bovine samples were reported previously [12]. Primers targeting *BbCP2*, *BbSBP-4* and *BbβTUB* genes were created with Primer-BLAST program of the NCBI using reference sequences BBOV_IV007730 (GenBank accession number XM_001610645), BBOV_IV005390 (XM_001610418) and BBOV_III004850 (XM_001611566), respectively. All primers shown in Table 1 were synthesized by Inqaba Biotechnical Industries (Pretoria, South Africa).

Amplification of genes

PCR was performed in a 25-μl reaction containing 2.5 μl of the extracted DNA template, 0.6 μM of each primer and 12.5 μl of 2× DreamTaq Green PCR Master Mix (Inqaba Biotechnical Industries). The reactions were subjected to thermal conditions in a Bio-Rad T100™ thermal cycler (Bio-Rad Laboratories, Johannesburg, South Africa) with the following temperature profiles: 94 °C for 3 min, followed by 35 cycles of 94°C for 30 s, 55–65 °C for 45 s and 72 °C for 1 min. This was followed by a final extension at 72 °C for 10 min. The specific annealing temperatures are shown in Table 1. For nested PCR, 1 μl of the amplified PCR products was used as a template. Nested PCR products were subjected to gel electrophoresis in 1.2% (*w*/*v*) agarose gels stained with Biotium GelRed Acid

Table 1 Primer sets used to amplify DNA fragments specific for *Babesia bovis*

Gene	Assay	Primer name	Oligonucleotide primers (5′ → 3′)	Annealing	Product size[a]	Reference
BbRAP-1	PCR	BoF	F-CACGAGGAAGGAACTACCGATGTTGA	55 °C	360 bp	[12]
		BoR	R-CCAAGGAGCTTCAACGTACGAGGTCA			[12]
	nPCR	BoFN	F-TCAACAAGGTACTCTATATGGCTACC	57 °C	298 bp	[12]
		BoRN	R-CTACCGAGCAGAACCTTCTTCACCAT			[12]
BbCP2	PCR	CpBovF	F-TGCATCGGACCTATCCAACC	57 °C	960 bp	This study
		CpBovR	R-TCAGCAGCCAAATAAGGCCA			This study
	nPCR	CpBov3	F-ATCGGAAGAAGTCGCCGTTG	65 °C	829 bp	This study
		CpBov4	R-AAGCGTAGTCGCTGTAACCA			This study
BbSBP-4	PCR	BbSBP1	F-AGTTGTTGGAGGAGGCTAAT	57 °C	887–905 bp	This study
		BbSBP2	R-CTTCTCGGCGTCCTTTTC			This study
	nPCR	BbSBP3	F-CCGCATTCTTAAGACTTCTGA	60 °C	726–744 bp	This study
		BbSBP4	R-GTTACCATTTCATCGTTGTCA			This study
BbβTUB	PCR	BTbovA	F-AGAGCGGTACTTACCACGGA	61 °C	1203 bp	This study
		BTbovB	R-CGTCGTCGATGGTTGCTTCT			This study
	nPCR	BTbovC	F-GTTCCACGCGCTGTACTCAT	65 °C	954 bp	This study
		BTbovD	R-CATGTCCTGGATGGCGGTAG			This study

[a]Theoretical product sizes based on nucleotide gene sequences of several *B. bovis* strains used as templates for primer design

Stain (Anatech Instruments, Johannesburg, South Africa) and visualized under ultraviolet illumination. GeneRuler 100-bp DNA Ladder (Inqaba Biotechnical Industries) was used as the standard molecular weight marker.

DNA sequencing and phylogenetic analysis

Nested PCR products of positive samples, and whose GenBank accession numbers appear in Table 2, were selected for subsequent sequencing of *BbCP2*, *BbSBP-4* and *BbβTUB* genes. To corroborate correct amplification of *BbRAP-1* genes, 12 positive samples were sequenced. Nucleotide sequences were determined with ABI 3130XL Genetic Analyzer (Applied Biosystems, Johannesburg, South Africa) using a Big Dye Terminator Kit (Applied Biosystems). For each gene, DNA sequencing was performed on both strands using the corresponding forward and reverse primers. Multiple sequence alignments were performed using a Biological Sequence Alignment Editor [13]. Neighbour-joining trees were created using MEGA v5.0 software [14]. Molecular distances were estimated with Kimura two-parameter model [15], and the robustness of branches was determined using bootstrapping analysis with 1000 replicates [16]. Pairwise comparisons of nucleotide sequences were performed with EMBOSS Needle program (version 6.3.1) of the European Bioinformatics Institute (http://www.ebi.ac.uk/tools/psa/emboss_needle). Nucleotide sequences were translated to protein sequences using ExPASy translate tool (http://web.expasy.org/translate).

Table 2 GenBank accession numbers of nucleotide sequences generated in this study

Province	Sample ID	GenBank accession number		
		BbCP2	*BbSBP-4*	*BbβTUB*
KwaZulu-Natal	KZN-C1	–	KF626629	–
	KZN-C2	KF626619	KF626630	KF626639
	INDIA	KF626620	KF626631	KF626640
Mpumalanga	MP-C16	KF626621	–	–
	MP-C17	–	–	KF626641
	MP-C18	KF626622	KF626632	KF626642
Western Cape	WC-10270	KF626623	KF626633	KF626643
Gauteng	GP-C7	KF626624	KF626634	KF626644
	GP-C15	–	KF626635	–
	GP-C17	KF626625	KF626636	KF626645
Eastern Cape	EC-23A	KF626626	–	–
North West	NW-C2	KF626627	KF626637	KF626646
	NW-C4	KF626628	KF626638	KF626647

(–) No sequences generated

Nucleotide sequence accession numbers

Nucleotide sequences determined in this study were deposited in GenBank under the accession numbers KF626619 – KF626647.

Results

Amplification of target genes by PCR

The nested PCR primers specifically designed to detect *B. bovis* DNA in bovine samples yielded single amplicons of 298 bp for *BbRAP-1*, 829 bp for *BbCP2*, 726–744 bp for *BbSBP-4* and 954 bp for *BbβTUB*. Nested PCR assays with primers targeting four different genes were able to detect *B. bovis* DNA from some of the tested bovine samples. For example, BoFN/BoRN primers detected the *BbRAP-1* genes in 32 out of 54 samples tested (59.3%). On the other hand, a total of 15 (27.8%), 20 (37.0%) and 16 (29.6%) samples possessed *BbCP2*, *BbSBP-4* and *BbβTUB* fragments, respectively. In testing the specificity of PCR and nested PCR assays, purified DNA samples of *B. bigemina*, *Anaplasma centrale*, *Ehrlichia ruminantium* and *Theileria parva* were employed as negative controls, and as such, they yielded no PCR amplifications.

In order to corroborate if the correct PCR fragments were amplified, 12 samples possessing the *BbRAP-1* gene and representing seven provinces were sequenced. The resulting nucleotide sequences were subjected to homology searches in GenBank. The *BbRAP-1* sequences determined in this study exhibited 99–100% identity with published sequences of *B. bovis* strains originating from Philippines (JX860283), Brazil (FJ588009 to FJ588013 and AF030057 to AF030058), Uruguay (AF030060 to AF030061), Argentina (AF030053 and AF030056), USA (AF030054 and AF030059) and Cuba (JF279443).

In silico analysis of *B. bovis* sequences

Among the samples showing positive PCR amplifications, samples whose GenBank accession numbers appear in Table 2 were selected for sequencing. Alignment of 10 *BbCP2* gene sequences determined in this study revealed the existence of single nucleotide polymorphisms (SNPs) between the sequences. The sequences from NW-C4, GP-C7, GP-C17 and MP-C16 shared 100% identity, and contained 5 nucleotide differences in relation to MP-C18 sequence. Similarly, the sequences from EC-23A, NW-C2 and WC-10270 shared 100% identity, while the highest identity recorded with sequences from KZN-C2 and INDIA was 98.9% (9 nucleotide differences). A *blastn* search in GenBank exhibited that the sequences determined in this study were most closely related to *B. bovis* strains identified in cattle from other parts of the world. In particular, our sequences exhibited 99% identity with sequences of *B. bovis* strains R1A (GQ412131), M3P (GQ412133), S2P (GQ412136), Veracruz (GQ412135), Uruguay (GQ412134) and Brazil (GQ412132).

Pairwise comparison of the *BbSBP-4* sequences using EMBOSS Needle program indicated a close genetic similarity between sequences of South African *B. bovis* isolates and world strains. As shown in Table 3, the *BbSBP-4* sequences from samples designated KZN-C2 and WC-10270 shared 100% identity with sequences of *B. bovis* strains previously identified in cattle from Ghana (AB569301) and South Africa (AB569303). The *BbSBP-4* sequence of GP-C17 indicated 99.9% identity with the sequence of INDIA sample and 100% identity with that of KZN-C1. In an in silico analysis of *BbSBP-4* gene sequences derived from MP-C18, NW-C4, reference strain (XM_001610418) and other world strains (Fig. 1a), it was worth noting that these sequences possessed a gap with 18 nucleotides missing in relation to sequences originating from KZN-C2, WC-10270 and two other published sequences (AB569301 and AB569303). A similar trend was observed after translating nucleotide sequences to protein sequences; the latter strains also possessed a gap with six amino acid residues missing (Fig. 1b). Similarly, the *BbSBP-4* sequences from NW-C2, GP-C7, GP-C15, GP-C17, INDIA and KZN-C1 had 9 nucleotides missing (Fig. 1a), sharing between 98.1 and 98.8% sequence identities. Despite the high percentage identities observed among closely related sequences, there were SNPs occurring at different positions across the length of *BbSBP-4* gene sequences (Fig. 1a).

A multiple sequence alignment of *BbβTUB* sequences revealed the presence of SNPs among the South African *B. bovis* isolates and GenBank strains. The *BbβTUB* sequence from MP-C17 sample showed 97% identity with corresponding sequences from Texas (AK440534) and Samford (L00978) strains. MP-C17 sequence was also compared to other *BbβTUB* sequences determined in this study and the highest sequence identities recorded were between 97.2 and 97.5%. Sequences derived from other South African bovine samples (GP-C7, GP-C17, KZN-C2, INDIA, MP-C18, NW-C2, NW-C4 and WC-10270) showed 99% sequence identity when compared to those of Texas (AK440534) and Samford (L00978) strains.

Phylogenetic tree analyses

In order to study the phylogenetic relationship among the sequences of tested *B. bovis* isolates, nested PCR-amplified fragments of selected samples were sequenced in both strands. A neighbour-joining tree constructed with the *BbCP2* sequences showed a clear phylogenetic separation of sequences derived from geographical isolates of *B. bovis* (Fig. 2). The *BbCP2* sequences determined in this study were found in four different clusters. The first cluster grouped the reference strain (XM_001610645) with sequences from NW-C4, GP-C7, GP-C17 and MP-C16. Sequences of EC-23A, NW-C2 and WC-10270 formed a cluster clearly distinct from that of other sequences, with a high bootstrap support of 97%. While MP-C18 sequence clustered with that of R1A strain (GQ412131), the *BbCP2* sequences of INDIA and KZN-C2 exhibited a close phylogenetic relationship with the sequence of S2P strain (GQ412136).

A phylogram created with neighbour-joining method based on *BbSBP-4* nucleotide gene sequences is shown in Fig. 3. The sequences obtained in this study fell into three clades that resulted from the existence of SNPs across the lengths of *BbSBP-4* genes. The sequences of MP-C18 and NW-C4 were clearly distinct from other

Table 3 Pairwise comparisons of the *BbSBP-4* nucleotide gene sequences of South African *Babesia bovis* isolates and GenBank strains

Isolate origin		01	02	03	04	05	06	07	08	09	10	11	12	13	14	15	16	17	18	19	20	21	22
South Africa	01	100	100	94.5	94.5	94.2	94.4	94.4	93.7	94.4	94.5	94.5	94.5	94.8	94.8	98.3	98.1	98.3	98.1	98.3	98.8	100	100
Ghana	02		100	94.5	94.5	94.2	94.4	94.4	93.7	94.4	94.5	94.5	94.5	94.8	94.8	98.3	98.1	98.3	98.1	98.3	98.8	100	100
Brazil	03			100	100	99.7	99.9	99.9	99.2	99.9	100	100	100	98.6	98.6	96.1	95.9	96.1	96.2	96.2	95.6	94.5	94.5
Japan	04				100	99.7	99.9	99.9	99.2	99.9	100	100	100	98.6	98.6	96.1	95.9	96.1	96.2	96.2	95.6	94.5	94.5
Mongolia	05					100	99.6	99.6	99.2	99.6	99.7	99.7	99.7	98.3	98.3	95.8	95.6	95.8	95.9	95.9	95.4	94.2	94.2
Syria	06						100	99.7	99.0	99.7	99.9	99.9	99.9	98.5	98.5	95.9	95.8	95.9	96.1	96.1	95.5	94.4	94.4
Syria	07							100	99.0	99.7	99.9	99.9	99.9	98.5	98.5	95.9	95.8	95.9	96.1	96.1	95.5	94.4	94.4
Thailand	08								100	99.0	99.2	99.2	99.2	97.9	97.9	95.2	95.1	95.2	95.4	95.4	94.8	93.7	93.7
Thailand	09									100	99.9	99.9	99.9	98.5	98.5	95.9	95.8	95.9	96.1	96.1	95.5	94.4	94.4
Thailand	10										100	100	100	98.6	98.6	96.1	95.9	96.1	96.2	96.2	95.6	94.5	94.5
USA	11											100	100	98.6	98.6	96.1	95.9	96.1	96.2	96.2	95.6	94.5	94.5
USA	12												100	98.6	98.6	96.1	95.9	96.1	96.2	96.2	95.6	94.5	94.5
MP-C18	13													100	100	96.3	96.2	96.3	96.5	96.5	95.9	94.8	94.8
NW-C4	14														100	96.3	96.2	96.3	96.5	96.5	95.9	94.8	94.8
GP-C17	15															100	99.9	100	99.9	99.7	99.5	98.3	98.3
INDIA	16																100	99.9	99.7	99.6	99.3	98.1	98.1
KZN-C1	17																	100	99.9	99.7	99.5	98.3	98.3
NW-C2	18																		100	99.9	99.3	98.1	98.1
GP-C7	19																			100	99.5	98.3	98.3
GP-C15	20																				100	98.8	98.8
KZN-C2	21																					100	100
WC-10270	22																						100

Accession numbers of *BbSBP-4* sequences extracted from GenBank are (01 through 12): AB569303, AB569301, AB569300, AB594813, AB569302, AB617639, AB617641, AB571871, AB586125, AB594814, AF486506 and AF486507, respectively. Accession numbers of sequences generated in this study are (13 through 22): KF626632, KF626638, KF626636, KF626631, KF626629, KF626637, KF626634, KF626635, KF626630, KF626633

```
a
XM_001610418    GTCAGAAGAGGATGGAGAGGAAGCCGAGGG------------------CGCTGATGAAGCCGCCCCGCTATACTCCACG 62
01. S. Africa   ..............................TGCCGAGGGTGCCGAGGG...........................T.... 80
02. Ghana       ..............................TGCCGAGGGTGCCGAGGG...........................T.... 80
03. Brazil      ..............................------------------................................ 62
04. Japan       ..............................------------------................................ 62
05. Mongolia    ..............................------------------................................ 62
06. Syria       ..............................------------------................................ 62
07. Syria       ..............................------------------................................ 62
08. Thailand    ..............................------------------...A.C.......................... 62
09. Thailand    ..............................------------------................................ 62
10. Thailand    ..............................------------------................................ 62
11. USA         ..............................------------------................................ 62
12. USA         ..............................------------------................................ 62
13. MP-C18      ..............................------------------......................G......... 62
14. NW-C4       ..............................------------------......................G......... 62
15. GP-C17      ..............................TACCGAGGG---------...........................T.... 71
16. INDIA       ..............................TACCGAGGG---------...........................T.... 71
17. KZN-C1      ..............................TACCGAGGG---------...........................T.... 71
18. NW-C2       ..............................TACCGAGGG---------...........................T.... 71
19. GP-C7       ..............................TGCCGAGGG---------...........................T.... 71
20. GP-C15      ..............................TGCCGAGGG---------...........................T.... 71
21. KZN-C2      ..............................TGCCGAGGGTGCCGAGGG...........................T.... 80
22. WC-10270    ..............................TGCCGAGGGTGCCGAGGG...........................T.... 80

b
XM_001610418    EETETKSEEDGEEAE------GADEAAPAILHADLQNKFIDEVVVFRNCFDTAVSVNVDGKQIYFTATGNEAEDFEEVEA 74
01. S. Africa   ...............GAEGAE................................I...................N...... 80
02. Ghana       ...............GAEGAE................................I...................N...... 80
03. Brazil      ...............------........................................................... 74
04. Japan       ...............------........................................................... 74
05. Mongolia    ...............------........................................................... 74
06. Syria       ...............------........................................................... 74
07. Syria       ...............------...................E....................................... 74
08. Thailand    ...............------..N..............................T......................... 74
09. Thailand    ...............------........................................................... 74
10. Thailand    ...............------........................................................... 74
11. USA         ...............------........................................................... 74
12. USA         ...............------........................................................... 74
13. MP-C18      ...............------........V.................................................. 74
14. NW-C4       ...............------........V.................................................. 74
15. GP-C17      ..............GTEG---....................................................N...... 77
16. INDIA       ..............GTEG---....................................................N...... 77
17. KZN-C1      ..............GTEG---....................................................N...... 77
18. NW-C2       ..............GTEG---....................................................N...... 77
19. GP-C7       ..............GAEG---....................................................N...... 77
20. GP-C15      ..............GAEG---................................I...................N...... 77
21. KZN-C2      ...............GAEGAE................................I...................N...... 80
22. WC-10270    ...............GAEGAE................................I...................N...... 80
```

Fig. 1 Multiple sequence alignments of partial *BbSBP-4* nucleotide gene sequences (**a**) and ceduced amino acid sequences (**b**) of 12 GenBank strains and 10 South African isolates of *Babesia bovis*. The dots and dashes respectively indicate sequence identities and gaps in relation to a reference sequence (accession number XM_001610418). Accession numbers of sequences extracted from GenBank (01 to ˙4) correspond to those given in Table 3

sequences. The *BbSBP-4* gene sequences from GP-C7, GP-C17, KZN-C1, INDIA and NW-C2 all formed a separate grouping. Similarly, GP-C15, WC-10270 and KZN-C2 sequences showed a very close phylogenetic relationship with sequences of *B. bovis* strains published in GenBank (AB569301 and AB569303), and were supported by a high bootstrap value.

The phylogenetic tree inferred with *BbβTUB* sequences is reflected in Fig. 4. In the phylogeny, it was observed that the sequences from GP-C7, GP-C17, INDIA, MP-C18, NW-C2 and NW-C4 clustered together. The DNA sequences derived from KZN-C2 and WC-10270 showed a grouping with Texas (AK440534) and T2Bo (XM_001611566) strains. Furthermore, it was noted that the *BbβTUB* sequence of MP-C17 isolate formed a separate cluster clearly distinct from that of other South African isolates, with a bootstrap support of 100%. Phylogenetic analysis of *BbβTUB* gene also indicated that *Babesia ovata* (AB634844) is genetically related to *B. bigemina* Argentina strain (AB634846).

Discussion

The search for *B. bovis* vaccine that could confer absolute protective immunity against bovine babesiosis has been the subject of many studies over the last decades. To date, no recombinant subunit vaccines are available to eliminate babesial infections in cattle globally because of extensive antigenic variations displayed by heterologous parasitic strains. As a result, many research groups have intensified their efforts in an endeavour to search for novel vaccine candidates with potential to offer complete protective immune response against a challenge by heterologous strains.

In particular, many studies have focused on functionally important proteins that are believed to play a pivotal role in parasite survival and growth [17, 18]. For example, the RAP-1 protein is involved in the process of invasion of bovine red blood cells by merozoites [19, 20]. Peptidases, such as cysteine peptidase 2, possess enzymatic activities identified as virulence factors for Apicomplexan parasites [21]. The BbSBP is involved in stabilizing the environment after parasite invasion and plays a role in parasite growth

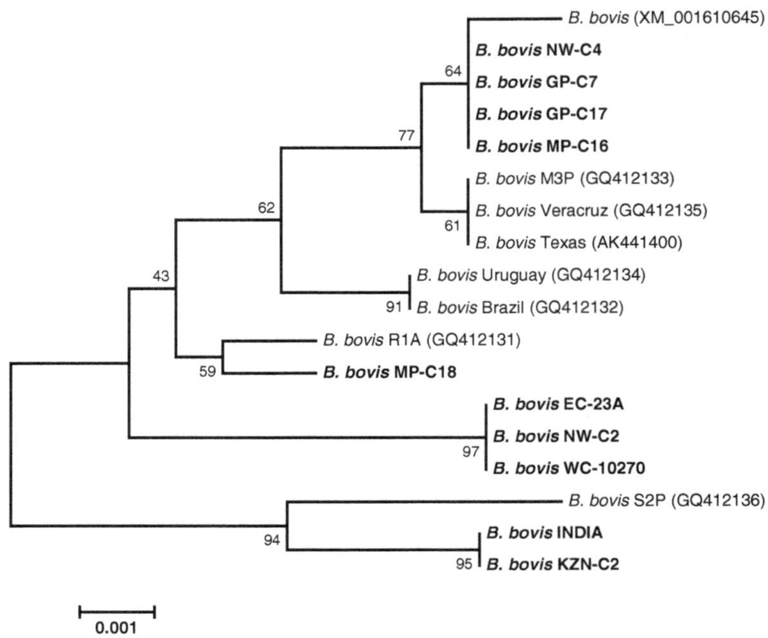

Fig. 2 Phylogenetic tree inferred with *BbCP2* gene sequences (809 *nt*) of several *B. bovis* isolates from bovine samples collected at various geographical regions in South Africa, together with corresponding sequences retrieved from GenBank. Accession numbers are given in parentheses. Bootstrap values calculated as percentages of 1000 replicates are indicated at branching points. The horizontal scale bar shows the number of base substitutions per site

[22]. In addition, BbSBP has been documented as a new serological antigen for global epidemiological research [23]. Likewise, the β-tubulin gene of *Babesia* parasites has been used as an informative marker for species discrimination [24].

The fight against bovine babesiosis in southern Africa has always relied on the use of live attenuated vaccines which are more prone to cross-contamination [6]. Furthermore, the practical application of these vaccines is hampered by genetic heterogeneities observed among field isolates [25]. Therefore, it remains imperative to document the genetic profiles of *B. bovis* parasitic field isolates in an endeavour to develop effective control strategies with potential to curtail infection of susceptible bovines by *Babesia* parasites.

In the present study, we describe the successful development and application of three nested PCR assays for the specific detection of *B. bovis* DNA in field bovine samples. The *BbRAP-1* nested PCR assay developed previously [12] was employed as the control for the newly developed nested PCR assays. Due to the high number of samples tested positive with *BbRAP-1* nested PCR-based assay, it appears that this assay was more sensitive than *BbCP2*, *BbSBP-4* and *BbβTUB* assays developed in the present study. However, it is reported in the literature that the high number of positive samples detected by *BbRAP-1* nested PCR may be attributed to the presence of several nearly identical copies of *B. bovis BbRAP-1* genes in the genome [26, 27].

To corroborate the specificities of nested PCR assays, PCR-generated amplicons from randomly selected positive samples were sequenced. Sequence analysis revealed high genetic conservation among the *BbRAP-1* DNA fragments of South African *B. bovis* isolates and those published in GenBank, with identities ranging between 99 and 100%. The high conservation of *BbRAP-1* genes in *B. bovis* field isolates is comparable to previous studies that observed significant similarities in *BbRAP-1* sequences of isolates from countries other than South Africa [10, 28].

Accordingly, in silico analysis of *BbCP2* sequences indicated a high degree of sequence conservation between South African *B. bovis* isolates and GenBank strains. In the BLAST search for homologous sequences in GenBank, the highest *BbCP2* sequence identities (99%) were recorded with *B. bovis* strains originating from Argentina, Mexico, Uruguay and Brazil. This suggested high conservation of *BbCP2* gene sequences among *B. bovis* strains from geographically distinct regions of the world. Although cysteine peptidases of *B. bovis* have not been well characterized [29], the evidence of the importance of peptidases for parasite growth and survival was obtained when specific inhibitors of these enzymes impaired merozoite growth in vitro [30]. Recent findings on in vitro and in vivo expression of bovipain-2, a cysteine protease, in *B. bovis* also suggest that peptidases might potentially be considered as important

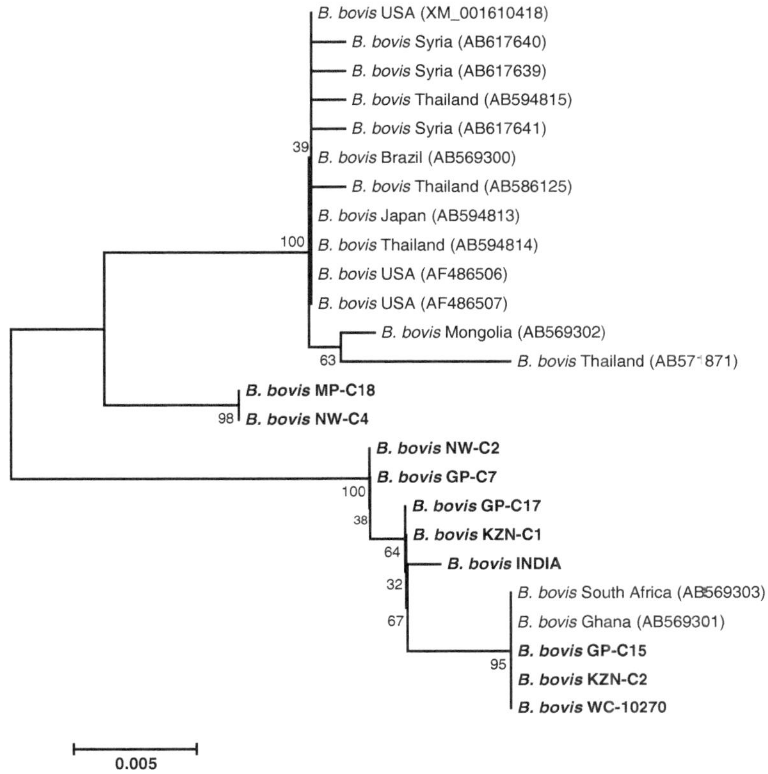

Fig. 3 A neighbour-joining tree generated with *BbSBP-4* nucleotide gene sequences (726–744 *nt*) of South African *B. bovis* isolates (in bold type), together with sequences previously published in GenBank. Accession numbers are given in parentheses. Bootstrap values calculated as percentages of 1000 replicates are indicated at branching points. The horizontal scale bar shows the number of base substitutions per site

targets for the development of effective control strategies against bovine babesiosis [29].

Sequencing of *BbSBP-4* genes from *B. bovis* isolates examined in this study demonstrated the existence of gaps in some isolates, a feature commensurate with base-pair insertion or deletion events. These insertions and deletions of nucleotide bases within the open reading frames (ORFs) may result in frame shift mutations, depending on whether the nucleotides that are added to (insertion event) or deleted from (deletion event) the ORF are a multiple of three or not. To further investigate whether there were any significant differences between the protein sequences as well as the possibility of frame shift mutations among *B. bovis* isolates possessing gaps, the determined nucleotide sequences were translated to protein sequences in silico and aligned with corresponding sequences of *B. bovis* strains published in GenBank. Analysis of aligned protein sequences revealed high conservation between sequences, albeit there were amino acid differences observed along the stretch of the protein sequences. The conservation of BbSBP sequences among geographical isolates of *B. bovis* has also been observed elsewhere [31, 32].

In studying the phylogenetic relationship among *B. bovis* isolates based on *BbCP2, BbSBP-4* and *BbβTUB* gene sequences, neighbour-joining trees were inferred. The analyses of phylogenies indicated a close phylogenetic relationship between the South African *B. bovis* isolates and geographical strains originating from cattle in other countries, albeit the sequences showed varying phylogenetic groupings because of the existence of SNPs across the lengths of nucleotide gene sequences. However, the observed clustering of *BbCP2* and *BbSBP-4* sequences incorporated in the phylogenies should be interpreted with caution given that the trees were not rooted. Furthermore, the current dearth of *B. bovis BbβTUB* sequences in GenBank could not allow for a better discrimination of the phylogenetic relatedness between *B. bovis* isolates of South African origin and those of countries other than South Africa. Given the importance of β-tubulin protein-encoding gene as the molecular marker for species identification and discrimination [24], it is of paramount importance that more *BbβTUB* genes of geographical *B. bovis* strains are sequenced and made available in GenBank.

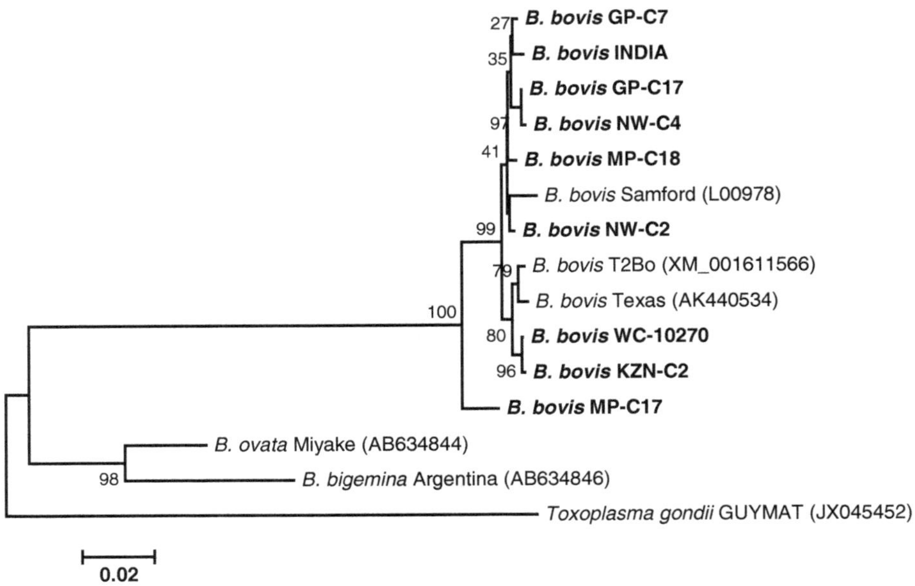

Fig. 4 Phylogenetic tree based on *BbβTUB* nucleotide gene sequences (920 *nt*) derived from blood samples collected from South African cattle (in bold type), together with sequences previously published in GenBank (accession numbers in parentheses). Bootstrap values calculated as percentages of 1000 replicates are indicated at branching points. The horizontal scale bar shows the number of base substitutions per site. *Toxoplasma gondii* GUYMAT (accession no. JX045452) was used as an outgroup

Conclusion

In this study, we have described the development and application of three newly developed nested PCR assays for the specific detection and genetic characterization of *B. bovis* isolates in field bovine samples. Although only few sequences were incorporated in the phylogenetic analyses, it must be acknowledged that the findings from this study provide valuable information regarding the genetic conservation among *B. bovis* isolates of South African origin in comparison to those previously published in GenBank. Taken together, the data presented in this study has given an indication that immunologically important proteins encoded by the genes examined in this study could potentially be considered for exploitation as viable candidates for inclusion in recombinant subunit vaccines.

Acknowledgements

The authors are indebted to the farmers who participated during bovine blood sample collection. The technical assistance of Lerato Dlamini and Veronica Phetla is gratefully acknowledged. This work is based upon the research supported financially by the National Research Foundation (NRF) and the National Zoological Gardens of South Africa (NZG). Any opinion, finding and conclusion or recommendation expressed in this material is that of the authors and the NRF does not accept any liability in this regard.

Funding

This research was supported by the National Research Foundation (NRF) (Moses Sibusiso Mtshali, grant number 69090) and the National Zoological Gardens of South Africa. The funders played no role in study design, data collection and interpretation, or the decision to submit this work for publication.

Authors' contributions

PS conceived the study. PS and MS participated in study design and coordination. PS carried out laboratory assays, performed data analysis and interpretation, constructed phylogenetic trees and drafted the manuscript. PS and MS critically reviewed the manuscript. All authors read and approved the final version of the manuscript.

Ethics approval and consent to participate

Ethics approval was granted by the National Zoological Gardens of South Africa Research Ethics and Scientific Committee, project number NZG/RES/P/001/F/01 for the national research project on the epidemiology and genetic diversity of bovine anaplasmosis in South Africa. The NZG Research Ethics and Scientific Committee approved the collection of blood samples from animals. Animal owners gave verbal informed consent for the collection of the samples for the epidemiological survey, and animals were not involved in any clinical trials or treatments.

Consent for publication

Not applicable.

Competing interests

The authors declare that they have no competing interests.

References

1. Jongejan F, Uilenberg G. The global importance of ticks. Parasitology. 2004; 129:S3–14.
2. de Vos AJ, Potgieter FT. Bovine babesiosis. In: JAW C, Thomson GR, Tustin RC, editors. Infectious diseases of livestock. South Africa: Oxford University Press; 1994. p. 278–94.

3. OIE. Bovine babesiosis: OIE Terrestrial Manual [Internet]. Available from: http://www.oie.int/fileadmin/Home/eng/Health_standards/tahm/2.04.02_bovine_babesiosis.pdf (2010). Accessed 29 Aug 2013.
4. Bock R, Jackson L, de Vos AJ, Jorgensen W. Babesiosis of cattle. Parasitology. 2004;129:S247–69.
5. Ristic M. Babesiosis. In: Ristic M, McIntyre I, editors. Disease of cattle in the tropics. The Netherlands: Martinus Nijhof Publishers; 1981. p. 443–68.
6. de Vos A, Bock RE. Vaccination against bovine babesiosis. Ann N Y Acad Sci. 2000;916:540–5.
7. Ojeda JJ, Orozco L, Flores R, Figueroa JV, Alvarez JA. Validation of an attenuated live vaccine against babesiosis in native cattle in an endemic area. Transbound Emerg Dis. 2010;57(1–2):84–6.
8. Callow LL, Dalgliesh RJ, de Vos AJ. Development of effective living vaccines against bovine babesiosis: the longest field trial? Int J Parasitol. 1997;27(7):747–67.
9. Torina A, Agnone A, Sireci G, Mosqueda JJ, Blanda V, Albanese I, La Farina M, Cerrone A, Cusumano F, Caracappa S. Characterization of the apical membrane antigen-1 in Italian strains of *Babesia bigemina*. Transbound Emerg Dis. 2010;57(1–2):52–6.
10. Ramos CAN, Araújo FR, Alves LC, de Souza IIF, Guedes DS Jr, Soares CO. Genetic conservation of potentially immunogenic proteins among Brazilian isolates of *Babesia bovis*. Vet Parasitol. 2012;187(3–4):548–52.
11. Brayton KA, Lau AOT, Herndon DR, Hannick L, Kappmeyer LS, Berens SJ, Bidwell SL, Brown W, Crabtree J, Fadrosh D, Feldblum T, Forberger HA, Haas BJ, Howell JM, Khouri H, Koo H, Mann DJ, Norimine J, Paulsen IT, Radune D, Nene VM. Genome sequence of *Babesia bovis* and comparative analysis of apicomplexan hemoprotozoa. PLoS Pathog. 2007;3(10):1401–13.
12. Figueroa JV, Chieves LP, Johnson GS, Buening GM. Multiplex polymerase chain reaction based assay for the detection of *Babesia bigemina*, *Babesia bovis* and *Anaplasma marginale* DNA in bovine blood. Vet Parasitol. 1993;50(1–2):69–81.
13. Hall TA. BioEdit: a user-friendly biological sequence alignment editor and analysis program for windows 95/98/NT. Nucleic Acids Symp Ser. 1999;41:95–8.
14. Tamura K, Peterson D, Peterson N, Stecher G, Nei M, Kumar S. MEGA5: molecular evolutionary genetics analysis using maximum likelihood, evolutionary distance, and maximum parsimony methods. Mol Biol Evol. 2011;28(10):2731–9.
15. Kimura M. A simple method for estimating evolutionary rate of base substitutions through comparative studies of nucleotide sequences. J Mol Evol. 1980;16(2):111–20.
16. Felsenstein J. Confidence limits on phylogenies: an approach using the bootstrap. Evolution. 1985;39(4):783–91.
17. Yokoyama N, Okamura M, Igarashi I. Erythrocyte invasion by *Babesia* parasites: current advances in the elucidation of the molecular interactions between the protozoan ligands and host receptors in the invasion stage. Vet Parasitol. 2006;138(1–2):22–32.
18. Florin-Christensen M, Schnittger L, Dominguez M, Mesplet M, Rodriguez A, Ferreri L, Asenzo G, Wilkowsky S, Farber M, Echaide I, Suarez C. Search for *Babesia bovis* vaccine candidates. Parassitologia. 2007;1:9–12.
19. Suarez CE, Palmer GH, Hötzel I, Hines SA, McElwain TF. Sequence and functional analysis of the intergenic regions separating babesial rhoptry-associated protein-1 (rap-1) genes. Exp Parasitol. 1998;90(2):189–94.
20. Gaffar FR, Yatsuda AP, Franssen FF, Vries EA. A *Babesia bovis* merozoite protein with a domain architecture highly similar to the thrombospondin-related anonymous protein (TRAP) present in *Plasmodium* sporozoites. Mol Biochem Parasitol. 2004;136(1):25–34.
21. Mesplet M, Palmer GH, Pedroni MJ, Echaide I, Florin-Christensen M, Schnittger L, Lau AOT. Genome-wide analysis of peptidase content and expression in a virulent and attenuated *Babesia bovis* strain pair. Mol Biochem Parasitol. 2011;179(2–2):111–3.
22. Goo YK, Jia H, Aboge GO, Terkawi MA, Kuriki K, Nakamura C, Kumagai A, Zhou J, Lee EG, Nishikawa Y, Igarashi I, Fujisaki K, Xuan X. *Babesia gibsoni*: serodiagnosis of infection in dogs by an enzyme-linked immunosorbent assay with recombinant BgTRAP. Exp Parasitol. 2008;118(4):555–60.
23. Terkawi MA, Huyen NX, Wibowo PE, Seuseu FJ, AbouLaila M, Ueno A, Goo YK, Yokoyama N, Xuan X, Igarashi I. Spherical body protein 4 is a new serological antigen for global detection of *Babesia bovis* infection in cattle. Clin Vaccine Immunol. 2011;18(2):337–42.
24. Cacciò S, Cammà C, Onuma M, Severini C. The β-tubulin gene of *Babesia* and *Theileria* parasites is an informative marker for species discrimination. Int J Parasitol. 2000;30(11):1181–5.
25. Berens SJ, Brayton KA, Molloy JB, Bock RE, Lew AE, McElwain TF. Merozoite surface antigen 2 proteins of *Babesia bovis* vaccine breakthrough isolates contain a unique hypervariable region composed of degenerate repeats. Infect Immun. 2005;73(11):7180–9.
26. Norimine J, Suarez CE, McElwain TF, Florin-Christensen M, Brown WC. Immunodominant epitopes in *Babesia bovis* rhoptry-associated protein 1 that elicit memory CD4^{+}-T-lymphocyte responses in *B. bovis*-immune individuals are located in the amino-terminal domain. Infect Immun. 2002;70(4):2039–48.
27. AbouLaila M, Yokoyama N, Igarashi I. Development and evaluation of two nested PCR assays for the detection of *Babesia bovis* from cattle blood. Vet Parasitol. 2010;172(1–2):65–70.
28. Silva MG, Henriques G, Sánchez C, Marques PX, Suarez CE, Oova A. First survey for *Babesia bovis* and *Babesia bigemina* infection in cattle from central and southern regions of Portugal using serological and DNA detection methods. Vet Parasitol. 2009;166(1–2):66–72.
29. Mesplet M, Echaide I, Dominguez M, Mosqueda JJ, Suarez CE, Schnittger L, Florin-Christensen M. Bovipain-2, the falcipain-2 ortholog, is expressed in intraerythrocytic stages of the tick-transmitted hemoparasite *Babesia bovis*. Parasit Vectors. 2010;3:113.
30. Okubo K, Yokoyama N, Govind Y, Alhassan A, Igarashi I. *Babesia bovis*: effects of cysteine protease inhibitors on *in vitro* growth. Exp Parasitol. 2007;117(2):214–7.
31. Ruef BJ, Dowling SC, Conley PG, Perryman LE, Brown WC, Jasmer DP, Rice-Ficht AC. A unique *Babesia bovis* spherical body protein is conserved among geographical isolates and localizes to the infected erythrocyte membrane. Mol Biochem Parasitol. 2000;105(1):1–12.
32. Terkawi MA, Seuseu FJ, Eko-Wibowo P, Huyen NX, Minoda Y, AbouLaila M, Kawai S, Yokoyama N, Xuan X, Igarashi I. Secretion of a new spherical body protein of *Babesia bovis* into the cytoplasm of infected erythrocytes. Mol Biochem Parasitol. 2011;178(1–2):40–5.

11

Epidemiological analysis of bovine ephemeral fever in 2012–2013 in the subtropical islands of Japan

Yoko Hayama[1*], Sachiko Moriguchi[1,2], Tohru Yanase[3], Moemi Suzuki[4,5], Tsuyoshi Niwa[5], Kazufumi Ikemiyagi[5], Yoshiki Nitta[4], Takehisa Yamamoto[1], Sota Kobayashi[1], Kiyokazu Murai[1] and Toshiyuki Tsutsui[1]

Abstract

Background: Bovine ephemeral fever (BEF) is a febrile disease of cattle that is transmitted by arthropod vectors such as mosquitoes and *Culicoides* biting midges. An outbreak of BEF recently occurred in Ishigaki Island and surrounding islands that are located southwest of Japan. In this study, an epidemiological analysis was conducted to understand the temporal and spatial characteristics of the outbreak. Factors associated with the disease spread within Ishigaki Island were investigated by hierarchical Bayesian models. The possibility of between-island transmission by windborne vectors and transmission by long-distance migration of infected vectors were examined using atmospheric dispersion models.

Results: In September 2012, the first case of the disease was detected in the western part of Ishigaki Island. In 1 month, it had rapidly spread to the southern part of the island and to surrounding islands, and led to 225 suspected cases of BEF during the outbreak. The dispersion model demonstrated the high possibility of between-island transmission by wind. Spatial analysis showed that paddy fields, farmlands, and slope gradients had a significant impact on the 1-km cell-level incidence risk. These factors may have influenced the habitats and movements of the vectors with regard to the spread of BEF. A plausible incursion event of infected vectors from Southeast Asia to Ishigaki Island was estimated to have occurred at the end of August.

Conclusion: This study revealed that the condition of a terrain and land use significantly influenced disease transmission. These factors are important in assessing favorable environments for related vectors. The results of the dispersion model indicated the likely transmission of the infected vectors by wind on the local scale and on the long-distance scale. These findings would be helpful for developing a surveillance program and developing preventive measures against BEF.

Keywords: Arboviral disease, Atmospheric dispersal modeling, Bovine ephemeral fever, Conditional autoregressive model, *Culicoides* biting midges, Epidemiology, Japan, Mosquito, Spatial analysis, Windborne spread

Background

Bovine ephemeral fever (BEF) is an arboviral (short for "arthropod-borne viral") disease of cattle and water buffalos that is caused by the BEF virus (BEFV), which is a member of the genus *Ephemerovirus* in the family *Rhabdoviridae*. Bovine ephemeral fever is geographically distributed from tropical to temperate zones such as parts of Australia, Asia, the Middle East, and Africa [1–6]. The characteristic clinical signs of BEF are the sudden onset of a high fever, anorexia, depression, ocular and nasal discharge, salivation, muscle stiffness, lameness, ruminal stasis, sternal recumbency, and other inflammatory responses [1, 2]. The disease can cause severe economic impact through the reduction of milk production in dairy cattle and the loss of condition in beef cattle. The symptoms of BEF usually subside within a few days [2]. Hematophagous arthropod vectors of BEF have not been clearly defined [7], although mosquitoes and

* Correspondence: hayama@affrc.go.jp
[1]Viral Disease and Epidemiology Research Division, National Institute of Animal Health, National Agriculture and Food Research Organization, 3-1-5 Kannondai, Tsukuba, Ibaraki 305-0856, Japan
Full list of author information is available at the end of the article

Culicoides biting midges are possible vectors that transmit the BEFV [1, 2, 7].

In Japan, the domestic animal infectious disease control law designates BEF as a notifiable infectious disease. The disease has not occurred for more than 20 years in the mainland of Japan [8]. The recent occurrences of BEF occurred only in Okinawa, which is a subtropical archipelago in the southwestern-most region of Japan. In 1989 and 2001 in Okinawa, large-scale outbreaks of BEF affected more than 1000 animals, and in 2002 and 2004 small-scale outbreaks occurred [8]. In 2012, an outbreak of BEF occurred in Okinawa after an 8-year absence [9]. This outbreak occurred in the Yaeyama Islands, which form an archipelago approximately 400 km southwest of the Okinawa Islands and 280 km east of Taiwan. During this outbreak, BEF was confirmed in Ishigaki Island (223 km^2), Iriomote Island (289 km^2), Kohama Island (7.8 km^2), and Kuroshima Island (10 km^2). In Ishigaki Island, in particular, the disease spread widely and affected more than 200 farms of 523 farms at risk.

In previous studies, BEFVs isolated in Japan were closely related to the Taiwanese strains, based on phylogenetic analysis of the glycoprotein gene. [10–12]. The BEFV isolated in 2012 in Japan was also classified in the same cluster of strains isolated in Taiwan and China in 1996–2004. The BEFV isolated during the large BEF epidemic in Taiwan in 2012 was also included in the same cluster and closely related to the strain isolated in China in 2002 [9, 13]. In addition, the recent outbreaks of BEF in the Yaeyama Islands were synchronized with the large epidemics in Taiwan, which suggested an epidemiological linkage between these regions [9, 10, 13]. These findings suggested that BEFVs were introduced from a gene pool in a lower latitude region and widely spread among East Asian countries during each epidemic. The incursion of BEFVs was supposedly caused by long-distance transmission by wind from lower latitude regions (which include southern China) to Taiwan and/or Japan [10].

The long-distance transport of insects by wind is considered a cause of outbreaks of agricultural pests or insect-borne plant and animal disease [14, 15]. Wind can disperse *Culicoides* biting midges, a major vector of arboviruses in ruminants, up to hundreds of kilometers [16], although the insect's usual movements are short and range from a few hundred meters to less than 2 km [17]. The possibility of long-distance distribution of biting midges has been well investigated in outbreaks of bluetongue in Europe and Australia by using atmospheric dispersion models to estimate the potential sources of the disease and to simulate the dispersion of biting midges from source sites [18–24]. Flights of more than 100 km by wind have been recorded for several species of mosquitoes, although flight activity varies greatly between species [25, 26]. A past outbreak of BEF in Australia reportedly spread nearly 2000 km over land along with the window direction [27].

Environmental and climatic conditions in a local area affect vector habitats and influence the spread of an arbovirus disease. Mosquitoes and *Culicoides* biting midges use a wide variety of aquatic and semiaquatic environments for breeding and growth; however, wetlands such as paddy fields and bogs provide a favorable habitat for some vector species of arboviruses [25, 28, 29]. Temperature, humidity, and rainfall reportedly affect adult survivorship and egg development in these vectors [28, 30, 31]. After the outbreaks of bluetongue in Europe, climatic conditions, environmental conditions such as landscape and farm husbandry, and host availability have been proven to influence biting midges abundance [32–36]. These investigations revealed a positive relationship between biting midges abundance and pasture cover [32], prairies and woodlands [36], cattle density, and dense vegetation [34, 35]. In addition, a relationship has been demonstrated between the spatial distribution of confirmed cases of West Nile virus (which is transmitted by mosquitoes) and landscapes such as shrubland, row crops, and wetland [37]. Topographical and climatic conditions also affect the habitats of mosquitoes [38].

In this study, an epidemiological analysis of the BEF outbreak in 2012 in Japan was conducted. First, the spatial and temporal features of the BEF epidemic were described. In this paper, we used an atmospheric dispersion model to examine the likelihood that windborne infected vectors were responsible for between-island transmission of the disease. Second, to clarify the risk factors associated with the disease spread, a spatial analysis was conducted to investigate the influence of landscape and topographical conditions on the disease spread within Ishigaki Island, where most BEF cases were confirmed. Third, the hypothesis that the long-distance dispersion of infected vectors occurred from surrounding Asian regions to Yaeyama was examined. Plausible incursion events and possible source sites of infected vectors were estimated using an atmospheric dispersion model.

Methods

Data and descriptive analysis

In this study, an "infected farm" was defined as a farm that had been notified of a BEF-suspected case by a farmer or by a private veterinarian and the disease was subsequently diagnosed by a local veterinary officer. For the first case on each island and some notified cases on a farm located distant from other infected farms, blood samples were collected from cattle and confirmed by virus isolation and a viral neutralization test conducted at the Okinawa Prefectural Institute of Animal Health (Okinawa, Japan). Other notified cases were diagnosed based on the clinical onset of the disease and the epidemiological situations.

Information on the infected farms, date of notification, details of clinical onset, farm type, farm size, and farm location (longitude and latitude) were collected by local veterinary officers. These data were used for spatial and temporal descriptive analysis. For Ishigaki Island, information on the noninfected farms such as farm type, farm size, and farm location (i.e., longitude and latitude) was also organized by local veterinary officers for the spatial analysis. These farm information was collected as a part of epidemiological investigation based on the domestic animal infectious disease control law and was permitted to be used in this study from the animal health authority of Okinawa Prefecture. This study did not include any experimental research on animals. Therefore, approval by an ethical committee was not required. Clinical inspection and blood sampling for confirmation diagnosis were performed by local veterinary officers in accordance with the law. All maps in this study were generated using Arc GIS 10 (Esri, Redlands, CA).

Atmospheric dispersion model

Two types of atmospheric dispersion models were applied to examine the possibility of between-island transmission by windborne infected vectors and to estimate the potential source site of infected vectors. The Hybrid Single Particle Lagrangian Integrated Trajectory (HYSPLIT) Model (National Oceanic and Atmospheric Administration [NOAA] Air Resources Laboratory, College Park, MD) is a computer model that is used to compute air parcel trajectories and the dispersion or deposition of atmospheric pollutants or particles (e.g. insects) [39]. The HYSPLIT (version 4) model has been previously used to model long-distance dispersal of *Culicoides* biting midges [18, 24, 40, 41] and other insects [42]. An overview of the HYSPLT model is described in detail in a paper by Draxler and Hess [43, 44]. In this study, back-trajectory analysis was conducted using the HYSPLIT model to estimate the potential source sites of infected vectors. The meteorological dataset used as input for the model was the Global Data Assimilation System (GDAS), which is available in 3-h intervals with a global resolution of 1° latitude/longitude (approximately 100 km^2).

The Meteorological Data Explorer (METEX) is also an atmospheric dispersion model used to calculate air trajectory; it was developed at the Centre for Global Environmental Research (CGER) in Tsukuba, Japan [45] and was used to examine the possibility of the between-island dispersion of infected vectors by wind. Because the distance between Ishigaki Island and neighboring islands is approximately 15 km, we believe it is plausible to examine the effect of local wind in relation to the transport of infected vectors. In comparison to the HYSPLIT model, the METEX model calculates trajectories by using a more detailed meteorological dataset with a resolution of 0.1 °latitude and 0.15 °longitude (approximately 10 km^2), based on grid point value data from the Japan Meteorological Agency. Thus, the METEX model is proper to examine short-distance vector dispersal between islands.

Evaluation of vector dispersal by wind between the islands

The possibility of windborne transmission of vectors from Ishigaki Island to surrounding islands was examined by forward trajectory analysis using the METEX model. Because of the spread of the disease in Ishigaki Island, two sites were set as the starting points of the trajectory: the first site was where the first case of BEF occurred in the western part of Ishigaki Island (i.e., Location 1) and the second site was where the first case of BEF occurred in the southern part of Ishigaki Island (i.e., Location 2), which was a major epidemic area with a high density of cattle farms (Fig. 1).

To examine the possibility of windborne transmission of vectors between the islands, the terms "potential source period" and "incursion risk period" were defined as follows:

Potential source period The period in which infected vectors have already invaded in an area and the infected vectors can disperse into other areas. After BEF is first detected in an area, it is assumed to be in the potential source period. This period is assumed to continue at the end of the epidemic because of the possibility that infected vectors survive in the area.

Incursion risk period The period during which the incursion event is most likely to have occurred. The duration of this period was set 14 days before the detection of the first case of BEF in an area. This period was based on the incubation period of the BEFV (usually 2–4 days with a maximum of 10–11 days) [2, 46], and on the estimated lifespan of adult insects in the field (1–2 weeks for mosquitoes and *Culicoides* biting midges) [31, 47, 48].

Based on these definitions, the potential source period of Location 1 and Location 2 on Ishigaki Island was determined as beginning on September 10, 2012 and September 16 2012, respectively (Table 1). The incursion risk period of each island was September 1–14, 2012 for Iriomote and Kohama Islands and September 12–25, 2012 for Kuroshima Island.

Using the METEX model, 24-h forward trajectories were generated at hourly intervals from Location 1 and

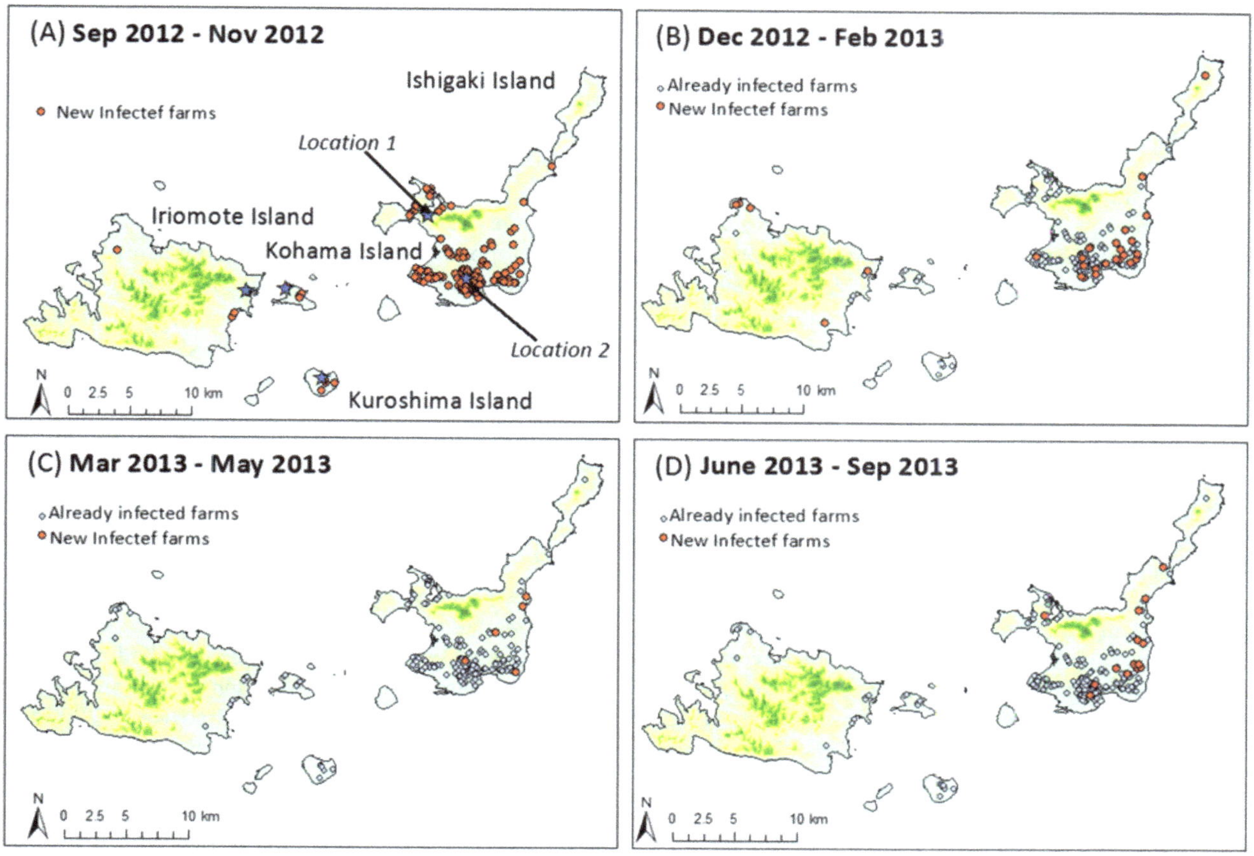

Fig. 1 Distribution of infected farms in the Yaeyama Islands during the BEF outbreak in 2012–2013. The blue stars indicate the first case of BEF on each island and the starting points of the trajectory (on Location 1 and Location 2). The red dots show new infected farms during the period September 2012 to November 2012 (**a**), December 2012 to February 2013 (**b**), March 2013 to May 2013 (**c**), and June 2013 to September 2013 (**d**)

Location 2, and the likely dates of windborne transmission of vectors to the surrounding islands within the incursion risk period were explored.

Estimation of the potential sources of the vectors

Potential sources of the infected vectors were estimated by backward trajectory analysis using the HYSPLIT model. The location of the first case in Ishigaki Island (i.e., Location 1) was set as the starting point of the trajectory. During the incursion risk period in Location 1 (August 27, 2012–September 9, 2012), 72-h back trajectories were generated at hourly intervals. The length of the trajectory was based on the assumption that the vectors travelled the approximately 2000-km distance between Southeast Asia and Ishigaki Island in 3 days. With regard to the longevity of the vectors, female mosquitoes and *Culicoides* biting midges reportedly survive 3–5 days without sugar or a blood meal [49–51]; therefore, the 72 h-length of the trajectory is supposed to represent the possible situation of infected vectors reaching the islands through a windborne flight across the sea.

Table 1 First notification date, potential source period, and incursion risk period of each island

Island	First notification date	Potential source period	Incursion risk period
Ishigaki			
Location 1	Sep 10 2012	After Sep 10 2012	Aug 27–Sep 9 2012
Location 2	Sep 16 2012	After Sep 16 2012	—
Kohama	Sep 15 2012	—	Sep 1–14 2012
Iriomote	Sep 15 2012	—	Sep 1–14 2012
Kuroshima	Sep 26 2012	—	Sep 12–25 2012

Spatial analysis

Data

Spatial statistical modeling was conducted to explore the factors associated with vector transmission within Ishigaki Island. The incidence risk on 1-km grid cells of the island, which was defined as the proportion of the cumulative number on infected farms to the total number of cattle farms within the grid cell, was analyzed as the dependent variable. The terrain and land use data were analyzed as the explanatory variable. The grid cell size was determined by taking into account the spatial dependency of infected and noninfected farm distribution. This spatial dependency of farm distribution was checked by a semivariogram, which defines the spatial scales over which the pattern are dependent [52]. In plotting a semivariogram, a saturated state indicates a pattern that lacks special dependencies [52]. In this study, the semivariograms were calculated by a farm's status (i.e., 0, noninfected; 1, infected) and by the distance between farms. Visual inspection of the semivariogram plots detected a saturated pattern of semivariogram when the distance was greater than 0.8 km. Thus, the 1-km grid cell size was considered an appropriate size to exclude farm spatial dependency.

Environmental information such as elevations and slope gradients, land use information, and farm density (i.e., the number of cattle farms in a 1-km grid cell) was selected as the potential predictors of disease transmission on the island. Data on the elevations and slope gradients in each 1-km cell were obtained from a free publicly accessible database, the National Land Numerical Information (NLNI) by the Ministry of Land, Infrastructure, Transport and Tourism (MLIT) in Tokyo, Japan [53]. The average value, minimum value, and maximum value of the evaluations and slope gradients in each cell were used for the analysis. The 100-m grid cell sized land use data, obtained from the NLNI [53], were used to calculate the proportion of each land use classification for each 1-km cell. Land use was classified as paddy fields; farmland (except for paddy fields), which mostly included sugar cane and pasture in the island; forest; wasteland; building use; inland water (i.e., rivers and lakes); and others.

Statistical analysis

The number of BEF cases and the number of farms in a cell i are y_i and n_i, respectively; therefore, the expected incidence risk, p_i, in cell i can be described by the following logistic regression formula:

$$y_i \sim Binominal\,(p_i, n_i)\ \mathrm{log}it\,(p_i) = \log\left(\frac{p_i}{1-p_i}\right) = \beta_0 + Z\beta + \varepsilon$$

in which β_0 represents the intercept, $Z\beta$ represents a series of explanatory variables, and ε represents the residual term (assumed to have an approximately normal distribution).

In spatial analysis, unknown factors often vary in space and induce a spatial correlation between the observed disease counts in each area and its neighbors [54]. To account for this correlation, it is assumed that the unexplained variation comprises two parts: a structured component (i.e., spatially correlated) and an unstructured component (i.e., spatially random). In this context, the aforementioned model was parameterized as follows:

$$\mathrm{log}it\,(p_i) = \log\left(\frac{p_i}{1-p_i}\right) = \beta_0 + Z\beta + S_i + U_i$$

in which S_i and U_i correspond to the structured and unstructured random effects, respectively, for cell i,. The unstructured heterogeneity term, U_i, was assumed to have a normal distribution with mean 0 and precision (inverse variance) τ_u. The structured heterogeneity term, S_i, was assumed to have a conditional intrinsic Gaussian autoregressive (CAR) structure, which was described in 1991 by Besag et al. [55]. It has been applied in previous spatial modeling studies in epidemiology and ecology [56–59]. The inclusion of the CAR structure allows the incidence risk of cell i to be modeled by taking into account the spatial structured effects from cell i's neighbors. In this paper, we specified that cell j is a neighbor of cell i, if they share the same boundaries. In the CAR structure, the spatial component S_i is assumed to depend on a conditional distribution that is a normal distribution with a mean equal to the average of the spatial component in the set of cells (i.e., neighbors) adjacent to cell i and precision proportional to the number of neighbors (this precision is defined as τ_s). Non-informative prior distributions were given for the priors of the intercept and coefficients of explanatory variables, assuming normal distribution with a mean of 0 and a variance of 10^{-5}. The precisions of the unstructured and structured spatial components were also given non-informative distribution by gamma distribution (shape, 0.5; scale, 0.0005) [60].

In the spatial analysis, all explanatory variables were first subjected to univariable logistic regression. Only variables with a p value less than 0.15 in the univariable analysis were then included in the multivariable logistic regression model. In multivariable analysis, all possible combinations of explanatory variables were examined, and the model with the smallest Akaike information criterion (AIC) was determined as the best-fitting model without taking into consideration spatial correlation [61]. Finally, the explanatory variables selected in multivariable analysis were included for the CAR model, which took into consideration the unstructured and structured spatial components (Model 1). To evaluate the influences of unstructured and structured random effects, we also compared three other models: Model 2, which included only the structured random effect; Model 3, which included only the unstructured random effect; and Model 4, which did not include the structured random effect or the unstructured random effect. Spatial autocorrelations of residuals in these models were assessed using Moran's *I* index [62] and the goodness of fit for the models was compared using the deviance information criterion (DIC). These hierarchal spatial models were run by the Markov chain Monte Carlo algorithm implemented Bayesian Inference Using Gibbs Sampling software (WinBUGS 1.4) [63]. R2WinBUGS package [64] and R version 3.10 (R Core Team, 2014) were used to run the model in WinBUGS. In the model, three chains were simulated, and each chain had 500,000 iterations after a burn-in of 20,000 iterations. After storing every 10th iteration from each chain, 150,000 iterations were used for the posterior parameter estimates. The explanatory variables were scaled to a mean of zero and standard deviation of one prior to the model to facilitate the convergence of model estimate. Convergence was assessed by the visual inspection of the plots of the sampled parameters and values of R-hat by the Gelman-Rubin convergence diagnostic, which indicate convergence when the values are close to 1 [65].

Results

Descriptive analysis and transmission between islands

The first case of BEF was detected on a beef-breeding farm in the western part of Ishigaki Island on September 10, 2012 (Figs. 1 and 2). By the middle of September, the disease had spread to the southern part of Ishigaki Island; it was also confirmed on Iriomote and Kohama Islands on September 15, 2012. The disease was then confirmed on Kuroshima Island on September 26, 2012. Between October 2012 and January 2013, BEF cases were detected sporadically in the southern and eastern parts of Ishigaki Island. The last case of BEF was reported on Ishigaki Island on September 17, 2013. Further suspected cases have not been observed. All 225 cases of BEF were detected on beef cattle farms. The farm-level incidence risk on each island was the following: Ishigaki Island, 39 % (204/523, 95 % confidence interval [CI], 35 %–43 %), Iriomote Island, 20 % (10/49, 95 % CI, 9 %–32 %); Kohama Island, 19 % (5/26, 95 % CI, 4 %–34 %); and Kuroshima Island, 11 % (6/55, 95 % CI, 3 %–19 %).

The distributions of forward trajectories that originated from Ishigaki Island are shown in Fig. 3. During the potential source period of Location 1 on Ishigaki Island, dispersal by air to Iriomote and Kohama Islands occurred on September 10, 11, and 13—dates that were within the incursion risk period of these islands. In addition, during the potential source period of Location 2 on Ishigaki Island, dispersal by air to Kuroshima Island occurred on September 19 and September 25, which was within the incursion risk period on Kurohama Island. Wind dispersal from Ishigaki Island occurred 1 week before the first detection of the disease on each island. Except for these wind events, no typical wind blew from Ishigaki Islands to the surrounding islands within the incursion risk period of each island.

Estimation of the potential source of the vectors

Results of backward trajectory analysis showed that the source of trajectories reaching Ishigaki Island were Viet Nam, Laos, and the Philippines during the incursion risk period (August 28, 2012–September 1, 2012); a few trajectories were observed from Taiwan on August 28, 2012 (Fig. 4). However, during September 2–9, 2012 (i.e., 1 week before the first detection of the disease), no back

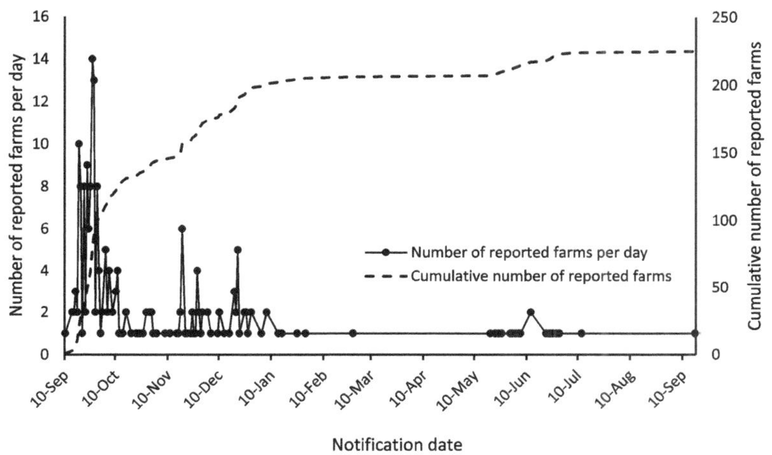

Fig. 2 The number of infected farms during the bovine ephemeral fever outbreak in 2012–2013

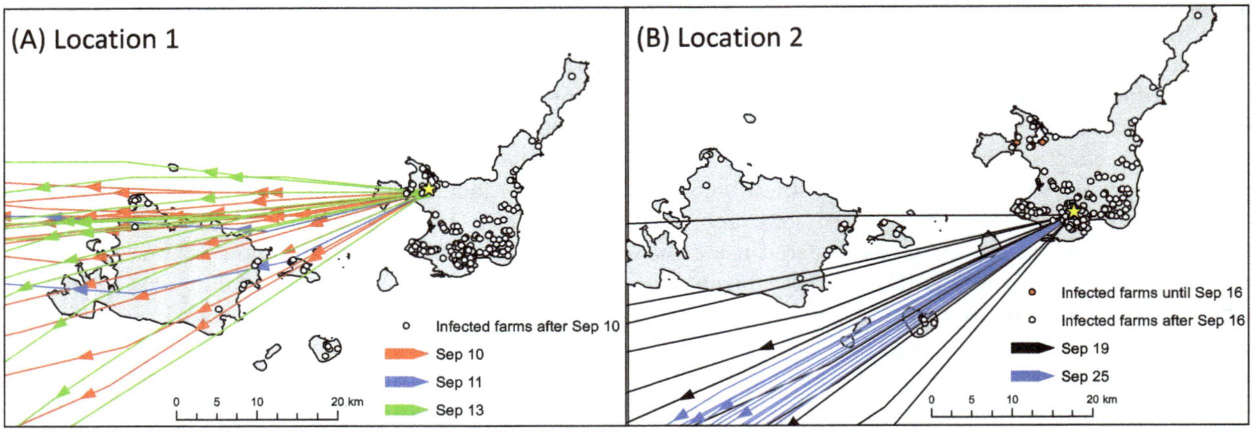

Fig. 3 Forward trajectories from Ishigaki Island to neighboring islands. The yellow stars indicate the starting point of trajectory, (i.e., Location 1 and Location 2) on Ishigaki Island

trajectories extended to Southeast Asia, and the terminal points of the trajectories were distributed over the sea to the east coast of the island (Fig. 4).

Spatial analysis

The distribution of infected farms with the kernel density of cattle farms, elevation and topography and the land use of the island is shown in Fig. 5a–c, respectively. There were 122 grid cells, which included cattle farms. The median number of cattle farms per cell was four farms (range, 1–33 farms). As a result of univariable and multivariable analyses, the 1-km cell-level incidence risk was best explained by the model, which included the minimum slope gradient ($p = 0.01$), the proportion of paddy fields ($p = 0.01$), and the proportion of farmlands ($p < 0.01$). The results of the assessment of residuals and the goodness of fit for the hierarchal spatial models, which include these three variables, are shown in Table 2. In Models 3 and 4, which did not include the structure random effect, autocorrelations of residuals were marginally detected ($p = 0.07$) and the values of DIC were larger than those of Models 1 and 2, which included the structure random effect. Among the four models, Model 2 gave a better fit in terms of a lower DIC value; thus, the results of Model 2 were used for the final analysis (Table 3). The posterior distribution of

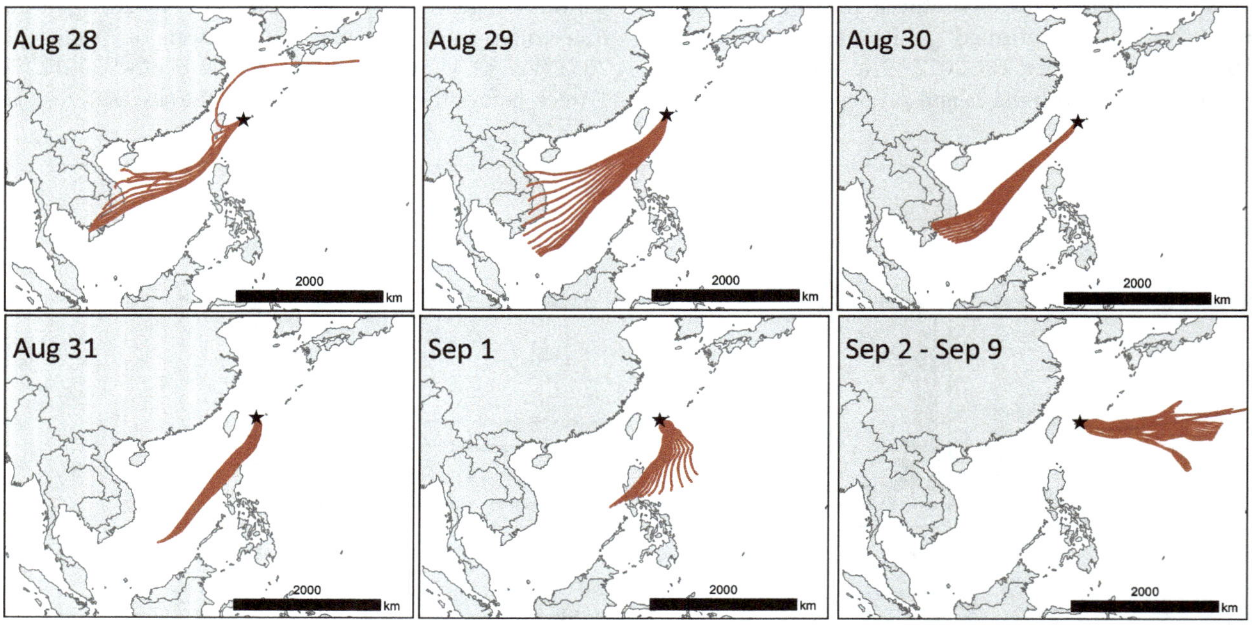

Fig. 4 Backward trajectories from Ishigaki Island. The black star indicates the starting point of the trajectory at Location 1 on Ishigaki Island

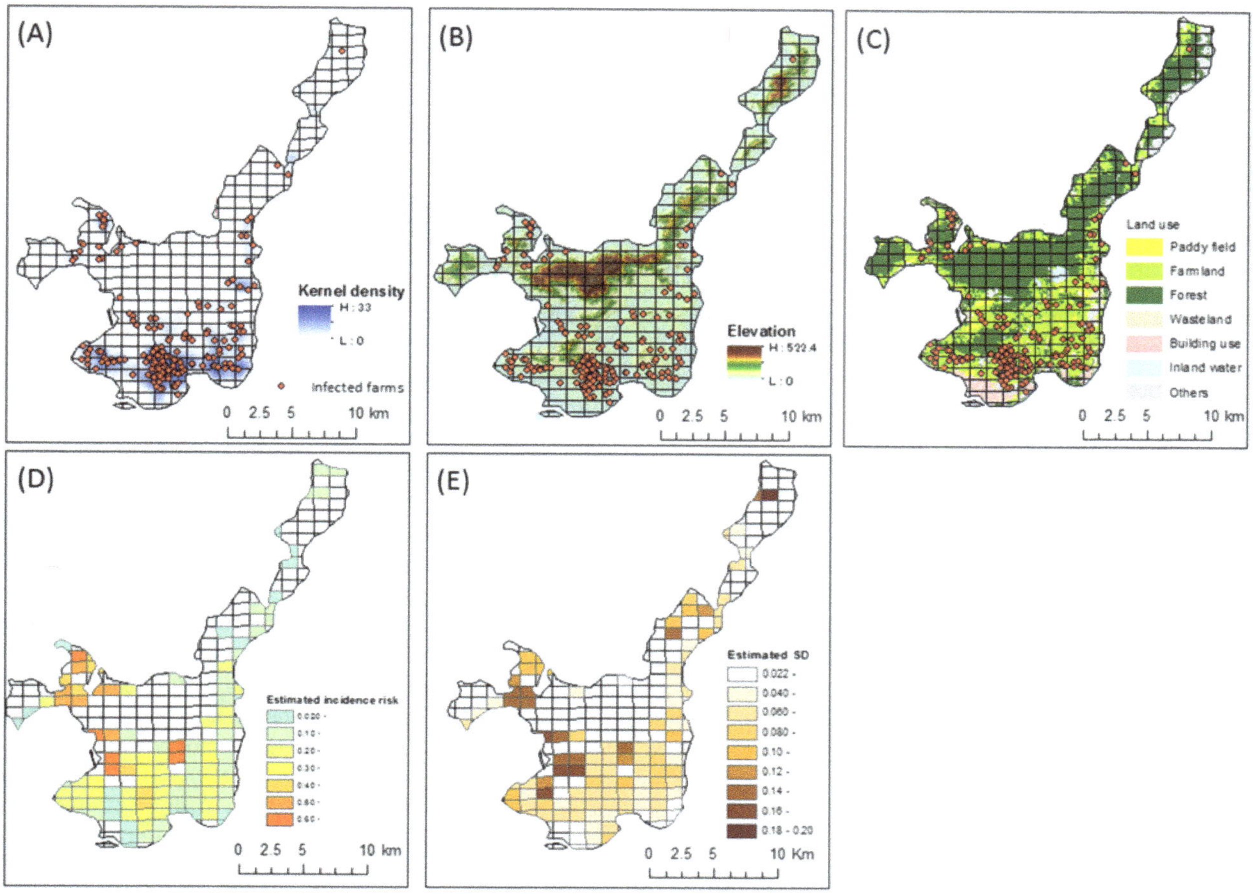

Fig. 5 The spatial analysis results. **a** The distribution of infected farms and kernel density of cattle farms on Ishigaki Island. **b** Elevation and topography of Ishigaki Island. **c** Land use on Ishigaki Island. **d** The estimated incidence risk in each 1-km cell. **e** The estimated standard deviations of each 1-km cell

parameters in the model was converged (i.e., the value of R-hat was nearly equal to 1). With regard to the factor of land use, the proportion of paddy fields and the proportion of farmlands showed a positive impact on the 1-km cell-level incidence risk, although the proportion of paddy fields was a little less than 0 in the 2.5 % credible value, which was significant in the multivariable logistic mode. With regard to the terrain factor, the minimum slope gradient was a significant predictor for the 1-km cell-level incidence risk (i.e., a cell with a lager minimum slope gradients tended to have a higher incidence risk). The predicted 1-km cell-level incidence risk and its estimated standard deviation are shown Fig. 5d, e. Relatively high incidence risk areas were predicted in the western to southwestern region of Ishigaki Island. In some grid cells with a small number of cattle farms (i.e., fewer than five farms), the estimated standard deviations of predicted incidence risk were a little higher than in the other grid cells.

Table 2 Moran's *I* index for residuals and the deviance information criterion of four hierarchical spatial models

Models	Parameters[a]	Moran's *I* (p value)	DIC
Model 1	Fixed effects, S, U	−0.1031 (0.9157)	306.385
Model 2	Fixed effects, S	−0.1193 (0.9467)	301.918
Model 3	Fixed effects, U	0.0923 (0.0721)	323.569
Model 4	Fixed effects	0.0888 (0.0794)	331.492

DIC deviance information criterion

[a]Fixed effects indicate variables that were significant in univariable and multivariable analyses and included in the hierarchical spatial models. The letters "S" and "U" indicate the structured and unstructured heterogeneity term, respectively

Discussion

The present epidemiological analysis clarified the spatial and temporal characteristics of the 2012–2013 BEF outbreak in the Yaeyama Islands. The first BEF case was detected on a beef cattle farm in the western part of Ishigaki Island. In 1 month, the disease had spread to the southern part of the island and was transmitted to neighboring islands. Analysis using an atmospheric dispersion model showed that the forward trajectories from

Table 3 The posterior means and standard deviations of the regression coefficients in Model 2

Variables	Mean	SD	95 % CI	R-hat
Minimum slope gradients[a]	0.2941	0.1453	0.0049, 0.5777	1.0459
Proportion of paddy fields[a]	0.1556	0.1493	−0.1320, 0.4565	1.0074
Proportion of farmland[a]	0.4603	0.1413	0.1863, 0.7469	1.0341
Structured heterogeneity term[b]	0.0014	0.0008	0.0002, 0.9042	1.1295

Model 2 is the hierarchical spatial model which included structured heterogeneity term. 95 % CI, 95 % credible interval; *SD* standard deviation
[a]Each estimated regression coefficient is the standardized coefficient, which indicates the relative contribution to the incidence risk of bovine ephemeral fever
[b]The standard deviation of the structured heterogeneity term

Ishigaki Island dispersed to the neighboring islands 1 week before the disease was detected on each island. This result suggested that wind dispersion of infected vectors could occur from Ishigaki Island to neighboring islands during the high risk incursion period for each island. The potential of introducing BEF *via* infected cattle movements from Ishigaki Island to neighboring islands was negligible, based on the cattle movement data during the early phase of the outbreak. Furthermore, the introduction of infected cattle from surrounding Asian countries was negligible because the importation of cloven-hoofed animals and their products are prohibited from these countries on account of the outbreaks of foot-and-mouth disease. Therefore, atmospheric transport of infected vectors is presumable in the transmission of the disease between islands.

The windborne spread of bluetongue virus infection and Schmallenberg virus infection has also been reported in the recent emergence of these diseases in European countries [18–23, 66]. In the United Kingdom and Sweden, analysis using atmospheric dispersion models well demonstrates the possibility that infected vectors were likely to have reached over the sea from affected regions in Europe [19, 20]. In comparison to the transmission distance in Europe (approximately 100–200 km), the distance between Ishigaki Island and neighboring islands are extremely short (approximately 15 km); thus between-island transmission of infected vectors *via* wind could have readily occurred.

The BEF outbreak continued in Ishigaki Island for 1 year, which included the winter. The BEFV gene from blood samples from febrile cattle in April 2013 shared the identical sequence of the virus isolated in 2012. In infected cattle, the viremic period of BEFV usually lasts 4–5 days [67]; therefore, it is probable that the virus had been maintained in a cycle between the vector and the host, even in the winter. The winter season in Yaeyama Island is milder and shorter (average temperature is approximately 20 °C); as a result, the maintenance of BEFV would be possible, even in the winter.

The influence of landscape on an outbreak of arbovirus infection or the abundance of the related vectors has been investigated in previous studies. The abundance of *Culicoides* biting midges is positively associated with pasture cover [32]. Woodland, open prairies, and impervious surface areas have been associated with the risk of bluetongue infection [36]. Furthermore, row crops, shrublands, soil, and wetlands are positively associated with West Nile virus transmission by mosquitoes [37]. The BEFV has been isolated from field-caught mosquitoes and biting midges [2, 67]. In addition, viral replication is also evident in both insects by experimental feeding on infected blood [2, 67]. In the present study, spatial analysis showed that the proportion of paddy fields and farmlands was significantly associated with the incidence risk within Ishigaki Island. Biting midges and mosquitoes require wet soil or semiaquatic habitats for breeding; therefore, the areas covered with paddy fields or farmlands are suitable for the growth and survival of the vectors. A previous field study in Japan demonstrated that the larvae of some species of *Culicoides* biting midges such as *C. oxystoma*, which has a high potential to transmit ruminant arboviruses [68], were recovered from paddy fields. This finding suggests that paddy fields contribute to the breeding and maintenance of biting midges [69]. Furthermore, it is important to note that farmlands on Ishigaki Island are primarily used for pastures and sugar cane. Larvae of *C. asiana*, which is a recently recognized cryptic species of *C. brevitarsis* [70, 71], have been collected from cattle dung in pastures in the Yaeyama Islands in a previous field survey [69]. Previous entomological surveillance in Ishigaki Island also shows that these species are dominant or subdominant in cowsheds [72, 73]. Meanwhile, the larvae of Anopheline and Culicine mosquitoes are frequently collected from paddy fields in the Yaeyama Islands [74, 75]. Several species such as *Anopheles sinensis* and *Culex tritaeniorhynchus*, which breed in paddy fields, obtain their blood meal from cattle [76]. If one or more of these hematophagous insects contribute to the transmission of BEFV, paddy fields and farmlands could be a high risk factor for disease spread. Little information on the vectors of BEF has been available in this region; however, the spatial analysis in this study showed that farmlands and paddy fields would be logical search areas if studies were conducted to identify BEF vectors in this area, and it would support an understanding of the ecological mechanism of BEFV circulation.

Spatial analysis also showed that the explanatory variable of the minimum slope gradient was positively associated with the incidence risk. This result indicates that a sloping area tended to have a higher incidence risk. In general, the nature of air flow is complex and a variety of local winds arise in complex terrains such as a hilly or mountainous terrain [14, 77]. Local winds may influence the movement and concentration of flying insects [14, 77]. Some insects such as grasshoppers or moths move up and down the slopes by using the updraft or downdraft from the terrains; in addition, rotor waves or lee waves deposit insects in an area and produce localized outbreaks of a pest species [14, 77–79]. The western part of Ishigaki Island is a mountainous region; therefore, the complicated condition of its terrain may concentrate the vectors and lead to a BEF outbreak.

The backward trajectory analysis in this study estimated the possible source of infected vectors in Southeast Asian regions such as Viet Nam, Laos, and the Philippines. Mitochondrial phylogeography analysis reveals that *C. oxystoma* specimens captured in Japan is closely related to specimens captured in Southeast Asia [80]. A few backward trajectories from Taiwan were also observed, which suggested that Taiwan was not negligible as a potential source. A previous study demonstrated that the Japanese and Taiwanese strains of the BEFV, which were isolated in the outbreaks of 1996, 1984–1989, and 1996–2004, were classified in the same clusters and were closely related, based on their nucleotide sequences [10]. As in Japan in 2012, an outbreak of BEF was reported in Taiwan, which is adjacent to the Yaeyama Islands [13]. The BEFV isolated in the 2012 outbreak was classified in the same cluster [9]. With regard to other arbovirus infections, Japanese encephalitis virus, which is transmitted by mosquitoes, was isolated from pigs on Ishigaki Island and was most closely related to the Taiwanese strains [81]. These findings support that the arbovirus infections in Japan and Taiwan have an epidemiological linkage and are exposed from the enzootic lower latitude regions *via* long-distance movements of infected vectors carried by wind. Rice planthoppers, a major rice pest in Japan, can fly more than 2000 km by wind from Southeast Asia or from southern China to Japan [82]. Therefore, the windborne long-distance migration of BEF-infected vectors would be possible, even for *Culicoides* biting midges (1–3 mm), which are smaller than rice planthoppers (4–6 mm). Overseas migration of *Culex* mosquitoes, which are the vector for the Japanese encephalitis virus, has also been suggested in Asia and Oceania [83–85]. The possibility of BEF introduction by the infected mosquitoes from lower latitude regions could not be ruled out at present.

This study clarified the spatiotemporal characteristics of a BEF outbreak in Japan and revealed the risk factors associated with the disease transmission in Ishigaki Island. However, because of the following limitations of this study, some degree of caution is needed in interpreting these results. First, the outbreak data used for the analysis in this study focused on BEF cases that were based on clinical and epidemiological observations. Because of the possibility of subclinical infection, the disease may have in actuality spread wider. Second, the present analysis did not take into account the effect of vaccination. After the outbreak of BEF, emergency vaccinations with a single dose of inactivated vaccine were administered to the cattle in the region; vaccination was especially mandatory for cattle that were shipped to market and 8182 cattle (24 % of cattle in the region) were vaccinated. However, because serological surveillance had not been conducted, we did not explore the effect of vaccination in the current study. The routine vaccination of dairy cattle and beef heifers has been also encouraged in the Yaeyama region as a preventive measure of BEF. However, the vaccination coverage of all cattle population in this region was low in past 3 years: the vaccine coverage and the number of vaccinated animals were 2.6 % and 875 animals in 2010, 2.5 % and 808 animals in 2011, and 1.3 % and 410 animals in 2012 (except for emergency vaccination). Therefore, the influence of vaccination in this region seems to have a limited effect on BEF infection.

In this study, the potential sources of infected vectors were estimated in Southeast Asia. The prediction of the migration of infected vectors to Japan will be useful to prevent and control BEF. However, further investigations are still needed to achieve this. First, although BEF is a disease that occurs in tropical, subtropical, and temperate regions in Asia [2], the current situation of BEF in Southeast Asia has not been investigated well. With the evidence that BEF has been confirmed in the southeast region of China [12, 86], it is highly probable that the disease is enzootic in Southeast Asia. Second, the air temperature at flying height was not considered in the trajectory analysis. To refine the prediction of infected vector immigration, more detailed information on meteorological conditions such as temperature, humidity, and wind speed would need to be considered. In Japan, the migration simulation model for rice planthoppers has been developed by incorporating a numerical weather prediction model and a particle dispersion model, and it has been put to practical use [87, 88]. This approach would be a useful reference to predict the migration of infected vectors in relation to BEF. Third, the prediction of infected vector migration is difficult to validate. As discussed in a previous study on the dispersal model of *Culicoides* biting midges in Australia [24], areal collections, use of entomological radars, or recapture technics are not feasible for biting midges because of its smallness and fragileness. Therefore, a mitochondrial genome phylogeographic analysis has been established to distinguish between invasive and indigenous species of biting midges [80]. A further knowledge and understanding of these factors will refine the prediction of migrating infected vectors.

Conclusions

The epidemiological analysis in this study demonstrated that the condition of topography and landscape had a significant influence on the spatial distribution of BEF within Ishigaki Island. There is a complex interaction between hosts, vectors, and viruses in arbovirus infection outbreaks. Therefore, the landscape components that affect the distribution of vectors and their habitats would be important when assessing the favorable environments for arbovirus infections such as BEF. Furthermore, trajectory analysis using atmospheric dispersion models demonstrated that the long-distance migration of infected vectors would have occurred from Southeast Asia and that the local-scale between-island transmission by wind would have occurred during the outbreak. These findings would be helpful in developing a surveillance program and preventive measures against BEF.

Abbreviations

AIC: Akaike information criterion; BEF: bovine ephemeral fever; CAR: conditional intrinsic Gaussian autoregressive; CGER: Centre for Global Environmental Research; DIC: deviance information criterion.; GDAS: global data assimilation system; HYSPLIT: hybrid single particle lagrangian integrated trajectory model; METEX: Meteorological Data Explorer; MLIT: Ministry of Land, Infrastructure, Transport and Tourism; NLNI: National Land Numerical Information.

Competing interests

The authors declare that they have no competing interests.

Authors' contributions

YH performed all epidemiological analysis and wrote the manuscript. SM assisted in performing spatial analysis and helped to draft the manuscript. TY performed the field investigation and helped to draft manuscript by giving suggestions concerning the vectors of arbovirus disease. MS and YN performed the field investigation, took charge of clinical inspection during the epidemic, and collected the farm data. TN and KI took charge of performing confirmation diagnosis. TY contributed to the interpretation of results and helped to draft the manuscript. SK and KM assisted in performing data analysis and contributed to interpreting the results. TT conceived of the study, and participated in its design, and coordinated and helped to draft the manuscript. All authors have read and approved the manuscript.

Acknowledgements

We thank all staff members of the Yaeyama livestock hygiene service centers of the Okinawa Prefecture for their help in conducting field investigations and organizing farm information. We extend to our appreciation to Yumie Zeniya and Naoko Mastumoto for their assistance. The authors gratefully acknowledge the National Oceanic and Atmospheric Administration (NOAA) Air Resources Laboratory (ARL) for the provision of the HYSPLIT transport and dispersion model and/or the READY website (http://www.ready.noaa.gov) used in this publication. This study was supported by the Research Project for Improving Food Safety and Animal Health of the Ministry of Agriculture, Forestry and Fisheries (Tokyo, Japan).

Author details

[1]Viral Disease and Epidemiology Research Division, National Institute of Animal Health, National Agriculture and Food Research Organization, 3-1-5 Kannondai, Tsukuba, Ibaraki 305-0856, Japan. [2]Department of Environmental Science Graduate School of Science and Technology, Niigata University, Niigata, Japan. [3]Kyushu Research Station, National Institute of Animal Health, National Agriculture and Food Research Organization, Kagoshima, Japan. [4]Yaeyama Livestock Hygiene Service Center, Okinawa Prefectural Government, Okinawa, Japan. [5]Okinawa Prefectural Institute of Animal Health, Okinawa, Japan.

References

1. St. George TD. Bovine ephemeral fever: a review. Trop Anim Health Prod. 1988;20:194–202.
2. Walker PJ. Bovine ephemeral fever in Australia and the world. Curr Top Microbiol Immunol. 2005;292:57–80.
3. Tonbak S, Berber E, Yoruk MD, Azkur AK, Pestil Z, Bulut H. A large-scale outbreak of bovine ephemeral fever in Turkey, 2012. J Vet Med Sci. 2013;75:1511–4.
4. Bai WB, Jiang CL, Davis SS. Preliminary observations on the epidemiology of bovine ephemeral fever in China. Trop Anim Health Prod. 1991;23:22–6.
5. Liao YK, Inaba Y, Li NJ, Chain CY, Lee SL, Liou PP. Epidemiology of bovine ephemeral fever virus infection in Taiwan. Microbiol Res. 1998;153:289–95.
6. Yeruham I, Van Ham M, Stram Y, Friedgut O, Yadin H, Mumcuoglu KY, et al. Epidemiological investigation of bovine ephemeral fever outbreaks in Israel. Vet Med Int. 2010. doi:10.4061/2010/290541.
7. Nandi S, Negi BS. Bovine ephemeral fever: a review. Comp Immunol Microbiol Infect Dis. 1999;22:81–91.
8. Ministry of Agriculture, Forestry and Fisheries (MAFF). Data on animal hygiene. 2014.
9. Niwa T, Shirafuji H, Ikemiyagi K, Nitta Y, Suzuki M, Kato T, Yanase T. Occurrence of bovine ephemeral fever in Okinawa Prefecture, Japan, in 2012 and development of a reverse-transcription polymerase chain reaction assay to detect bovine ephemeral fever virus gene. J Vet Med Sci. 2015;77: 455–60.
10. Kato T, Aizawa M, Takayoshi K, Kokuba T, Yanase T, Shirafuji H, Tsuda T, Yamakawa M. Phylogenetic relationships of the G gene sequence of bovine ephemeral fever virus isolated in Japan, Taiwan and Australia. Vet Microbiol. 2009;137:217–23.
11. Aizawa M, Takayoshi K, Kokuba T, Kato T, Yanase T, Yamakawa M, Tsuda T. Molecular epidemiological analysis of bovine ephemeral fever viruses isolated in Okinawa Prefecture (In Japanese, with English abstract). J Jpn Vet Med Assoc. 2008;63:363–6.
12. Zheng OF, Qiu C. Phylogenetic relationships of the glycoprotein gene of bovine ephemeral fever virus isolated from mainland China, Taiwan, Japan, Turkey, Israel and Australia. Virol J. 2012;9:268.
13. Ting LJ, Lee MS, Lee SH, Tsai HJ, Lee F. Relationships of bovine ephemeral fever epizootics to population immunity and virus variation. Vet Microbiol. 2014;173:241–8.
14. Drake VA, Farrow RA. The Influence of atmospheric structure and motions on insect migration. Annu Rev Entomol. 1988;33:183–210.
15. Pedgley DE. Windborne pests and diseases: meteorology of airborne organisms. Chichester: Ellis Horwood Ltd.; 1982. p. 250.
16. Sellers RF, Pedgley DE, Tucker MR. Possible spread of African horse sickness on the wind. J Hyg (Lond). 1977;79:279–98.
17. Lillie TH, Marquardt WC, Jones RH. The flight range of *Culicoides variipennis* (Diptera, Ceratopogonidae). Can Entomol. 1981;113:419–26.
18. Garcia-Lastra R, Leginagoikoa I, Plazaola JM, Ocabo B, Aduriz G, Nunes T, Juste RA. Bluetongue virus serotype one outbreak in the Basque Country (Northern Spain) 2007–2008. Data support a primary vector windborne transport. PLoS One. 2012;7, e34421.
19. Agren EC, Burgin L, Lewerin SS, Gloster J, Elvander M. Possible means of introduction of bluetongue virus serotype 8 (BTV-8) to Sweden in August 2008: comparison of results from two models for atmospheric transport of the *Culicoides* vector. Vet Rec. 2010;167:484–8.
20. Gloster J, Burgin L, Witham C, Athanassiadou M, Mellor PS. Bluetongue in the United Kingdom and northern Europe in 2007 and key issues for 2008. Vet Rec. 2008;162:298–302.

21. Hendrickx G, Gilbert M, Staubach C, Elbers A, Mintiens K, Gerbier G, Ducheyne E. A wind density model to quantify the airborne spread of *Culicoides* species during north-western Europe bluetongue epidemic. 2006. Prev Vet Med. 2008;87:162–81.
22. Ducheyne E, De Deken R, Becu S, Codina B, Nomikou K, Mangana-Vougiaki O, Georgiev G. 596 Purse BV, Hendickx G. Quantifying the wind dispersal of *Culicoides* species in Greece and Bulgaria. Geospat Health. 2007;1:177–89.
23. Alba A, Casal J, Domingo M. Possible introduction of bluetongue into the Balearic Islands, Spain, in 2000, *via* air streams. Vet Rec. 2004;155:460–1.
24. Eagles D, Melville L, Weir R, Davis S, Bellis G, Zalucki MP, Walker PJ, Durr PA. Long-distance aerial dispersal modelling of *Culicoides* biting midges: case studies of incursions into Australia. BMC Vet Res. 2014;10:135.
25. Kettle DS. *Culicidae* (mosquitoes). In: Kettle DS, editor. Medical and veterinary entomology. 2nd ed. Cambridge: CABI Publishing; 1995. p. 142–3.
26. Service MW. Mosquito (Diptera: Culicidae) dispersal—the long and short of it. J Med Entomol. 1997;34:579–88.
27. Murray MD. The spread of ephemeral fever of cattle during the 1967–68 epizootic in Australia. Aust Vet J. 1970;46:77–82.
28. Mellor PS, Boorman J, Baylis M. *Culicoides* biting midges: their role as arbovirus vectors. Annu Rev Entomol. 2000;45:307–40.
29. Kettle DS. Ceratopogonidae (biting midges). In: Kettle DS, editor. Medical and veterinary entomology. 2nd ed. Cambridge: CABI Publishing; 1995. p. 152–76.
30. Impoinvil DE, Cardenas GA, Gihture JI, Mbogo CM, Beier JC. Constant temperature and time period effects on *Anopheles gambiae* egg hatching. J Am Mosq Control Assoc. 2007;23:124–30.
31. Borkent A. The biting midges, the Ceratopogonidae (Diptera). In: Marquardt WC, editor. Biology of disease vectors. 2nd ed. Burlington: Elsevier Academic Press; 2004. p. 113–26.
32. Purse BV, Falconer D, Sullivan MJ, Carpenter S, Mellor PS, Piertney SB, Mordue Luntz AJ, Albon S, Gunn GJ, Blackwell A Impacts of climate, host and landscape factors on *Culicoides* species in Scotland. Med Vet Entomol. 2012;26:168–77.
33. De Liberato C, Farina F, Magliano A, Rombola P, Scholl F, Spallucci V, Scaramozzino P. Biotic and abiotic factors influencing distribution and abundance of *Culicoides obsoletus* group (Diptera: Ceratopogonidae) in central Italy. J Med Entomol. 2010;47:313–8.
34. Calvete C, Estrada R, Miranda MA, Borras D, Calvo JH, Lucientes J. Ecological correlates of bluetongue virus in Spain: predicted spatial occurrence and its relationship with the observed abundance of the potential *Culicoides* spp. vector. Vet J. 2009;182:235–43.
35. Conte A, Goffredo M, Ippoliti C, Meiswinkel R. Influence of biotic and abiotic factors on the distribution and abundance of *Culicoides imicola* and the *Obsoletus* Complex in Italy. Vet Parasitol. 2007;150:333–44.
36. Guis H, Tran A, de La Rocque S, Baldet T, Gerbier G, Barrague B, Biteau-Coroller F, Roger F, Viel JF, Mauny F. Use of high spatial resolution satellite imagery to characterize landscapes at risk for bluetongue. Vet Res. 2007;38:669–83.
37. DeGroote JP, Sugumaran R, Ecker M. Landscape, demographic and climatic associations with human West Nile virus occurrence regionally in 2012 in the United States of America. Geospat Health. 2014;9:153–68.
38. Mughini-Gras L, Mulatti P, Severini F, Boccolini D, Romi R, Bongiorno G, Khoury C, Bianchi R, Montarsi F, Patregnani T, Bonfanti L, Rezza G, Capelli G, Busani L. Ecological niche modelling of potential West Nile virus vector mosquito species and their geographical association with equine epizootics in Italy. Ecohealth. 2014;11:120–32.
39. Draxler RR, Rolph GD. National Oceanic and Atmospheric Administration (NOAA) Air Resources Laboratory (ARL; College Park, MD) READY website. HYSPLIT—Hybrid Single Particle Lagrangian Integrated Trajectory Model. http://www.arl.noaa.gov/HYSPLIT.php. Accessed 10 June 2015.
40. Eagles D, Walker PJ, Zalucki MP, Durr PA. Modelling spatio-temporal patterns of long-distance Culicoides dispersal into northern Australia. Prev Vet Med. 2013;110:312–22.
41. Kedmi M, Herziger Y, Galon N, Cohen RM, Perel M, Batten C, Braverman Y, Gottlieb Y, Shpigel N, Klement E. The association of winds with the spread of EHDV in dairy cattle in Israel during an outbreak in 2006. Prev Vet Med. 2010;96:152–60.
42. Zhu M, Radcliffe EB, Ragsdale DW, MacRae IV, Seeley MW. Low-level jet streams associated with spring aphid migration and current season spread of potato viruses in the U.S. northern Great Plains. Agric For Meteorol. 2006;138:192–202.
43. Draxler RR, Hess GD. An overview of the HYSPLIT_4 modelling system for trajectories, dispersion and deposition. Aust Meteorol Mag. 1988;47:295–308.
44. Draxler RR, Hess GD. An overview of the HYSPLIT_4 modelling system for trajectories, dispersion and deposition. Aust Meteorol Mag. 1998;47:295–308.
45. Zeng J. Centre for Global Environmental Research (CGER). National Institute for Environmental Studies (Tsukuba, Japan). CGER–METEX (Meteorological Data Explorer) model. 2002. http://db.cger.nies.go.jp/metex/index.html. Accessed 10 June 2015.
46. Tzipori S. The susceptibility of young and newborn calves to bovine ephemeral fever virus. Aust Vet J. 1975;51:251–3.
47. Centers for Disease Control and Prevention (CDC). Anopheles mosquitoes. 2012. http://www.cdc.gov/malaria/about/biology/mosquitoes. Accessed on 10 June 2015.
48. Gerry AC, Mullens BA. Seasonal abundance and survivorship of *Culicoides sonorensis* (Diptera: Ceratopogonidae) at a southern California dairy, with reference to potential bluetongue virus transmission and persistence. J Med Entomol. 2000;37:675–88.
49. Kaufmann C, Mathis A, Vorburger C. Sugar-feeding behaviour and longevity of European *Culicoides* biting midges. Med Vet Entomol. 2015;29:17–25.
50. Jamnback H. Observation on *Culicoides obsoletus* (Meigen) in the laboratory (Diptera: Ceratopogonidae). Mosq News. 1961;21:48–53.
51. Zhou G, Scaraffia PY, Wells MA. Vector nutrition and energy metabolism. In: Marquardt WC, editor. Biology of disease vectors. 2nd ed. Burlington: Elsevier Academic Press; 2004. p. 311–5.
52. Turner MG, Gardner RH, O'Neill RV. Landscape ecology in theory and practice: pattern and process. New York: Springer; 2001.
53. Ministry of Land, Infrastructure, Transport and Tourism (MLIT; Tokyo, Japan). National Land Numerical Information (NLNI) 2011. http://nlftp.mlit.go.jp/ksj-e/index.html Accessed 10 June 2015.
54. Pfeiffer DU, Robinson TP, Stevenson M, Stevens KB, Rogers DJ, Clements AC. Identifying factors associated with the spatial distribution of disease. In: Spatial analysis in epidemiology. New York: Oxford University Press; 2008. p. 81–109.
55. Besag J, York J, Mollie A. Bayesian image restoration with applications in spatial statistics. Ann Inst Stat Math. 1991;43:1–20.
56. Richardson S, Abellan JJ, Best N. Bayesian spatio-temporal analysis of joint patterns of male and female lung cancer risks in Yorkshire (UK). Stat Methods Med Res. 2006;15:385–407.
57. Allepuz A, Casal J, Napp S, Saez M, Alba A, Vilar M, Domingo M, Gonzalez MA, Duran-Ferrer M, Vicente J, Alvarez J, Munoz M, Saez JL. Analysis of the spatial variation of bovine tuberculosis disease risk in Spain (2006–2009). Prev Vet Med. 2011;100:44–52.
58. Stevenson MA, Morris RS, Lawson AB, Wilesmith JW, Ryan JB, Jackson R. Area-level risks for BSE in British cattle before and after the July 1988 meat and bone meal feed ban. Prev Vet Med. 2005;69:129–44.
59. Latimer AM, Wu S, Gelfand AE, Silander JA. Building statistical models to analyze species distributions. Ecol Appl. 2006;16:33–50.
60. Kelsall JE, Wakefield JC. Discussion of Bayesian models for spatially correlated disease and exposure data. In: Bernardo JM, Berger JO, Dawid AP, Smith AFM, editors. Bayesian statistics 6. Oxford: Oxford University Press; 1999. p. 151.
61. Burnham KP, Anderson DR. Model selection and multimodel inference: a practical information–theoretic approach. 2nd ed. New York: Springer; 2002.
62. Moran PAP. Notes on continuous stochastic phenomena. Biometrika. 1950;37:17–23.
63. Lunn DJ, Thomas A, Best N, Spiegelhalter D. WinBUGS—a Bayesian modelling framework: concepts, structure, and extensibility. Stat Comput. 2000;10:325–37.
64. Sturtz S, Ligges U, Gelman A. R2WinBUGS: A Package for Running WinBUGS from R. J Stat Softw. 2005;12:1–16.
65. Gelman A, Rubin DB. Inference from iterative simulation using multiple sequences. Stat Sci. 1992;7:457–511.
66. Sedda L, Rogers DJ. The influence of the wind in the Schmallenberg virus outbreak in Europe. Sci Rep. 2013;3:3361.
67. St. George TD. Bovine ephemeral fever. In: Coetzer JAW, Tustin RC, editors. Infectious diseases of livestock. Cape Town: Oxford University Press; 2004. p. 1183–98.
68. Yanase T, Kato T, Kubo T, Yoshida K, Ohashi S, Yamakawa M, Miura Y, Tsuda T. Isolation of bovine arboviruses from Culicoides biting midges (Diptera: Ceratopogonidae) in southern Japan: 1985–2002. J Med Entomol. 2005;42:63–7.
69. Yanase T, Matsumoto Y, Matsumori Y, Aizawa M, Hirata M, Kato T, Shirafuji H, Yamakawa M, Tsuda T, Noda H. Molecular identification of field-collected *Culicoides* larvae in the southern part of Japan. J Med Entomol. 2013;50:1105–10.

70. Bellis G, Dyce A, Gopurenko D, Yanase T, Garros C, Labuschagne K, Mitchell A Revision of the *Culicoides (Avaritia) imicola* complex Khamala & Kettle (Diptera: Ceratopogonidae) from the Australasian region. Zootaxa. 2014;3768:401–27.
71. Bellis G, Halling L, Anderson SJ. Pictorial key to adult female *Culicoides* Latreille, 1809 (Diptera: Ceratopogonidae) from the Northern Territory, Western Australia and South Australia. Austral Entomol. 2015;54:28–59.
72. Hoshino C. Notes on biting midges collected by light traps at a cowshed in Ishigaki-jima, Ryukyu Islands [in Japanese with English summary]. Med Entomol Zool. 1985;36:55–8.
73. Yanase T, Kato T, Katagiri Y, Aizawa M, Nakamura K, Kokuba T, Araki M, Shirafuji H, Yamakawa M, Tsuda T. Isolation and characterization of bluetongue virus from *Culicoides brevitarsis* (Diptera: Ceratopogonidae) in Okinawa. Med Entomol Zool. 2010;61:85–91.
74. Miyagi I, Toma T. Studies on the mosquitoes in the Yaeyama Islands—1. Appearances of anopheline mosquitoes, especially *Anopheles minimus minimus* Theobald in Ishigaki and Iriomotejima [in Japanese with English Summary]. Med Entomol Zool. 1978;29:243–50.
75. Miyagi I, Toma T. Studies on the mosquitoes in Yaeyama Islands, Japan—5. Notes on the mosquitoes collected in forest areas of Iriomotejima [in Japanese with English summary]. Med Entomol Zool. 1980;31:81–91.
76. Tamashiro M, Toma T, Mannen K, Higa Y, Miyagi I. Bloodmeal identification and feeding habitats of mosquitoes (Diptera: Culicidae) collected at five islands in the Ryukyu Archipelago. Japan Med Entomol Zool. 2011;62:53–70.
77. Burt PJA, Pedgley DE. Nocturnal insect migration: effects of local winds. Adv Ecol Res. 1997;27:61–92.
78. Joyce RJV. Aerial transport of pests and pest outbreaks. EPPO Bull. 1983;13:111–9.
79. Noda T, Kiritani K. Landing places of migratory planthoppers, *Nilaparvata lugens* (STÅL) and *Sogatella furcifera* (HORVATH) (Homoptera : Delphacidae) in Japan. Appl Entomol Zool. 1989;24:59–65.
80. Yanase T, Matsumoto Y, Bellis G, Gopurenko D, Wardhana A, Lee F, et al. Mitochondrial phylogeography of *Culicoides oxystoma* in East and Southeast Asia, and Australia. Potsdam: 8th International Congress of Dipterology; 2014. p. 408–9.
81. Nidaira M, Kyan H, Taira K, Okano S, Oshiro T, Kato T, Kudo N, Azama Y, Mahoe Y, Kudaka J, Tamanaha K, Takasaki T. Survey of Japanese encephalitis virus in pigs and wild boars on Ishigaki and Iriomote Islands in Okinawa. Japan Epidemiol Infect. 2014;142:856–60.
82. Otuka A. Migration of rice planthoppers and their vectored re-emerging and novel rice viruses in East Asia. Front Microbiol. 2013;4:309.
83. Asahina S. Transoceanic flight of mosquitoes on the Northwest Pacific. Jpn J Med Sci Biol. 1970;23:255–8.
84. Ritchie SA, Rochester W. Wind-blown mosquitoes and introduction of Japanese encephalitis into Australia. Emerg Infect Dis. 2001;7:900–3.
85. Hemmerter S, Slapeta J, van den Hurk AF, Cooper RD, Whelan PI, Russell RC, Johansen CA, Beebe NW. A curious coincidence: mosquito biodiversity and the limits of the Japanese encephalitis virus in Australasia. BMC Evol Biol. 2007;7:100.
86. Li Z, Zheng F, Gao S, Wang S, Wang J, Liu Z, Du J, Yin 759 H. Large-scale serological survey of bovine ephemeral fever in China. Vet Microbiol. 2015;176:155–60.
87. Otuka A, Zhou Y, Lee GS, Matsumura M, Zhu Y, Park HH, Liu Z, Sanada-Morimura S. Prediction of overseas migration of the small brown planthopper, *Laodelphax striatellus* (Hemiptera: Delphacidae) in East Asia. Appl Entomol Zool. 2012;47:379–88.
88. Otuka A, Watanabe T, Suzuki Y, Matsumura M, Furuno A, Chino M. Real-time prediction system for migration of rice planthoppers *Sogatella furcifera* (Horvath) and *Nilaparvata lugens* (Stal) (Homoptera: Delphacidae). App Entemol Zool. 2005;40:221–9.

Selenium ameliorates *Staphylococcus aureus*-induced inflammation in bovine mammary epithelial cells by inhibiting activation of TLR2, NF-κB and MAPK signaling pathways

Heng Wang[1,2†], Chongliang Bi[1,2,3†], Yinjie Wang[1,2], Jun Sun[1,2], Xia Meng[1,2] and Jianji Li[1,2*]

Abstract

Background: *Staphylococcus aureus* (*S. aureus*) internalization into bovine mammary epithelial cells (bMECs) is considered an important pathogenic mechanism for the establishment of mastitis. Given the interesting link between selenium (Se) status and mastitis, our objective was to prove that Se was essential to suppress pro-inflammatory mediators, in part, by modulation of Toll-like receptor2 (TLR2), nuclear factor kappaB (NF-κB) and mitogen activated protein kinase (MAPK) signal transduction pathway in bMECs.

Results: Results showed that Se (0~ 16 μM) did not affect the growth of bMECs. The mRNA expression of TLR2, Myeloid differentiation factor 88 (Myd88), Interleukin-1 receptor-associated kinase4 (Irak4), Interleukin-1 receptor-associated kinase1 (Irak1) and TNF receptor-associated factor6 (Traf6) in TLR2 signal pathway were increased or significantly increased by *S. aureus*. Se played an important role in regulating the genes expression of TLR2, Myd88, Traf6 but not in controlling the expression of Irak4 and Irak1. In addition, Se exerted strong inhibitory effects on the genes expression of tumor necrosis factor-alpha (TNF-α), interleukin-1β (IL-1β) and interleukin-6 (IL-6) induced by *S. aureus*. To further investigate the possible signaling mechanisms involved in the processes, we analyzed the role of MAPK and NF-κB signaling pathway in inflammation response in *S. aureus*-stimulated bMECs in vitro. Results showed that the phosphorylation of inhibitory kappaB alpha (*IκBα*), *p65*, *p38* and extracellular regulated protein kinase (*Erk*) were significantly increased in *S. aureus*-stimulated bMECs. It indicated that *S. aureus* activated NF-κB and MAPK signaling pathway. We also examined the effects of Se on the phosphorylation of *IκBα, p65, p38* and *Erk* in NF-κB and MAPK signaling pathway, which have well been proved to control the synthesis and release of pro-inflammatory mediators during inflammation. The findings are exciting, that pretreatment with Se (4, 8 μM) significantly suppressed the phosphorylation of *IκBα*, *p65*, *p38* and *Erk*.

Conclusions: These results suggest that Se down-regulates inflammatory mediators TNF-α, IL-1β and IL-6 gene expressions via TLR2, NF-κB and MAPK signaling pathway in *S. aureus*-stimulated bMECs, which may be responsible for the anti-inflammatory effect of Se.

Keywords: Se, TLR2, NF-κB, MAPK, Mammary

* Correspondence: yzjjli@163.com
†Heng Wang and Chongliang Bi contributed equally to this work.
[1]College of Veterinary Medicine, Yangzhou University, Yangzhou 225009, Jiangsu, China
[2]Jiangsu Co-innovation Center for Prevention and Control of Important Animal Infectious Diseases and Zoonoses, Yangzhou 225009, Jiangsu, China
Full list of author information is available at the end of the article

Background

Bovine mastitis is a frequent and costly disease in the dairy industry [1]. *S. aureus* internalization into bMECs is considered an important pathogenic mechanism for the establishment of mastitis. In contrast to clinical mastitis, *S. aureus*-induced mastitis may manifest very diverse degrees of severity, from fulminating gangrenous mastitis with nervous systemic signs to mild local infection with only local signs [2, 3]. Therefore, it is of prime importance to determine how to detect and eradicate bacteria earlier and control the inflammation [4]. Antibiotics as an effective treatment of bovine mastitis existed many limits such as drug resistance and food safety concerns [5]. Thus, innate immune defense in local against pathogenic microorganisms has already attracted extensive attention.

The epithelium is an important line of defense against pathogenic microorganisms. Beyond the function of milk production, bMECs also equipped with a battery of receptors sensing the presence molecular components of pathogens, which has been verified that these cells are capable of initiating an in vitro innate immune response to pathogenic bacteria [6, 7]. Among these pattern recognition receptors (PPRs), 13 different TLRs have been well described in mammalian [8]. Some of these receptors span across the cell membrane and bind bacterial ligands with their extracellular domain. TLR2, for example, has been confirmed to be indispensable for *S. aureus* recognition [9]. Successful TLR2 signaling mostly involves the activation of the factor Myd88. Myd88 possesses two remarkable domains, the N-terminal death domain and C-terminal Toll/IL-1R domain (TIR) domain [10]. Ligand binding to the TLR family results in the recruitment of Myd88 to TIR domains of receptors. And the death domain of Myd88 is known to interact with Irak, a serine/threonine kinase harbors a death domain in N-terminal portion by homophilic interaction. Subsequently, another adaptor protein Traf6 is phosphorylated and recruited to Irak [11]. Further, the TLR2-*S. aureus* interaction leads to the rapid and coordinated activation of various intracellular signaling pathways such as NF-κB and MAPK [12]. NF-κB and MAPK signaling pathways, responsible for regulating the expression of cytokines, chemokines, are essential immune mediators during inflammation [13].

Se is an essential micronutrient, which has been investigated for various medical applications such as anti-bacterial, anti-oxidant, anti-inflammatory, and anti-cancer growth [14, 15]. Previous studies have shown the correlation between Se and LPS-induced mammary epithelial cells inflammatory response. Results demonstrated that Se exert beneficial effects to mammary epithelial cells, after the treatment of cells with the LPS. Result also showed that Se could inhibit *LPS*-induced inflammation response of mammary epithelial cells through the inhibition of NF-κB and MAPK activation [16]. However, the effect of Se in *S. aureus*-induced bovine mastitis is still unclear. The aim of this study was to investigate the protective effect of Se against *S. aureus*-induced inflammation injury in bMECs and to clarify the associated signaling pathways of Se supplement in *S. aureus*-infected bMECs.

Methods

bMECs isolation, cell culture, and treatment

bMECs were isolated from udders of lactating cows as previously described and cryopreserved in liquid nitrogen [17, 18]. Cows were from the University of Yangzhou herd and the protocol was approved by the Animal Care and Ethics Committee of the Yangzhou University (Approval ID: SYXK [Su] 2012–0029). Cells were cultured in Dulbecco's modified Eagle's medium/Ham's F-12 nutrient mixture (DMEM/F12), supplemented with 10% fetal bovine serum (Gibco, Grand island), 5 μg/mL of insulin, 1 μg/mL of hydrocortisone, and 10 ng/mL of epidermal growth factor (Sigma, US).

Sodium selenite was diluted in DMEM/F12 medium. *S. aureus* (29,213, ATCC) was grown overnight at 37 °C in 10 mL Luria-Bertani. The number of *S. aureus* was determined by dilution method of plate counting. Bacteria was then diluted to achieve a multiplicity of infection (MOI) of 1:1 (bacteria:cell) in DMEM/F12. All cells were washed with serum-free medium and serum starved for 1 h before incubation with Se or *S. aureus*.

Cell viability assay

To measure cell viability, 1×10^5 cells of bMECs were seeded in 96-well multiplies and cultured in 100 μL DMEM/F12 medium at 37 °C and 5% CO_2. When cells grew to 90% confluence, all cells were washed twice with phosphate buffer saline (PBS) and serum starved for 1 h before incubation with Se in different concentrations for 12 h, and then 10 μL of 3-(4,5-dimethylthiazol-2-yl)-2,5-diphenyltetrazolium bromide (Amresco, US) was added to each well and incubated for another 4 h. The formazan product was dissolved using dimethyl sulfoxide (Amresco, US). The optical density was measured at 570 nm using a microplate reader (Tecan, Austria) [19].

RNA extraction and genes expression analysis

Total RNA was extracted from infected cells using Trizol reagent (Amresco, US) according to the manufacturer's instructions. Integrity of RNA and reverse transcription were performed as previously described [20]. Reverse transcription-generated cDNA encoding β-actin, TLR2, Myd88, Irak4, Irak1, Traf6, IL-1β, TNF-α and IL-6 were amplified by RT-PCR using selective primers listed in Table 1. Quantitative PCR analysis was carried out as previously described [21]. The PCR reaction system

Table 1 Primers used in experiment

Gene	Sequence
β-actin	F:ACATCCGCAAGGACCTCTA R:CCATGCCAATCTCATCTCGTT
TNF-α	F:CTGCTGACGGGCTTTACC R:GACTGCAATGCGGCTGAT
IL-1β	F:GCTATGAGCCACTTCGTGAGGAC R:GATTGAGGGCGTCGTTCAGGAT
IL-6	F:TGATGACTTCTGCTTTCCCTACCC R:ATCTTTGCGTTCTTTACCCACTCG
TLR2	F:GATGACTACCGCTGTGAC R:GGTTTTGTGGCTCTTTTC
Myd88	F:AGCAGCATAACTCGGATAA R:CAGACACGCACAACTTCA
Irak4	F:TGGCAAAGACAGGACATCTG R:CACAACTCCCAAACCCTCCTT
Irak1	F:GAGTTCCAACGTCCTTCTGG R:CTCCCGGTCTTCACGTACTG
Traf6	F:CGGTGACTCTCTCCAGGTGT R:TGGACATTTGTGACCTGCAT

contained 10 μL of SYBR Green PCR mix (Takara, Japan), 0.8 μL of each primer, 2 μL of cDNA template, and 6.4 μL of diethylpyrocarbonate water.

Western blot analysis

Total protein was extracted from bMECs using a total protein extraction kit (BioChain, US) and the protein concentrations were determined by bicinchoninic acid protein assay kit (BioChain, US). All cells were respectively pretreated with Na_2SeO_3 (2, 4, and 8 μM) or left untreated for 12 h and infected with *S. aureus* (MOI = 1:1) for 0.5 h. Cell lysates were prepared as described previously [2]. Proteins were loaded into 10% SDS polyacrylamide gel for electrophoresis, and transferred using sodium phosphate buffer to polyvinylidene fluoride membrane metastasis (Merck Millipore, Germany). The membrane was then hybridized with specific antibodies. Antibodies included β-actin, phosphor-*IκBα* (*p-IκBα*), phospho-*p65* (*p-p65*), phosphor-*p38* (*p-p38*), and phosphor-*Erk* (*p-Erk*) (Cell Signaling Technology, US).

Statistical analysis

All data were presented as *mean ± standard error of mean* (sem). The groups were compared by using one-way ANOVA and Dunnett's test. A *p*-value< 0.05 was considered statistically significant. Unless indicated otherwise, all data were obtained from at least 3 independent experiments.

Results

The cytotoxicity of se on bMECs

Results showed that there was no significant effect of 1~ 16 μmol/L selenium on cell activity. As selenium concentrations increased further, cell activity was significantly suppressed, compared with the control group ($p < 0.001$). Activity of bMECs fell by 33% with 32 μmol/L selenium, and by 84% with 64 μmol/L selenium, which shew cytotoxicity (Fig. 1).

Se inhibits the activation of TLR2 pathway

As shown in Fig. 2a, the expression of TLR2 were up-regulated after *S. aureus* infection. This effect was significantly blocked by Se at 8 and 10 h in all group ($p < 0.01$). However at 6 h no statistically significant differences were shown between Se-pretreatment and control groups.

The genes expression of Myd88 induced by *S.aureus* were significantly up-regulated ($p < 0.001$) at 8 h and this effect was blocked by Se in all group ($p < 0.001$) (Fig. 2b). but at 6 h and 10 h there was no difference in statistics between all groups.

The gene expression of Irak4 induced by *S. aureus* were increased or significantly increased ($p < 0.01$ *or* $p < 0.001$) at all time point, but Se showed no blocking effect to the mRNA expression of Irak4 (Fig. 2c). Similar to Irak4, the mRNA expression of Irak1 were all up-regulated at any time points ($p < 0.05$ *or* $p < 0.001$) after *S. aureus* infection, and Se showed no blocking effect to the mRNA expression of Irak1 (Fig. 2d).

Compared to the control group, the Traf6 levels increased or significantly increased after *S. aureus* infection ($p < 0.05$ *or* $p < 0.001$) and this effect was blocked by Se in all group ($p < 0.001$) (Fig. 2e) at 6 h. So, the blocking effect of Se on TLR2 signal pathway in the inflammation response of bMECs induced by *S. aureus* was confirmed initially.

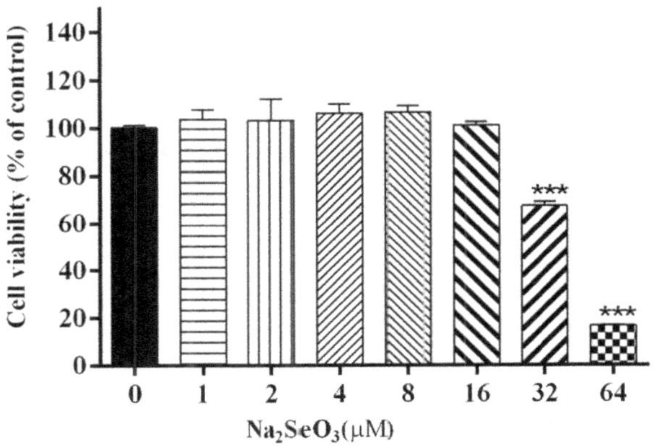

Fig. 1 The cytotoxicity of Se on bMECs. Cell viability was measured by MTT following treatment with various concentrations (0, 1, 2, 4, 8, 16, 32 and 64 μM) of Se for 12 h. Cell proliferation was not inbitited by Se in concentration lower than 16 μM. The data are *mean ± sem* ($n = 6$). ***$p < 0.001$ vs. 0 μM

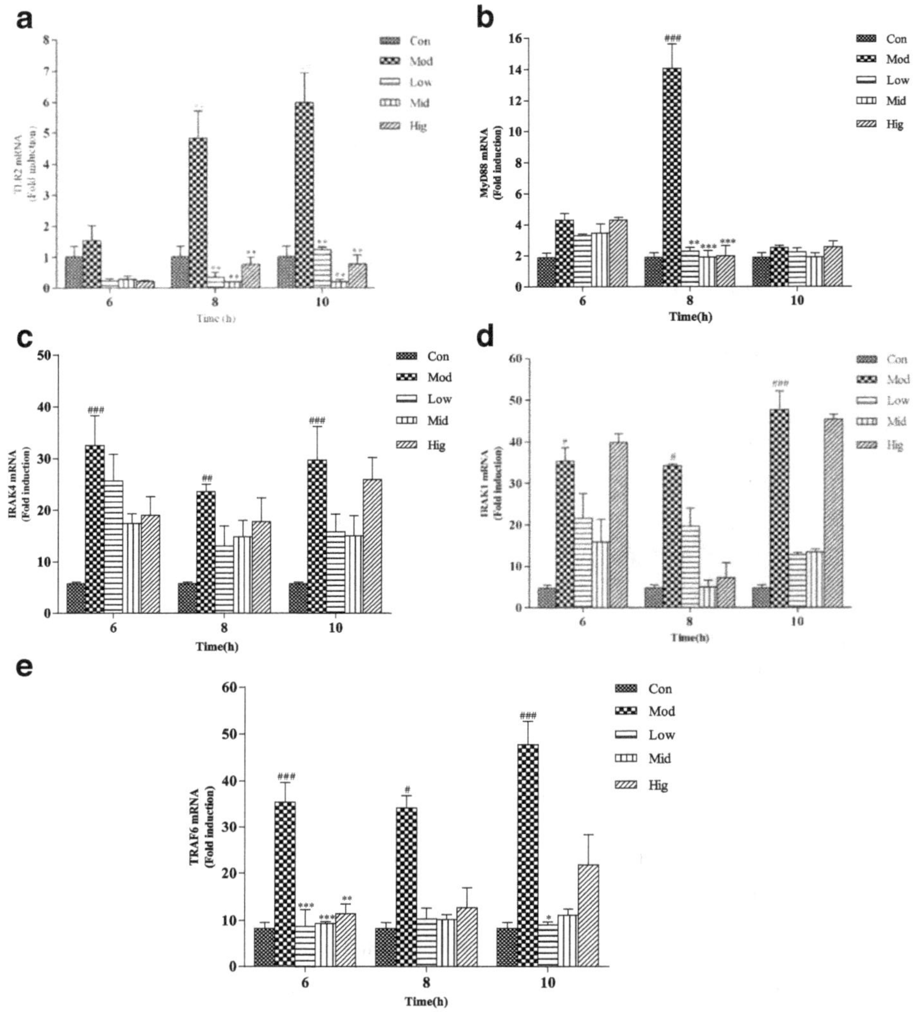

Fig. 2 The effect of Se on TLR2 signaling pathway associate genes induced by *S. aureus* in bMECs. Cells were incubated with different concentrations of Se or serum-free medium for 12 h and subsequently treated with *S. aureus* (MOI = 1:1) for 0, 6, 8 and 10 h. Total RNA was prepared at the indicated time points after *S. aureus* treated. The TLR2 (**a**) , Myd88 (**b**) , Irak4 (**c**) , Irak1 (**d**) and Traf6 (**e**) mRNA expression levels were assayed using qRT-PCR. con = control cells without any treatment; mod = cells treated with *S. aureus* (MOI = 1:1) only; low = Se (2 μM) + *S. aureus* (MOI = 1:1); mid = Se (4 μM) + *S. aureus* (MOI = 1:1); high = Se (8 μM) + *S. aureus* (MOI = 1:1). The data are shown as *mean* ± *sem* (*n* = 3). ###: $p < 0.001$ vs. Con; *: $p < 0.05$ vs. Mod; **: $p < 0.01$ vs. Mod; ***: $p < 0.001$ vs. Mod

Se weakens the inflammation injury of bMECs induced by *S. aureus*

The protective effect of Se against *S. aureus*-induced inflammation injury in bMECs was analyzed by qRT-PCR. *S. aureus* could significantly up-regulate the gene expression of TNF-α, IL-1β, and IL-6 at the various time points. But the effect was markedly inhibited by Se (Fig. 3a, b and c). Thus, the anti-inflammatory effect of Se was confirmed in the inflammation response of bMECs induced by *S. aureus*.

Se inhibits the activation of NF-κB pathway

Protein expression of *p-IκBα* and *p-p65* were up-regulated significantly ($p < 0.001$) by innoculation with *S. aureus* for 0.5 h (Fig. 4), which indicated that NF-κB signaling pathway was activated. However, the phosphorylation of *IκBα* and *p65* were suppressed by the addition of 4 μM and 8 μM Se. So, the higher Se concentration could suppress the inflammatory response by NF-κB pathway to some extent.

Se inhibits the activation of MAPK pathway

The phosphorylation of *p38* and *Erk* increased significantly with *S. aureus* or associated with 2 μM Se innoculation for 0.5 h, while phosphorylation of *p38* and *Erk* were markedly suppressed by Se at 4 and 8 μM (Fig. 5), which suggesting that higher concentration of Se could inhibit

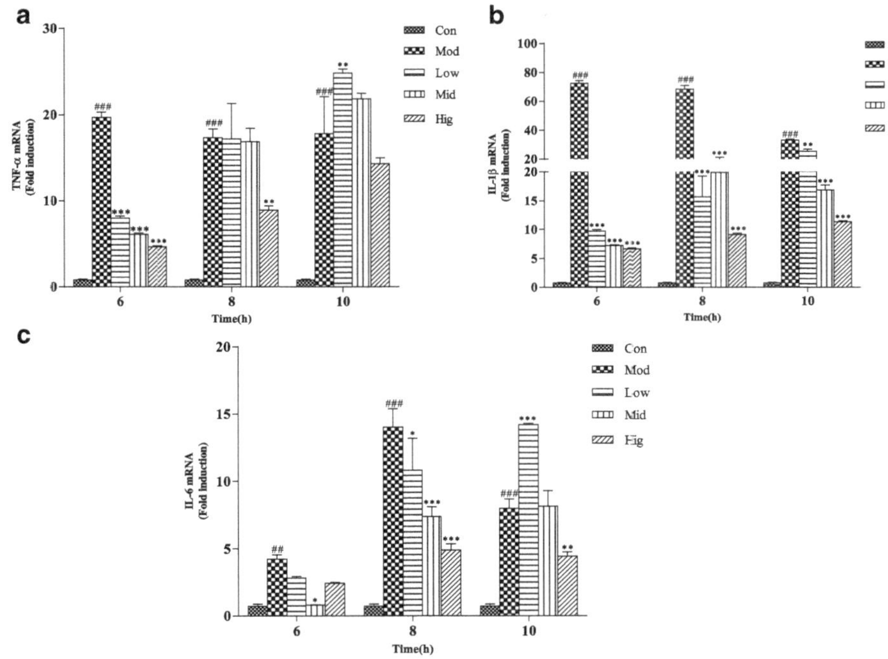

Fig. 3 The effect of Se on gene expression of pro-inflammatory cytokines induced by *S. aureus* in bMECs. Cells were incubated with various concentrations of Se or serum-free medium for 12 h and subsequently challenged with *S. aureus* (MOI = 1:1) for 0, 6, 8, and 10 h. Total RNA was prepared at the indicated time points after *S. aureus* injection. The TNF-α, IL-1β and IL-6 mRNA expression were quantified using qRT-PCR. con = control cells without any treatment; mod = cells treated with *S. aureus* (MOI = 1:1) only; low = Se (2 μM) + *S. aureus* (MOI = 1:1); mid = Se (4 μM) + *S. aureus* (MOI = 1:1); high = Se (8 μM) + *S. aureus* (MOI = 1:1). The data are shown as *mean ± sem* (*n* = 3). ##: *p < 0.01* vs. Con; ###: *p < 0.001* vs. Con; *: *p < 0.05* vs. Mod; **: *p < 0.01* vs. Mod; ***: *p < 0.001* vs. Mod

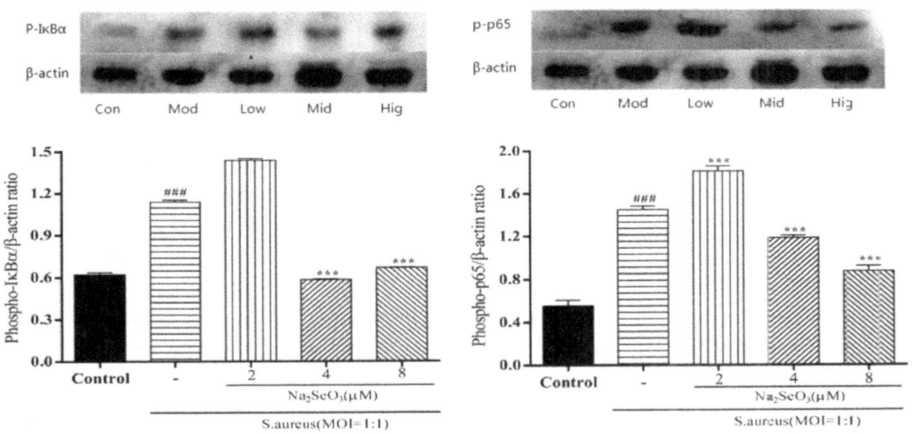

Fig. 4 Effect of Se on *S. aureus*-induced IκBα and p65 phosphorylation in bMECs. Cells were pretreated with various concentrations (0, 2, 4 and 8 μM) of Se or serum-free medium for 12 h before stimulated with *S. aureus* (MOI = 1:1) for 0.5 h and then washing twice with PBS. Total proteins were prepared at the indicated time points and subjected to Western blotting. Con = control cells without any treatment; mod = cells treated with *S. aureus* (MOI = 1:1) only; low = Se (2 μM) + *S. aureus* (MOI = 1:1); mid = Se (4 μM) + *S. aureus* (MOI = 1:1); high = Se (8 μM) + *S. aureus* (MOI = 1:1). The data are shown as *mean ± sem* (n = 3). ###: *p < 0.001* vs. Con; *: *p < 0.05* vs. Mod; **: *p < 0.01* vs. Mod; ***: *p < 0.001* vs. Mod. One out of 3 independent experiments is shown

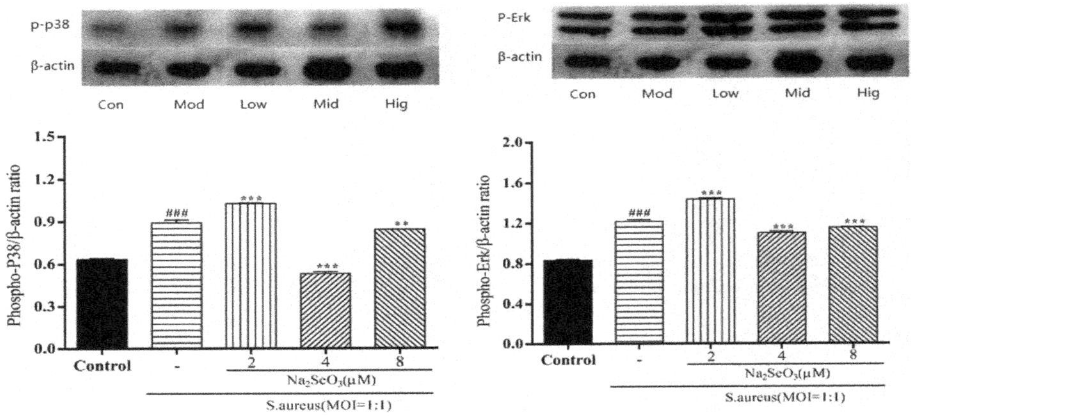

Fig. 5 Effect of Se on *S. aureus*-induced p38 and Erk phosphorylation in bMECs. Cells were pretreated with various concentrations (0, 2, 4 and 8 μM) of Se or serum-free medium for12 h before stimulated with *S. aureus* (MOI = 1:1) for 0.5 h and then washing twice with PBS. Total proteins were prepared at the indicated time points and subjected to Western blotting. Con = control cells without any treatment; mod = cells treated with *S. aureus* (MOI = 1:1) only; low = Se (2 μM) + *S. aureus* (MOI = 1:1); mid = Se (4 μM) + *S. aureus* (MOI = 1:1); high = Se (8 μM) + *S. aureus* (MOI = 1:1). The data are shown as *mean ± sem* (n = 3). $^{###}$: $p < 0.001$ vs. Con; *: $p < 0.05$ vs. Mod; **: $p < 0.01$ vs. Mod; ***: $p < 0.001$ vs. Mod. One out of 3 independent experiments is shown

the activation of MAPK signaling pathway by suppression of phosphorylation of *p38* and *Erk*.

Discussion

Se is an essential micronutrient that play an important role in regulating the immune function [22]. Many studies have indicated that Se is involved in several biological activities, including the regulation of inflammation and immunological reaction [23]. The acute and sub-actue toxicity of Se were studies in bMECs, and these results showed that when the concentrations of Se is lower than 16 μM, the cell viability was not affected, which is also within the normal range of selenium in the dairy cow.

Our previous study supports the hypothesis that TLR2 plays an important role at the early inflammation induced by *S. aureus* [24]. In the meanwhile, Irak was activated via an adaptor protein Myd88 in TLR2 signalling pathway [25, 26]. In this study, proteins expression of TLR2 signaling pathway were examined by qRT-PCR. Accompanied by the activation of Irak, another adaptor protein Traf 6 is phosphorylated and recruited to Irak in model group. Then, NF-κB and MAPK signaling pathway were triggered, which were characterized by the releasing of a large number proinflammatory cytokines [27]. Appropriate inflammation response is beneficial for immune cells to fight against infection, but excessive inflammation response will injure the tissues and cells. So the releasing of proinflammatory cytokines must be tightly regulated during the inflammatory response [28]. Our study found that a strong activity of TLR2 signaling pathway could be triggered by *S. aureus* at about 10 h. Moreover, the gene expression of TNF-α, IL-1β, and IL-6 were significantly increased in bMECs induced by *S. aureus* at any time point, which indicated a strong inflammatory response. Se obviously suppressed the mRNA expression of TLR2, Myd88, and Traf6 induced by *S. aureus* at 6, 8, 10 h. The results support the hypothesis that Se could protect bMECs from *S. aureus* injury by inhibiting the expression of TNF-α, IL-6 and IL-1β. Furthermore the effect of Se on TLR2 signaling pathway is mainly regulated by the gene expression of TLR2, Myd88 and Traf6.

NF-κB and MAPK signaling pathways are two classical pathways associated with inflammation, which are important in numerous processes such as immune processes, cell survival and inflammation [29, 30]. As an accelerant of NF-κB and MAPK, *S. aureus* could strongly enhance the phosphorylation of *IκBα, p65, p38,* and *Erk*, leading to a conformational change of NF-κB and MAPK that evokes NF-κB and MAPK signaling activity. The different members of NF-κB and MAPK have different downstream targets, and thus play distinct roles in cellular responses. Our results showed that the phosphorylation of *IκBα, p65, p38,* and *Erk* were markedly increased after stimulation with *S. aureus* for 0.5 h., which demonstrated a significant activation of NF-κB and MAPK and subsequently lead to a high expression of pro-inflammation cytokines. Se suppressed the phosphorylation of *IκBα, p65, p38, Erk,* which indicating an inhibitory effect of NF-κB and MAPK activity. Therefore, the releasing of pro-inflammatory cytokines were inhibited. Ultimately, the protective effect of Se was validated through blocking TLR2, NF-κB and MAPK signaling pathways against bMECs inflammatory injury induced by *S. aureus*.

Conclusions

This study proved the protective effect of Se on *S. aureus*-induced inflammation in bMECs. This effect was at least partly achieved by the blocking of TLR2 signaling pathway. On the other hand, Se could decrease the gene expression of pro-inflammation cytokines through mediating the phosphorylation of IκBα and p65 in NF-κB pathway and inhibiting the phosphorylation of p38 and Erk in the MAPK pathway. Se reveal potential benefit for the adjuvant therapy of mastitis induced by *S. aureus*. But other anti-inflammatory associated pathways and targets of Se need to be studied in the future.

Abbreviations

bMECS: Bovine mammary epithelial cells; MAPK: Mitogen-activated protein kinase; NF-κB: Nuclear factor kappa-light-chain-enhancer of activated B cells.; Se: Selenium.; TLR2: Toll-like receptor 2.

Funding

Natural Science Foundation of Jiangsu Province (No. BK20160062, BK2012265), The investigation was supported by the National Natural Science Foundation of China (No. 31302151,31672614), Priority Academic Program Development of Jiangsu Higher Education Institutions (PAPD) and Outstanding Young Backbone Teacher Foundation of Yangzhou University.

Authors' contributions

HW, CB, and JL conceived, designed and performed the majority of the experiments and drafted the manuscript. YW and JS helped with experiments, provided valuable discussion and modified the final manuscript. XM participated in experimental procedures and data analysis. HW, JL, and XM conceived the study, participated in its coordination and helped to revise the manuscript. All authors read and approved the final manuscript.

Competing interests

The authors declare that they have no competing interests.

Author details

[1]College of Veterinary Medicine, Yangzhou University, Yangzhou 225009, Jiangsu, China. [2]Jiangsu Co-innovation Center for Prevention and Control of Important Animal Infectious Diseases and Zoonoses, Yangzhou 225009, Jiangsu, China. [3]College of Agriculture Forestry Science, Linyi University, Linyi 276000, Shandong, China.

References

1. Günther J, Liu S, Esch K, Schuberth HJ, Seyfert HM. Stimulated expression of TNF-α and IL-8, but not of lingual antimicrobial peptide reflects the concentration of pathogens contacting bovine mammary epithelial cells. Vet Immunol Immunopathol. 2010;135:152–7.
2. Günther J, Kathrin E, Seyfert HM. Comparative kinetics of *Escherichia coli* and *Staphylococcus aureus*-specific activation of key immune pathways in mammary epithelial cells demonstrates that *S.aureus* elicits a delayed response dominated by Interleukin-6 (IL-6) but not by IL-1α or tumor necrosis factor alpha. Infect Immun. 2011;79:695–707.
3. Sutra LB, Poutrel B. Virulence factors involved in the pathogenesis of bovine intramammary infections due to Staphylococcus aureus. J Med Microbiol. 1994;40:79–89.
4. Quesnell RR, Klaessig S, Watts JL, Schukken YH. Bovine intramammary *Escherichia coli* challenge infections in late gestation demonstrate a dominant antiinflammatory immunological response. J Dairy Sci. 2012;95: 117–26.
5. Dego OK, Oliver SP, Almeida RA. Host-pathogen gene expression profiles during infection of primary bovine mammary epithelial cells with *Escherichia coli* strains associated with acute or persistent bovine mastitis. Vet Microbiol. 2011;155:291–7.
6. Schukken YH, Günther J, Fitzpatrick J, Fontaine MC, Goetze L, Holst O, et al. Host response patterns of intramammary infections in dairy cows. Vet Immunol Immunopathol. 2011;144:270–89.
7. Rinaldi M, Li RW, Capuco AV. Mastitis associated transcriptomic disruptions in cattle. Vet Immunol Immunopathol. 2010;138:267–79.
8. Akira S, Takeda K. Toll-like receptor. Curr Protoc Immunol. 2015;109:1–14.
9. Yang W, Zerbe H, Petzl W, Brunner RM, Günther J, Draing C. Bovine TLR2 and TLR4 properly transduce signals from *Staphylococcus aureus* and *E. coli*, but *S. aureus* fails to both activate NF-κB in mammary epithelial cells and to quickly induce TNF-α and interleukin-8 (CXCL8) expression in the udder. Mol Immunol. 2007;45:1385–97.
10. Takeuchi O, Akira S. Toll-like receptors; their physiological role and signal transduction system. Int Immunopharmacol. 2001;1:625–35.
11. Meads MB, Li ZW, Dalton WS. A novel TNF receptor-associated factor 6 (Traf6) binding domain mediates NF-κB signaling by the common cytokine receptor β subunit. J Immunol. 2010;185:1605–15.
12. Hines DJ, Choi HB, Hines RM, Phillips AG, MacVicar BA. Prevention of LPS-induced microglia activation, cytokine production and sickness behavior with TLR4 receptor interfering peptides. PLoS One. 2013;8:e60388.
13. Calzado MA, Bacher S, Schmitz ML. NF-kappaB inhibitors for the treatment of inflammatory diseases and cancer. Curr Med Chem. 2007;14:367–76.
14. Rayman MP. Selenium in cancer prevention: a review of the evidence and mechanism of action. Proc Nutr Soc. 2005;64:527–42.
15. Clark LC, Combs GFJ, Turnbull BW, Slate EH, Chalker DK, Chow J, et al. Effects of selenium supplementation for cancer prevention in patients with carcinoma of the skin. A randomized controlled trial. Nutritional prevention of Cancer study group. J Am Med Assoc. 1996;276:1957–63.
16. Zhang W, Zhang R, Wang T, Jiang H, Guo M, Zhou E, et al. Selenium inhibits LPS-induced pro-inflammatory gene expression by modulating MAPK and NF-kappa B signaling pathways in mouse mammary epithelial cells in primary culture. Inflammation. 2014;37:478–85.
17. Lahouassa H, Moussay E, Rainard P, Riollet C. Differential cytokine and chemokine responses of bovine mammary epithelial cells to *Staphylococcus aureus* and *Escherichia coli*. Cytokine. 2007;38:12–21.
18. Porcherie A, Cunha P, Trotereau A, Roussel P, Gilbert FB, Rainard P, Germon P. Repertoire of Escherichia coli agonists sensed by innate immunity receptors of the bovine udder and mammary epithelial cells. Vet Res. 2012; 43:14–22.
19. Shimohashi N, Nakamuta M, Uchimura K, Sugimoto R, Lwamoto H, Enjoji M, Nawata H. Selenoorganic compound, ebselen, inhibits nitric oxide and tumor necrosis factor-alpha production by the modulation of Jun-nterminal kinase and NF-kappa B signaling pathway in rat kupffer cells. J Cell Biochem. 2000;78:595–606.
20. Yu J, Yin P, Liu F, Cheng G, Guo K, Lu A, et al. Effect of heat stress on the porcine small intestine: a morphological and gene expression study. Comp Biochem Physiol. 2010;156:119–28.
21. Yu J, Yin P, Liu F, Cheng G, Guo K, Lu A, et al. Involvement of ERK1/2 signalling and growth-related molecule expression in response to heat stress-induced damage in rat jejunum and IEC-6 cells. Int J Hyperth. 2010;26:538–55.
22. Hoffmann PR, Berry MJ. The influence of selenium on immune responses. Mol Nutr Food Res. 2008;52:1273–80.
23. Kim SH, Johnson VJ, Shin TY, Sharma RP. Selenium attenuates lipopolysaccharide-induced oxidative stress responses through modulation of p38 MAPK and NF-kappa B signaling pathways. Exp Biol Med. 2004;229: 203–13.
24. Wang H, Yu G, Yu H, Gu M, Zhang J, Meng X, et al. Characterization of TLR2, NOD2, and related cytokines in mammary glands infected by Staphylococcus aureus in a rat model. Acta Vet Scand. 2015;57:25–31.

25. Medzhitov R, Hurlburt PP, Kopp E, Stadlen A, Chen C, Ghose H. Myd88 is an adaptor protein in the toll/IL-1 receptor family signaling pathways. Mol Cell. 1998;2:253–8.
26. Muzio M, Ni J, Feng P, Dixit VM. IRAK (Pelle) family member IRAK-2 and Myd88 as proximal mediators of IL-1 signaling. Science. 1997;278:1612–5.
27. Strandberg Y, Gray C, Vuocolo T, Donaldson L, Broadway M, Tellam R. Lipopolysaccharide and lipoteichoic acid induce different innate immune responses in bovine mammary epithelial cells. Cytokine. 2005;31:72–86.
28. Scheibel M, Klein B, Merkle H, Schulz M, Fritsch R, Greten FR, Arkan MC, Schneider G, Schmid RM. IκBβ is an essential co-activator for LPS-induced IL-1β transcription in vivo. J Exp Med. 2010;207:2621–30.
29. Lee Y, Shin DH, Kim JH, Hong S, Choi D, Kim YJ, Kwak MK, Jung Y. Caffeic acid phenethyl ester-mediated Nrf2 activation and IκB kinase inhibition are involved in NF-κB inhibitory effect: structural analysis for NFκB inhibition. Eur J pharmacol. 2010;643:21–8.
30. Gehart H, Kumpf S, Ittner A, Ricci R. MAPK signalling in cellular metabolism: stress or wellness? EMBO Rep. 2010;11:834–40.

MiR-139 suppresses β-casein synthesis and proliferation in bovine mammary epithelial cells by targeting the GHR and IGF1R signaling pathways

Yingjun Cui[1,2], Xia Sun[1], Lianfeng Jin[1], Guangpu Yu[1], Qingzhang Li[1], Xuejun Gao[1], Jinxia Ao[2] and Chunmei Wang[1*]

Abstract

Background: MicroRNAs have important roles in many biological processes. However, the role of miR-139 in healthy mammary gland remains unclear. The objective of this study was to investigate the effects of miR-139 on lactation in dairy cows.

Results: Here, we found that miR-139 was down-regulated in mid-lactation dairy cow mammary tissues compared with mid-pregnancy tissues. Then, we prioritized two of potential target genes of miR-139 in cow growth hormone receptor (*GHR*) and type I insulin-like growth factor receptor (*IGF1R*) for further functional studies based on their roles in lactation processes. Dual luciferase reporter assays validated direct binding of miR-139 to the 3'-untranslated region (UTR) of *GHR* and *IGF1R*. Moreover, over-expression or silencing of miR-139 affected mRNA levels of GHR and IGF1R in cultured bovine mammary epithelial cells (BMECs). Furthermore, over-expression of miR-139 decreased protein levels of β-casein, proliferation in mammary epithelial cell, and the protein levels of IGF1R and key members of the GHR or IGF1R pathways as well, whereas silencing miR-139 produced the opposite result. Among these signal molecules, signal transducer and activator of transcription-5 (STAT5), protein kinase B (also known as AKT1), mammalian target of rapamycin (mTOR), and p70-S6 Kinase (p70S6K) are involed in β-casein synthesis, and Cyclin D1 is involved in cell proliferation. In addition, silencing *GHR* decreased protein levels of β-casein, IGF1R, and key members of the IGF1R pathway, whereas co-silencing miR-139 and *GHR* rescued the expression of *GHR* and reversed *GHR* silencing effects.

Conclusions: Our results demonstrate that *GHR* and *IGF1R* are target genes of miR-139 in dairy cow. MiR-139 suppresses β-casein synthesis and proliferation in BMECs by targeting the GHR and IGF1R signaling pathways.

Keywords: miR-139, Mammary gland, β-casein, Growth hormone receptor, Type I insulin-like growth factor receptor

Background

MicroRNA-139-5p (miR-139-5p) and miR-139-3p are mature miRNAs generated from a miR-139 precursor [1, 2]. The knowledge about miR-139-3p function in bovine mammary epithelium is very limited, but it is worth noting that miR-139-3p has been identified in bovine milk [3]. It is a widely used assumption that there is only one type of mature bta-miR-139, and it has the same sequence as hsa-miR-139-5p. MicroRNAs regulate a wide variety of biological processes, including cell proliferation, apoptosis, developmental timing, and signal transduction [4]. Previous studies about miR-139 have focused on its antioncogenic and antimetastatic activities [5]. It has been shown that miR-139-5p suppresses proliferation, migration, and invasion in esophageal cancer [6], colorectal cancer [7], non-small cell lung cancer [8], hepatocellular carcinoma [9] and breast cancer [5, 10]. Moreover, miR-139-5p inhibits the epithelial-mesenchymal transition of hepatocellular carcinoma cells [2]. Although some

* Correspondence: wangcm-1@163.com
[1]Key Laboratory of Dairy Science of Education Ministry, Northeast Agricultural University, Harbin, Heilongjiang 150030, People's Republic of China
Full list of author information is available at the end of the article

microarray studies show that miR-139 expression is down-regulated in the mammary tissue during the transition period between pregnancy and lactation [11], little is known about effects of miR-139 in healthy mammary glands.

Growth hormone (GH) is a pituitary hormone that exerts a galactopoietic effect on the bovine mammary gland and controls milk protein synthesis [12, 13]. In addition to the pituitary gland, GH is produced in an autocrine manner by the mammary gland [14]. The effects of GH are mediated through interaction with growth hormone receptor (GHR), whose expression is regulated by GH [14, 15]. Localization of GHR is strong on the membrane as well as in the cytoplasm of the bovine mammary epithelial cell (BMEC) [15, 16]. GHR immunostaining within the nucleus is rare or absent [17]. GHR may be involved in milk protein secretion in BMECs [12]. The most abundant milk protein is β-casein, which makes up approximately 30% of the total protein in cows' milk [18].

Type I insulin-like growth factor (IGF1) is the major mediator of GH effects in many tissues. Previous studies have indicated that GH can act indirectly on the mammary gland by stimulating IGF1 secretion from the liver [19]. Evidence has also shown that GH induces the expression of IGF1 mRNA in mammary gland [20, 21]. The functions of IGF1 are mainly mediated through the type I insulin-like growth factor receptor (IGF1R) [22]. Interestingly, some of the IGF1R downstream signaling members are shared with GH [20]. IGF1R signaling can promote cell proliferation, survival, differentiation, and protein synthesis [19, 20].

In this study, *GHR* and *IGF1R* were prioritized as two of potential target genes of miR-139 in cow. Combining their roles in lactation processes, and the down-regulation of miR-139 in the mammary tissue during the transition period between pregnancy and lactation, we hypothesized that miR-139 is also involved in regulation of lactation. The aim of this study was to investigate the effects of miR-139 on lactation in dairy cows.

Methods

Animals and mammary gland samples

Samples were collected from mammary glands of Holstein cows. All animals were clinically healthy. The average weights of the dairy cows were 609 ± 9.08 kg (mean ± SEM). The cows were separated into two groups by developmental stage: mid-pregnancy ($n = 3$) or mid-lactation (n = 3). Three pregnant cows went through a dry period and then were pregnant again. Lactating cows were at 90 DIM. The cows were slaughtered by exsanguination, and the mammary glands were removed immediately after slaughtering. Mammary gland samples were frozen in liquid nitrogen and stored at −80 °C. In our study, all animal experimental protocols were approved by the Institutional Animal Care and Use Committee of Northeast Agricultural University (China).

Plasmid construction

The wild-type and mutated sequences of the 3′- untranslated region (UTR) of *GHR* (Cow *GHR*, NCBI Accession # NC_007318.5) and *IGF1R* (Cow *IGF1R*, NCBI Accession # AC_000178.1) with specific restriction sites *XhoI* and *NotI* were constructed by Sangon Biotech Company (Shanghai, China).

The 214-bp fragment from *GHR* 3′-UTR contained a predicted bta-miR-139 binding region (**5′-ACACG**GTG TAC**TGTAG-3′**). The binding site of the mutated 3′-UTR sequence of *GHR* was **5′-TGTGC**GTGTACA **CATC-3′**. The 242-bp fragment from *IGF1R* 3′-UTR contained a predicted bta-miR-139 binding region (**5′-ACTGTAGA-3′**). The binding site of the mutated 3′-UTR sequence of *IGF1R* was **5′-TGACATCT-3′**. All sequences were confirmed by sequence analysis. The wild-type or mutant 3′-UTR was subcloned into the *XhoI-NotI* site of the psiCHECK-2 vector (Promega, Madison, WI, USA).

HeLa cell culture and dual luciferase reporter assay

The HeLa cell line was purchased from the American Type Culture Collection (ATCC, Rockville, MD, USA). The cell line was maintained in Dulbecco's modified Eagle's medium (DMEM) (High Glucose) (Invitrogen, Carlsbad, CA, USA) and supplemented with 10% fetal bovine serum (FBS) (Gibco, Rockville, Maryland, USA), penicillin (100 units/mL), and streptomycin (100 μg/mL) at 37 °C in a 5% CO_2 humidified incubator. Cells were seeded at 1×10^5 cells per well in a 12-well plate the day before transfection. Cells were co-transfected with a total of 500 ng of the psiCHECK-2 luciferase reporter construct or empty psiCHECK-2 vector, and 40 pmol of negative control of bta-miR-139 mimic or bta-miR-139 mimic (RiboBio Company, Guangzhou, China). Transfections were performed using Lipofectamine 2000. At 24 h post-transfection, the medium was changed. The cells were grown for an additional 24 h before the assay was performed.

Firefly and Renilla luminescent signals arising from psiCHECK-2 transfected cells were quantified according to the manufacturer's instructions for the Dual-Luciferase Reporter Assay System (Promega, Madison, WI, USA) with a VICTOR Multilabel Counter luminometer (PerkinElmer, Waltham, MA). Independent experiments were performed 3–5 times.

BMECs culture and transfection

BMECs were prepared and identified as previously described [23]. In brief, the tissue samples from lactating

Holstein cows were minced with surgical scissors and transferred to cell culture bottles coated with collagen. Mammary tissue pieces were cultured in Dulbecco's modified Eagle's medium F-12 (DMEM/F12) (Gibco, Rockville, Maryland, USA) and supplemented with 10% FBS, penicillin (100 units/mL), and streptomycin (100 μg/mL) at 37 °C in a 5% CO_2 humidified incubator. BMECs and fibroblasts were separated by selective trypsinization (0.25% trypsin). Pure BMECs were obtained after four passages and identified by immunofluorescence for Cytokeratin-18 and β-casein.

The BMECs were seeded at 3×10^5 cells per well in a 6-well plate and grown for 24 h. Then, the cells were transfected with 100 pmol of negative control of bta-miR-139 mimic (Mimic NC), bta-miR-139 mimic, negative control of bta-miR-139 inhibitor (Inhibitor NC) or bta-miR-139 inhibitor (RiboBio Company, Guangzhou, China) using Lipofectamine 2000 (Invitrogen Life Technologies, Carlsbad, CA, USA) according to the manufacturer's instructions. The control group was only transfected with Lipofectamine 2000. Opti-MEM (Reduced Serum Medium) (Gibco, Rockville, Maryland, USA) was used as medium. Approximately 5 h after transfection, the medium was changed to DMEM/F12 supplemented with 10% FBS.

RNA extraction and quantitative real-time polymerase chain reaction assay

Total RNA was extracted from frozen tissues or BMECs using Trizol reagent (Invitrogen, Carlsbad, CA, USA) according to the manufacturer's instructions. RNA extraction from BMECs was performed 24 h post-transfection. RNA integrity was assessed by electrophoresis on 1% (*w*/*v*) agarose gels. The ratio of the optical densities measured at 260 and 280 nm by an ND-1000 spectrophotometer (NanoDrop Technologies, USA) was >1.8 for all RNA samples.

To determine the relative amount of miR-139 or U6 transcripts, cDNA was synthesized using M-MLV reverse transcriptase (Invitrogen, Carlsbad, CA, USA) according to the manufacturer's instructions. Primer sets used in reverse transcription and quantitative Real-time Polymerase Chain Reaction(qPCR) for bta-miR-139 or U6 were purchased from GenePharma Company (Shanghai, China). To determine the relative amount of *GHR* or *IGF1R* transcripts, cDNA was synthesized using the PrimeScript™ RT reagent kit (TaKaRa, Ostu, Japan). QPCR reactions were performed using SYBR Premix Ex Taq™ (TaKaRa, Ostu, Japan) and the ABI PRISM 7300 Real-Time PCR System (Applied Biosystems, Foster City, CA, USA). The primers were designed by Primer Premier 5.0 software. The primers used were as follows—*GHR*: forward 5′-CGTGGACAACGCTTACT -3′ and reverse 5′-AAGGGTTTCTGTGGTGAT -3′; *IGF-IR*: forward 5′-AGAAGCAGGCGGAGAAGGA-3′ and reverse 5′-AAGGGTTTCTGTGGTGAT -3′; *β-actin*: forward 5′-TTAGCTGCGTTACACCCTT -3′ and reverse 5′-GTCACCTTCACCGTTCCA -3′. All reactions were performed in triplicate. The expression of miR-139 was normalized to U6. Gene expression was normalized to β-actin. The stability of U6 and β-actin were confirmed under the experimental conditions. The relative levels of miRNA or mRNA were determined using the $2^{-\Delta\Delta Ct}$ method.

Western blotting analysis

Western blotting analysis was performed as previously described [24]. Briefly, BMECs were harvested on ice using RIPA buffer (Beyotime Biotechnology, Shanghai, China) to which protease inhibitors had been added (2 mM PMSF, 5 mM Na_3PO_4, 5 mM NaF, and complete protease inhibitor) at 48 h post-transfection and then homogenized by ultrasonication. The BCA protein assay was used to measure protein concentration in the samples. Approximately 50 μg total protein was subjected to a 10% SDS-PAGE. The separated proteins were transferred to a nitrocellulose membrane and incubated in blocking buffer. Membranes were then incubated with primary antibodies overnight at 4 °C, followed by incubation with horseradish peroxidase-conjugated secondary antibodys against mouse, rabbit or goat (ZSGB-BIO, Beijing, China) at room temperature for 1 h. Protein bands were visualized using an ECL system. The following primary antibodies were purchased from Santa Cruz Biotechnology: antibodies for phosphorylated signal transducer and activator of transcription-5 (p-STAT5) (1:200 dilution, sc-11,761), signal transducer and activator of transcription-5 (STAT5) (1:200 dilution, SC-836), protein kinase B (also known as AKT1) (1:200 dilution, SC-1618), phosphorylated AKT1 (1:200 dilution, sc-135,650), phosphorylated p70-S6 Kinase (1:200 dilution, p-p706SK) (sc-11,759), p70-S6 Kinase (p706SK) (1:200 dilution, sc-230), Cyclin D1 (1:200 dilution, sc-718), and β-actin (1:400 dilution, sc-47,778); from Cell Signaling Technology: antibodies for IGF1R (1:1000 dilution, #3027), phosphorylated mammalian target of rapamycin (p-mTOR) (1:1000 dilution, #2971) and mammalian target of rapamycin (mTOR) (1:1000 dilution, #2972); and from Abbiotec Company: β-casein antibody (1:200 dilution, #251309). β-actin was used as an endogenous reference gene. All experiments were performed in triplicate. Western blotting data were scanned and quantified using Bandscan5.0 software.

3-(4,5-Dimethylthiazol-2-yl)-2,5- diphenyltetrazolium bromide assay

BMECs were cultured in 96-well plates (1×10^4 cells per well). At 24, 48, 72, or 96 h post-transfection with Lipofectamine 2000 (Control), negative control of bta-miR-

139 mimic (Mimic NC), bta-miR-139 mimic, negative control of bta-miR-139 inhibitor (Inhibitor NC) or bta-miR-139 inhibitor, cell proliferation was assayed using (3-(4,5-Dimethylthiazol-2-yl)-2,5- diphenyltetrazolium bromide) (MTT) dye (Amresco, Colorado, USA). MTT (5 mg/ml) was added to plates and incubated for 4 h. After that, the medium was discarded and cells were lysed in dimethyl sulfoxide (DMSO) (Amresco, Colorado, USA). Absorbance was measured at 490 nm using the Bio-Rad iMark 680 microplate reader (Bio-Rad, USA).

Co-transfection of *GHR* siRNA and miR-139 inhibitor

Small interfering RNA (siRNA) duplexe targeting bovine *GHR* mRNA and a negative control were designed and synthesized by RiboBio Company (Guangzhou, China). The siRNA sequences were as follows: forward 5′-CCA GUCCUAGAGACAAAUU dTdT -3′ and reverse -3′ dTdT GGUCAGGAUCUCUGUUUAA 5′. The targeting sequence in GHR was as follow: CCAGTCCTAGAGA CAAATT. BMECs were seeded in a 6-well plate at a density of 3×10^5 cells per well in DMEM/F12 without antibiotics at ~80–90% confluence. They were co-transfected with negative control of bta-miR-139 inhibitor or bta-miR-139 inhibitor, and negative control of *GHR* siRNA or *GHR* siRNA (2 μg per 10^5 cells). Lipofectamine 2000 was used according to the manufacturer's protocol. Approximately 6 h after transfection, the medium was changed to DMEM/F12. RNA extraction from BMECs was performed 24 h post-transfection, and protein extraction was performed 48 h post-transfection.

Statistical analysis

Statistical analyses were performed using SPSS19.0 software. All data are reported as the mean ± SEM of three independent experiments. Comparisons between treatments were made by *t* tests for two groups or ANOVA if there were more than two groups. Statistical significance was considered at $P<0.05$.

Results

Expression of miR-139 in dairy cow mammary tissues

To determine the expression of miR-139 in dairy cow mammary glands, we used qPCR to measure levels of the mature miR-139 in mid-pregnancy and mid-lactation mammary tissues of dairy cows. U6 was used for normalization. The result showed that miR-139 expression in mid-lactation bovine mammary tissues was significantly reduced compared with that in mid-pregnancy tissues ($P < 0.05$) (Fig. 1). This result suggested that down-regulation of miR-139 may be important in lactation of dairy cows.

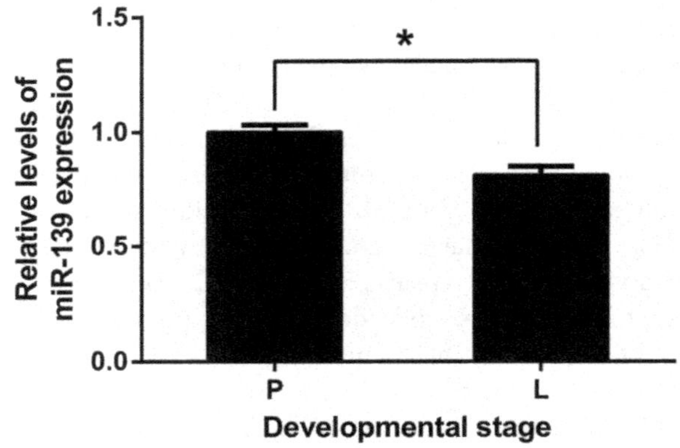

Fig. 1 Expression of miR-139 in Holstein cow mammary gland. Mammary tissues were from mid-pregnancy (P) ($n = 3$) or mid-lactation (L) (n = 3) cows. MiR-139 expression was normalized to U6. Results are shown as means ± SEM from three independent experiments. Statistical analysis was conducted using the *t* test."*", statistical significance was considered at $P<0.05$

MiR-139 directly targets 3′-UTRs of *GHR* and *IGF1R* in dairy cow

Through a target prediction algorithm (TargetScan, http://www.targetscan.org), we found that *GHR* and *IGF1R* are potential target genes of miR-139 in cow. It is known that miRNAs function by binding to the 3′-UTR of their target mRNAs and inhibiting their expression. Then, to verify the binding of miR-139 to *GHR* and *IGF1R*, we performed a dual luciferase reporter assay in HeLa cells using the psiCHECK-2 vector and engineered luciferase reporter constructs containing the wild-type (WT) or mutant (Mut) 3′-UTR of the GHR or IGF1R gene, separately (Fig. 2a and b). Compared with co-transfection of negative control of miR-139 mimic with the luciferase reporter gene linked to the wild-type 3′-UTR of *GHR* or *IGF1R*, co-transfection of miR-139 mimic with the wild-type construct of *GHR* or *IGF1R* 3′-UTR strongly inhibited the luciferase activity. Luciferase activity was decreased in these cells by 53.5% or 51.7%, respectively ($P < 0.05$) (Fig. 2c and d). In addition, luciferase activity was not altered by co-transfection of negative control of miR-139 mimic/miR-139 mimic with the mutant construct of *GHR* or *IGF1R* 3′-UTR in which the miR-139 binding sequence was mutated ($P > 0.05$) (Fig. 2c and d). These results revealed that miR-139 directly binds to the 3′-UTRs of *GHR* and *IGF1R*.

MiR-139 decreases mRNA levels of *GHR* and *IGF1R* in BMECs

To investigate whether expression of *GHR* and *IGF1R* is regulated by miR-139, we measured mRNA levels of miR-139, GHR and IGF1R by qPCR, following over-expression or silencing of miR-139 in cultured BMECs. BMECs were transfected with negative control of miR-

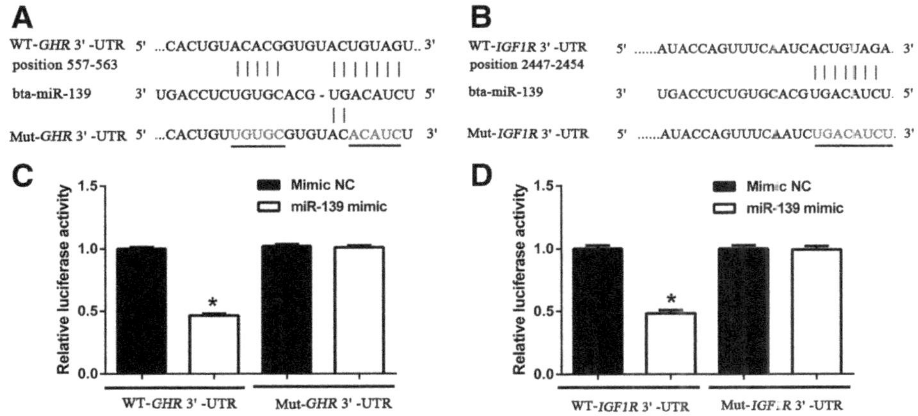

Fig. 2 Identifying target genes of miR-139 via the dual luciferase reporter assay. **a** Bta-miR-139 binding sites in the 3'-UTR of *GHR*. Ten nucleotides (underlined) were mutated in luciferase reporter plasmids carrying *GHR* 3'-UTR. **b** Bta-miR-139 binding sites in the 3'-UTR of *IGF1R*. Eight nucleotides (underlined) were mutated in the luciferase reporter plasmids carrying *IGF1R* 3'-UTR. **c** Luciferase activity of reporter plasmids carrying wild-type or mutant *GHR* 3'-UTR in HeLa cells, in response to co-transfection with miR-139. **d** Luciferase activity of reporter plasmids carrying wild-type or mutant *IGF1R* 3'-UTR in HeLa cells, in response to co-transfection with miR-139. Results are shown as means ± SEM from three independent experiments. Statistical analysis was conducted using one-way ANOVA."*", statistical significance was considered at $P < 0.05$

139 mimic, miR-139 mimic, negative control of miR-139 inhibitor or miR-139 inhibitor, separately. The Control group was transfected with Lipofectamine 2000. As expected, compared with the Control group, over-expression of miR-139 significantly increased the level of miR-139 ($P < 0.05$) (Fig. 3a), whereas silencing miR-139 decreased it ($P < 0.05$) (Fig. 3b). Then, we examined mRNA levels of *GHR* or *IGF1R* with each treatment. Our qPCR results revealed that over-expression of miR-139 inhibited *GHR* expression by approximately 32% compared with the Control group ($P < 0.05$) (Fig. 3c). However, miR-139 inhibitor treatment increased the level of *GHR* by approximately 37% compared with the Control group ($P < 0.05$) (Fig. 3d). Our qPCR results also showed that over-expression of miR-139 significantly decreased the expression of *IGF1R* by approximately 21% compared with the Control group ($P < 0.05$) (Fig. 3e), whereas loss of miR-139 increased the expression of *IGF1R* by approximately 73% compared with the Control group ($P < 0.05$) (Fig. 3f). Taken together, these results confirmed that miR-139 negatively regulates mRNA levels of *GHR* and *IGF1R*.

Effects of miR-139 in BMECs

The mammary gland in female mammals is responsible for milk production. To determine the role of miR-139 in milk production, we measured the protein levels of β-casein after over-expression or silencing of miR-139 in cultured BMECs. We found that over-expression of miR-139 decreased the protein level of β-casein compared with the Control group ($P < 0.05$) (Fig. 4a and c), whereas silencing miR-139 increased it ($P < 0.05$) (Fig. 4b and d).

Milk production is determined by the number of secretory mammary epithelial cell [25]. Then, we assessed the role of miR-139 on the proliferation of BMECs. The MTT assay revealed that miR-139 significantly decreased the number of BMECs at 48 and 72 h post-transfection with miR-139 mimic in comparison with the Control and Mimic NC groups ($P < 0.05$) (Fig. 5a), whereas silencing miR-139 increased the proliferation of BMECs at 48 and 72 h post-transfection in comparison with the Control and Inhibitor NC groups ($P < 0.05$) (Fig. 5b). These results revealed that miR-139 inhibits cell growth in BMECs.

Next, to explore the underlying molecular mechanism of miR-139, we examined the protein levels of key members of the GHR and IGF1R signaling pathways after over-expression or silencing of miR-139 in cultured BMECs. Western blotting analysis showed that, compared with the Control and Mimic NC groups, over-expression of miR-139 reduced protein levels of p-STAT5 and STAT5, which are key members in the GHR signaling pathway ($P < 0.05$) (Fig. 6a and c); IGF1R, p-AKT1, AKT1 and Cyclin D1, which are key members in the IGF1R signaling pathway ($P < 0.05$) (Fig. 6a and c); and p-mTOR, mTOR, p-p70S6K and p70S6K, which are key members in both GHR and IGF1R signaling pathways ($P < 0.05$) (Fig. 6a and c). Moreover, compared with the Control and Ihibitor NC groups, silencng miR-139 increased the levels of these proteins ($P < 0.05$) (Fig. 6b and d). These results demonstrated that miR-139 down-regulates β-casein synthesis and mammary epithelial cells proliferation by influencing the GHR and IGFIR signaling pathways in BMECs.

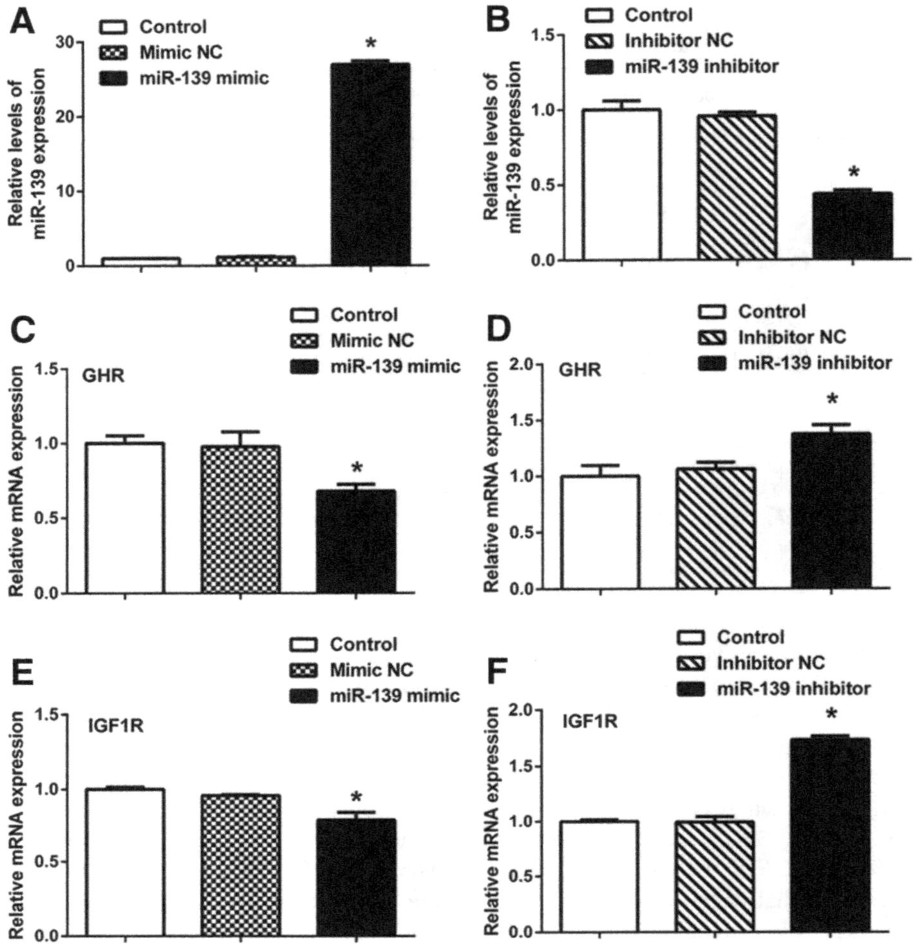

Fig. 3 *GHR* and *IGF1R* are target genes of miR-139. BMECs were transfected with negative control of miR-139 mimic (Mimic NC), miR-139 mimic, negative control of miR-139 inhibitor (Inhibitor NC) or miR-139 inhibitor using Lipofectamine 2000. The Control group was only transfected with Lipofectamine 2000. MRNA levels of miR-139 (**a**, **b**), *GHR* (**c**, **d**) and *IGF1R* (**e**, **f**) were examined by qPCR at 24 h post-transfection. MiR-139 expression was normalized to U6. *GHR* and *IGF1R* expression was normalized to β-actin. Results are shown as means ± SEM from three independent experiments. Statistical analysis was conducted using one-way ANOVA."*", statistical significance was considered at $P<0.05$

MiR-139 also regulates β-casein synthesis and IGF1R signaling by influencing *GHR*

We next sought to determine the relationship among miR-139, GHR, and IGF1R. As we have shown, silencing miR-139 significantly increased mRNA levels of *GHR* ($P < 0.05$) (Fig. 7a), and protein levels of IGF1R, p-AKT1, AKT1, and β-casein in comparison with the Control group ($P < 0.05$) (Fig. 7b and c). While, silencing *GHR* by siRNA significantly decreased the mRNA levels of *GHR* in comparison with the Control group ($P < 0.05$) (Fig. 7a). Moreover, the loss of *GHR* expression also contributed to decreased protein levels of IGF1R, p-AKT1, AKT1, and β-casein in comparison with the Control group ($P < 0.05$) (Fig. 7b and c). In addition, when *GHR* and miR-139 were both silenced, mRNA level of *GHR* and protein levels of IGF1R, p-AKT1, AKT1, and β-casein increased relative to those of the group with silenced *GHR* ($P < 0.05$) (Fig. 7a–c). These results indicated that IGF1R signaling is also regulated by *GHR*. However, the expression and effects of *GHR* can be influenced by miR-139.

Discussion

The mammary gland gains the function of milk production during lactation [26]. Our previous results from microRNA microarrays showed that the expression of some miRNAs, such as miR-139, is down-regulated on transition from pregnancy to lactation in mammary tissues from mouse [11] and dairy cow (data unpublished). Since miRNAs can trigger inhibition of protein translation [4, 27, 28], down-regulation of certain miRNAs during lactation indicates that they may play important roles related to lactation [29]. We observed that the expression of miR-139 is reduced in dairy cow mammary gland from pregnancy to lactation. Therefore, we

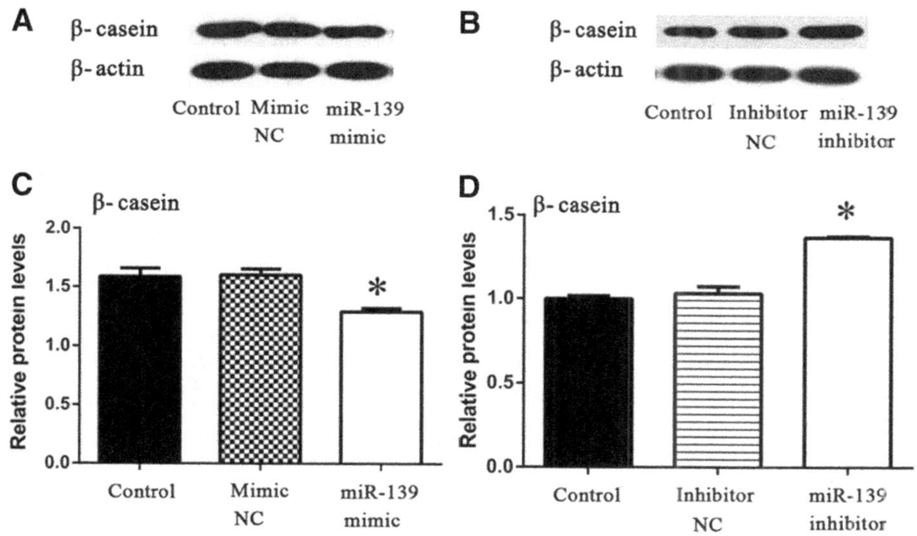

Fig. 4 MiR-139 inhibits protein levels of β-casein in BMECs. **a** BMECs were transfected with Lipofectamine 2000 (Control), negative control of miR-139 mimic (Mimic NC) or miR-139 mimic. Western blotting analysis showed the protein levels of β-casein and β-actin at 48 h post-transfection. **b** BMECs were transfected with Lipofectamine 2000 (Control), negative control of miR-139 inhibitor (Inhibitor NC) or miR-139 inhibitor. Western blotting analysis showed the protein levels of β-casein and β-actin at 48 h post-transfection. **c** Relative protein levels were quantified by analyzing scanned blots in panel **a** using Bandscan5.0 software. β-actin was used as a loading control. **d** Relative protein levels were quantified by analyzing scanned blots in panel **b** using Bandscan5.0 software. β-actin was used as a loading control. For **c** and **d**, results are shown as means ± SEM from three independent experiments. Statistical analysis was conducted using one-way ANOVA. "*", statistical significance was considered at $P<0.05$

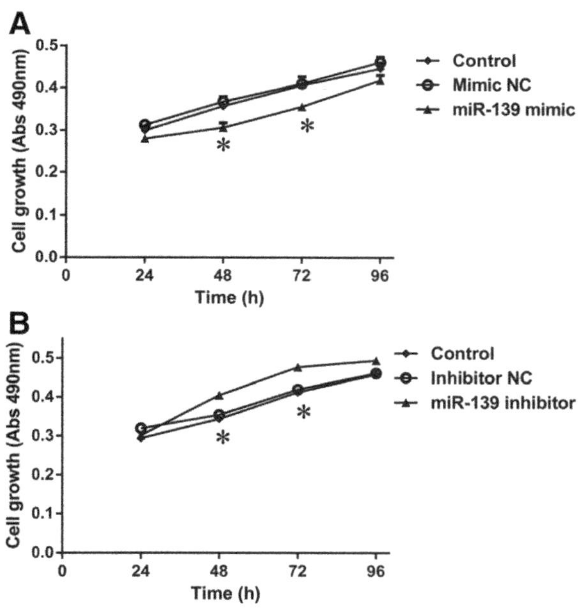

Fig. 5 MiR-139 inhibits proliferation of BMECs. **a** BMECs were transfected with Lipofectamine 2000 (Control), negative control of miR-139 mimic (Mimic NC) or miR-139 mimic. Cell proliferation was measured by the MTT assay at 24, 48, 72, or 96 h post-transfection. **b** BMECs were transfected with Lipofectamine 2000 (Control), negative control of miR-139 inhibitor (Inhibitor NC) or miR-139 inhibitor. Cell proliferation was measured by the MTT assay at 24, 48, 72, or 96 h post-transfection. Results are shown as means ± SEM from three independent experiments. Statistical analysis was conducted using one-way ANOVA."*", statistical significance was considered at $P<0.05$

hypothesized that miR-139 may be involved in lactation of dairy cows and tested this hypothesis. Out of potential target genes for miR-139, we prioritized *GHR* and *IGF1R* for further studies based on their roles in lactation processes. Our dual luciferase reporter assay indicated that miR-139 binds to *GHR* and *IGF1R* by their 3′-UTRs. Furthermore, we observed that mRNA levels of GHR and IGF1R were inversely correlated with miR-139 expression in cultured BMECs. These results confirmed that *GHR* and *IGF1R* are target genes of miR-139 in dairy cow mammary gland.

GHR activates signaling pathways including the Janus kinase2/signal transducer and activator of transcription (JAK2/STAT), mitogen activated protein kinase (MAPK), and the phosphatidylinositol-3-kinase (PI3K) pathways [14]. In particular, the JAK-STAT5 pathway is the main pathway through which GH influences the expression of genes encoding milk proteins such as β-casein, an important differentiation marker in mammary epithelial cells [16, 30, 31]. Moreover, GH influences protein metabolism through changes in the mTOR signaling pathway in bovine mammary gland [9]. It is worth noting that the mTOR signaling pathway can also be influenced by IGF1R. There are two classical signaling pathways regulated by IGF1R, the PI3K-AKT and RAS/RAF/MAPK pathways [32]. IGF1R regulates protein synthesis through the PI3K-AKT1-mTOR pathway [33]. After phosphorylation of mTOR, the mTOR pathway regulates the translation process by directly

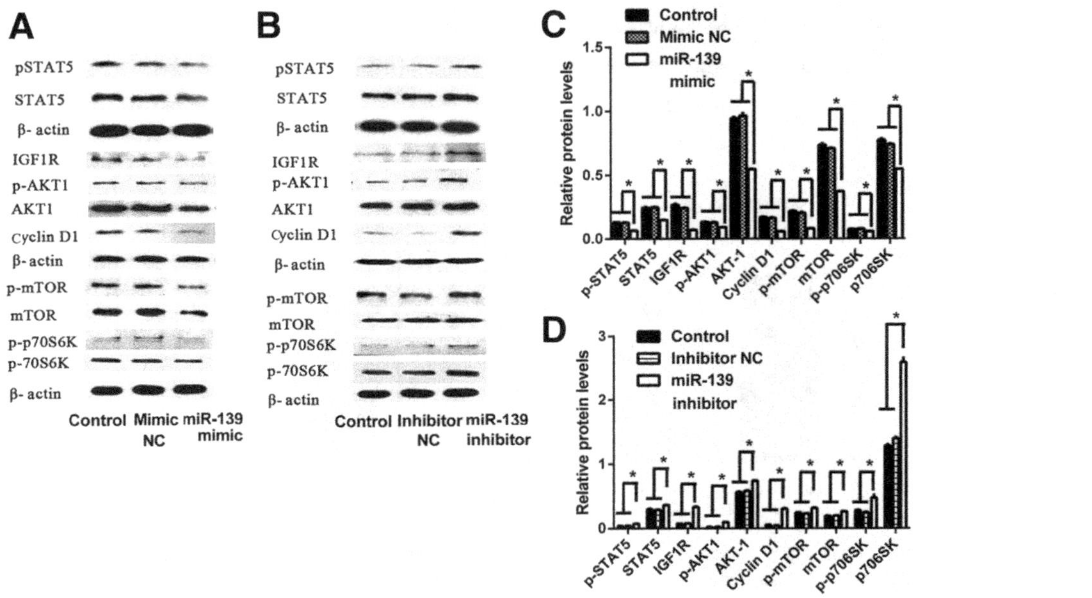

Fig. 6 MiR-139 reduces protein levels of major downstream members of GHR and IGF1R signaling in BMECs. **a** BMECs were transfected with Lipofectamine 2000 (Control), negative control of miR-139 mimic (Mimic NC) or miR-139 mimic. Western blotting analysis showed the protein levels of p-STAT5, STAT5, IGF1R, p-AKT1, AKT1, Cyclin D1, p-mTOR, mTOR, p-p70S6K, p70S6K and β-actin at 48 h post-transfection. **b** BMECs were transfected with Lipofectamine 2000 (Control), negative control of miR-139 inhibitor (Inhibitor NC) or miR-139 inhibitor. Western blotting analysis showed the protein levels of p-STAT5, STAT5, IGF1R, p-AKT1, AKT1, Cyclin D1, p-mTOR, mTOR, p-p70S6K, p70S6K and β-actin at 48 h post-transfection. **c** Relative protein levels were quantified by analyzing scanned blots in panel **a** using Bandscan5.0 software. β-actin was used as a loading control. **d** Relative protein levels were quantified by analyzing scanned blots in panel **b** using Bandscan5.0 software. β-actin was used as a loading control. For **c** and **d**, results are shown as means ± SEM from three independent experiments. Statistical analysis was conducted using one-way ANOVA. "*", statistical significance was considered at $P<0.05$

phosphorylating the translational regulators eukaryotic translationinitiation factor 4E (eIF4E) binding protein 1 (4E–BP1) and S6 kinase 1 (S6 K1), which in turn promote protein synthesis [19, 34]. In our study, we revealed that miR-139 reduced protein levels of β-casein. In addition, we found that miR-139 inhibited not only the activity of downstream signaling molecules of the GHR and IGF1R pathways, but also the total protein levels of key molecules of these pathways. This phenomenon has also been found by others [24, 35]. These observations suggest that miR-139 likely inhibits synthesis of β-casein through GHR and IGF1R signaling in BMECs.

In general, the number of secretory mammary epithelial cells determines milk production in a mammary gland, and the balance between proliferation and apoptosis controls the number of secretory mammary epithelial cells. Both proliferation and apoptosis produce effects gradually throughout the lactation period [25]. Previous studies showed that IGF1R can stimulate cell proliferation and inhibit apoptosis through the PI3K/AKT and MAPK pathways [36]. Our study revealed that miR-139 down-regulated expression of IGF1R and PI3K/AKT members. Moreover, in our cell proliferation assay, miR-139 significantly inhibited the growth of BMECs. Cyclin D is a known cell cycle regulator which indirectly stimulates the expression of various cell cycle promoters [37]. Previous studies showed that IGF1R induces elevated protein levels of Cyclin D1 through binding of the lymphoid Enhancer-Binding Factor 1 (LEF1) transcription factor in the nucleus [38]. Then, we determined the expression of Cyclin D1 by western blotting analysis. Our results showed that miR-139 decreased the protein level of Cyclin D1 in cultured BMECs. These results suggest that miR-139 also reduces the number of BMECs via IGF1R signaling.

In this study, we determined that *GHR* and *IGF1R* are target genes of miR-139 and that miR-139 inhibits synthesis of β-casein through down-regulating both GHR and IGF1R signaling. However, there is another connection between GHR and IGF1R. As we know, the binding of GHR to its ligand regulates IGF1 production by activating the STAT5b signaling cascade [39, 40]. Moreover, postnatal IGF1 production is predominantly regulated by GH [41]. These data indicate that the effect of GHR on the mammary gland may be exerted via IGF1R. Then, we investigated the relationship among miR-139, GHR, and IGF1R. As a result, we revealed that GHR is a regulator of IGF1R signaling because silencing *GHR* decreased protein levels of β-casein, IGF1R, and key

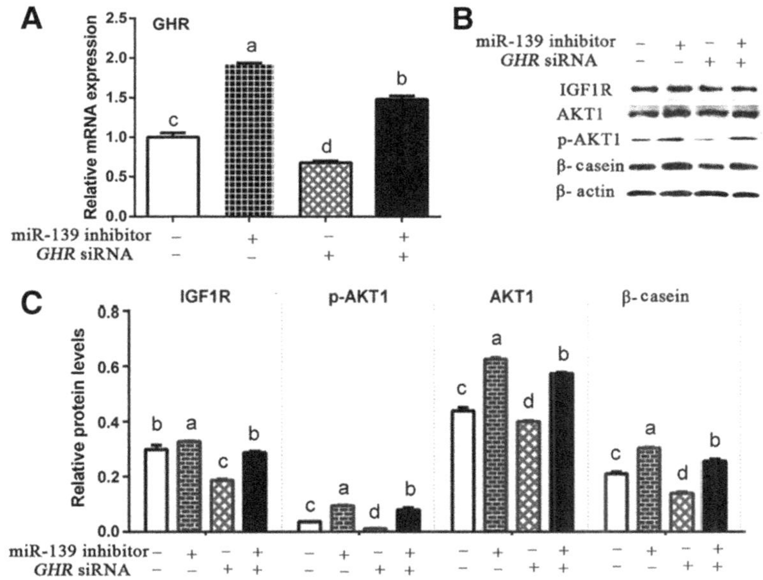

Fig. 7 MiR-139 also regulates synthesis of β-casein and IGF1R signaling by influencing *GHR*. BMECs were transfected with (without) *GHR* siRNA and (or) miR-139 inhibitor. **a** GHR mRNA levels were examined by qPCR at 24 h post-transfection in cultured BMECs. GHR expression was normalized to β-actin. **b** Western blotting analysis showed the levels of IGF1R, p-AKT1, AKT1, β-casein, and β-actin at 48 h post-transfection in cultured BMECs. **c** Relative protein levels were quantified by analyzing scanned blots in panel **b** using Bandscan5.0 software. β-actin was used as a loading control. For **a** and **c**, results are shown as means ± SEM from three independent experiments. Statistical analysis was conducted using one-way ANOVA. Bars with different lowercase letters are significantly different ($P < 0.05$)

members of the IGF1R pathway. Additionally, we found that co-silencing miR-139 and *GHR* rescued the expression of *GHR* and *GHR* silencing effects. These data suggest that miR-139 also regulates synthesis of β-casein and IGF1R signaling by influencing GHR.

Conclusions

In conclusion, we have revealed that miR-139 is downregulated in lactating dairy cow mammary glands and that miR-139 inhibits β-casein synthesis and proliferation by targeting the GHR and IGF1R signaling pathways in BMECs. This finding suggests that miR-139 may act as a potent inhibitor in lactation.

Abbreviations

AKT1: Protein kinase B; BMEC: Bovine mammary epithelial cell; DIM: Day in milk; DMEM: Dulbecco's modified Eagle's medium; DMSO: Dimethyl sulfoxide; eIF4E: Eukaryotic translationinitiation factor 4E; FBS: Fetal bovine serum; GH: Growth hormone; GHR: Growth hormone receptor; IGF1: Type I insulin-like growth factor; IGF1R: Type I insulin-like growth factor receptor; JAK: Janus kinase; LEF1: Lymphoid Enhancer-Binding Factor 1; MAPK: Mitogen activated protein kinase; mTOR: Mammalian target of rapamycin.; MTT: 3-(4,5-Dimethylthiazol-2-yl)-2,5- diphenyltetrazolium bromide.; Mut: Mutant.; p70S6K: p70-S6 Kinase.; PI3K: Phosphatidylinositol-3-kinase.; qPCR: Quantitative Real-time Polymerase Chain Reaction.; SDS-PAGE: Sodium dodecyl sulfate polyacrylamide gel electrophoresis.; SEM: Standard error of mean.: STAT5: Signal transducer and activator of transcription-5.; UTR: Untranslated region.; WT: Wild-type.

Acknowledgements

Not applicable.

Funding

This work was supported by the National Natural Science Foundation of China (31401093), the Scientific Research Project of Heilongjiang Province Department of Education (12541018) the "Academic Backbone" Project of Northeast Agricultural University (16XG17), and the Open Research Fund for Key Laboratory of Dairy Science (Northeast Agricultural University), Ministry of Education, Heilongjiang Province,China (2015KLDSDF-02).

Authors' contributions

YC designed the experiments and wrote the manuscript. XS conducted most of the experiments, and analyzed the results. LJ performed dual luciferase reporter assay. GY and JA helped XS analyzed the results. QL and XG made the figures and revised the manuscript. CW conceived the idea for the project, and finalized the manuscript. All authors read and approved the final manuscript.

Consent for publication

Not applicable.

Competing interests

The authors declare that they have no competing interests.

Author details

[1]Key Laboratory of Dairy Science of Education Ministry, Northeast Agricultural University, Harbin, Heilongjiang 150030, People's Republic of China. [2]College of Life Science, Northeast Agricultural University, Harbin, Heilongjiang 150030, People's Republic of China.

References

1. Yonemori M, Seki N, Yoshino H, Matsushita F, Miyamoto K, Nakagawa M, Enokida H. Dual tumor-suppressors miR-139-5p and miR-139-3p targeting matrix metalloprotease 11 in bladder cancer. Cancer Sci. 2016;107:1233–42.

2. Qiu G, Lin Y, Zhang H, Wu D. miR-139-5p inhibits epitheliale mesenchymal transition, migration and invasion of hepatocellular carcinoma cells by targeting ZEB1 and ZEB2. Biochem Biophys Res Commun. 2015;463:315–21.
3. Chen X, Gao C, Li H, Huang L, Sun Q, Dong Y, Tian C, Gao S, Dong H, Guan D, Hu X, Zhao S, Li L, Zhu L, Yan Q, Zhang J, Zen K, Zhang CY. Identification and characterization of microRNAs in raw milk during different periods of lactation, commercial fluid, and powdered milk products. Cell Res. 2010;20:1128–37.
4. Hasseine LK, Hinault C, Lebrun P, Gautier N, Paul-Bellon R, Van Obberghen E. miR-139 impacts FoxO1 action by decreasing FoxO1 protein in mouse hepatocytes. Biochem Biophys Res Commun. 2009;390:1278–82.
5. Zhang HD, Sun DW, Mao L, Zhang J, Jiang LH, Li J, WuY JH, Chen W, Wang J, Ma R, Cao HX, Wu JZ, Tang JH. MiR-139-5p inhibits the biological function of breast cancer cells by targeting Notch1 and mediates chemosensitivity to docetaxel. Biochem Biophys Res Commun. 2015;465:702–13.
6. Liu R, Yang M, Meng Y, Liao J, Sheng J, Pu Y, Yin L, Kim SJ. Tumor-suppressive function of miR-139-5p in esophageal squamous cell carcinoma. PLoS One. 2013; https://doi.org/10.1371/journal.pone.0077068.
7. Zhang L, Dong Y, Zhu N, Tsoi H, Zhao Z, Wu CW, Wang K, Zheng S, Ng SS, Chan FK, Sung JJ, Yu J. microRNA-139-5p exerts tumor suppressor function by targeting NOTCH1 in colorectal cancer. Mol Cancer. 2014; doi:10.1186/1476-4598-13-124.
8. Xu W, Hang M, Yuan CY, FL W, Chen SB, Xue K. MicroRNA-139-5p inhibits cell proliferation and invasion by targeting insulin-like growth factor 1 receptor in human non-small cell lung cancer. Int J Clin Exp Pathol. 2015;8: 3864–70.
9. Wong CC, Wong CM, Tung EK, SL A, Lee JM, Poon RT, Man K, Ng IO. The microRNA miR-139 suppresses metastasis and progression of hepatocellular carcinoma by down-regulating rho-kinase 2. Gastroenterology. 2011;140: 322–31.
10. Krishnan K, Steptoe AL, Martin HC, Pattabiraman DR, Nones K, Waddell N, Mariasegaram M, Simpson PT, Lakhani SR, Vlassov A, Grimmond SM, Cloonan N. miR-139-5p is a regulator of metastatic pathways in breast cancer. RNA. 2013;19:1767–80.
11. Wang C, Li Q. Identification of differentially expressed microRNAs during the evelopment of Chinese murine mammary gland. J Genet Genomics. 2007; 34:966–73.
12. Hayashi AA, Nones K, Roy NC, McNabb WC, Mackenzie DS, Pacheco D, McCoard S. Initiation and elongation steps of mRNA translation are involved in the increase in milk protein yield caused by growth hormone administration during lactation. J Dairy Sci. 2009;92:1889–99.
13. Lombardi S, Honeth G, Ginestier C, Shinomiya I, Marlow R, Buchupalli B, Gazinska P, Brown J, Catchpole S, Liu S, Barkan A, Wicha M, Purushotham A, Burchell J, Pinder S, Dontu G. Growth hormone is secreted by normal breast epithelium upon progesterone stimulationand increases proliferation of stem/progenitor cells. Stem Cell Reports. 2014;2:780–93.
14. Perry JK, Mohankumar KM, Emerald BS, Mertani HC, Lobie PE. The contribution of growth hormone to mammary neoplasia. J Mammary Gland Biol Neoplasia. 2008;13:131–45.
15. Sakamoto K, Komatsu T, Kobayashi T, Rose MT, Aso H, Hagino A, Obara Y. Growth hormone acts on the synthesis and secretion of alpha-casein in bovine mammary epithelial cells. J Dairy Res. 2005;72:264–70.
16. Postel-Vinay MC, Kelly PA. Growth hormone receptor signalling. Bailliere Clin Endocrinol Metab. 1996;10:323–36.
17. Ilkbahar YN, Thordarson G, Camarillo IG, Talamantes F. Differential expression of the growth hormone receptor and growth hormone-binding protein in epithelia and stroma of the mouse mammary gland at various physiological stages. J Endocrinol. 1999;161:77–87.
18. Pal S, Woodford K, Kukuljan S, Ho S. Milk intolerance, Beta-casein and lactose. Nutrients. 2015;7:7285–97.
19. Sciascia Q, Pacheco D, McCoard SA. Increased milk protein synthesis in response to exogenous growth hormone is associated with changes in mechanistic (mammalian) target of rapamycin (mTOR)C1-dependent and independent cell signaling. J Dairy Sci. 2013;96:2327–38.
20. Divisova J, Kuiatse I, Lazard Z, Weiss H, Vreeland F, Hadsell DL, Schiff R, Osborne CK, Lee AV. The growth hormone receptor antagonist pegvisomant blocks both mammary gland development and MCF-7 breast cancer xenograft growth. Breast. Cancer Res Treat. 2006;98:315–27.
21. Felice DL, El-Shennawy L, Zhao S, Lantvit DL, Shen Q, Unterman TG, Swanson SM, Frasor J. Growth hormone potentiates 17β-estradiol-dependent breast cancer cell proliferation independently of IGF-I receptor signaling. Endocrinology. 2013;154:3219–27.
22. Fürstenberger G, Morant R, Senn HJ. Insulin-like growth factors and breast cancer. Onkologie. 2003;26:290–4.
23. Cui Y, Liu Z, Sun X, Hou X, Qu B, Zhao F, Gao X, Sun Z, Li Q. Thyroid hormone responsive protein spot 14 enhances lipogenesis in bovine mammary epithelial cells. In Vitro Cell Dev Biol Anim. 2015;51:586–94.
24. Zhao F, Liu C, Hao YM, Qu B, Cui YJ, Zhang N, Gao XJ, Li QZ. Up-regulation of integrin α6β4 expression by mitogens involved in dairy cow mammary development. In Vitro Cell Dev Biol Anim. 2015;51:287–99.
25. Murney R, Stelwagen K, Wheeler TT, Margerison JK, Singh K. The effects of milking frequency in early lactation on milk yield, mammary cell turnover, and secretory activity in grazing dairy cows. J Dairy Sci. 2015;98:305–11.
26. Knight CH, Peaker M. Development of the mammary gland. J ReprodFertil. 1982;65:521–36.
27. Zhang HD, Jiang LH, Sun DW, Li J, Tang JH. MiR-139-5p:promising biomarker for cancer. Tumour Biol. 2015;36:1355–65.
28. Ruelas DS, Chan JK, Oh E, Heidersbach AJ, Hebbeler AM, Chavez L, Verdin E, Rape M, Greene WC. MicroRNA-155 reinforces HIV latency. J Biol Chem. 2015;290:13736–48.
29. Zhou Y, Gong W, Xiao J, Wu J, Pan L, Li X, Wang X, Wang W, Hu S, Transcriptomic YJ. Analysis reveals key regulators of mammogenesis and the pregnancy-lactationcycle. Sci China Life Sci. 2014;57:340–55.
30. Chiba T, Maeda T, Sanbe A, Kudo K. Serotonin suppresses β-casein expression via PTP1B activation in human mammary epithelial cells. Biochem Biophys Res Commun. 2016;473:323–8.
31. Postel-Vinay MC, Finidori J. Growth hormone receptor: structure and signal transduction. Eur J Endocrinol. 1995;133:654–9.
32. Chitnis MM, Yuen JS, Protheroe AS, Pollak M, Macaulay VM. The type 1 insulin-like growth factor receptor pathway. Clin Cancer Res. 2008;14:6364–70.
33. Iams WT, Lovly CM. Molecular pathways: clinical applications and future direction of insulin-like growth Factor-1 receptor pathway blockade. Clin Cancer Res. 2015;21:4270–7.
34. Laplante M, Sabatini DM. mTOR signaling in growth control and disease. Cell. 2012;149:274–93.
35. Ao J, Wei C, Si Y, Luo C, Lv W, Lin Y, Cui Y, Gao X. Tudor-SN Regulates milk synthesis and proliferation of bovine mammary epithelial cells. Int J Mol Sci. 2015;16:29936–47.
36. de Groot S, Charehbili A, van Laarhoven HW, Mooyaart AL, Dekker-Ensink NG, van de Ven S, Janssen LG, Swen JJ, Smit VT, Heijns JB, Kessels LW, van der Straaten T, Böhringer S, Gelderblom H, van der Hoeven JJ, Guchelaar HJ, Pijl H, Kroep JR, Dutch Breast Cancer Research Group. Insulin-like growth factor 1 receptor expression and IGF1R 3129G > T polymorphism are associated with response to neoadjuvant chemotherapy in breast cancer patients: results from the NEOZOTAC trial (BOOG 2010-01). Breast Cancer Res. 2016;18:3.
37. Park JH, Darvin P, Lim EJ, Joung YH, Hong DY, Park EU, Park SH, Choi SK, Moon ES, Cho BW, Park KD, Lee HK, Kim MJ, Park DS, Chung IM, Yang YM. Hwanggeumchal sorghum induces cell cycle arrest, and suppresses tumor growth and metastasis through Jak2/STAT pathways in breast cancer xenografts. PLoS One. 2012; doi:10.1371/journal.pone.0040531.
38. Warsito D, Sjöström S, Andersson S, Larsson O, Sehat B. Nuclear IGF1R is a transcriptional co-activator of LEF1/TCF. EMBO Rep. 2012;13:244–50.
39. Hwa V, Nadeau K, Wit JM, Rosenfeld RG. STAT5b deficiency: lessons from STAT5b gene mutations. Best Pract Res Clin Endocrinol Metab. 2011;25:61–75.
40. Feigerlova E, Hwa V, Derr MA, Rosenfeld RG. Current issues on molecular diagnosis of GH signaling defects. Endocr Dev. 2013;24:118–27.
41. Hwa V, Fang P, Derr MA, Fiegerlova E, Rosenfeld RG. IGF-I in human growth: lessons from defects in the GH-IGF-I axis. Nestle. NutrInst workshop. Ser. 2013;71:43–55.

14

Illumina MiSeq 16S amplicon sequence analysis of bovine respiratory disease associated bacteria in lung and mediastinal lymph node tissue

Dayle Johnston[1,2], Bernadette Earley[1], Paul Cormican[1], Gerard Murray[3], David Anthony Kenny[1], Sinead Mary Waters[1], Mark McGee[4], Alan Kieran Kelly[2] and Matthew Sean McCabe[1*]

Abstract

Background: Bovine respiratory disease (BRD) is caused by growth of single or multiple species of pathogenic bacteria in lung tissue following stress and/or viral infection. Next generation sequencing of 16S ribosomal RNA gene PCR amplicons (NGS 16S amplicon analysis) is a powerful culture-independent open reference method that has recently been used to increase understanding of BRD-associated bacteria in the upper respiratory tract of BRD cattle. However, it has not yet been used to examine the microbiome of the bovine lower respiratory tract. The objective of this study was to use NGS 16S amplicon analysis to identify bacteria in post-mortem lung and lymph node tissue samples harvested from fatal BRD cases and clinically healthy animals. Cranial lobe and corresponding mediastinal lymph node post-mortem tissue samples were collected from calves diagnosed as BRD cases by veterinary laboratory pathologists and from clinically healthy calves. NGS 16S amplicon libraries, targeting the V3-V4 region of the bacterial 16S rRNA gene were prepared and sequenced on an Illumina MiSeq. Quantitative insights into microbial ecology (QIIME) was used to determine operational taxonomic units (OTUs) which corresponded to the 16S rRNA gene sequences.

Results: *Leptotrichiaceae, Mycoplasma, Pasteurellaceae*, and *Fusobacterium* were the most abundant OTUs identified in the lungs and lymph nodes of the calves which died from BRD. *Leptotrichiaceae, Fusobacterium, Mycoplasma, Trueperella* and *Bacteroides* had greater relative abundances in post-mortem lung samples collected from fatal cases of BRD in dairy calves, compared with clinically healthy calves without lung lesions. *Leptotrichiaceae, Mycoplasma* and *Pasteurellaceae* showed higher relative abundances in post-mortem lymph node samples collected from fatal cases of BRD in dairy calves, compared with clinically healthy calves without lung lesions. Two *Leptotrichiaceae* sequence contigs were subsequently assembled from bacterial DNA-enriched shotgun sequences.

Conclusions: The microbiomes of the cranial lung lobe and mediastinal lymph node from calves which died from BRD and from clinically healthy H-F calves have been characterised. Contigs corresponding to the abundant *Leptotrichiaceae* OTU were sequenced and found not to be identical to any known bacterial genus. This suggests that we have identified a novel bacterial species associated with BRD.

Keywords: Bovine respiratory disease, lung microbiome, 16S sequencing, diagnostics

* Correspondence: matthew.mccabe@teagasc.ie
[1]Animal and Bioscience Research Department, Animal & Grassland Research and Innovation Centre, Teagasc Grange, Dunsany, Co. Meath, Ireland
Full list of author information is available at the end of the article

Background

Bovine respiratory disease (BRD) is associated with significant morbidity and mortality in cattle worldwide, and contributes to substantial economic losses [1–3]. Clinical signs associated with BRD typically include elevated rectal temperature, increased respiratory rate, nasal and ocular discharges, cough, dyspnea, decreased appetite and depression [2, 4, 5]. In Ireland, BRD is a leading cause of mortality in calves between one and 5 months of age [6].

BRD results from a multifactorial aetiology of infectious agents, host factors, environmental stress factors and their interactions [7–9]. Primary pathogens including bovine herpesvirus 1 (Bo-HV1), bovine respiratory syncytial virus (BRSV), bovine parainfluenza 3 virus (BPIV-3), bovine viral diarrhoea virus (BVDV), bovine coronavirus (BCoV) and *Mycoplasma bovis,* are thought to be generally responsible for the onset of BRD [1, 4, 10–12] although recent viral metagenomic NGS studies suggest that there are many more uncharacterised BRD-associated viruses than was previously thought [13, 14]. BRD-associated viral and *Mycoplasmal* pathogens damage the lungs by causing immunosuppression, ciliary dysfunction and cellular necrosis [15, 16]. This damage allows proliferation and colonisation by secondary bacterial pathogens, commonly including *Mannheimia haemolytica, Pasteurella multocida, Histophilus somni, Mycoplasma bovis* and *Trueperella pyogenes,* which are normally commensal in the nasopharyngeal region of cattle [1, 7, 11, 17–19]. These bacteria evade the lung's remaining immune defences and their virulence factors cause progression of the disease if left untreated [7, 11, 15, 16].

Currently available vaccinations and antibiotic treatments are targeted against the known viruses and bacteria associated with BRD. Poor efficacy of vaccination and antimicrobial treatments against BRD associated bacteria [20–22] may partially be due to the involvement of unknown bacterial pathogens in the disease.

The methods that are currently used for identification of specific bacteria associated with fatal cases of BRD are culture, immunohistochemistry, in-situ hybridisation and multiplex and uniplex polymerase chain reaction (PCR) [23]. However, these techniques are time consuming and they have several limitations. Although culture is considered the gold standard for pathogen identification [24], the main limitation of this technique is that many bacterial species associated with BRD are difficult to culture [25, 26]. PCR has been demonstrated to be a more sensitive method than culture for identification of bacteria in bovine pneumonic lung tissue [27, 28]. Although real-time qPCR is commonly used in veterinary diagnostic laboratories, only known bacteria can be identified using this "closed reference" technique and each qPCR assay is generally designed to detect one individual bacterial species.

Next generation sequencing of 16S ribosomal RNA gene PCR amplicons (NGS 16S amplicon analysis) has been used for identification of bacteria present in diverse sample types including clinical isolates [29, 30], the bovine rumen [31], human nasal lavage [32] and nasopharyngeal swabs from feedlot cattle [26, 33]. As primers bind to conserved regions of the 16S ribosomal RNA (rRNA) gene [34] and phylogenetically variable regions are amplified and subsequently sequenced (typically generating 10,000–100,000 sequences per sample), identification of the bacteria present (both known and unknown) in the sample is possible at unprecedented depth [35].

The aim of this study was to use NGS 16S amplicon analysis to identify unculturable and previously unknown bacteria which may play a pathogenic role in BRD. For this we analysed DNA from post-mortem cranial lung lobe and mediastinal lymph node tissue from beef and dairy calves with BRD diagnosed as the cause of death, and from clinically healthy Holstein-Friesian (H-F) calves. We found highly abundant 16S sequence for which the closest match was *Leptotrichiaceae.* This putative *Leptotrichiaceae* 16S sequence was present in lung and lymph node tissue from fatal BRD cases and in lung lesions from clinically healthy calves but was absent in lesion-free lungs from clinically healthy calves. To our knowledge this is the first report of detection of this putative *Leptotrichiaceae* species in bovine lung lesions in cattle with BRD and also the first report of NGS 16S amplicon analysis of lung tissue and lung-associated lymph nodes in cattle with BRD.

Methods

Post-mortem tissue sample collection

Thirty-eight cranial lung lobe tissue samples were collected post-mortem from 32 beef calves and 6 dairy calves which were submitted from farms in three different regions in Ireland. Mediastinal lymph node tissue was also collected from 32 of these animals. BRD was diagnosed on gross examination at three regional veterinary laboratories (RVLs) (Athlone, Kilkenny and Sligo) by experienced pathologists. Bacteriological culture, virological and/or bacteriological PCR and histology for identification of aetiological agents (Table 1 and Additional file 1) were performed at the RVLs. In all cases, lung tissue samples were harvested from lesions (lesions were defined as macroscopic consolidation or abscessation of lung tissue) present on the cranial lobes of the lung. Approximately 1 g of each of these tissues was collected from each calf (comprising 13 beef and dairy breeds) (Table 1). Six of these post-mortem lung tissue samples were frozen at -80 °C immediately following collection. The remaining lung and lymph node post-mortem tissue samples were

Table 1 Description of post-mortem tissue samples collected at RVLs

Calf ID	Tissue types collected	Preservation method	Age (months)	Sex	Breed	County of farm of origin	RVL location	Lesions observed	Histology	RVL diagnosis
1	lung	frozen	6	F	SIX	Donegal	Sligo	✓	✓	Pneumonia (BRSV suspected)
2	lung	frozen	1	M	FRX	Donegal	Sligo	✓	x	Pneumonia and enteritis
3	lung	frozen	12	M	PTX	Donegal	Sligo	✓	✓	Pneumonia - IBR and *M. bovis*
4	lung	frozen	12	M	BBX	Donegal	Sligo	✓	✓	Pneumonia - IBR and *M. bovis*
5	lung	frozen	7	M	CHX	Donegal	Sligo	✓	✓	Pneumonia - *H. somni*
6	lung	frozen	6	F	CHX	Leitrim	Sligo	✓	x	Pneumonia - *M. haemolytica* and BPIV-3 virus
7	lung and lymph node	frozen	1	F	LM	Sligo	Sligo	✓	x	Pneumonia and navel infection - *M. bovis*, *Pseudomonas* spp.
8	lung and lymph node	RNALater	8	M	FR	Leitrim	Sligo	✓	x	Pneumonia - *T. pyrogenes*
9	lung and lymph node	RNALater	0	M	RBX	Donegal	Sligo	✓	x	Pneumonia - IBR, *H. somni*, *T. pyrogenes*
10	lung and lymph node	RNALater	3.5	M	FR	Leitrim	Sligo	✓	x	Pneumonia- *P. multocida* and *S. dublin*
11	lung and lymph node	RNALater	2.5	F	LM	Sligo	Sligo	✓	x	Pneumonia
12	lung and lymph node	RNALater	0	F	CHX	Carlow	Kilkenny	✓	x	Pneumonia
13	lung and lymph node	RNALater	3	F	AAX	Galway	Athlone	✓	✓	Pneumonia - *M. haemolytica*
14	lung and lymph node	RNALater	2	F	LMX	Westmeath	Athlone	✓	✓	Pneumonia and bacteraemia- *P. multocida*
15	lung and lymph node	RNALater	0	F	AAX	Offaly	Athlone	✓	✓	Pneumonia - IBR and necrotic laryngitis
16	lung and lymph node	RNALater	0	F	AAX	Offaly	Athlone	✓	✓	Pneumonia and pleurisy - *Pasteurella* spp., IBR and BRSV
17	lung and lymph node	RNALater	0	M	CHX	Longford	Athlone	✓	✓	Pneumonia and rotavirus enteritis
18	lung and lymph node	RNALater	1	M	CHX	Roscommon	Athlone	✓	✓	Pneumonia and navel ill - *T pyogenes* (suspected virus and *Pasteurella*)
19	lung and lymph node	RNALater	0	M	WAX	Waterford	Kilkenny	✓	x	Pneumonia and rotavirus enteritis
20	lung and lymph node	RNALater	1.5	F	FR	Tipperary	Kilkenny	✓	✓	Pneumonia - *H. somni* and *M. bovis*
21	lung and lymph node	RNALater	3	M	LM	Kilkenny	Kilkenny	✓	✓	Pneumonia - *H. somni* and *M. bovis*
22	lung and lymph node	RNALater	0	F	CHX	Kilkenny	Kilkenny	✓	✓	Pneumonia - *P. multocida / H. somni* bronchopneumonia
23	lung and lymph node	RNALater	0	M	LMX	Laois	Kilkenny	✓	✓	Pneumonia - *H. somni* bronchopneumonia
24	lung and lymph node	RNALater	3	M	LMX	Sligo	Sligo	✓	x	Pneumonia
25	lung and lymph node	RNALater	2	M	CH	Mayo	Sligo	✓	x	Pneumonia - *Proteus* spp.
26	lung and lymph node	RNALater	3	F	CHX	Leitrim	Sligo	✓	x	Pneumonia - Endocarditis, enzootic pneumonia, inhalation pneumonia
27	lung and lymph node	RNALater	1.5	F	LMX	Sligo	Sligo	✓	x	Pneumonia - IBR

Table 1 Description of post-mortem tissue samples collected at RVLs *(Continued)*

28	lung and lymph node	RNALater	1.5	F	AAX	Sligo	Sligo	✓	x	Pneumonia - IBR and *Proteus* spp.
29	lung and lymph node	RNALater	12	M	CHX	Donegal	Sligo	✓	✓	Pneumonia - (possible IBR) and meningitis
30	lung and lymph node	RNALater	1	M	AA	Sligo	Sligo	✓	x	Pneumonia - *M. bovis*
31	lung and lymph node	RNALater	2.5	F	LMX	Donegal	Sligo	✓	x	Pneumonia - *M. bovis*
32	lung and lymph node	RNALater	3	F	LMX	Kilkenny	Kilkenny	✓	✓	Pneumonia - interstitial pneumonia
33	lung and lymph node	RNALater	2.5	M	FR	Laois	Kilkenny	✓	x	Pneumonia - *P. multocida*
34	lung and lymph node	RNALater	5	M	AAX	Kilkenny	Kilkenny	✓	✓	Pneumonia - *P. multocida, T. pyrogenes* chronic bronchopneumonia
35	lung and lymph node	RNALater	4.5	F	LMX	Sligo	Sligo	✓	✓	Pneumonia - Pasteurellosis
36	lung and lymph node	RNALater	1	M	CHX	Longford	Athlone	✓	✓	Pneumonia - suppurative bronchial pneumonia.
37	lung and lymph node	RNALater	1.5	M	CHX	Galway	Athlone	✓	✓	Pneumonia - *M. haemolytica*
38	lung and lymph node	RNALater	3.5	F	AAX	Offaly	Athlone	✓	✓	Pneumonia - *H. somni, M. bovis, M. haemolytica, P. multocida, T. pyogenes*

Lesions were defined as macroscopic consolidation or abscessation of lung tissue.
M male, *F* female, *AA* Aberdeen Angus, *AAX* Aberdeen Angus cross, *BBX* Belgium Blue cross, *CH* Charolais, *CHX* Charolais cross, *FR* Friesian, *FRX* Friesian cross, *LM* Limousin, *LMX* Limousin cross, *PTX* Parthenaise cross, *RBX* Rotbunt cross, *SIX* simmental cross, *WAX* wagyu cross, ✓ = performed and confirmed bovine respiratory disease, x = not performed, *H. somni* = *Histophilus somni*, *M. bovis* = *Mycoplasma bovis*, *M. haemolytica* = *Mannheimia haemolytica*, *P. multocida* = *Pasteurella multocida*, *S. dublin* = *Salmonella dublin*, *T. pyrogenes* = *Trueperella pyrogenes*, BRSV = bovine respiratory syncytial virus, IBR = infectious bovine rhinotracheitis, BPIV-3 = bovine parainfluenza 3 virus.

cut into slices less than 0.5 cm thick, placed in RNALater RNA Stabilization Reagent (Qiagen, Manchester, UK), stored at 4 °C overnight, and subsequently stored at -20 ° C, according to the manufacturer's instructions (Table 1).

Bacteriology, virology and histology performed at RVLs

Aerobic bacteriology of swab samples from pneumonic lungs was performed on blood agar and McConkey agar at 37 °C for 2 days (n = 36) (Additional file 1), as described by Murray et al. [36]. Culture on chocolate agar under 8% CO_2 for 3 days and on xylose lysine desoxycholate agar (following selenite enrichment) for 2 days at 37 °C was also conducted for the identification of *Histophilus somni* (n = 13) and *Salmonella* species (n = 24), respectively (Additional file 1) [36].

Lung and tracheal mucosa were submitted for detection of *Mycoplasma bovis* (n = 15), *Histophilus somni* (n = 11), *Mannheimia haemolytica* (n = 4) and *Pasteurella multocida* (n = 1), by real-time qPCR analyses (Additional file 1), which were performed as previously described [28, 37–39]. Real-time qPCR was also used to identify Bo-HV1 (n = 36) and reverse transcriptase qPCR was used to identify BRSV (n = 38), BPIV-3 (n = 35) and BCoV (n = 34) (Additional file 1) as previously described [12]. Positive and negative (no template) controls were included in each qPCR assay.

Sections for histology were taken from the border of grossly visible lesions on the cranial lobe (n = 21) (Table 1 and Additional file 1). Sections were fixed by placing them in 10% neutral-buffered formalin for 4 days, embedding them in paraffin wax, cutting them with a microtome and staining them with hematoxylin and eosin, as previously described by Murray et al. [36].

Clinically healthy calves: health assessments

To serve as a comparison, 20 lung (cranial lobe) and 20 corresponding mediastinal lymph node tissue samples were also sourced from clinically healthy H-F calves which were slaughtered at approximately 2.5 months of age. These calves all recorded good performance prior to slaughter and achieved an average daily weight gain within a 0.25 standard deviation of their expected average daily gains.

Clinical health assessments of these calves were performed on the morning before slaughter using the Wisconsin calf health scoring criteria (https://www.vetmed.wisc.edu/dms/fapm/fapmtools/8calf/calf_respiratory_scoring_chart.pdf) to determine a respiratory score. A calf was considered to have respiratory disease if it had a respiratory score greater than or equal to 5 as it was then showing at least two signs of respiratory disease [5]. A full clinical history was available for these calves including a record of veterinary treatments for BRD.

Clinically healthy control calves: collection of post-mortem tissue samples

The lungs were harvested from the calves immediately following slaughter at Teagasc Ashtown Research Centre. All surfaces and forceps were cleaned with 20% Domestos extended germ kill bleach (1% final sodium hypochlorite solution) (Unilever, Surrey, UK Ltd) Virusolve® + (Amity International Healthcare; Barnsley, UK), 70% ethanol and RNaseZAP™ (Sigma-Aldrich® Ireland Ltd., Wicklow, Ireland) initially and between samples.

The lungs were visually examined and the presence and number of lesions was recorded. Tissue samples from the cranial lobe and mediastinal lymph node were removed using sterile scalpel blades and forceps. Tissue samples were cut into slices less than 0.5 cm thick, placed in RNALater RNA Stabilization Reagent, stored at 4 °C overnight, and subsequently stored at -20 °C, according to the manufacturer's instructions. When lesions were present on the cranial lobe, the lesions, rather than the lesion-free regions, were sampled.

DNA extraction

DNA extraction from post-mortem tissue samples was carried out in a class II biosafety cabinet. Forceps, homogeniser and all work surfaces were cleaned initially and between samples using 20% sodium hypochlorite solution, Virusolve®+, 70% ethanol and RNaseZAP™. Homogeniser blades were sonicated for 10 min at 60 °C in molecular grade water (Sigma, Ireland), then rinsed by running while submerged in 75% ethanol and molecular grade water. DNA was extracted from post-mortem tissue samples using the Qiagen QIAamp Cador pathogen mini kit (with pre-treatments T2 (enzymatic digestion of tissue) and B1 (for difficult-to-lyse bacteria in pre-treated tissue)) (Qiagen, Manchester, UK) according to the manufacturer's instructions with some modifications to pre-treatment T2.

A small piece of each tissue sample was removed using sterile scalpel blades and forceps, placed in a sterile Petri-dish, weighed, immediately submerged in buffer ATL (Qiagen, Manchester, UK) (360 μl per 50 mg tissue) and homogenised using a hand-held homogeniser (PRO 200, Bio-Gen Series; PRO Scientific Inc. Oxford, USA). Following homogenisation, 205 μl homogenised tissue was transferred to a 1.5 ml microcentrifuge tube (sterile) and 20 μl proteinase K was added. The microcentrifuge tube was placed in a shaking incubator overnight (300 rpm, 56 °C).

Pre-treatment B1 and the subsequent purification of pathogen nucleic acids from fluid samples were carried out according to the manufacturer's instructions. Following nucleic acid extraction, RNA was removed using RNaseA solution, 4 mg/ml (Promega, Southampton, UK). This was achieved by adding 5 μl RNaseA solution to 100 μl of the sample's purified nucleic acid eluate and incubating at 37 °C for 20 min. Subsequently, the DNA was purified using a Zymo genomic DNA clean & concentrator™-10 kit (Zymo Research Corp, Irvine, CA, USA), according to the manufacturer's instructions. A Nanodrop spectrophotometer (NanoDrop Technologies, Wilmington, DE, USA) was used to quantify the DNA. All waste was autoclaved appropriately prior to disposal.

16S amplicon library preparation and sequencing

One hundred and sixteen 16S rRNA gene amplicon libraries (including 6 water control libraries) were prepared by PCR amplification of an approximate 467 bp region within the hypervariable (V3-V4) region of the 16S rRNA gene in bacteria, from 50 ng of each of the extracted and purified DNA from lung and lymph node tissue, and molecular grade water (non-template control), respectively, according to the Illumina 16S metagenomic sequencing library protocol, with modifications.

PCR was initially performed with broad spectrum 16S rRNA primers (forward primer: 5′-TCGTCGGCAGCG TCAGATGTGTATAAGAGACAG*CCTACGGGNGGCW GCAG*-3′, reverse primer: 5′-GTCTCGTGGGCTCGGA GATGTGTATAAGAGACAGGACTACHVGGGTATCT AATCC-3′) [34], using Kapa HiFi HotStart 2× ReadyMix DNA polymerase (Kapa Biosystems Ltd., London, UK). Cycle conditions were 95 °C (3 min), then 35 cycles of 95 °C (30 s), 63 °C (30 s), 72 °C (30 s), then a final extension of 72 °C (5 min). Libraries were purified using AMPure XP beads (LABPLAN; Naas, Ireland) according to the Illumina 16S metagenomic sequencing library protocol. Dual indices and Illumina sequencing adapters from the Illumina Nextera XT index kits v2 B and C (Illumina, San Diego, USA) were added to the target amplicons in a second PCR step using Kapa HotStart HiFi 2× ReadyMix DNA polymerase (Kapa Biosystems Ltd., London, UK). Cycle conditions were 95 °C (3 min), then 9 cycles of 95 °C (30 s), 55 °C (30 s), 72 °C (30 s), then a final extension of 72 °C (5 min). Libraries were again purified using AMPure XP beads (LABPLAN; Naas, Ireland) according to the Illumina 16S metagenomic sequencing library protocol.

Libraries were measured for purity and quantity on a Nanodrop 1000 spectrophotometer. The barcoded amplicon libraries were combined in equal concentrations into a single pool according to their Nanodrop quantification measurement. Two μl of each negative control library was added to the pool. The library pool was then quantified using the KAPA SYBR FAST Universal qPCR kit with Illumina Primer Premix (Kapa Biosystems Ltd., London, UK) and the size was assessed with an Agilent DNA 1000 Kit (Agilent Technologies Ireland Ltd., Dublin, Ireland) on an

Agilent 2100 Bioanalyser (Agilent Technologies Ireland Ltd., Dublin, Ireland).

The library pool was diluted and denatured according to the Illumina MiSeq library preparation guide. The amplicon library (8 pM) was spiked with 30% denatured and diluted PhiX Illumina control library version 3 (12.5 pM). The sequencing run was conducted on the Illumina MiSeq using the 500 cycle MiSeq reagent kit (version 2) with paired 250 bp reads. All sequence data produced in this study has been deposited to NCBI SRA repository and are available through series accession number SRP080306.

Bioinformatic analysis of amplicon library sequences

Raw sequence reads for all samples in the study were quality controlled using the BBduk (https://sourceforge.net/projects/bbmap/) Java package. This was used to trim low quality bases (<20 Phred score) from the 3′ end of sequence read pairs and identify and remove adaptor sequences. Illumina paired reads with an insert size (length of template molecule) that was shorter than the sum of the lengths of read 1 and read 2 were merged into a single, longer read. Size selection of 467 bp ±20 bp sequences was performed with an in-house Perl script.

The wrapper package Quantitative Insights Into Microbial Ecology (QIIME) [40] was used to determine the operational taxonomic units (OTU)s which corresponded to the 16S rRNA gene sequences in each sample. Sequences were clustered into individual OTUs at a default similarity level of 97% using an open reference picking strategy, and subsequently, a single representative sequence from each clustered OTU was used to align to the Greengenes database. The RDP Classifier [41], using a minimum confidence cut off of 0.8, was used to determine the taxonomic classification for each OTU. Any OTUs with fewer than 50 sequences across all samples were excluded from further analysis. All OTUs with only a single read count in any sample were removed from the analysis.

Statistical analysis

Differences between relative abundances and the presence of bacterial OTUs between post-mortem lung tissue frozen at -80 °C upon collection and post-mortem lung tissue preserved with RNA-Later, from beef calves which died from BRD, were calculated in GraphPad Prism 6 (version 6.04) using the Mann-Whitney U test and the Fisher's exact test, respectively.

The Mann-Whitney U test and the Fisher's exact test in GraphPad Prism 6 (version 6.04) were used to determine if differences existed between the relative abundances and the presence, respectively, of bacterial OTUs in the lung and lymph node tissues between dairy calves which died from BRD and clinically healthy dairy calves without lung lesions present at slaughter.

Stacked bar charts displaying relative abundances of bacterial OTUs in the specific tissue types were prepared in GraphPad Prism 6 (version 6.04).

Microbial DNA enrichment and metagenomics shotgun sequencing

A lung sample from calf number 23 was chosen for shotgun sequencing as it had a high prevalence of a genus of interest (*Leptotrichiacea*) and did not contain many other different bacterial genera. DNA was suspended in Tris-EDTA buffer and re-quantified using the Nanodrop spectrophotometer. One µg of the DNA was enriched for microbial DNA by selective binding and removal of the CpG-methylated host DNA using the NEBNext® Microbiome DNA Enrichment Kit (New England Biolabs (UK) Ltd., Hitchin, Herts, UK). The microbial-enriched DNA sample was diluted and quantified with an Agilent high sensitivity DNA kit (Agilent Technologies Ireland Ltd., Dublin, Ireland) on an Agilent 2100 Bioanalyser.

Shotgun library preparation and sequencing

One nanogram of microbial-enriched DNA was used to prepare a library using the Illumina Nextera®XT DNA Library Preparation Kit, according to the manufacturer's instructions. Estimation of library size was performed using an Agilent high sensitivity DNA kit on an Agilent 2100 Bioanalyser and the library was quantified using the KAPA SYBR FAST Universal qPCR kit with Illumina Primer Premix. The library was diluted and denatured according to the Illumina MiSeq library preparation guide. The 8 pM shotgun library was spiked with 1% denatured and diluted PhiX Illumina control library version 3 (12.5 pM). A 250 bp paired end sequencing run was conducted on an Illumina MiSeq using a 500 cycle MiSeq reagent kit (version 2).

Bioinformatic analysis of microbial DNA enriched shotgun sequence

The BBduk (https://sourceforge.net/projects/bbmap/) Java package was used to trim low quality bases (<20 Phred score) from the 3′ end of raw sequence read pairs and to identify and remove adaptor sequence. All surviving read pairs were mapped to the bovine genome (v.UMD3.1) using bwa [42] to identify host sequences. Approximately 100,000 paired-end sequences with no full-length alignment to the bovine genome were retained for *de novo* assembly. Contig assemblies were generated using OMEGA metagenome assembler (V1.0.2) with default settings. BLAST (BLASTN 2.3.0+) searches against the non-redundant nucleotide collection database on the NCBI website [43, 44] were conducted to determine known bacterial sequences that were most similar to the contig assemblies.

Results

Health assessments of clinically healthy calves

All of the clinically healthy H-F calves were assessed as clinically healthy on the day of slaughter and had respiratory scores based on the Wisconsin calf health scoring criteria [5] of less than 5 (Additional file 2).

Lung lesions in clinically healthy calves

Lesions (macroscopic consolidation or abscessation of lung tissue) were observed on lungs from 12 H-F calves from the 'clinically healthy' group immediately post-slaughter (Additional file 3). Seven of these calves had lesions only on the cranial lobes, two had lesions on the middle lobe, two had lesions on both cranial and middle lobes and one calf had lesions on both the cranial and caudal lobes (Additional file 3). Eight calves from the 'clinically healthy' group had healthy lungs with no lesions present (Additional file 3).

In total, 5 out of the 20 H-F calves from the 'clinically healthy' group had recorded incidents of BRD (Additional file 3). These calves were all treated with Nuflor (Merck Animal Health, New Jersey) and Metacam (Boehringer Ingelheim Vetmedica GmbHm, Germany) and one calf was also treated with Dexamethasone (Norbrook, UK) and Zuprevo (Merck Animal Health, New Jersey). These antibiotic treatments were received at least 41 days before slaughter. All calves with previous recorded incidents of BRD had lung lesions present at slaughter and 7 calves with no recorded incidents of BRD also had lung lesions observed at slaughter (Additional file 3). Furthermore, one calf with lung lesions received Primidoxine (Norbrook, UK) and ASGold (Volac, UK) for treatment of enteritis 70 days before slaughter and one calf with lung lesions present received Dexamethasone and Nuflor 10 days before slaughter due to a reaction to vaccination.

Negative control amplicon library PCR

To test for contaminating 16S DNA in the PCR reagents that we used for generation of amplicon libraries, we conducted six negative (non-template) control amplicon library reactions by substituting template DNA for molecular grade water. Following PCR amplification and agarose gel electrophoresis, no amplicon bands were observed in the gel (Additional file 4 (A)) and no peaks were observed on the electropherogram images obtained from the DNA 1000 chip on an Agilent 2100 Bioanalyser (Additional file 4 (C)). In contrast, bands of the expected amplicon size (467 bp) were observed on the gel for the selected lung tissue DNA libraries and the pooled lung and lymph node tissue DNA libraries (Additional file 4 (A)). Furthermore, the electropherogram images for the selected lung tissue DNA libraries and the pooled lung and lymph node tissue DNA libraries also confirmed that these libraries contained DNA fragments corresponding to the expected amplicon size (Additional file 4 (B)).

Taxonomic classification

One hundred and fifteen bacterial OTUs were identified overall. Seventy-two were identified to genus level. Additionally, 32 OTUs could only be identified as far as family level, 7 OTUs could only be identified to order, 2 to class level and 2 only to phylum level (Additional files 5 and 6).

Low numbers of classifiable reads in clinically healthy animals

Even though equimolar amounts of each library were added to the pool that was sequenced on the MiSeq, the number of reads that were assigned to bacterial OTUs that could be classified by QIIME were much higher in lung and lymph node tissue from fatal BRD cases than from clinically healthy animals (Fig. 1). Unexpectedly, the PCR amplicon library yields were not different between BRD cases and clinically healthy animals. This indicates that in the clinically healthy animals, the 16S primers were amplifying a sequence in the lung and lymph node that was not on the 16S Greengenes database.

OTU abundance in lung tissue

The top 5 most abundant OTUs in the post-mortem lung samples from the beef calves which died from BRD were classified by QIIME as *Pasteurellaceae* ((mean relative abundance (S.E.M)) 22.4 (5.84)%), *Mycoplasma* (15.1 (5.03)%), *Leptotrichiaceae* (14.9 (4.40)%), *Clostridium* (6.4 (4.04)%) and *Fusobacterium* (5.1 (2.14)%). The top 5 most abundant OTUs in the post-mortem lung tissue samples from dairy calves which died from BRD were classified as *Leptotrichiaceae* (26.0 (14.0)%), *Mycoplasma* (22.0 (11.00)%), *Pasteurellaceae* (16.0 (7.40)%), *Fusobacterium* (15.0 (8.70)%) and *Bacteroides* (8.1 (6.00)%). The most abundant OTUs within the lung tissue samples from the clinically healthy H-F calves with lung lesions were classified as *Leptotrichiaceae* (20.0 (9.90)%), *Mycoplasma* (15.5 (7.42)%), *Prevotella* (12.3 (4.31)%) *Pasteurellaceae* (10.2 (6.44)%), and *Actinobacillus* (4.6 (4.59)%). *Leptotrichiaceae* and *Fusobacterium* were undetectable in the lesion-free lung samples from the clinically healthy H-F calves. The most abundant OTUs in lesion-free samples were *Prevotella* (30.7 (7.56)%), *Bacteroides* (7.4 (7.38)%), *Pasteurellaceae* (6.6 (5.03)%), *S24–7* (6.0 (5.24)%), and *Clostridium* (5.5 (3.78)%).

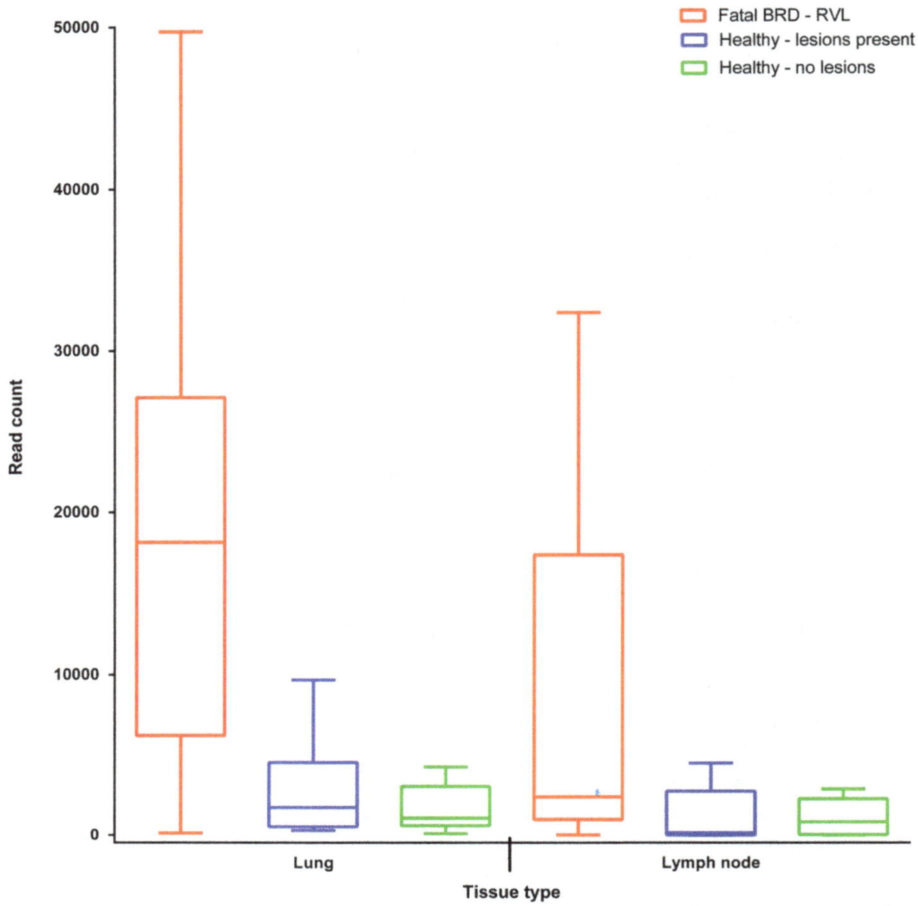

Fig. 1 Number of reads (classified as bacterial) within post-mortem lung and mediastinal lymph node tissues corresponding to each sample type; calves which died from the BRD ($n = 38$), and healthy Holstein-Friesian calves (with ($n = 12$) and without ($n = 8$) lung lesions). Fatal BRD - RVL = samples from calves with the bovine respiratory disease complex collected at regional veterinary laboratories. Healthy – lesions present = samples from healthy Holstein-Friesian calves with lung lesions. Healthy – no lesions = samples from healthy Holstein-Friesian calves without lung lesions. Boxplot = Tukey boxplot (lowest datum (whisker) is within a 1.5 interquartile range of the lower quartile, highest datum (whisker) is within a 1.5 interquartile range of the upper quartile, outliers (individual points) fall above and below these whiskers)

OTU abundance in lymph node tissue

The most abundant OTUs in lymph node tissue from beef calves which died from BRD were classified as *Pasteurellaceae* (18.0 (5.66)%), *Clostridium* (9.6 (5.30)%), *Fusobacterium* (7.3 (2.84)%), *Leptotrichiaceae* (6.8 (2.66)%) and *Prevotella* (6.0 (2.90)%). *Clostridium* (21.9 (19.11)%), *Fusobacterium* (21.7 (14.81)%), *Mycoplasma* (21.3 (19.67)%), *Leptotrichiaceae* (13.7 (10.68)%) and *Pasteurellaceae* (8.1 (5.46)%) were the most abundant OTUs in post-mortem lymph node samples from dairy calves which died from BRD. The most abundant OTUs in post-mortem lymph node samples from the clinically healthy H-F calves with lung lesions were classified as *Prevotella* (21.9 (10.40)%), *Lysinibacillus* (16.7 (11.24)%), *Cupriavidus* (8.4 (8.10)%), *Clostridium* (7.5 (5.64)%) and *Leptotrichiaceae* (6.8 (3.79)%). Notably, *Leptotrichiaceae* and *Fusobacterium* OTUs were not detected in the lymph node samples from the clinically healthy H-F calves without lung lesions. *Prevotella* (42.2 (11.63)%), *Enterobacteriaceae* (12.5 (12.50)%), *Bacteroides* (10.0 (9.96)%), *Succinivibrionaceae* (7.9 (4.73)%), and *Clostridiales* (3.9 (2.27)%) were the most abundant OTUs that were detected in these lymph nodes.

Differences between lung and lymph node microbiomes

Although OTU relative abundances in lung and lymph node were similar in some calves, the microbiomes of these two tissues were quite different in most of the animals. For example, more than half of the OTUs were identified as *Clostridium* in the lymph node of calf number 34 whereas no *Clostridium* was detected in the lung of this animal. Furthermore, *Ureaplasma* was the main genera detected in the lung of calf number 36 but this genera was not detected in the lymph node of this animal (Fig. 2).

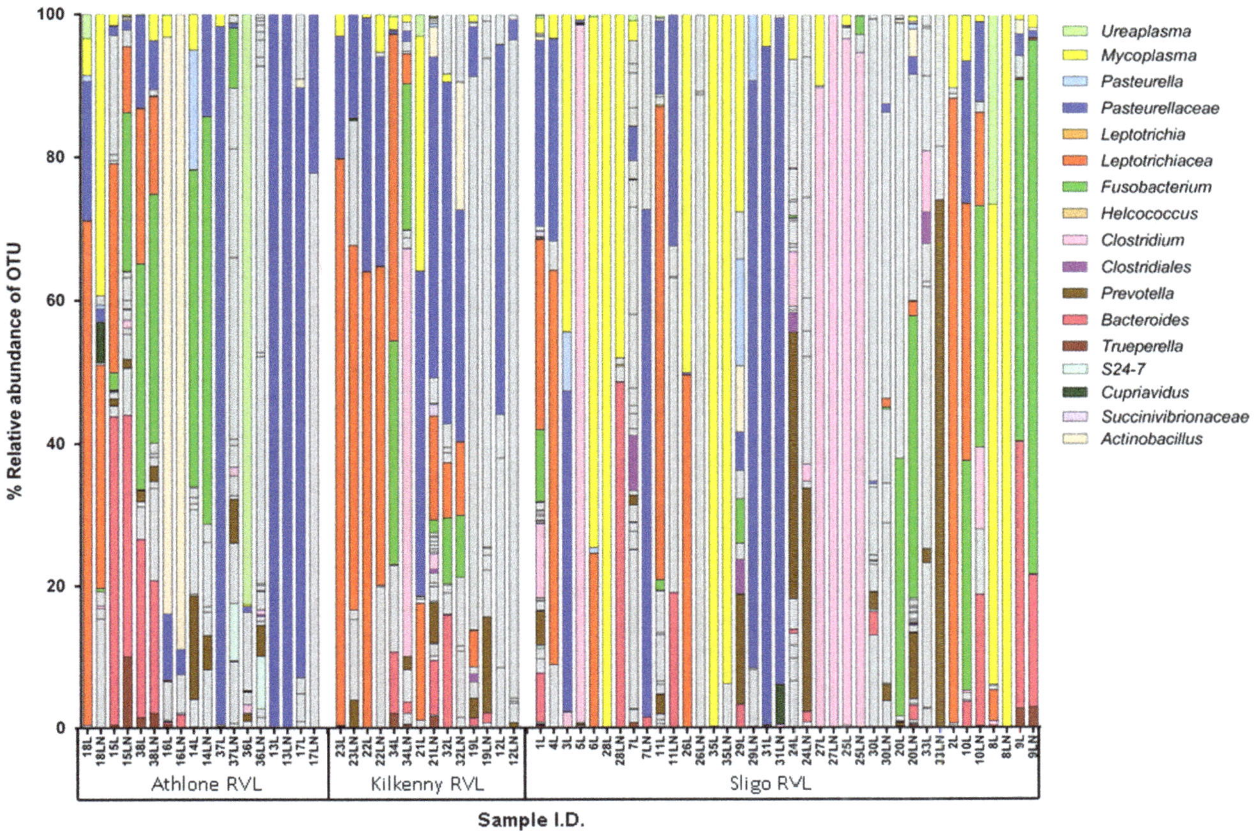

Fig. 2 Percentage relative abundance of bacteria in post-mortem lung (L) and corresponding lymph node (LN) samples from calves which died from bovine respiratory disease. Adjacent profiles of L and LN are from the same animal. Athlone = sample collected at Athlone regional veterinary laboratory (RVL). Kilkenny = sample collected at Kilkenny RVL. Sligo = sample collected at Sligo RVL. Grey bars represent infrequently occurring OTUs (see Additional file 6 for full details of all bacterial OTU classifications)

Undetected and detected genera in clinically healthy lesion-free lungs and lymph nodes

OTUs that were classified as *Leptotrichiaceae, Fusobacterium, Pasteurella, Trueperella, Helcococcus,* and *Ureaplasma* were abundant in lung and lymph node tissue samples from both beef and dairy calves that died from BRD, but these genera were not detected in either lung or lymph node tissue samples from the subset of clinically healthy H-F calves which had no observable lung lesions (n = 8) (Figs. 2 and 3).

At least two putative BRD-associated genera were detected in the lesion-free lungs. *Mycoplasma* was detected in three lung (6L, 19L and 13L) and one lymph node tissue sample (5LN) (Fig. 3). Although relative abundances of *Mycoplasma* were reasonably high in 6 L and 19L, the read counts of this genera were negligable (6L = 308 reads) compared to the fatal BRD cases, several of which had read counts of >10,000 (Additional file 5). Sequences that were classified as *Pasteurellaceae,* a family containing species that are commonly associated with BRD were detected in three lung tissue and one lymph node tissue sample from the lesion-free calves (Fig. 3) but, again, compared to the fatal BRD cases these were negligable. The most abundant bacterial genus detected in the lesion-free samples was *Prevotella* which is more commonly associated with the rumen. However, the average raw read counts for *Prevotella* were not significantly different ($P > 0.05$) between the fatal BRD (average 212, standard deviation 446) cases and the lesion-free animals (average 498, standard deviation 610).

Comparison of OTU abundance between lung samples preserved with RNALater and frozen lung samples

There were no differences in the relative abundances or the presence of bacterial OTUs within post-mortem lung tissue samples which were frozen at -80 °C immediately following collection and post-mortem lung tissue samples preserved with RNALater.

Comparison of OTU abundance between dairy calves which died from BRD and clinically healthy calves

Bacterial OTUs associated with BRD including *Fusobacterium, Mycoplasma, Trueperella* and *Bacteroides,* and an

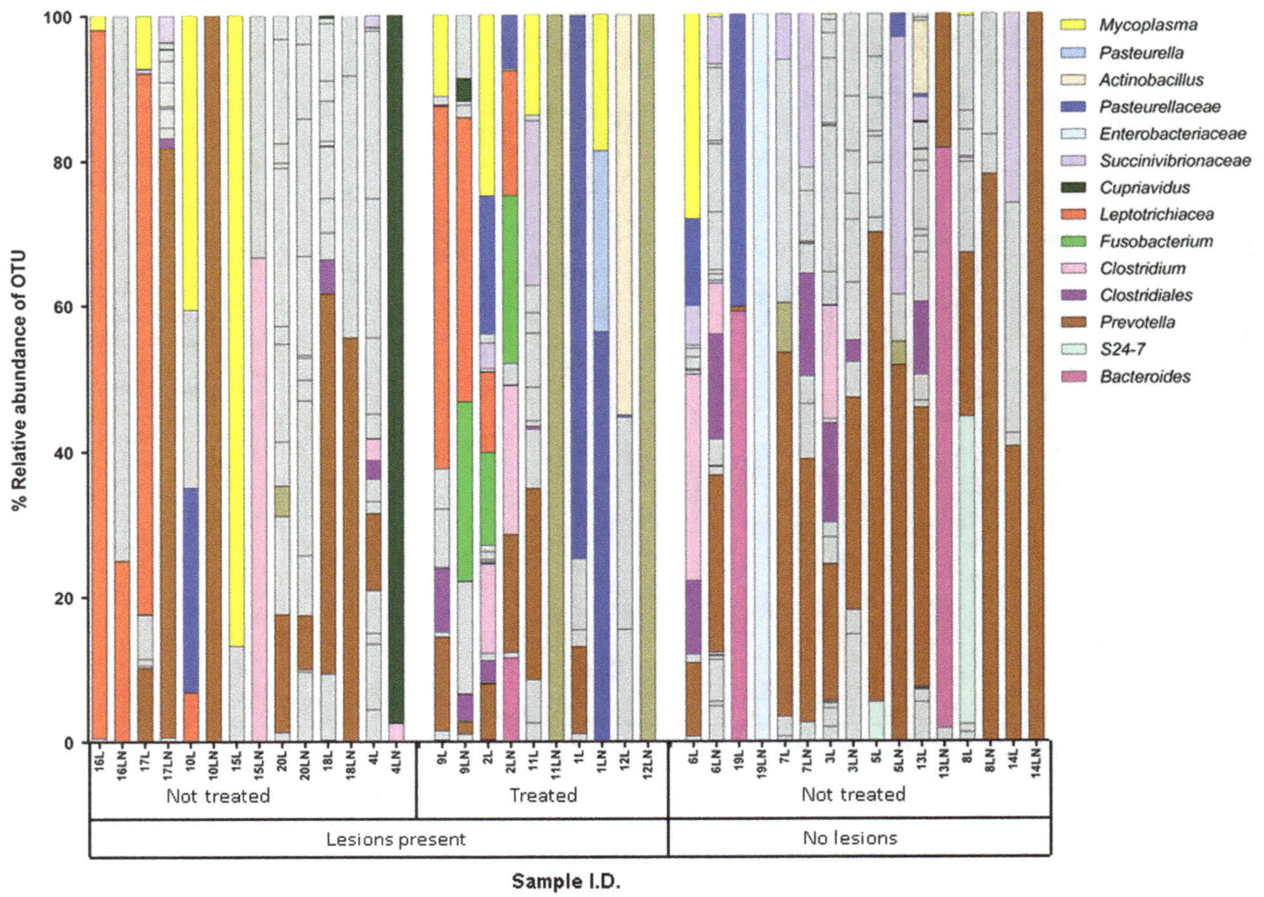

Fig. 3 Percentage relative abundance of bacteria in post-mortem lung (L) and corresponding lymph node (LN) samples from clinically healthy H-F calves with lung lesions (n = 12) and without lung lesions (n = 8). Adjacent profiles of L and LN are from the same animal. The first seven calves received antibiotic treatment during their lifetimes. Grey bars represent infrequently occurring OTUs (see Additional file 6 for full details of all bacterial OTU classifications)

OTU not yet associated with BRD (*Leptotrichiaceae*), had greater relative abundances and were present more often, among the lung tissue samples collected from the dairy calves which died from BRD compared with the lung tissue samples collected from the clinically healthy H-F calves with no lung lesions ($P < 0.05$) (Additional file 7).

Leptotrichiaceae, *Mycoplasma* and *Pasteurellaceae* had greater relative abundances ($P < 0.05$) (Additional file 8) and were present more often ($P < 0.05$) among the lymph node tissue samples collected from the dairy calves which died from BRD compared with the lymph node tissue samples collected from the clinically healthy H-F calves with no observable lung lesions.

Comparison of 16S rRNA gene amplicon sequencing and RVL qPCR

This 16S rRNA gene amplicon sequencing assay identified many more bacteria present in post-mortem lung and lymph node tissue from calves which died from BRD than were identified from the same calves at the RVLs using both culture and uniplex PCRs on swab samples from the pneumonic lungs (Additional file 9). An OTU representing the species detected by PCR in RVLs was identified using the 16S rRNA gene amplicon sequencing assay in all but one case (calf I.D. = 30) (Additional file 9). However, in seven calves (calf I.D. = 9, 19, 22, 23, 32, 35, 37) the *Mycoplasma* OTU was identified using the 16S rRNA gene amplicon sequencing assay even though a PCR test at the RVLs had confirmed no *Mycoplasma bovis* present (Additional file 9).

The 16S rRNA gene amplicon sequencing assay identified bacterial OTUs in all ten calves (calf I.D. = 1, 5, 11, 12, 17, 30, 31, 32, 35, 36) which were culture negative at the RVLs (Additional file 9). Two cases of *Escherichia coli* (calf I.D. = 4, 27), one case of *Pseudomonas* species (calf I.D. = 7), one case of *Trueperella pyogenes* (calf I.D. = 18) and one case of *Salmonella dublin* (calf I.D. = 3) were cultured at RVLs but were not identified by the 16S rRNA gene amplicon sequencing assay (Additional file 9).

Metagenomic shotgun sequencing of a microbial DNA enriched post-mortem lung tissue sample

One of the post-mortem lung DNA samples (from calf number 23) was enriched for microbial DNA and completely sequenced. However, despite microbial DNA enrichment, 99% of the reads in the run mapped to the bovine genome. Approximately 100,000 sequences did not map to the bovine genome and were assembled into contigs. Most of these contigs aligned to the PhiX174 bacteriophage genome but three contigs (contig 1 = 2647 bp, contig 2 = 1376 bp, contig 3 = 744 bp) aligned to bacterial sequences. PhiX sequence was from the pre-prepared non-indexed PhiX V3 library (supplied by Illumina) which was added, as a quality control, to the microbial DNA-enriched library prior to sequencing on the MiSeq. Fluorescence from the bases in the non-indexed PhiX clusters bleeds into the fluorescence in the adjacent indexed clusters. Additional file 10 contains the sequences of the contigs which aligned to bacterial sequences. These contigs were blasted against the non-redundant nucleotide collection database on the NCBI website using the BLASTN 2.3.0+ [45, 46] programme in order to determine the most similar known bacterial sequences.

The top 10 blast hits for each contig are shown in Table 2. No sequences on the database were found to be 100% identical to any of the complete assembled contigs (Table 2). The top hit for contig number 1 was *Sneathia amnii* strain SN35 (GenBank: CP011280.1) (Table 2). It was 92% identical to 99% of contig number 1 (Table 2). The top hit for contig number 2 was also *Sneathia amnii* strain SN35 (GenBank: CP011280.1) (Table 2). It was 93% identical to 99% of contig number 2 (Table 2). Interestingly, contig number 2 was 100% identical to two identical partial 16S rRNA gene sequences (GenBank: KR514404.1) obtained from uncultured bacterial clones in the bovine reproductive tract of farm animals at University College Dublin (Table 2). Contig number 3 was 99% identical to 100% of *Histophilus somni* strain 2336 23S ribosomal RNA gene, complete sequence (Table 2).

Discussion

At the time of writing there was a paucity of reports on high throughput 16S amplicon sequencing and metagenomic shotgun sequencing in lung tissue in cattle and sheep. A detailed recent study was conducted on the lung microbiome in sheep [42] but, to our knowledge, the present report is the first high throughput 16S amplicon sequencing study in lung and corresponding mediastinal lymph nodes in multiple cattle with BRD. The cranial lung lobe tissue was chosen for investigation as it is the most common site of BRD lesions [43, 44]. Mediastinal lymph node tissue was also examined as respiratory disease causing viruses and bacteria often disseminate to these lymph nodes from the lungs [47–50]. To gain an understanding of the bacteria associated with BRD cases in Ireland, we analysed lung tissue from 'real' BRD fatalities on a number of farms in three different regions of the country. Obtaining lung and lymph node tissue from healthy 'matched' controls (i.e. same breed, sex, sire, age, farm) was not feasible in this study as it would have required slaughtering a healthy animal on the same farm as every BRD case. Instead, we had access to healthy calves which were being slaughtered as part of another study from which we took lung and lymph node tissue. In the present study, the composition of bacteria in the lungs and lymph nodes were very different between animals. In several cases, bacterial genera were different in lung and mediastinal lymph node tissues from the same calf.

In humans, the lungs of clinically healthy individuals were originally thought to be sterile [51]. However, recent studies have demonstrated that small numbers of bacteria inhabit the lungs of clinically healthy humans and sheep [44, 51]. The current study also indicated that there are low numbers of bacteria in the lungs and additionally in the lymph nodes of clinically healthy calves. *Prevotella* was the most prevalent genus in terms of relative abundance in the lesion-free lungs but in terms of raw read counts, similar numbers of reads were detected in fatal BRD cases. This is a highly abundant anaerobic genus in the rumen so unlikely to actively grow in aerobic lung tissue and probably passes into the upper regions of the lung by inhalation when rumen regurgitation occurs. A possible explanation for the greater number of bacterial reads found in fatal cases of BRD compared with the clinically healthy calves (with and without lung lesions) in both tissues, is that the disease may cause a proliferation of bacteria that can overcome the natural "equilibrium" in healthy individuals.

Although the 20 H-F calves in the "clinically healthy" group displayed no clinical signs of disease at slaughter and only 5 of these calves had been previously treated for BRD, lung lesions were observed in 12 of these 20 animals (60%). This is similar to observations by Schneider et al. [52] and Wittum et al. [53], who reported that 61% and 68%, of feedlot steers with no recorded history of BRD presented with lung lesions at slaughter, respectively [53]. These authors suggested that many cases of BRD can be missed or may be sub-clinical [52].

Leptotrichiaceae, *Fusobacterium*, *Mycoplasma*, *Trueperella* and *Bacteroides* were more abundant among post-mortem lung tissue samples from dairy calves which died from BRD compared to the lesion-free lung

Table 2 Assembled bacterial contigs description and top BLAST hits

Contig number	Top 10 BLAST hits	Query cover	Percentage identity
1 (2647 bp)	1.*Sneathia amnii* strain SN35, complete genome CP011280.1	99%	92%
	2. *Streptobacillus moniliformis* DSM 12112, complete genome CP001779.1	96%	90%
	3. *Streptobacillus moniliformis* strain DSM 12112 23S ribosomal RNA gene, complete sequence NR_076688.1	96%	90%
	4. *Sebaldella termitidis* strain ATCC 33386 23S ribosomal RNA gene, complete sequence NR_076681.1	96%	89%
	5. *Sebaldella termitidis* ATCC 33386, complete genome CP001739.1	96%	89%
	6. *Leptotrichia buccalis* strain C-1013-b 23S ribosomal RNA gene, complete sequence NR_076664.1	96%	88%
	7. *Leptotrichia buccalis* DSM 1135, complete genome CP001685.1	96%	88%
	8. *Leptotrichia* sp. oral taxon 212 strain W10393, complete genome CP012410.1	96%	87%
	9. *Fusobacterium hwasookii* ChDC F206, complete genome CP013336.1	96%	83%
	10. *Propionigenium maris* 23S rRNA gene, strain DSM 9537 T AJ307979.1	93%	83%
2 (1376 bp)	1. *Sneathia amnii* strain SN35, complete genome CP011280.1	99%	93%
	2. Uncultured bacterium clone T21VE9_4 16S ribosomal RNA gene, partial sequence KR514404.1	67%	100%
	3. Uncultured bacterium clone T21UE13_2 16S ribosomal RNA gene, partial sequence KR514401.1	67%	100%
	4. Uncultured bacterium clone T21VE9_24 16S ribosomal RNA gene, partial sequence KR514494.1	67%	99%
	5. Uncultured bacterium clone T21VE9_36 16S ribosomal RNA gene, partial sequence KR514405.1	67%	99%
	6. Uncultured bacterium clone T21UE13_23 16S ribosomal RNA gene, partial sequence KR514403.1	67%	99%
	7. Uncultured bacterium clone T21UE13_12 16S ribosomal RNA gene, partial sequence KR514402.1	67%	99%
	8. Uncultured bacterium clone H94 16S ribosomal RNA gene, partial sequence KC894542.1	69%	99%
	9. Uncultured bacterium clone H35 16S ribosomal RNA gene, partial sequence KC894531.1	69%	99%
	10. Uncultured bacterium clone T21UE060212_22 16S ribosomal RNA gene, partial sequence KR514400.1	67%	99%
3 (744 bp)	1. *Histophilus somni* strain 2336 23S ribosomal RNA gene, complete sequence NR_103965.1	100%	99%
	2. *Histophilus somni* strain 129P 23S ribosomal RNA gene, complete sequence NR_076444.1	100%	99%
	3. *Haemophilus somnus* 2336, complete genome CP000947.1	100%	99%
	4. *Haemophilus somnus* 129PT, complete genome CP000436.1	100%	99%
	5. *Pasteurella multocida* subsp. *multocida* OH4807, complete genome CP004391.1	100%	94%
	6. *Pasteurella multocida* subsp. *multocida* str. HN06, complete genome CP003313.1	100%	94%
	7. *Pasteurella multocida* subsp. *multocida* PMTB2.1, complete genome CP007205.1	100%	94%
	8. *Pasteurella multocida subsp. multocida* strain Pm70 23S ribosomal RNA gene, complete sequence NR_103956.1	100%	94%
	9. *Pasteurella multocida subsp. multocida* str. Pm70, complete genome AE004439.1	100%	94%
	10. *Pasteurella multocida strain* Pm-3, complete genome CP014618.1	100%	94%

Database = Non redundant (nr) Nucleotide collection (nt).
Program = BLASTN 2.3.0+ [45, 46]

tissue samples from clinically healthy H-F calves. Additionally, *Leptotrichiaceae*, *Mycoplasma* and *Pasteurellaceae* had significantly greater relative abundances among post-mortem lymph node tissue samples from dairy calves which died from BRD relative to the clinically healthy, lung lesion-free H-F calves. It is also possible that other bacterial OTUs were more abundant and present more often within tissue samples from BRD-affected relative to clinically healthy dairy calves, however, as this study lacked power due to restricted sample sizes of BRD-affected dairy calves and lung lesion-free, clinically healthy dairy calves, these differences were not statistically different.

It is possible that the bacterial OTUs present among the samples obtained from the RVLs were the result of contaminating bacteria which propagated post-mortem. However, this is unlikely as most bacterial OTUs found among these samples were also found in the samples from the clinically healthy calves with lung lesions, in which the samples were obtained immediately following slaughter.

Leptotrichiaceae

The *Leptotrichiaceae* OTU was more abundant within post-mortem lung and lymph node tissue samples from dairy calves which died from BRD relative to post-mortem lung and lymph node tissue samples from clinically healthy, lung lesion-free, H-F calves. Additionally, it was one of the most abundant OTUs identified within tissue samples from beef and dairy calves which died from BRD and was absent in samples from clinically healthy H-F calves which had no lung lesions.

The prevalence of OTUs that were classified as the bacterial family *Leptotrichiaceae* in lung and lymph node tissue from fatal BRD cases and lung lesions from clinically healthy cattle was of particular interest as members of this family were recently proposed to be associated with lung disease in humans. *Leptotrichiaceae* species are not currently associated with BRD and have not been previously described in lungs or mediastinal lymph nodes of cattle. All members of this bacterial family are facultative to obligate anaerobic Gram-negative rods [54]. They can occur in anoxic environments as well as oral and intestinal environments [54]. Although little is known about their role in disease, mainly due to the difficulties associated with their isolation and identification, they have been suggested as emerging pathogens [55]. A member of this family within the genus *Leptotrichia* was identified in bronchoalveolar lavage fluid from an elderly man with pneumonia and was hypothesized to be responsible for the disease [56]. Additionally, a member of the genus *Sneathia* was hypothesised to be responsible for late-onset bronchiolitis obliterans syndrome in a lung transplant recipient [57]. Furthermore, species within the *Leptotrichia* genus have been isolated from blood cultures of patients with lesions in the oral mucosa [55] and from blood cultures from patients with anaerobic bloodstream infection receiving high-dose chemotherapy [58].

As the OTU sequence for *Leptotrichiaceae* found in the present study was not identical to any known genus we wanted to achieve better classification with longer DNA sequences than was possible with the 472 bp V3-V4 16S sequence. To do this we partially sequenced the genome of this unknown species of bacteria by metagenomic shotgun sequencing and de novo assembly of a bacterial DNA enriched post-mortem lung tissue sample. From this we obtained three bacterial sequence contigs which were 2647 bp, 1376 bp and 744 bp long. The 744 bp contig corresponded to a known BRD-associated bacterial species, *Histophilus somni*. A BLAST search against the NCBI cultured bacteria database showed the 2647 bp and 1376 bp contigs were most similar (92 and 93% identity respectively) to *Sneathia amnii*. A BLAST search against the nr/nt collection showed that part of one of the *Leptotrichiaceae* contigs (67%) was 100% identical to an uncultured clone. As this uncultured clone (GenBank: KR514404.1, submitted by Lu, J) was obtained from the bovine reproductive tract of farm animals at University College Dublin, it appears to be a novel species that is present in at least two microbiomes in cattle. From the present study it is not possible to infer whether this novel *Leptotrichiaceae* species is pathogenic and causing lung lesions in cattle or wheteher it is merely able to grow opportunistically in the relatively anaerobic lung lesions (some *Leptotrichiaceae* are facultative anaerobes) which have been caused by known pathogens. In lung tissue samples from the calves in this study, the *Leptotrichiaceae* OTU always co-occurred with either *Pasteurellaceae*, *Mycoplasma* or *Fusobacterium* OTUs.

Pasteurellaceae

Pasteurellaceae was one of the most abundant OTUs identified overall and was consistently more abundant in post-mortem lymph node samples from dairy calves which died from BRD compared with those from clinically healthy, lung lesion-free, H-F calves. Many bacterial species implicated in BRD, including *Mannheimia haemolytica*, *Histophilus somni*, *Bibersteinia trehalosi* and *Pasteurella multocida*, belong to the *Pasteurellaceae* family. Indeed, these bacterial species possess many virulence factors which enable them to become pathogenic [17–19, 38, 59, 60]. Furthermore they have been commonly isolated from the lungs and respiratory tracts of cattle with BRD and healthy cattle [11, 17, 19, 22, 61–64].

Fusobacterium

Fusobacterium was one of the most abundant OTUs identified. Furthermore, within the post mortem lung tissue samples, it was found to be more abundant among samples from dairy calves which died from BRD relative to the samples from the clinically healthy, lung lesion-free, H-F calves. Additionally, it was not present within any of the tissue samples from the calves that had no lung lesions. This was not surprising as *Fusobacterium* species are commonly isolated from chronic, abscessing lung lesions in cattle with BRD [11]. Furthermore, this genus contains the anaerobic species *Fusobacterium necrophorum*, which is a significant opportunistic animal pathogen with several virulence factors [65] and it has been previously isolated from ruminant respiratory tracts [63, 66] and pneumonic bovine lungs [67].

Mycoplasma

Mycoplasma was one of the most abundant OTUs present in the post-mortem lung and lymph node samples. It was found to be more abundant among the tissue samples from dairy calves which died from BRD relative to the tissue samples from the clinically healthy, lung lesion-free, H-F calves. This is consistent with previous studies which reported *Mycoplasma* to be one of the dominant genera in nasopharyngeal swab samples from cattle at feedlot [26, 33], despite being infrequent in cattle at feedlot entry [26]. Additionally, this result is concordant with previous observations which report that *Mycoplasma* species *bovis, dispar* and *bovirhinis,* were identified more often in pneumonic lungs and respiratory tracts compared with clinically healthy lungs and respiratory tracts [25, 62, 68, 69].

Although *Mycoplasma bovis* is a recognised BRD pathogen [70] and is commonly screened for in veterinary diagnostic laboratories [71, 72], the other major *Mycoplasma* species are not generally screened. However, they may be responsible for BRD as *Mycoplasma dispar* is a recognised pathogenic *Mycoplasma* species [10], capable of colonising the lower respiratory tract and caused pneumonia when inoculated into gnotobiotic calves [73]. Moreover, it has been cultured from the respiratory tracts of calves presenting with BRD [63, 74] and has been isolated from lavage fluids of calves with recurrent respiratory disease [68]. Furthermore, although *Mycoplasma arginine* and *Mycoplasma bovirhinis* did not cause pneumonia following inoculation into gnotobiotic calves, these species have also been isolated from lavage fluids of calves with recurrent respiratory disease [68] and pneumonic lungs [68, 69] and have been suggested to act as co-pathogens which may intensify respiratory disease symptoms [69, 74].

Ureaplasma

Ureaplasmas, also belong to the same family as the *Mycoplasmas,* and are pathogenic bacteria which were initially associated with urogenital tract infections but have also been isolated from pneumonic bovine lungs [10, 68, 75]. The species *Ureaplasma diversum* has been associated with clinical respiratory disease [75, 76]. As *Ureaplasma* was found to be present in pneumonic lung tissue samples from calves which died from BRD, this genus may be an important contributor to BRD which is often overlooked.

Bacterioides

Bacterioides species are associated with bacterial pneumonia [1, 18]. They had high relative abundances within the post-mortem lung and lymph node tissue samples taken from beef and dairy calves which died from BRD. Furthermore, they were more abundant among samples from dairy calves which died from BRD compared with clinically healthy lesion-free dairy calves. This result was expected as *Bacterioides* species have been commonly isolated from chronic, abscessing lung lesions in cattle with BRD [11] and have previously been cultured from pneumonic bovine lungs [67].

NGS 16S compared to RVL results

The bacterial 16S rRNA gene amplicon sequencing assay identified many more bacteria from calves which died from BRD than the culture and PCR tests carried out at the RVLs. However, at the RVLs, there were several cases where bacterial species were identified by culture, and one case where a bacterial species was identified by PCR, which were not identified by the bacterial 16S rRNA gene amplicon sequencing assay. This may be because only a small part of the cranial lobe region of the lung and the mediastinal lymph node were examined with the 16S sequencing assay, whereas culture was performed on swab samples covering the whole lung area at RVLs. In the present study, the 16S rRNA gene amplicon assay showed that many bacteria which are not currently screened for by PCR or cultured at RVLs were found to be present within the cranial lung lobes and mediastinal lymph nodes from calves which died from BRD, including *Leptotrichiaceae, Fusobacterium, Helcococcus, Mycoplasma, Ureaplasma,* and *Bacteroides.*

Although *Mycoplasma bovis* is currently screened for by PCR in RVLs, the bacterial 16S rRNA gene amplicon sequencing assay found the *Mycoplasma* OTU to be present in seven calves which tested negative for *Mycoplasma bovis* by PCR at RVLs. This is most likely because other species belonging to the *Mycoplasma* genus, other than *Mycoplasma bovis*, were present within these samples. Despite *Helcococcus* species not being currently associated with BRD, *Helcococcus ovis* has been isolated from sheep with respiratory disease [77], a calf with valvular endocarditis [78] and from a horse with a pulmonary abscess [79]. Therefore, implementation of this 16S rRNA amplicon sequencing assay at veterinary diagnostic laboratories would enable discovery of more of the bacteria responsible for each case of BRD as the present study has highlighted that this assay can identify more known bacteria (both culturable and non-culturable) than culture, and can also identify yet unknown and unculturable bacteria in tissue samples, which cannot be identified by culture and PCR tests currently carried out at veterinary diagnostic laboratories.

Next generation sequencing can revolutionise BRD bacterial diagnostics. By using a single 16S rRNA amplicon sequencing assay, the bacteria present in a tissue sample can be accurately identified. A limitation of the Illumina MiSeq based bacterial 16S rRNA gene amplicon sequencing assay is that currently, it is unable to identify bacterial OTUs to species level due to the fact that the maximum read length is <550 base pairs. However, the entire 16S rRNA gene can be sequenced with Pacific Biosciences' single molecule, real-time sequencing technology but this is expensive and the error rate for individual reads are high [80].

Conclusions

In conclusion, we have shown that a convenient, single universal bacterial 16S rRNA gene amplicon sequencing assay can detect the bacterial OTUs present in a BRD-affected lung or lymph node sample. Using this assay, we have characterised the microbiomes of the cranial lung lobe and mediastinal lymph node from calves which died from BRD and from clinically healthy H-F calves. We have confirmed that the cranial region of bovine lungs are not sterile environments and that some bacteria associated with BRD can be present within the lung and lymph node tissues of clinically healthy calves as well as those calves which were suffering from BRD. However, the frequency of the detection of bacteria associated with BRD is lower in the lungs and lymph nodes of clinically healthy calves compared with calves which died from BRD.

Furthermore, we have identified bacterial sequences corresponding to an unidentified species, which is classified as a member of the bacterial family *Leptotrichiaceae*, that was a dominant species in bovine lung lesions in BRD cases and absent in healthy lesion-free lung tissue. Therefore, this 16S rRNA gene amplicon sequencing assay has potential to expedite BRD diagnosis and identify as of yet unknown bacteria which may be key players in BRD development and progression. Furthermore, results from the 16S rRNA gene amplicon sequencing assay, presented in this paper, highlight that continually focusing on bacterial agents that have been commonly associated with BRD could lead to common commensals that may offer a pathogenic threat being neglected. This could result in increased morbidity, increased mortality, and decreased performance in beef and dairy calves.

The present study shows that further NGS study of large numbers of healthy and BRD lung and lymph node tissue samples to generate a comprehensive view of the microbiome of healthy and diseased bovine lungs is warranted.

Additional files

Additional file 1: Description of post-mortem tissue samples collected, sample preservation methods and the diagnostics tests performed on these samples at regional veterinary laboratories (RVL)s.

Additional file 2: Clinical assessment report from the clinically healthy calves on the morning before slaughter.

Additional file 3: Description of the lungs from the clinically healthy calves observed following slaughter.

Additional file 4: Agilent 2100 bioanalyzer DNA Electrophoresis assay results

Additional file 5: Operational taxonomic unit absolute read counts table.

Additional file 6: Operational taxonomic unit relative abundance table.

Additional file 7: Comparison of OTU abundance between post-mortem lung tissue samples from dairy calves which died from BRD (n = 6) and clinically healthy calves without lung lesions (n = 8).

Additional file 8: Comparison of OTU abundance between post-mortem lymph node tissue samples from dairy calves which died from BRD (n = 5) and clinically healthy calves without lung lesions (n = 8).

Additional file 9: Description of the results of the PCR and culture tests carried out at the regional veterinary laboratories and the corresponding results of the OTUs identified by 16S rRNA amplicon sequencing.

Additional file 10: Assembled bacterial contig sequences.

Abbreviations

BCoV: Bovine coronavirus; Bo-HV1: Bovine herpesvirus 1; BPIV-3: Bovine parainfluenza 3 virus; BRD: Bovine respiratory disease; BRSV: Bovine respiratory syncytial virus; BVDV: Bovine viral diarrhoea virus; H-F: Holstein-Friesian; NGS 16S amplicon analysis: Next generation sequencing of 16S ribosomal RNA gene PCR amplicons; OTU: Operational taxonomic unit; QIIME: Quantitative insights into microbial ecology; rRNA: Ribosomal RNA; RVL: Regional veterinary laboratory

Acknowledgements

The authors would like to acknowledge the veterinary pathlogogists and technicians at the regional veterinary laboratories for sample acquisition and collection.

Funding

This research, including all experimental procedures, was funded by the Irish Government under the National Development Plan 2007–2013, Department of Agriculture, Food and the Marine (DAFM) Research Stimulus Fund 11/S/131 (B. Earley, Principal Investigator) and EU project: 311,825 (B. Earley, Principal Investigator). The healthy calves were part of a study funded by DAFM Research Stimulus Fund 11/S/322 (D.A. Kenny Principal Investigator). The funding bodies were not involved in the design of the study and collection, analysis, and interpretation of data or in writing of the manuscript.

Authors' contributions
BE, MSM, DAK, MM, SW, AKK, PC and DJ designed the study. GM obtained the samples from fatal BRD cases at the regional veterinary laboratories (RVL) and performed culture and PCR at the RVL. DJ and MSM performed the NGS experiments. PC performed the bioinformatics analysis. DJ and MSM wrote the manuscript. All authors contributed to data interpretation and approved the final version of the manuscript.

Competing interests
The authors declare that they have no competing interests.

Consent for publication
Not applicable.

Ethics approval and consent to participate
Tissue samples from healthy calves were harvested from a cohort of slaughtered calves in an EU licenced abattoir as part of a separate study examining the effect of early life nutrition on adipogenesis in calves. This latter study was licenced (project authorisation number: AE19132/P014) by the Irish Health Products Regulatory Authority in accordance with the European Union (Protection of Animals used for Scientific Purposes) Regulations 2012 (SI 543/2012), the European Union (Protection of Animals used for Scientific Purposes) (Amendment) Regulations 2013 (SI 434/2013) and the European Union (Protection of Animals used for Scientific Purposes) (Amendment) Regulations 2014 (SI 174/2014). As the tissue samples used in the current study were obtained post-mortem, this study, therefore, did not require a separate licence.
Tissue samples from calves which died from BRD were sourced from calves which succumbed to disease on-farm and were submitted for post-mortem examination. No permissions or licences were required to sample these animals as they were being sampled as part of a diagnostic process by the Department of Agriculture to achieve a diagnosis for the herd. None of the sick animals were euthanised for the purposes of this study.

Author details
[1]Animal and Bioscience Research Department, Animal & Grassland Research and Innovation Centre, Teagasc Grange, Dunsany, Co. Meath, Ireland. [2]School of Agriculture Food Science and Veterinary Medicine, University College Dublin, DublinBelfield, Dublin 4, Ireland. [3]Department of Agriculture, Food and the Marine, Regional Veterinary Laboratory, Sligo, Co. Sligo, Ireland. [4]Livestock Systems Research Department, Animal & Grassland Research and Innovation Centre, Teagasc Grange, Dunsany, Co. Meath, Ireland.

References
1. Griffin D, Chengappa MM, Kuszak J, McVey DS. Bacterial pathogens of the bovine respiratory disease complex. Vet Clin N Am Food Anim Pract. 2010;26:381–94.
2. Taylor JD, Fulton RW, Lehenbauer TW, Step DL, Confer AW. The epidemiology of bovine respiratory disease: What is the evidence for preventive measures? Can. Vet. J. 2010;51:1351–9.
3. Brooks KR, Raper KC, Ward CE, Holland BP, Krehbiel CR, Step DL. Economic effects of bovine respiratory disease on feedlot cattle during backgrounding and finishing phases. Prof. Anim. Sci. 2011;27:195–203.
4. Arcangioli M-A, Duet A, Meyer G, Dernburg A, Bézille P, Poumarat F, Le Grand D. The role of Mycoplasma bovis in bovine respiratory disease outbreaks in veal calf feedlots. Vet J. 2008;177:89–93.
5. McGuirk SM, Peek SF. Timely diagnosis of dairy calf respiratory disease using a standardized scoring system. Anim Health Res Rev. 2014;15:145–7.
6. DAFM/AFBI. All-Ireland animal disease surveillance report 2014. https://www.agriculture.gov.ie/media/migration/animalhealthwelfare/labservice/rvlreports/2014_All_Island_Disease_Surveillance_Report.pdf.
7. Edwards TA. Control methods for bovine respiratory disease for feedlot cattle. Vet Clin N Am Food Anim Pract. 2010;26:273–84.
8. Hay KE, Barnes TS, Morton JM, Clements ACA, Mahony TJ. Risk factors for bovine respiratory disease in Australian feedlot cattle: Use of a causal diagram-informed approach to estimate effects of animal mixing and movements before feedlot entry. Prev. Vet. Med. 2014;117:160–9.
9. Neibergs HL, Seabury CM, Wojtowicz AJ, Wang Z, Scraggs E, Kiser JN, Neupane M, Womack JE, Van Eenennaam A, Hagevoort GR, et al. Susceptibility loci revealed for bovine respiratory disease complex in pre-weaned holstein calves. BMC Genomics. 2014;15:1164.
10. Howard CJ. Mycoplasmas and bovine respiratory disease: studies related to pathogenicity and the immune response–a selective review. Yale J. Biol. Med. 1983;56:789–97.
11. Callan R, Garry F. Biosecurity and bovine respiratory disease. Veterinary Clinics: Food Animal Practice. 2002;18:57–77.
12. O'Neill R, Mooney J, Connaghan E, Furphy C, Graham DA. Patterns of detection of respiratory viruses in nasal swabs from calves in Ireland: a retrospective study. Vet Rec. 2014;175:351.
13. Ng TFF, Kondov NO, Deng X, Van Eenennaam A, Neibergs HL, Delwart E. A metagenomics and case-control study to identify viruses associated with bovine respiratory disease. J Virol. 2015;89:5340–9.
14. Mitra N, Cernicchiaro N, Torres S, Li F, Hause BM. Metagenomic characterization of the virome associated with bovine respiratory disease in feedlot cattle identified novel viruses and suggests an etiologic role for influenza D virus. J Gen Virol. 2016;97:1771–84.
15. Caswell JL. Failure of respiratory defenses in the pathogenesis of bacterial pneumonia of cattle. Vet Pathol. 2014;51:393–409.
16. Gershwin LJ, Van Eenennaam AL, Anderson ML, McEligot HA, Shao MX, Toaff-Rosenstein R, Taylor JF, Neibergs HL, Womack J. Single pathogen challenge with agents of the bovine respiratory disease complex. PLoS One. 2015;10:e0142479.
17. Dabo SM, Taylor JD, Confer AW. Pasteurella multocida and bovine respiratory disease. Anim Health Res Rev. 2007;8:129–50.
18. Panciera RJ, Confer AW. Pathogenesis and pathology of bovine pneumonia. Vet Clin N Am Food Anim Pract. 2010;26:191–214.
19. Griffin D. Bovine pasteurellosis and other bacterial infections of the respiratory tract. Vet Clin N Am Food Anim Pract. 2010;26:57–71.
20. McVey DS. BRD research needs in the next 10–20 years. Anim Health Res Rev. 2009;10:165–7.
21. Larson RL, Step DL. Evidence-based effectiveness of vaccination against Mannheimia haemolytica, Pasteurella multocida, and Histophilus somni in feedlot cattle for mitigating the incidence and effect of bovine respiratory disease complex. Vet Clin N Am Food Anim Pract. 2012;28:97–106.e107.
22. Gagea MI, Bateman KG, van Dreumel T, McEwen BJ, Carman S, Archambault M, Shanahan RA, Caswell JL. Diseases and pathogens associated with mortality in Ontario beef feedlots. J Vet Diagn Investig. 2006;18:18–28.
23. Fulton RW, Confer AW. Laboratory test descriptions for bovine respiratory disease diagnosis and their strengths and weaknesses: Gold standards for diagnosis, do they exist? Can. Vet. J. 2012;53:754–61.
24. Padmanabhan R, Mishra AK, Raoult D, Fournier P-E. Genomics and metagenomics in medical microbiology. J Microbiol Methods. 2013;95:415–24.
25. Marques LM, Buzinhani M, Yamaguti M, Oliveira RC, Ferreira JB, Mettifogo E, Timenetsky J. Use of a polymerase chain reaction for detection of Mycoplasma Dispar in the nasal mucus of calves. J Vet Diagn Investig. 2007;19:103–6.
26. Holman DB, Timsit E, Alexander TW. The nasopharyngeal microbiota of feedlot cattle. Sci. Rep. 2015;5:15557.
27. Tegtmeier C, Angen Ø, Ahrens P. Comparison of bacterial cultivation, PCR, in situ hybridization and immunohistochemistry as tools for diagnosis of Haemophilus somnus pneumonia in cattle. Vet Microbiol. 2000;76:385–94.
28. Bell CJ, Blackburn P, Elliott M, Patterson TIAP, Ellison S, Lahuerta-Marin A, Ball HJ. Investigation of polymerase chain reaction assays to improve detection of bacterial involvement in bovine respiratory disease. J Vet Diagn Investig. 2014;26:631–4.
29. Woo PCY, Lau SKP, Teng JLL, Tse H, Yuen KY. Then and now: use of 16S rDNA gene sequencing for bacterial identification and discovery of novel bacteria in clinical microbiology laboratories. Clin Microbiol Infect. 2008;14:908–34.
30. Taylor JD, Doyle DJ, Blackall PJ, Confer AW. Use of REP-PCR and 16S rRNA gene sequencing for comparison of Mannheimia haemolytica isolates obtained from fatal cases of bovine respiratory disease in the USA and Australia. Aust Vet J. 2014;92:15–23.
31. McCabe MS, Cormican P, Keogh K, O'Connor A, O'Hara E, Palladino RA, Kenny DA, Waters SM. Illumina miSeq phylogenetic amplicon sequencing shows a large reduction of an uncharacterised *Succinivibrionaceae* and an

increase of the *Methanobrevibacter gottschalkii* clade in feed restricted cattle. PLoS One. 2015;10:e0133234.

32. Allen EK, Koeppel AF, Hendley JO, Turner SD, Winther B, Sale MM. Characterization of the nasopharyngeal microbiota in health and during rhinovirus challenge. Microbiome. 2014;2:22.
33. Timsit E, Workentine M, Schryvers AB, Holman DB, van der Meer F, Alexander TW. Evolution of the nasopharyngeal microbiota of beef cattle from weaning to 40 days after arrival at a feedlot. Vet Microbiol. 2016;187:75–81.
34. Klindworth A, Pruesse E, Schweer T, Peplies J, Quast C, Horn M, Glöckner FO. Evaluation of general 16S ribosomal RNA gene PCR primers for classical and next-generation sequencing-based diversity studies. Nucleic Acids Res. 2013;41:e1.
35. Sontakke S, Cadenas MB, Maggi RG, Diniz PPVP, Breitschwerdt EB. Use of broad range16S rDNA PCR in clinical microbiology. J Microbiol Methods. 2009;76:217–25.
36. Murray GM, More SJ, Sammin D, Casey MJ, McElroy MC, O'Neill RG, Byrne WJ, Earley B, Clegg TA, Ball H, et al. Pathogens, patterns of pneumonia, and epidemiologic risk factors associated with respiratory disease in recently weaned cattle in Ireland. J Vet Diagn Investig. 2017;29:20–34.
37. Sachse K, Salam HSH, Diller R, Schubert E, Hoffmann B, Hotzel H. Use of a novel real-time PCR technique to monitor and quantitate Mycoplasma bovis infection in cattle herds with mastitis and respiratory disease. Vet J. 2010;186:299–303.
38. Klima CL, Alexander TW, Hendrick S, McAllister TA. Characterization of Mannheimia haemolytica isolated from feedlot cattle that were healthy or treated for bovine respiratory disease. Can J Vet Res. 2014;78:38–45.
39. Liu D, Lawrence ML, Austin FW. Specific PCR identification of Pasteurella multocida based on putative transcriptional regulator genes. J Microbiol Methods. 2004;58:263–7.
40. Caporaso JG, Kuczynski J, Stombaugh J, Bittinger K, Bushman FD, Costello EK, Fierer N, Pena AG, Goodrich JK, Gordon JI, et al. QIIME allows analysis of high-throughput community sequencing data. Nat Methods. 2010;7:335–6.
41. Wang Q, Garrity GM, Tiedje JM, Cole JR. Naïve bayesian classifier for rapid assignment of rRNA sequences into the new bacterial taxonomy. Appl Environ Microbiol. 2007;73:5261–7.
42. Glendinning L, Wright S, Pollock J, Tennant P, Collie D, McLachlan G. Variability of the Sheep Lung Microbiota. Appl Environ Microbiol. 2016;82:3225–38.
43. Epperson WB. A preliminary assessment of lung lesion distribution in fed cattle, South Dakota Beef Report, paper 4. Department of Veterinary Science, South Dakota State University, Brookings, SD.; 2003. http://openprairie.sdstate.edu/sd_beefreport_2003/4.
44. Prohl A, Ostermann C, Lohr M, Reinhold P. The bovine lung in biomedical research: Visually guided bronchoscopy, intrabronchial inoculation and in vivo sampling techniques. J Vis Exp. 2014;89:51557. doi:10.3791/51557.
45. Zhang Z, Schwartz S, Wagner L, Miller W. A greedy algorithm for aligning DNA sequences. J Comput Biol. 2000;7:203–14.
46. Morgulis A, Coulouris G, Raytselis Y, Madden TL, Agarwala R, Schaffer AA. Database indexing for production MegaBLAST searches. Bioinformatics. 2008;24:1757–64.
47. Valarcher J-F, Bourhy H, Lavenu A, Bourges-Abella N, Roth M, Andreoletti O, Ave P, Schelcher F. Persistent infection of b lymphocytes by bovine respiratory syncytial virus. Virology. 2001;291:55–67.
48. Bashiruddin JB, de Santis P, Persson A, Ball H, Regalla J. Detection of Mycoplasma mycoides subspecies mycoides SC in bovine lung and lymph node tissues by culture, sandwich ELISA and polymerase chain reaction systems. Res Vet Sci. 2005;78:199–205.
49. Bosio CM, Bielefeldt-Ohmann H, Belisle JT. Active suppression of the pulmonary immune response by Francisella tularensis Schu4. J Immunol. 2007;178:4538–457.
50. Rosendahl A, Bergmann S, Hammerschmidt S, Goldmann O, Medina E. Lung dendritic cells facilitate extrapulmonary bacterial dissemination during pneumococcal pneumonia. Front Cell Infect Microbiol. 2013;3:PMC3689026.
51. Beck JM, Young VB, Huffnagle GB. The microbiome of the lung. Transl Res. 2012;160:258–66.
52. Schneider M, Tait R, Busby W, Reecy J. An evaluation of bovine respiratory disease complex in feedlot cattle: Impact on performance and carcass traits using treatment records and lung lesion scores. J Anim Sci. 2009;87:1821–7.
53. Wittum TE, Woollen NE, Perino LJ, Littledike ET. Relationships among treatment for respiratory tract disease, pulmonary lesions evident at slaughter, and rate of weight gain in feedlot cattle. J Am Vet Med Assoc. 1996;209:814–8.
54. Gupta RS, Sethi M. Phylogeny and molecular signatures for the phylum Fusobacteria and its distinct subclades. Anaerobe. 2014;28:182–98.
55. Eribe ERK, Olsen I. Leptotrichia species in human infections. Anaerobe. 2008;14:131–7.
56. Kawanami T, Fukuda K, Yatera K, Kido T, Yoshii C, Taniguchi H, Kido M. Severe pneumonia with Leptotrichia sp. detected predominantly in bronchoalveolar lavage fluid by use of 16S rRNA gene sequencing analysis. J Clin Microbiol. 2009;47:496–8.
57. Charlson ES, Diamond JM, Bittinger K, Fitzgerald AS, Yadav A, Haas AR, Bushman FD, Collman RG. Lung-enriched organisms and aberrant bacterial and fungal respiratory microbiota after lung transplant. Am J Respir Crit Care Med. 2012;186:536–45.
58. Couturier MR, Slechta ES, Goulston C, Fisher MA, Hanson KE. Leptotrichia bacteremia in patients receiving high-dose chemotherapy. J Clin Microbiol. 2012;50:1228–32.
59. Rice JA, Carrasco-Medina L, Hodgins DC, Shewen PE. Mannheimia haemolytica and bovine respiratory disease. Anim Health Res Rev. 2007;8:117–28.
60. Corbeil LB. Histophilus somni host–parasite relationships. Anim Health Res Rev. 2007;8:151–60.
61. Welsh RD, Dye LB, Payton ME, Confer AW. Isolation and antimicrobial susceptibilities of bacterial pathogens from bovine pneumonia: 1994–2002. J Vet Diagn Investig. 2004;16:426–31.
62. Allen J, Viel L, Bateman K, Rosendal S, Shewen P, Physick-Sheard P. The microbial flora of the respiratory tract in feedlot calves: associations between nasopharyngeal and bronchoalveolar lavage cultures. Can J Vet Res. 1991;55:341–6.
63. Nikunen S, Härtel H, Orro T, Neuvonen E, Tanskanen R, Kivelä SL, Sankari S, Aho P, Pyörälä S, Saloniemi H, Soveri T. Association of bovine respiratory disease with clinical status and acute phase proteins in calves. Comp Immunol Microbiol Infect Dis. 2007;30:143–51.
64. Taylor JD, Holland BP, Step DL, Payton ME, Confer AW. Nasal isolation of Mannheimia haemolytica and Pasteurella multocida as predictors of respiratory disease in shipped calves. Res Vet Sci. 2015;99:41–5.
65. Nagaraja TG, Narayanan SK, Stewart GC, Chengappa MM. Fusobacterium necrophorum infections in animals: Pathogenesis and pathogenic mechanisms. Anaerobe. 2005;11:239–46.
66. Jang SS, Hirsh DC. Characterization, distribution, and microbiological associations of Fusobacterium spp. in clinical specimens of animal origin. J Clin Microbiol. 1994;32:384–7.
67. Chirino-Trejo JM, Prescott JF. The identification and antimicrobial susceptibility of anaerobic bacteria from pneumonic cattle lungs. Can. J. Comp. Med. 1983;47:270–5.
68. Thomas A, Dizier I, Trolin A, Mainil J, Linden A, Ball H, Bell C. Isolation of Mycoplasma species from the lower respiratory tract of healthy cattle and cattle with respiratory disease in Belgium. Vet Rec. 2002;151:472–6.
69. Gagea MI, Bateman KG, Shanahan RA, van Dreumel T, McEwen BJ, Carman S, Archambault M, Caswell JL. Naturally occurring Mycoplasma bovis—associated pneumonia and polyarthritis in feedlot beef calves. J Vet Diagn Investig. 2006;18:29–40.
70. Bürki S, Frey J, Pilo P. Virulence, persistence and dissemination of Mycoplasma bovis. Vet Microbiol. 2015;179:15–22.
71. Blackburn P, Brooks C, McConnell W, Ball HJ. Isolation of Mycoplasma bovis from cattle in Northern Ireland from 1999 to 2005. Vet Rec. 2007;161:452–3.
72. Byrne WJ, McCormack R, Egan J, Brice N, Ball HJ, Markey B. Isolation of Mycoplasma bovis from bovine clinical samples in the Republic of Ireland. Vet Rec. 2001;148:331–3.
73. Gourlay RN, Howard CJ, Thomas LH, Wyld SG. Pathogenicity of some Mycoplasma and Acholeplasma species in the lungs of gnotobiotic calves. Res Vet Sci. 1979;27:233–7.
74. Miles K, McAuliffe L, Ayling RD, Nicholas RAJ. Rapid detection of Mycoplasma dispar and M. bovirhinis using allele specific polymerase chain reaction protocols. FEMS Microbiol Lett. 2004;241:103–7.
75. Larsen LE, Tegtmeier C, Pedersen E. Bovine respiratory syncytial virus (BRSV) pneumonia in beef calf herds despite vaccination. Acta Vet Scand. 2001;42:113–21.
76. Autio T, Pohjanvirta T, Holopainen R, Rikula U, Pentikäinen J, Huovilainen A, Rusanen H, Soveri T, Sihvonen L, Pelkonen S. Etiology of respiratory disease in non-vaccinated, non-medicated calves in rearing herds. Vet Microbiol. 2007;119:256–65.
77. Zhang Y, Cui J, Parkinson A, Hayes J, Ott K, Byrum B. Isolation of Helcococcus Ovis from Sheep with Pleuritis and Bronchopneumonia. J Vet Diagn Investig. 2009;21:164–6.

78. Post KW, Rushton SD, Billington SJ. Valvular endocarditis associated with Helcococcus ovis infection in a bovine. J Vet Diagn Investig. 2003;15:473–5.
79. Rothschild CM, Oaks JL, Schaupp JK, Rurangirwa FR, Sellon DC, Hines MT. Helcococcus ovis Isolated from a Pulmonary Abscess in a Horse. J Clin Microbiol. 2004;42:2224–6.
80. Roberts R, Carneiro M, Schatz M. The advantages of SMRT sequencing. Genome Biol. 2013;14:405.

Biofilm production and other virulence factors in *Streptococcus* spp. isolated from clinical cases of bovine mastitis in Poland

Edyta Kaczorek*, Joanna Małaczewska, Roman Wójcik and Andrzej Krzysztof Siwicki

Abstract

Background: Mastitis is a common disease in dairy cattle throughout the world and causes considerable economic losses each year. An important aetiological agent of this disease is bacteria of the genus *Streptococcus*; hence, exploring the mechanisms of virulence in these bacteria is an extremely important step for the development of effective prevention programmes. The purpose of our study was to determine the ability to produce biofilm and the occurrence of selected invasiveness factors among bacteria of the genus *Streptococcus* isolated from cattle with the clinical form of mastitis in northeastern Poland.

Results: Most of the isolates analysed demonstrated an ability to produce biofilm (over 70%). Virulence genes were searched for in the three most common streptococci in our experiment: *S. agalactiae*, *S. uberis* and *S. dysgalactiae*. For *S. agalactiae*, only four genes were confirmed: *rib* (33%), *cylE* (78%), *bca* (37%), and *cfb* (100%). The genes *pavA*, *scpB*, *bac* and *lmb* were not present in any of the tested strains. The dominant serotypes of the species were Ia ($n = 8$) and II ($n = 8$), in addition to some strains that were not classified in any of the groups ($n = 6$). Out of the eight selected genes for *S. uberis* (*sua*, *pauA/skc*, *gapC*, *cfu*, *lbp*, *hasA*, *hasB*, *hasC*), only one was not found (*lbp*). Finally, two genes were chosen for *S. dysgalactiae* (*eno* and *napr*), and their presence was confirmed in 76% and 86% of the strains, respectively.

Conclusions: The experiment showed that strains of *Streptococcus* spp. isolated from dairy cattle with clinical cases of mastitis in the northeastern part of Poland possess several invasiveness factors that can substantially affect the course of the disease, and this should be considered when developing targeted prevention programmes.

Keywords: *Streptococcus*, Mastitis, Biofilm, Virulence genes

Background

Mastitis in dairy cattle is a globally widespread disease that is responsible for large economic losses each year due to lower milk yield and reduced milk quality [1]. One of the aetiological factors mentioned most often are bacteria of the genus *Streptococcus*, where pathogens classified as both contagious (e.g., *Streptococcus agalactiae)* and environmental (e.g., *Streptococcus uberis*) can be distinguished [2–4].

It is common knowledge that antibiotics are among the major tools in combating this disease [1]. However, to avoid development and spread of antibiotic resistance, the use of the antibiotics in the treatment of mastitis should be limited to situations where clinical and bacteriological findings justify their use. Sometimes, in spite of using an active substance that shows efficacy under in vitro conditions, antibiotic therapy is not effective. These situations are associated with the presence of various host and bacterial factors, including the ability of bacteria to produce biofilm [5, 6]. 'Biofilm' is defined as a matrix-enclosed microbial accretions which can adhere both to biological or non-biological surfaces. By producing various types of substances, the formation of biofilm is a significant factor in the pathogenesis of numerous diseases, both in humans and in animals [7–9].

By forming such a structure, bacteria are more likely to survive in an environment that is hostile to them, and after invading an organism, they can be better protected against the action of the host immune system while becoming less sensitive to the activity of antibiotics or disinfectants [7, 10]. In addition to the ability to produce biofilm, *Streptococcus*

* Correspondence: edyta.kaczorek@uwm.edu.pl
Department of Microbiology and Clinical Immunology, Faculty of Veterinary Medicine, University of Warmia and Mazury in Olsztyn, Oczapowskiego 13, 10-719 Olsztyn, Poland

spp. possess other invasiveness factors, for example those that provide protection against the host immune system (e.g., plasminogen activator, lactoferrin binding protein, or CAMP factor) [11, 12]. For years, the presence of specific virulence factors in pathogens has drawn the attention of research teams throughout the world because such research increases our understanding of the mechanisms responsible for inducing an illness and can therefore contribute to the development of optimal prevention programmes.

To date, several studies have evaluated the ability of *Streptococcus* spp. to produce biofilms as well as the presence of virulence factors in bacteria isolated from dairy cattle suffering from mastitis in different countries; however, we are the first to examine such phenomena in our region [8, 11, 13]. Hence, the purpose of our study was to identify the ability of bacteria to make biofilm and to detect the presence of selected virulence factors in bacteria of the genus *Streptococcus* isolated from cattle with the clinical form of udder inflammation in northeastern Poland.

Methods

Sample collection

A total of 135 previously described streptococcal isolates were used in this study [14]. All samples were collected from 65 different farms in north-eastern Poland from 2013 to 2015. To avoid testing of epidemiologically related isolates, only 1 isolate from one species per dairy farm was included. Prior to milk sampling, all animals were tested using the California mastitis test. Only milk from quarters presenting symptoms of infection was collected (i.e., slight thickening of the mixture; trace reaction seems to disappear with continued rotation of the paddle, CMT ≥ 4). After sampling, milk was kept in a container that was maintained a constant temperature of 6 to 8 °C and was delivered to the laboratory within 2 h.

Bacteriological identification

Milk samples were transferred with a calibrated loop (0.01 ml) onto Columbia agar (Oxoid, Great Britain) and Edwards medium (Oxoid, Great Britain), both supplemented with 5% defibrinated sheep blood. The plates were incubated at 37 °C for 48 ± 2 h under aerobic conditions. The grown cultures were examined microscopically after Gram staining, and the phenotypic traits were analysed (i.e., type of haemolysis, esculin hydrolysis, catalase production, CAMP reaction). For further analysis, only G+, catalase-negative cocci were selected. The final identification was performed using the commercial latex agglutination test Streptococcal Grouping Kit (Oxoid, Great Britain), API strep (bioMérieux, France) and PCR. All strains used in this study are summarized in Table 1.

Table 1 Strains used in this study

Species	*n*
S.uberis	53
S. dysgalactiae	41
S. agalactiae	27
Other *Streptococci*	14

DNA isolation

Bacterial DNA was extracted using the ExtractMe DNA bacteria kit (Blirt, Gdańsk, Poland) according to the manufacturer's protocols. Eluted DNA concentrations were measured using the BioSpectrometer® (Eppendorf, Hamburg, Germany) and stored at −20 °C for further analysis.

Detection of virulence genes of *S. agalactiae, S. uberis* and *S. dysgalactiae*

Virulence genes for *S. uberis (sua, pauA/skc, gap C, has C, lbp, cfu, has B, has A), S. agalactiae (pava, scpB, rib, bac, cylE, bca, cfb, lmb)* and *S. dysgalactiae (eno, napr)* were amplified using PCR. The confirmation of *S. agalactiae, S. uberis and S. dysgalactiae*, has been previously described [14]. Primer sequences, product sizes and annealing temperatures are summarized in Table 2. All primers were synthesized by Genomed S.A. (Warsaw, Poland). Amplification reactions were carried out with HotStarTaq Plus Master Mix Kit (Qiagen, Hilden, Germany) in a nexus gradient thermocycler (Eppendorf, Hamburg, Germany) using the same PCR protocol as described before [14]. All PCR reactions were carried out with positive and negative controls. Some PCR products of interest were randomly chosen and purified using a CleanUp kit (A&A Biotechnology, Gdynia, Poland) for sequencing (Genomed, Warsaw, Poland) to confirm the specificity of the obtained amplicons.

Biofilm assay

The experiment was performed using polystyrene microtiter plates with flat bottoms based on the techniques described by Ebrahimi et al. [13]. All isolates were grown in tryptic soy broth (TSB, Oxoid, Great Britain) at 37 °C for 16 h. The bacterial cells were centrifuged at 6000 g for 10 min. Supernatants were removed and the cell pellets were resuspended in 5 mL of fresh medium (TSB) to achieve an absorbance of 1.00 at 595 nm. The optical density (ODs) of the bacterial suspensions were measured using the BioSpectrometer® (Eppendorf, Hamburg, Germany). The suspensions were then diluted 1:40 in fresh TSB, and 200 μl of the diluted cell suspension was added to each well of the microtiter plate (8 wells in a single row for one strain). Plates were incubated at 37 °C for 24 h. The plates were then washed three times with sterile phosphate-buffered saline (PBS). The inverted plates were dried at ambient temperature for 1 h. Next, the plates were stained with 200 μl of 0.2% aqueous crystal violet solution for

Table 2 Primer sets used for the detection of virulence genes in *Streptococcus spp.*

Primer function	Putative function	Target gene	Primer sequence (5′–3′)	Amplicon size (bp)	Annealing temperature (°C)	Reference
Virulence genes						
S.uberis						
Adhesion molecue-	Adherence and invasion of mammary epithelial cells	*sua*	TCAACTTGACGAATCGCTTG TCAGCCATTGTTTCTGCTTG	480	47	[20]
Plasminogen activator	colonization	*pauA/skc*	*CGGGTTGAAGAACCTATCACTC* *TGGAAGTTGACCAAGAGAATTG*	255	50	[20]
Surfacedehydrogenase protein	colonization	*gapC*	GCTCCTGGTGGAGATGATGT GTCACCAGTGTAAGCGTGGA	200	51	[11]
CAMP factor	Forms pores in host-cell membran	*cfu*	*TATCCCGATTTGCAGCCTAC* *CCTGGTCAACTTGTGCAACTG*	205	50	[11]
Lactoferrin binding protein	Binding Lactoferrin	*lbp*	CGACCCTTCAGATTGGATTC TAGCAGCATCACGTTCTTCG	698	50	[11]
Hyaluronic acid capsule	Resistance to phagocytosis	*hasA*	*GAAAGGTCTGATGCTGATG* *TCATCCCCTATGCTTACAG*	319	44	[33]
		hasB	*TCTAGACGCCGATCAAGC* *TGAATTCCTATGCGTCGATC*	532	47	[33]
		hasC	TGCTTGGTGACGATTTGATG *GTCCAATGATAGCAAGGTCAC*	225	47	[33]
S.agalactiae						
Adherence and virulence protein A	Binding to immobilized fibronectin	*pavA*	*TTCCCATGATTTCAACAACAAG* *AACCTTTTGACCATGAATTGGTA*	495	47	[20]
Streptococcal C5a peptidase- adhesion	Prevents neutropil, promotes adherence	*scpB*	*AGTTGCTTCTTACAGCCCAGA* *GGCGCAGACATACTAGTTCCA*	567	51	[20]
Surface protein Rib-	Resistance to proteases	*rib*	CAGGAAGTGCTGTTACGTTAAAC CGTCCCATTTAGGGTCTTCC	369	51	[34]
C beta protein	Binds to the immuno-globulin A	*bac*	*CTATTTTTGATATTGACAATGCAA* *GTCGTTACTTCCTTGAGATGTAAC*	592	46	[35]
B-haemolisin	Promotes invasion of host cells	*cylE*	*TGACATTTACAAGTGACGAAG* *TTGCCAGGAGGAGAATAGGA*	248	47	[36]
C alfa protein	Adherence to epithelial cells	*bca*	TAACAGTTATGATACTTCACAGAC ACGACTTTCTTCCGTCCACTTAGG	535	49	[37]
CAMP factor	Forms pores in host-cell membran	*cfb*	ATGGGATTTGGGATAACTAAGCTAG AGCGTGTATTCCAGATTTCCTTAT	193	50	[38]
Lamining-binding protein	Promote adherence to host laminin	*lmb*	AGTCAGCAAACCCCAAACAG GCTTCCTCACCAGCTAAAACG	397	50	[39]
S.dysgalactiae						
α-enolase	Plasminogen binding	*eno*	ATGTCAATTATTACTGATGT CTATTTTTTTAAGTTATAGA	1308	36	[17]
Nephritis-associated plasminogen-binding receptor	Plasminogen binding	*napr*	GTTAAAGTTGGTATTAACGGT TTGAGCAGTGTAAGACATTTC	963	45	[17]

15 min. The plates were then washed three times with sterile PBS to remove excess dye. Crystal violet bound to the biofilms was extracted with 200 μl of an 80:20 (*v*/v) mixture of ethyl alcohol and acetone and the absorbance was measured at 595 nm using an ELISA plate reader (Sunrise absorbance reader, Tecan, Austria). Non-inoculated TSB wells stained with crystal violet were used as negative controls. All assays were performed in triplicate with 8 replicates for each strain. Interpretation of biofilm production was according to the criteria described by [15]. The mean optical density (OD) of the negative control +3 standard deviations of negative control was considered the cut-off (ODc = 0,2), and the biofilm producers were therefore categorized as follows:

- not a biofilm producer: OD ≤ ODc, (all strains which OD values were below 0,2)
- weak biofilm producer ODc: < OD ≤ 2 × ODc, (all strains which OD values were above 0,2 and below 0,4)

- moderate biofilm producer: 2 × ODc < OD ≤ 4 × ODc (all strains which OD values were above 0,4 and below 0,8)
- strong biofilm producer: OD > 4 × ODc. (all strains which OD values were above 0,8).

Molecular serotyping of *Streptococcus agalactiae*

The assay was performed by multiplex PCR using a protocol previously described by Poyart el al. [16]. The protocol is based on two multiplex PCRs, one containing the primer pairs specific for serotypes Ia, Ib, II, III, and IV and the other containing primer pairs specific for serotypes V, VI, VII, VIII. Serotype IX was not investigated using this method. Non-typeable isolates were designated 'NT'. To confirm the specificity of the obtained amplicons, some PCR products of interest were randomly chosen and purified using a CleanUp kit (A&A Biotechnology, Gdynia, Poland) for sequencing (Genomed, Warsaw, Poland).

Results

Biofilm production

Most of the analysed strains, which were classified into four groups (*S. agalactiae, S. uberis, S. dysgalactiae* and other streptococci), showed the ability to produce biofilm (over 70%). The occurrence of strains characterized as strong biofilm producers was noted in only two species (*S. uberis* and *S. agalactiae*; 6% and 7.5%, respectively) [Table 3].

Detection of virulence genes

Virulence genes were searched for in the three species of streptococci most frequently appearing in our study, i.e., *S. agalactiae, S. uberis* and *S. dysgalactiae*. For the remaining category of other streptococci (*n* = 14), invasiveness genes were not determined due to species diversity in this group (four different species).

Regarding *S. agalactiae* (*n* = 27), the eight most common virulence genes in this species were selected for analysis. Among the analysed isolates, the presence of only four genes was confirmed: *rib* (33%), *cylE* (78%), *bca* (37%), *cfb* (100%). The genes *pavA, scpB, bac* and l*mb* did not occur in any of the tested strains [Table 4].

As for the strains of *S. uberis* (*n* = 53), eight genes connected with virulence were selected for analysis. Only one gene, *lbp*, was not found in the isolates of this species. The other genes were quite abundant at70%. One exception was a gene of the has operon, *hasA*, which was identified in only 17% of the analysed strains [Table 4].

The last group submitted to analysis consisted of isolates of *S. dysgalactiae* (*n* = 41). In this group, only two genes, *eno* and *napr*, were selected for the tests, mainly because there is very little knowledge about the mechanisms of invasiveness in this species [17] Regarding our isolates, the presence of these two genes was confirmed in 76% and 86% of strains, respectively [Table 4].

Molecular serotyping of *Streptococcus agalactiae* and associated virulence genes

The presence of serotypes Ia, Ib, II, III, IV and V was confirmed among the analysed strains, and the most numerous group consisted of serotypes Ia and II (*n* = 8). In our experiment, there were 6 strains which could not be classified into any of the analysed serotypes (NT). In addition, an analysis was performed regarding the presence of virulence genes in the individual serotypes. In the case of serotype Ia, only one profile was observed: *rib, cylE, cfb*. The profile *cylE, bca, cfb* dominated in the second most numerous group, i.e., serotype II. In the NT strains, there was only one gene: *cfb* [Table 5].

Discussion

The presence or absence of virulence factors in pathogenic aetiological agent of a disease is an important variable that decides the course of the illness itself. The enzymes and toxins produced by bacteria or the ability of bacteria to produce biofilm help microorganisms survive in infected tissues either through direct impact on host stromal cells or by affecting host defence mechanisms [18]. In our experiment, most of the analysed isolates of *Streptococcus* spp. demonstrated an ability to produce biofilm (over 70%), many of which represented strains forming a weak structure. Such high abundance in this group can be explained by the fact that determinations in strains were made after a 24-h incubation period. Moliva et al. [19] recently showed that strains of *S. uberis* begin to form biofilm structure as early as after 2 h of incubation, but mature biofilm is not formed until after 48 h. It is possible that the relatively longer incubation of isolates in our study influenced the results. Nevertheless, we are convinced that the high occurrence of *Streptococcus* spp.

Table 3 Biofilm production capability and formation intensity

Species	No biofilm producers	Weak biofilm producers	Moderate biofilm produres	Strong biofilm producers
S.uberis	12 (23%)	33 (62%)	5 (9%)	3 (6%)
S.dysgalactiae	5 (13%)	26 (63%)	10 (24%)	0 (0%)
S.agalactiae	2 (7,5%)	20 (74%)	3 (11%)	2 (7,5%)
other	3 (21%)	10 (72%)	1 (7%)	0 (0%)

S. agalactiae (*n* = 27), *S. uberis* (*n* = 53), *S. dysgalactiae* (*n* = 41) and other streptococci (*n* = 14)

Table 4 Frequency of occurrence [no. (%)] of the chosen virulence genes

S.agalactiae								
	pavA	*scpB*	*rib*	*bac*	*cylE*	*bca*	*cfb*	*lmb*
n	0	0	9	0	21	10	27	0
%	0	0	33	0	78	37	100	0
S. uberis								
	sua	*pauA/skc*	*gapC*	*cfu*	*lbp*	*hasA*	*hasB*	*hasC*
n	51	50	52	10	0	9	42	44
%	96	94	98	19	0	17	79	83
S.dysgalactiae								
	eno	*naprl*						
n	31	34						
%	76	83						

Streptococcus uberis ($n = 53$), *Streptococcus agalactiae* ($n = 27$), *Streptococcus dysgalactiae* ($n = 41$), and other *Streptococcus* species ($n = 14$)

strains able to produce biofilm in the geographical area we investigated presents a serious challenge for both dairy farmers and veterinary doctors. As mentioned earlier, the production of this specific structure by bacteria can have a considerable impact upon treatment efficiency. From a clinical point of view, there is a significant relationship between the ability to create bacterial biofilm and antibiotic treatment [7]. Bacteria that form a 'biological membrane' can be characterized by up to 1000-fold lower sensitivity to the effects of some active substances compared to strains growing in planktonic form. In addition, some antibiotics, for example tetracyclines or erythromycin, can stimulate the formation of biofilm. This was observed in the case of *Staphylococcus epidermidis*, where following the administration of these antibiotics there was an observed increase in the expression of the gene responsible for the formation of biofilm (*ica*) [7]. In our earlier studies conducted on the same strains [14], we found a high level of resistance of these pathogens to tetracycline. This observation may indicate that the said active substance is overused in the analysed area, and simultaneously may

Table 5 Results of molecular serotyping of *S. agalactiae* strains ($n = 27$) (including virulence profiles)

Serotype	*n*	Profile			
		rib, cylE, cfb,	*cylE, bca, cfb*	*cylE, cfb*	*cfb*
Ia	8	8	0	0	0
Ib	2	2	0	0	0
II	8	0	7	1	0
III	1	0	1	0	0
IV	1	0	0	1	0
V	1	0	1	0	0
NT	6	0	1	0	5

explain the presence of such a high number of strains able to produce biofilm. However, we have not observed any correlation between biofilm formation ability and other virulence factors occurrence. This may provide that biofilm formation is not essential in the pathogenesis of mastitis in dairy cattle in the analysed area for now.

Next, we analysed bacteria searching for the presence of the selected virulence genes. Eight genes were selected or *S. agalactiae*, of which four (*rib, cylE, bca, cfb*) were determined to be present in the analysed strains. These results were unsurprising because their presence had been previously confirmed in bovine strains in countries such as Brazil, India or Egypt, and the frequency of occurrence of these genes is local in character [12, 19–21]. The situation differs with respect to the genes *scpB, lmb, pavA* and *bac,* whose presence was not detected in the strains we analysed. On the one hand, these genes are mainly associated with human strains, and therefore their absence is not puzzling [12, 20]. On the other hand, the genes *scpB, pavA* or *lmb* have been detected in isolates of *S. agalactiae* derived from cattle with mastitis in Asia and Africa [20–22]. Thus, our findings indicate that these four genes probably do not play important roles in the pathogenesis of udder inflammation in dairy cattle in the region, which may be connected with the different conditions and management practices for dairy cattle in Europe.

In the case of *S. agalactiae*, we performed additional molecular serotyping of the isolated strains. Such investigations are extremely important considering both epidemiology and prophylaxis, as they may aid the development of multivalent vaccines containing capsular polysaccharides [23]. Our isolates belonged to serotypes from Ia to V. The occurrence of these serotypes need not be surprising, as they were isolated previously in the United States and Europe; however, the dominance of serotype Ia in our study is quite puzzling because according to Delannoy et al. [24], this serotype is mostly present in humans. Serotype III is usually dominant in cattle but in our experiment it was confirmed in only one case. Nevertheless, the presence of serotype Ia in cattle has also been confirmed in the eastern part of China, Germany and the USA [23, 25, 26]. These observations collectively seem to support the claim that the presence of specific serotypes may be a local characteristic due to several factors (e.g., breed of cattle, geographic location, farm management), which highlights the importance of serotyping studies for selecting appropriate prevention measures [23, 25, 26]. In our study, we also found strains not classified to any serotype. This was not surprising because such strains are quite frequently observed among *S. agalactiae* isolated from cattle [25]. Nonetheless, we did not determine serotype IX in our experiment, and consequently, the number of strains in the NT group may be unduly high. In addition, we analysed of the presence of virulence genes in individual serotypes of *S. agalactiae*. Interestingly, despite the frequent presence of serotype IA that is typical of human diseases, we did not detect in this serotype genes characteristic for human strains of *S. agalactiae* (*scpB, lmb, pavA* or *bac*). In the two most often isolated serotypes IA and II, the dominance of two virulence profiles was observed: *rib, cylE, cfb,* and *bca, cylE, cfb,* respectively. These serotypes differed from each other by the presence of two genes: *rib* and *bca.* These genes belong to the same family, the alpha-like protein (Alp) family, and play important roles in the pathogenesis of illnesses caused by these bacteria, and they are also acknowledged as vaccine candidates [23]. Our results suggest that vaccines should contain at least two genes from this family because their presence may be correlated with the dominant serotype. However, there is a need to kept in mind that in the case of these bacteria there is a possibility of horizontal or lateral gene transfer. According to the Richards et al. [27] *S.agalactiae* can transfer genetic material both to their own species and other mastitis pathogens such as *S.uberis* or *S.dysgalactiae,* which is one of the mechanisms of these bacteria for adaptation to the bovine environment. However, our study was performed on a relatively small number of strains isolated from just one species, and further studies in this direction are necessary.

Eight genes (*sua, pauA/skc, gapC, cfu, lbp, hasA, hasB, hasC*) were selected for *S. uberis,* of which the following were most frequent: *gapC* (98%), *sua* (96%) and *pauA/skc* (94%). The presence of the gene *lbp* was not detected among the analysed strains. The three genes dominant in our study were previously confirmed at similar levels in Argentina, India, Great Britain, New Zealand and the USA [11, 28–31]. These genes are considered as good targets for vaccine development due to frequent occurrence and their highly conserved nature at the nucleotide and amino acid levels [11, 28, 32]. In our experiment, we also chose to analyse genes of the has operon (*hasABC*), which is responsible for capsule production. The key role in this process is played by the gene *hasA*, which was rather rare (17%) among the analysed strains. This finding suggests that in the region investigated, the ability of *S. uberis* to produce capsules does not play a key role in mastitis [11].

In *S. dysgalactiae,* we focused on two genes that encode proteins responsible for binding host plasminogen (*naprl* and *eno*). Both occurred quite frequently among the analysed strains (approximately 80%). Similar results for these two genes have been observed among *S. dysgalactiae* strains isolated from fish and pigs in Asian countries [17].

Conclusions

In summary, the experiment reported above showed that strains of *Streptococcus* spp. in northeastern Poland possess several invasiveness factors, which can considerably influence the course of disease and treatment. The data obtained during our study constitute a preliminary step towards further research targeting a better understanding of the dominant virulence mechanisms among these bacteria, and they may aid the development of target prevention programmes for this region of the country.

Acknowledgements

We would like to thank Wojciech Rękawek for collecting samples for this research.

Funding

Publication was supported by KNOW (Leading National Research Centre) Scientific Consortium "Healthy Animal-Safe Food," decision of the Ministry of Science and Higher Education No. 05-1/KNOW2/2015.

Authors' contributions

EK performed all PCR testing, bacterial identification and biofilm assay. JM was responsible for interpretation of data and study design. RW revised the manuscript, AKS contributed to the study design, conception, and interpretation of data. All authors read, revised, and approved the final manuscript.

Consent for publication

Not applicable.

Competing interests

The authors declare that they have no competing interests.

References

1. Thomas V, Jong A, Moyaert H, Simjee S, Garch FE, Morrissey I, et al. Antimicrobial susceptibility monitoring of *mastitis* pathogens isolated from acute cases of clinical *mastitis* in dairy cows across Europe: VetPath result. Int J Antimicrob Agents. 2015;46:13–20.
2. Neiwert O, Holst O, Duda KA. Structural investigation of rhamnose-rich polysaccharides from *Streptococcus dysgalactiae* bovine *mastitis* isolate. Carbohydr Res. 2014;389:192–5.
3. Bradley AJ. Bovine *Mastitis*: an evolving disease. Vet J. 2002;164:116–28.
4. Pieterse R, Todorov SD. Bacteriocins- exploring alternatives to antibiotics in *mastitis* teratment. Braz J Microbiol. 2010;41:542–62.
5. Preez JH. Bovine mastitis therapy and why it fails. J S Afr Vet Assoc. 2000;71:201–8.
6. Sordillo LM. Factors affecting mammary gland immunity and mastitis susceptibility. Livest Prod Sci. 2005;98:89–99.
7. Melchior MB, Vaarkamp H, Fink-Gremmels J. Biofilms: a role in recurrent mastitis infections? Vet J. 2006;171:398–407.
8. Boonyayatra S, Pata P, Nakharuthai P, Chaisri W. Antimicrobial resistance of biofilm-forming *Streptococcus agalactiae* isolated from bovine *mastitis.* J Vet Sci Technol. 2016; https://doi.org/10.4172/2157-7579.1000374.
9. Costerton JW, Stoodley P. Bacterial biofilms: from the natural environment to infectious diseases. Nat Rev Microbiol. 2004;2:95–108.
10. Felipe V, Morgante CA, Somale PS, Varroni F, Zingaretti ML, Bachetti RA, et al. Evaluation of the biofilm forming ability and its associated genes in *Staphylococcus* species isolates from bovine *mastitis* in Argentinean dairy farms. Microb Pathog. 2017;104:278–86.
11. Reinoso EB, Lasagno MC, Dieser SA, Odierno LM. Distribution of virulence-associated genes in *Streptococcus uberis* isolated from bovine *mastitis.* FEMS Microbiol Lett. 2011;318:183–8.
12. Carvalho-Castro GA, Silva JR, Paiva LV, Custódio DA, Moreira RO, Mian GF, et al. Molecular epidemiology of *Streptococcus agalactiae* isolated from mastitis in Brazilian dairy herds. Braz J Microbiol. 2017; https://doi.org/10.1016/j.bjm.2017.02.004.

13. Ebrahimi A, Moatamedi A, Lotfalian S, Mirshokraei P. Biofilm formation, hemolysin production and antimicrobial susceptibilities of *Streptococcus agalactiae* isolated from the mastitis milk of dairy cows in Shahrekord district, Iran. Vet Res Forum. 2013;4:269–72.
14. Kaczorek E, Małaczewska J, Wójcik R, Rękawek W, Siwicki AK. Phenotypic and genotypic antimicrobial susceptibility pattern of *Streptococcus spp.* isolated from cases of clinical *mastitis* in dairy cattle in Poland. J Dairy Sci. 2017;100:6442–53.
15. Stepanović S, Vuković D, Hola V, Di Bonaventura G, Djukić S, Cirković I, Ruzicka F. Quantification of biofilm in microtiter plates: overview of testing conditions and practical recommendations for assessment of biofilm production by staphylococci. APMIS. 2007;115:891–9.
16. Poyart C, Tazi A, Réglier-Poupet H, Billoët A, Tavares N, Raymond J, et al. Multiplex PCR assay for rapid and accurate capsular typing of group B Streptococci. J Clin Microbiol. 2007;45:1985–8.
17. Abdelsalam M, Fujino M, Eissa AE, Chen SC, Warda M. Expression, genetic localization and phylogenic analysis of NAPlr in piscine *Streptococcus dysgalactiae* subspecies dysgalactiae isolates and their patterns of adherence. J Adv Res. 2015;6:747–55.
18. Calvinho LF, Almeida RA, Oliver SP. Potential virulence factors of *Streptococcus dysgalactiae* associated with bovine mastitis. Vet Microbiol. 1998;15:93–110.
19. Moliva MV, Cerioli F, Reinoso EB. Evaluation of environmental and nutritional factors and sua gene on *in vitro* biofilm formation of *Streptococcus uberis* isolates. Microb Pathog. 2017;107:144–8.
20. Shome BR, Bhuvana M, Mitra SD, Krithiga N, Shome R, Velu D, et al. Molecular characterization of *Streptococcus agalactiae* and *Streptococcus uberis* isolates from bovine milk. Trop Anim Health Prod. 2012; https://doi.org/10.1007/s11250-012-0167-4.
21. El-Behiry A, Elsayed M, Marzouk E, Bathich Y. Detection of virulence genes in *Staphyococcus aureus* and *Streptococcus agalatctiae* isolated from mastitis in the middle east. Br Microbiol Res J. 2015;10:1–9.
22. Jain B, Tewari A, Bhandari BB, Jhala MK. Antibiotic resistance and virulence genes in *Streptococcus agalactiae* isolated from cases of bovine subclinical mastitis. Vet Arhiv. 2012;82:423–32.
23. Yang Y, Liu Y, Ding Y, Yi L, Ma Z, Fan H, Lu C. Molecular characterization of *Streptococcus agalactiae* isolated from bovine mastitis in Eastern China. PLoS One. 2013; https://doi.org/10.1371/journal.pone.0067755.
24. Delannoy CM, Crumlish M, Fontaine MC, Pollock J, Foster G, Dagleish MP, et al. Human *Streptococcus agalactiae* strains in aquatic mammals and fish. BMC Microbiol. 2013;13:1471–80.
25. Dogan B, Schukken YH, Santisteban C, Boor KJ. Distribution of serotypes and antimicrobial resistance genes among *Streptococcus agalactiae* isolates from bovine and human hosts. J Clin Microbiol. 2005;43:5899–906.
26. Merl K, Abdulmawjood A, Lämmler C, Zschöck M. Determination of epidemiological relationships of *Streptococcus agalactiae* isolated from bovine mastitis. FEMS Microbiol Lett. 2003;12:87–92.
27. Richards VP, Lang P, Bitar PD, Lefébure T, Schukken YH, Zadoks RN, Stanhope MJ. Comparative genomics and the role of lateral gene transfer in the evolution of bovine adapted *Streptococcus agalactiae*. Infect Genet Evol. 2011;11:1263–75.
28. Perrig MS, Veaute C, Renna MS, Pujato N, Calvinho L, Marcipar I, et al. Assessment of the potential utility of different regions of *Streptococcus uberis* adhesion molecule (SUAM) for mastitis subunit vaccine development. Microb Pathog. 2017;105:273–9.
29. Luther DA, Almeida RA, Oliver SP. Elucidation of the DNA sequence of *Streptococcus uberis* adhesion molecule gene (sua) and detection of sua in strains of *Streptococcus uberis* isolated from geographically diverse locations. Vet Microbiol. 2008;128:304–12.
30. Yuan Y, Dego OK, Chen X, Abadin E, Chan S, Jory L, et al. Conservation of *Streptococcus uberis* adhesion molecule and the *sua* gene in strains of *Streptococcus uberis* isolated from geographically diverse areas. J Dairy Sci. 2014;97:7668–73.
31. Ward PN, Leigh JA. Genetic analysis of *Streptococcus uberis* plasminogen activators. Indian J Med Res. 2004;119:136–40.
32. Perez-Casal J, Prysliak T, Potter AA. A GapC chimera retains the properties of the *Streptococcus uberis* wild-type GapC protein. Protein Expr Purif. 2004;33:288–96.
33. Field TR, Ward PN, Pedersen LH, Leigh JA. The hyaluronic acid capsule of Streptococcus uberis is not required for the development of infection and clinical mastitis. Infect Immun. 2003;71:132–9.
34. Wastfelt M, Stalhammar-Carlemalm M, Delisse AM, Cabezon T, Lindahl G. Identification of a family of streptococcal surface proteins with extremely repetitive structure. J Biol Chem. 1996;271:18892–7.
35. Jerlstrom PG, Chhatwal GS, Timmis KN. The IgA-binding beta antigen of the c protein complex of group B streptococci: sequence determination of its gene and detection of two binding regions. Mol Microbiol. 1991;5:843–9.
36. Bergseng H, Bevanger L, Rygg M, Bergh K. Real-time PCR targeting the sip gene for detection of group B Streptococcus colonization in pregnant women at delivery. J Med Microbiol. 2007;56:223–8.
37. Michel JL, Madoff LC, Olson K, Kling DE, Kasper DL, Ausubel FM. Large, identical, tandem repeating units in the C protein alpha antigen gene, bca, of group B streptococci. Proc Natl Acad Sci U S A. 1992;89:10060–4.
38. Dimitriev A, Shakleina E, Tkàčikova L, Mikula I, Totolian A. Genetic heterogeneity of the pathogenic potentials of human and bovine group B Streptococci. Folia Microbiol. 2002;47:291–5.
39. Pires R, Rolo D, Gama-Norton L, Morais A, Lito L, Salgado MJ, et al. Group A Streptococci from carriage and disease in Portugal: evolution of antimicrobial resistance and T antigenic types during 2000-2002. Microb Drug Resist. 2005;11:360–70.

16

Development of a novel immunochromatographic lateral flow assay specific for *Mycobacterium bovis* cells and its application in combination with immunomagnetic separation to test badger faeces

Linda D. Stewart[1], Nuria Tort[2], Paul Meakin[2], Jose M. Argudo[1], Ruramayi Nzuma[1], Neil Reid[1,3], Richard J. Delahay[4], Roland Ashford[5], W. Ian Montgomery[1,3] and Irene R. Grant[1*]

Abstract

Background: The European badger is an important wildlife reservoir of *Mycobacterium bovis* implicated in the spread of bovine tuberculosis in the United Kingdom and Ireland. Infected badgers are known to shed *M. bovis* in their urine and faeces, which may contaminate the environment. To aid bovine tuberculosis control efforts novel diagnostic tests for detecting infected and shedding badgers are needed. We proposed development of a novel, rapid immunochromatographic lateral flow device (LFD) as a non-invasive test to detect *M. bovis* cells in badger faeces. Its application in combination with immunomagnetic separation (IMS) to detect *Mycobacterium bovis* cells in badger faeces is reported here.

Results: A novel prototype LFD for *M. bovis* cells was successfully developed, with unique specificity for *M. bovis* and a limit of detection 50% ($LOD_{50\%}$) of 1.7×10^4 *M. bovis* cells/ml. When IMS was employed to selectively capture and concentrate *M. bovis* cells from badger faeces prior to LFD testing, the $LOD_{50\%}$ of the IMS-LFD assay was 2.8×10^5 *M. bovis* cells/ml faecal homogenate. Faeces samples collected from latrines at badger setts in a region of endemic bovine tuberculosis infection were tested; 78 (18%) of 441 samples tested IMS-LFD assay positive, whereas 140 (32%) tested IMS-qPCR positive (Kappa agreement -0.009 ± 0.044, $p = 0.838$). Subsequently, when 130 faeces samples from live captured, or captive, badgers of known infection status (on the basis of StatPak, interferon-γ and/or culture results) were tested, the IMS-LFD assay had higher relative diagnostic specificity (Sp 0.926), but poorer relative diagnostic sensitivity (Se 0.081), than IMS-qPCR (Sp 0.706, Se 0.581) and IMS-culture (Sp 0.794, Se 0.436).

Conclusions: The novel IMS-LFD assay, although very specific for *M. bovis*, has low analytical sensitivity (indicated by the $LOD_{50\%}$) and would only detect badgers shedding high numbers of *M. bovis* ($>10^{4-5}$ cells/g) in their faeces. The novel LFD would, therefore, have limited value as a non-invasive test for badger TB surveillance purposes but it may have value for alternative veterinary diagnostic applications.

Keywords: *Mycobacterium bovis*, European badger (*Meles meles*), Faeces, immunomagnetic separation, Lateral flow device, Non-invasive test, Diagnostic specificity, Diagnostic sensitivity

* Correspondence: i.grant@qub.ac.uk
[1]Institute for Global Food Security, School of Biological Sciences, Queen's University Belfast, Belfast, Northern Ireland, UK
Full list of author information is available at the end of the article

Background

Mycobacterium bovis is the causative agent of bovine tuberculosis (TB) in cattle, badgers and other wild and domestic mammals [1]. Bovine TB is the most serious endemic disease currently facing the livestock industry in the United Kingdom and Republic of Ireland [2]. Despite a systematic test and slaughter programme in cattle, which has been ongoing for many years within the United Kingdom, the incidence of bovine TB has continued to rise. This lack of success has been attributed in part to the presence of a reservoir of infection in the European badger (*Meles meles*) [3, 4]. Investigation of the dynamics of TB in wildlife and cattle herds using DNA fingerprinting of strains [5, 6] has revealed that badgers and cattle tend to have similar *M. bovis* spoligotypes, providing evidence of cross-species transmission [7]. In parts of the United Kingdom, herd incidence rates of TB in cattle more than doubled between 1998 and 2010, and although prevalence varies widely in badger populations, estimates of 6.3–33.9% infection (depending on county, overall 16.6%) were recorded in 2005 in endemic areas [3]. The ability to identify and monitor TB infection in the reservoir wildlife host may provide a valuable tool for targeting efforts to control risks of *M. bovis* transmission to cattle.

It is known that badgers can transmit *M. bovis* to cattle [8], but the precise route of transmission is unclear. A potential route if badgers and cattle come into close proximity is inhalation of aerosolised droplets; however, infected badgers are also known to shed *M. bovis* in their urine and faeces [9, 10], which may contaminate the environment. Badgers habitually defecate in clusters of shallow pits known as latrines which if accessible to cattle may act as a possible source of infection [11]. Infected badgers are known to intermittently shed *M. bovis* in their faeces in variable numbers. For example, King et al. [12] demonstrated heterogeneity in bacterial load for badgers in the Woodchester Park, Gloucestershire, study area, and reported shedding of 1×10^3-4×10^5 *M. bovis* cells per g of faeces. Faecal shedding is an indication of infectiousness, with shedding correlating with animals exhibiting more severe disease status [13]. *M. bovis* can persist in the environment for several months under certain conditions [14]. This environmental signal of the presence of *M. bovis* in a badger population was demonstrated by Courtenay et al. [15] who showed that the detectability of the bacterium at badger setts and latrines was strongly linked to the frequency of excretion detected in live-sampled badgers.

The *M. bovis* infection status of badgers in a given area may be assessed in various ways: by active surveillance involving the capture, anaesthesia and use of blood tests and microbiological culture of samples (invasive); by collecting and analysing badger faeces or other environmental samples (non-invasive); or, by the examination of badger carcasses after road traffic accidents (RTA) and tissue culture. The appropriate method to adopt depends on the question being asked and the geographical scale for which data are required. For example, RTA surveys have been used to provide coarse prevalence (or even presence/absence) data on a large geographical scale [16–19], whereas live capture and collection of clinical samples has been used to provide more detailed eco-epidemiological data over smaller areas [20]. The collection of faecal samples from latrines for TB surveillance in badgers has the potential to be used on a variety of geographical scales.

Since it is known that some infected badgers excrete *M. bovis* in their faeces [9, 10], we proposed the development of an immunochromatographic lateral flow device (LFD) and its use in combination with an existing immunomagnetic separation (IMS) technique [21, 22] as a non-invasive test for the presence of *M. bovis*. Immunochromatographic assays are easy to use, cheap to produce, and provide a rapid result (within 15 min), so are ideal for field use. The purpose of including IMS was to selectively capture and concentrate target mycobacterial cells from the faeces matrix before application to the LFD, to facilitate sample clean-up and improve detection sensitivity. Here, we report the successful development of a prototype *M. bovis*-specific LFD and its application in combination with IMS to test for evidence of *M. bovis* cells in badger faeces. We also assessed agreement between results of the field IMS-LFD assay and laboratory IMS-based methods (IMS-qPCR and IMS-culture) when faeces from badgers of unknown infection status were tested, and estimated relative diagnostic sensitivity (Se) and specificity (Sp) of the IMS-LFD assay by testing faeces from badgers for which we had independent information on their *M. bovis* infection status.

Methods

Bacterial cultures employed in the study

Mycobacterium bovis AF2122/97, *M. bovis* BCG NCTC 5692, *M. avium* subsp. *avium* NCTC 13034, *M. avium* subsp. *paratuberculosis* ATCC 19698, *M. fortuitum* NCTC 10394, *M. intracellulare* NCTC 10425, *M. kansasii* NCTC 10268, *M. xenopi* NCTC 10042, *M. terrae* NCTC 10856, *M. scrofulaceum* NCTC 10803, *M. marinum* NCTC 2275, *M. smegmatis* mc^2 155, *M. gordonae* NCTC 10267, *M. tuberculosis* H37Rv, and a field isolate of *M. hiberniae* were cultured in Middlebrook 7H9 broth containing 10% OADC supplement (both Difco) to stationary phase, harvested by centrifugation and washed in phosphate buffered saline, pH 7.2 (PBS, Sigma). Cell suspensions in PBS, containing 10^6–10^7 CFU/ml were subjected to a 10 kGy dose of gamma radiation using a Gammabeam 650 cobalt irradiator, in order to kill the bacteria without damaging cell surface antigens and to render them safe to use in a Containment Level 2 laboratory. Irradiated PBS bacterial suspensions were stored at −80 °C until required.

In addition, colonies of *M. tuberculosis* H37Rv grown on solid agar were emulsified in PBS and 80 μl tested directly on the LFD in a Containment Level 3 laboratory.

Development of a prototype lateral flow device (LFD) specific for *M. bovis*

A selection of previously produced [21] or locally sourced *M. bovis*-specific monoclonal and polyclonal antibodies was tested for their suitability for incorporation into the proposed LFD. In order to select the most appropriate antibodies to serve as capture and detector reagents, a series of trials were carried out. All the antibodies were conjugated to gold nanoparticles and also all were immobilised at the Test (T) line of different nitrocellulose membranes at different concentrations. A cocktail of commercial anti-mouse-IgG IgG and anti-rabbit-IgG IgG was immobilized at the Control (C) Line position. A two-step wet assay was performed to evaluate recognition of *M. bovis* whole cells using the different combinations of membranes (with the immobilized antibodies in the T Line) and gold conjugates. The combination of antibodies and membrane which gave the strongest T-line was selected in order to produce a batch of working prototype devices to be evaluated.

Assessment of detection specificity and cross-reactivity of the prototype LFD

PBS suspensions of the range of *Mycobacterium* spp. identified above and six different spoligotypes of *M. bovis* (SB140 (AF2122/97), SB129, SB273, SB142, SB263 and SB145) prepared as described above, were tested on the prototype LFD. Irradiated cultures were vortexed briefly before 80 μl were transferred to the sample well of the LFD. The presence or absence of a T-line on the LFD after 15 min at room temperature was assessed visually in each case.

Determination of the limit of detection of the prototype LFD

The 50% limit of detection ($LOD_{50\%}$) of the LFD was determined by testing 10-fold serial dilutions of a stock of irradiated *M. bovis* AF2122/97 (containing 5.3×10^6 CFU/ml) in PBS. Four replicate samples at each of four dilutions containing 10^5, 10^4, 10^3 and 0 CFU/ml were tested. The presence or absence of a T-line was assessed both visually and using an LFD reader (Forsite Diagnostics Limited, York, UK) after the sample had been run on the LFD for 15 min at room temperature. The $LOD_{50\%}$ was determined using the generalized Spearman-Kärber $LOD_{50\%}$ calculation for 4-level spiking protocols [23].

Coating of magnetic beads for immunomagnetic separation (IMS) and determination of *M. bovis* capture sensitivity and bead specificity

The MyOne tosylactivated Dynabeads (Life Technologies, Paisley, UK) previously used by Stewart et al. [22] for immunocapture of *M. bovis* from bovine lymph node tissue are 1 μm in diameter. These proved to be too large to run along the LFD, so smaller carboxylated magnetic beads, available in three sizes (200, 300 and 500 nm) were sourced (Ademtech, France). All three sizes of Ademtech bead were coated with the *M. bovis*-specific 11G3 monoclonal antibody and EEA302 biotinylated peptide [21] separately, and also with a mixture of the peptide and the antibody (dually coated), using the Carboxyl-Adembeads Coupling Kit (Ademtech 02820) according to the manufacturer's instructions. Tenfold serial dilutions (10^{-1} to 10^{-5}) of irradiated *M. bovis* AF2122/97 (10^6–10^7 CFU/ml) were prepared and 1 ml of each dilution was subjected to automated IMS using the Dynal BeadRetriever (Life Technologies) (21) using the different sized/coated Adembeads, with resuspension of the beads after IMS in 100 μl Tris-EDTA (TE) buffer. After extraction of DNA by heating at 100 °C for 25 min, the samples were analysed using *M. bovis* touchdown PCR [24] and visualised using agarose gel electrophoresis PCR, as described in Stewart et al. [21]. As controls, and to enable comparison of capture sensitivities achieved, dually coated MyOne Tosylactivated Dynabeads (Life Technologies) and a dilution series of irradiated *M. bovis* AF2122/97 in TE buffer not subjected to IMS were included.

Specificity of the 200 and 300 nm coated beads was assessed by IMS experiments involving the range of *Mycobacterium* spp. described above. Each species was tested on two separate occasions. Stationary phase broth cultures of each species were diluted to 10^3–10^4 CFU/ml in Middlebrook 7H9/OADC broth. A 100 μl sample of the dilutions was spread onto Middlebrook 7H10/OADC agar plates to determine CFU/ml before IMS and 1 ml of each dilution was then subjected to automated IMS using each of the coated beads. Following IMS, beads were resuspended in 1 ml Middlebrook 7H9/OADC broth (maintaining original sample volume in order to permit direct comparison of colony counts before and after IMS), 100 μl of which was spread onto Middlebrook 7H10/OADC agar plates. Agar plates were incubated at 30, 37 or 42 °C (as appropriate for the *Mycobacterium* sp. concerned) until colonies were evident. Mean colony count following IMS was expressed as a percentage of the number of CFU present in the original suspension before IMS to calculate the degree of non-specific binding by *Mycobacterium spp.* other than *M. bovis.*

Optimisation of faeces sample preparation protocol

Optimisation of the faeces sample preparation protocol is described in detail elsewhere [25]. Briefly, a number of factors in relation to application of IMS in the field needed to be considered before arriving at a finalised field IMS protocol. These included the volume of diluent required to homogenise the faecal samples, the effect of the faecal matrix on bead retrieval, the time needed to retrieve the beads, the dilution factor required, the quantity of beads required, the assessment of matrix effect on capture of *M. bovis* by coated beads, and the effect of nylon strainers on the recovery of *M. bovis*.

Limit of detection of IMS-LFD assay applied to faeces

The $LOD_{50\%}$ of the IMS-LFD assay was determined twice using two different *M. bovis* negative badger faeces samples as the spiking matrix. Four replicate samples were spiked at four cell concentrations (10^5, 10^4, 10^3 and 0 CFU/ml) before the field IMS-LFD assay was applied. The presence or absence of T-lines was assessed visually. The $LOD_{50\%}$ was, once again, estimated using the generalized Spearman-Kärber $LOD_{50\%}$ calculation for 4-level spiking protocols [23].

Ability of the novel IMS-LFD assay to detect *M. bovis* in naturally infected badger faeces

Badger faeces samples were collected from latrines at 110 setts throughout Northern Ireland. A random sample of 1 km squares containing main setts, located during the Northern Ireland Badger Survey 2007/08 [26], were selected to be visited for sampling purposes. These setts were located in geographic areas with high, moderate and low reported incidence of tuberculosis breakdowns in cattle, based on information supplied by the Department of Agriculture and Rural Development for Northern Ireland. On arrival at each main sett, a single latrine was located from which up to a maximum of five of the freshest appearing faecal samples were collected; each sample was taken from a different dropping.

The IMS-LFD procedure was performed in the field as summarised schematically in Fig. 1. Approximately 1 g of badger faeces was transferred to a tube containing 9 ml PBS pH 7.2 and the sample was shaken vigorously by hand. When a homogeneous suspension was obtained, the sample was filtered through a 70 μm cell strainer (Falcon) into a 50 ml centrifuge tube. A sub-sample of 6–8 ml of this homogenised, filtered faeces sample was poured into a tube containing 20 μl of antibody- and peptide- dually coated 300 nm carboxylated magnetic beads. The sample was incubated at ambient temperature for 30 min and shaken every 5 min. The tube was placed in a DynaMag™-15 magnetic rack (Life Technologies) for 10 min before the supernatant was carefully poured off, leaving the beads behind. Beads were washed three times by shaking in approx. 5 ml PBS-0.05% Tween 20 (PBS-T, Sigma) per wash with separation for 2 min on the magnetic rack between washes. After the third wash the beads were resuspended in 200 μl Detector™ block solution (KPL Inc., Gaithersburg, USA) and 80 μl was transferred to the test well of the LFD. After 15 min the IMS-LFD result was recorded as 'positive' if both Control (C) and Test (T) lines were visible or 'negative' if only the C line was observed. Digital photographs were taken to record test outcomes. The LFDs were retained and returned to the laboratory where the presence of a T line was subsequently verified using a Forsite LFD reader. Residual bead suspensions were also returned to the laboratory for Ziehl-Neelsen staining and examination by light microscopy, in order to verify the presence of large numbers of acid-fast cells in samples which had tested IMS-LFD positive in the field.

Laboratory IMS-based tests on residual faecal homogenates

The residual 1–2 ml portion of each homogenised, filtered badger faecal sample was returned to the laboratory where automated IMS followed by real-time qPCR (IMS-qPCR) and MGIT™ culture (IMS-culture) were carried out. One ml of each homogenised, filtered badger faecal sample was subjected to automated IMS with dually antibody- and peptide-coated MyOne tosylactivated Dynabeads [21] using a Dynal BeadRetriever (both Life Technologies). Following automated IMS, the beads plus any captured *M. bovis* cells were resuspended in 500 μl Middlebrook 7H9 broth which was then split between a 100 μl sample for qPCR (method of Sweeney et al. [27]) and 400 μl for BACTEC™ MGIT™ culture (Becton Dickinson). DNA was released from bead-bound *M. bovis* cells by boiling for 25 min and then purified by Zymoclean columns (ZymoResearch) before qPCR was performed using an Eco-PCR instrument (Illumina, Inc.). The reaction volume was 25 μl comprising 12.5 μl of TaqMan Gene expression ×2 master mix (Life Technologies), 1 μl (20 pmol/μl) forward RD4 flanking primer (5′ TGTGAATTCATACAAGCCGTAGTCG 3′), 1 μl (20 pmol/μl) reverse RD4 flanking primer (5′ CCCGTAGCGTTACTGAGAAATTGC 3′), 1 μl (10 pmol/μl) RD4 hydrolysis probe (5′ 6-FAM–AGCG CAACACTCTTGGAGTGGCCTAC–MGB 3′), 7 μl of nuclease-free sterile water and 2.5 μl of template DNA. The RD4 hydrolysis probe and qPCR primers were purchased from Life Technologies. Reaction conditions were: 50 °C for 2 min, 95 °C for 10 min, and 40 cycles of 95 °C for 15 s and 60 °C for 1 min. Duplicate 2.5 μl aliquots of DNA were tested for each faecal sample. Both aliquots had to report positive or negative for a definitive IMS-qPCR result to be recorded. In instances where there was disagreement between the duplicate results for any sample, the qPCR was repeated. If disagreement between duplicate results still existed after the second PCR then the sample was recorded as IMS-qPCR negative (interpretation adopted by Travis et al. [28]). A six point standard curve, generated

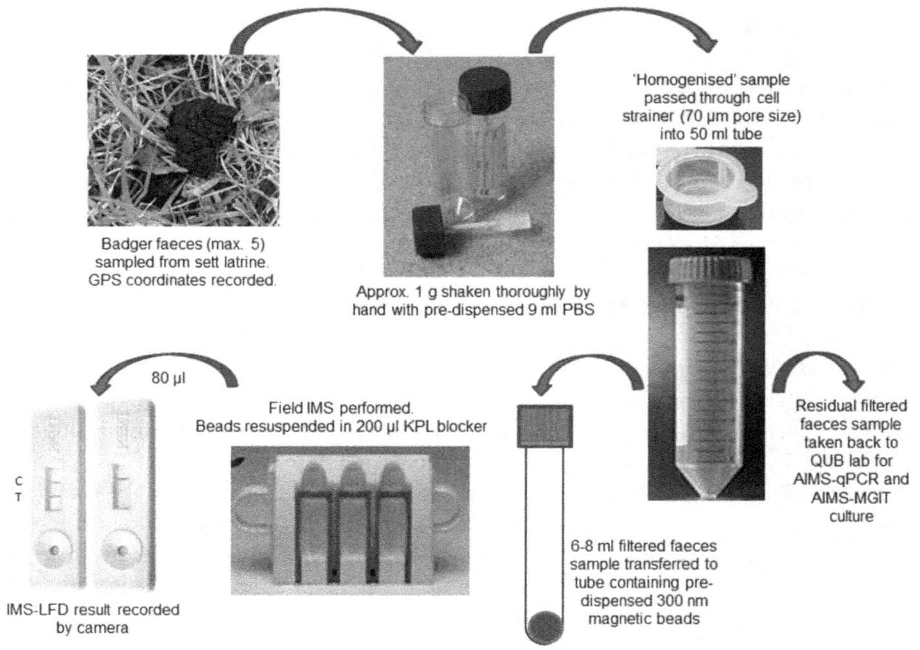

Fig. 1 Schematic outlining the field IMS-LFD testing procedure for testing badger faeces

using DNA from a dilution series (10^6–10 CFU/ml) of irradiated *M. bovis* AF2122/97, and a no template control (water only), were run in duplicate in each qPCR run.

For IMS-culture, after IMS the beads (400 µl) were inoculated directly into BACTEC™ MGIT™ culture tubes supplemented with 10% OADC supplement and PANTA antibiotic supplement (all Becton Dickinson). The MGIT cultures were observed visually (because no MGIT 960 instrument was available in the laboratory) at intervals over an incubation period of up to 12 weeks at 37 °C for signs of growth (turbidity change). After 4, 8 and 12 weeks of incubation 100 µl of each MGIT culture showing evidence of growth was removed, boiled at 100 °C for 25 min and checked for presence of *M. bovis* DNA by Touchdown PCR targeting the IS6110 element and employing INS1 and INS2 primers [24]. The Touchdown PCR was able to detect down to 50 *M. bovis* CFU/ml (Stewart and Grant, unpublished data). An IMS-culture positive result was declared if MGIT cultures showing evidence of growth (turbidity) tested Touchdown PCR positive. If no growth was observed after 12 weeks or if the final Touchdown PCR results for the MGIT positive cultures at 12 weeks were all negative, then a negative IMS-culture result was declared.

Assessment of the diagnostic specificity and sensitivity of the IMS-LFD assay by testing faeces from badgers of putative known infection status

In total, 130 faecal samples were collected from badgers for which independent live animal TB diagnostic test results were also available. The samples were tested by the IMS-LFD assay, IMS-qPCR and IMS-culture, as described above for the badger faecal samples collected from latrines, except that sample preparation and the IMS-LFD test were performed in the laboratory. Of the 130 faecal samples, 100 had been obtained, following administration of an enema, from badgers trapped as part of the long-term capture-mark-release project at Woodchester Park, Gloucestershire, England. In order to maximise the likelihood that a proportion of these samples came from *M. bovis*-infected animals, we targeted collection at badger social groups with evidence of current or recent live animal test positive results. Following collection all faeces samples were stored at -70 °C for up to 7 months prior to testing. BrockTB Stat-Pak® (Chembio Diagnostic Systems, Inc., Medford, NY), culture (of sputum, faeces, urine, wound/abscess swabs), and interferon-gamma enzyme immunoassay (IFN-γ EIA [29]) test results, obtained over the previous 1–2 years, were available for these animals. The remaining 30 faecal samples were obtained from captive badgers that were originally trapped in a part of the United Kingdom with very low incidence of TB in cattle. These 30 badgers had tested negative for *M. bovis* infection by the IFN-γ EIA test and bacteriological culture of clinical samples (sputum, urine and rectal swab) on three sequential occasions over a three month period. They were, therefore, considered putative 'non-infected'. All 130 faeces samples were blind tested by staff at Queen's University Belfast.

Statistical analysis

Descriptive statistics captured the prevalence of *M. bovis* positive results using the three IMS-based tests (IMS-LFD, IMS-qPCR and IMS-culture) on 441 badger faeces of unknown disease infection status collected in Northern Ireland, and 130 badger faecal samples collected from Woodchester Park (n = 100) and captive (n = 30) animals for which contemporaneous or previous live animal diagnostic test results were available. Venn diagrams were prepared to illustrate inter-relationships between the results obtained with each test. Cross-tabulation of results permitted determination of Kappa statistics, as a measure of the agreement between test results, which were interpreted according to Landis and Koch [30]. McNemar's test was performed on 2 × 2 contingency tables of results for the three IMS-based tests versus the badgers' putative TB infection status derived on the basis of the live animal diagnostic test results, to permit estimation of diagnostic sensitivity (Se) and specificity (Sp) of the field IMS-LFD, IMS-qPCR and IMS-culture tests applied to faeces. Since no gold standard diagnostic test for *M. bovis* in badgers exists, estimates of diagnostic specificity and sensitivity are relative to the live animal tests applied. All statistical analyses were performed using SPSS 21 (IBM), unless otherwise stated.

Results

Development of a prototype *M. bovis*-specific LFD

A specific monoclonal mouse anti-*M. bovis* antibody (Mab) and a rabbit anti-*M. bovis* polyclonal antibody (Pab) were successfully conjugated to the gold nanoparticles, and the resulting conjugates were found to be stable. Potential capture reagents were immobilised at the T-line position on the membranes and a cocktail of commercial anti-mouse-IgG and anti-rabbit-IgG IgG was immobilized at the C-line position. Following trials with different combinations and concentrations of capture and detector reagents, it was concluded that the working prototype LFD for the detection of *M. bovis* whole cells was comprised of 'membrane 1' with polyclonal antibody immobilised at the T-Line to act as the capture reagent and Mab conjugated to gold nanoparticles to act as the detector reagent. A batch of 1000 prototype LFDs was produced by Forsite Diagnostics Ltd., York, for evaluation at Queen's University Belfast. For commercial reasons, no additional detail about the membrane or antibodies used for the prototype LFD device can be provided here.

When the detection specificity of the prototype LFD was evaluated by testing a range of different *Mycobacterium* spp. diluted in PBS, the prototype LFD yielded a positive T-line for *M. bovis* (all six spoligotypes tested) and *M. bovis* BCG only (Fig. 2a), and gave a negative T-line with all other *Mycobacterium* spp. tested (Fig. 2b). In terms of detection sensitivity, the $LOD_{50\%}$ for *M. bovis* suspended in PBS was determined to be 1.7×10^4 *M. bovis* cells/ml.

IMS modification

Evaluation of the smaller Ademtech carboxylated magnetic beads indicated that, like the previously used MyOne Tosylactivated beads, dually coated beads (i.e. coated with both peptide and IgM antibody) produced the best *M. bovis* capture results. The dually coated 300 nm and 200 nm beads showed similar capture capability from both buffer and spiked faeces, with <3% non-specific binding with all the other non-target mycobacteria tested. It was, therefore, concluded that either sized bead could be used with the LFD, and we decided to use the 300 nm beads.

Combining field IMS with the LFD

After field IMS the beads were resuspended in 200 μl PBS for analysis on the LFD. However, it was found that uncoated beads, coated beads and the storage buffer recommended by Ademtech all produced a false positive T-line on the LFD after IMS. To resolve this issue an extra step of quenching the activated unused carboxyl groups present on the bead surface using ethanolamine was introduced during coating of the beads, and various blocking solutions were investigated as alternatives to the Ademtech storage buffer for resuspension of the coated beads. The false positive issue was resolved by resuspension of beads after IMS in KPL Detector™ block, a commercially available blocking solution (KPL Inc., Gaithersburg, Maryland). The finalised field IMS-LFD protocol was as illustrated in Fig. 1.

The $LOD_{50\%}$ of the field IMS-LFD was estimated to be 2.8×10^5 *M. bovis* cells/ml faeces homogenate (1:10 dilution), so the detection sensitivity of the LFD was reduced when IMS preceded LFD detection, and faeces homogenates rather than PBS suspensions were being tested.

Capability of the IMS-LFD test to detect *M. bovis* in badger faeces relative to the laboratory-based IMS-qPCR and IMS-culture tests

A total of 441 badger faecal samples, collected from 110 main setts throughout Northern Ireland were tested. A mean of four faeces samples were collected from a single latrine at each main sett. Using the individual faecal sample as the unit of analysis, 78 faecal samples (18%) tested positive with the field IMS-LFD test, 140 (32%) tested positive by IMS-qPCR, and 64 (15%) tested positive by IMS-culture, with only three faecal samples (0.7%) testing positive by all three tests (Fig. 3a). Given the $LOD_{50\%}$ of the IMS-LFD assay applied to badger faeces indicated above, a positive result with this assay should indicate the presence of ~10^5 *M. bovis* cells/ml, which should be visible microscopically. Acid-fast bacteria attached to the magnetic beads were observed for several of the IMS-LFD

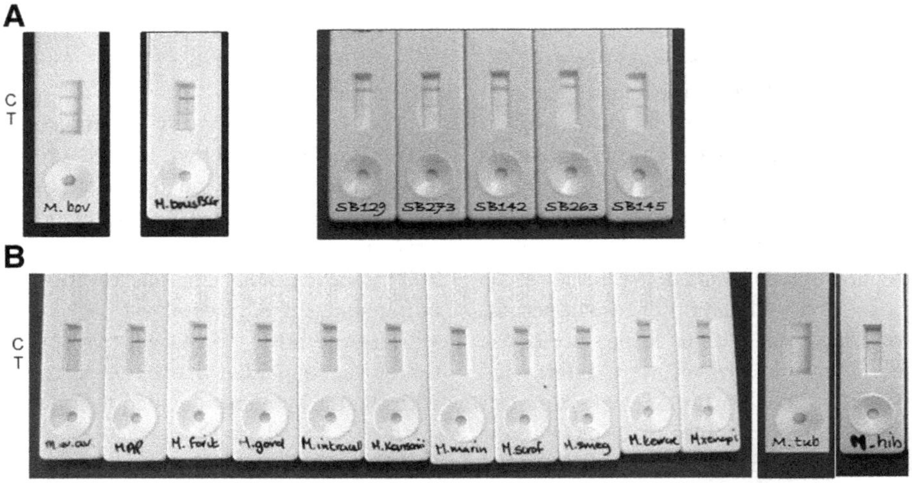

Fig. 2 Outcomes of specificity testing of the prototype lateral flow immunochromatographic device (LFD) demonstrating (**a**) the presence of a positive T-line with *Mycobacterium bovis* AF2122/97, *M. bovis* BCG NCTC 5692 and five other *M. bovis* spoligotypes and (**b**) only the presence of a C-line for all other *Mycobacterium* spp. tested

positive faecal samples, providing confirmation that high numbers of acid-fast bacteria (assumed to be *M. bovis*) were indeed present when an IMS-LFD positive result was obtained.

Field IMS-LFD results were compared with results of the two laboratory IMS-based methods; neither of which was being considered as the gold standard method for detecting *M. bovis* in faeces. There was no significant association between the results of field IMS-LFD, IMS-qPCR or IMS-culture ($P > 0.05$). Kappa statistics indicated 'poor' agreement between IMS-LFD and IMS-qPCR results (Kappa = −0.009, 95% CI: -0.095 to 0.077, $p = 0.838$) and 'slight' agreement (Kappa = 0.045, 95% CI: -0.054 to 0.144, $p = 0.342$) between IMS-LFD and IMS-culture results (Table 1A).

Estimation of the relative diagnostic specificity and sensitivity of the IMS-LFD assay by testing faeces from badgers of known infection status

The TB infection status of the 100 badgers from Woodchester Park that had contributed the faecal samples tested was only revealed to laboratory staff once results became available for the IMS-based tests. The badgers were categorised as putative 'TB infected' if a positive result had been obtained for Stat-Pak®, culture or IFN-γ EIA tests on any test occasion previously, and as putative 'non-

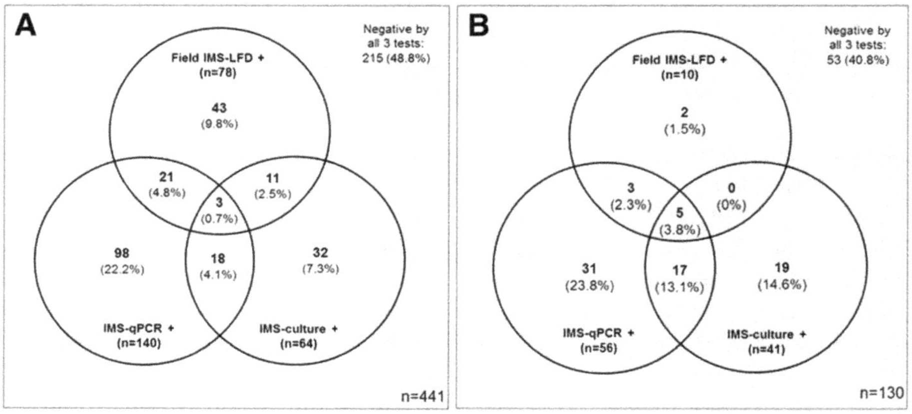

Fig. 3 Venn diagrams showing the numbers (percentage) of faeces samples that tested positive by field IMS-LFD, IMS-qPCR and IMS-culture from 441 badgers of unknown infection status collected from latrines at main setts in Northern Ireland (**a**) and from 100 live captured badgers and 30 captive putative TB negative badgers for which independent live animal diagnostic test data were available (**b**). Areas of overlap indicate positive test results in common

Table 1 Cross-tabulation of field IMS-LFD, IMS-qPCR and IMS-culture results for 441 badger faecal samples freshly collected from latrines at main setts in Northern Ireland (A), and 130 faecal samples obtained from live captured or captive badgers of putative known TB infection status (B)

(A)						
Field test result	Laboratory-based test results:					
	IMS-qPCR +	IMS-qPCR -	Kappa ± SE (significance)	IMS- culture +	IMS- culture -	Kappa ± SE (significance)
IMS-LFD +	24	54	−0.009 ± 0.044	14	64	0.045 ± 0.051
IMS-LFD -	116	247	(p = 0.838 [NS])	50	313	(p = 0.342[NS])
Total	140	301		64	377	
(B)						
Field test result	Laboratory-based test results:					
	IMS-qPCR +	IMS-qPCR -	Kappa ± SE (significance)	IMS- culture +	IMS- culture -	Kappa ± SE (significance)
IMS-LFD +	8	2	0.129 ± 0.056	5	5	0.083 ± 0.063
IMS-LFD -	48	72	(p = 0.014*)	36	84	(p = 0.083[NS])
Total	56	74		41	89	

[NS] no significant association, * P<0.05, significant association at the 95% level

infected' if a negative result had been obtained for all three live animal tests on each previous testing occasion. Overall, there were 62 faecal samples from putative 'TB infected' and 38 from putative 'non-infected' badgers in this cohort. The field IMS-LFD tested positive for 10% of faecal samples obtained by enema from these 100 live captured badgers, whilst IMS-qPCR and IMS-culture tested positive for 56% and 41% of samples, respectively. Five (3.8%) samples tested positive by all three IMS based tests (Fig. 3b). Two samples tested positive by the IMS-LFD test and not by either of the other two IMS-based tests. All of the 30 faeces from putative 'non-infected' captive badgers tested negative by field IMS-LFD, IMS-qPCR and IMS-culture, so no false positive IMS-LFD results were obtained. Overall, Kappa statistics indicated 'poor' agreement between IMS-LFD and IMS-qPCR results (Kappa = 0.129, 95% CI: 0.019 to 0.238, p = 0.014) and also between IMS-LFD and IMS-culture results (Kappa = 0.083, 95% CI: -0.056 to 0.221, p = 0.083) for the 130 faeces samples tested (Table 1B).

Cross-tabulation of badger infection status (on the basis of prior live animal diagnostic test results) with IMS-LFD, IMS-qPCR and IMS-culture results (Table 2) enabled estimates of relative diagnostic specificity (Sp) and sensitivity (Se) to be obtained using McNemar's test. IMS-qPCR and IMS-culture had much higher diagnostic Se (0.581 and 0.436, respectively) than the IMS-LFD test (0.081) (Table 2). However, the IMS-LFD test had greater diagnostic Sp (0.926) than either IMS-qPCR (0.706) or IMS-culture (0.794) (Table 2).

Discussion

The IMS-LFD test described here was developed with a view to it being a rapid and non-invasive test to detect the presence of whole *M. bovis* cells in badger faeces. To our knowledge, the prototype LFD developed is the first of its kind. Other *M. bovis* LFDs are available commercially, but these detect either serum antibodies to *M. bovis* (BrockTB Stat-Pak® assay or DPP® CervidTB assay, both Chembio Diagnostic Systems, Inc., Medford, NY), or the MPT64 antigen secreted by members of the *Mycobacterium tuberculosis* complex, which includes *M. bovis*, in liquid culture (BD MGIT™ TBc Identification Test, Becton, Dickinson and Company, NJ; SD Bioline TB Ag MPT 64, Standard Diagnostics, Inc., Gyeonggi-do, Republic of Korea; Capilia TB-Neo kit, TAUNS Laboratories, Inc., Shizuoka, Japan). The unique specificity of the LFD developed during this study is due to the particular monoclonal antibody conjugated to gold nanoparticles and used as the detector reagent in the novel LFD; for commercial reasons, no further details of this antibody can be provided. The novel *M. bovis*-specific LFD was used in combination with a modified IMS technique (involving smaller magnetic beads) in order to capture and concentrate *M. bovis* cells from the faeces matrix and remove gross faecal components that could potentially block movement of the beads along the LFD.

When 441 badger faeces samples collected from latrines at main setts throughout Northern Ireland were tested by the IMS-LFD assay, IMS-qPCR and IMS-culture, *M. bovis* was detected in 18%, 32% and 15% of faecal samples respectively (Fig. 3a). There was little agreement between the results of the three IMS-based tests. Whilst the same faecal homogenate was tested by all three methods, different volumes of material were tested in the field (by IMS-LFD) and in the laboratory (by IMS-qPCR and IMS-culture). Automated IMS in the laboratory was restricted to analysing 1 ml of sample whereas the field IMS was carried out on a 6–8 ml volume of filtered faecal homogenate. We estimate that there was the equivalent

Table 2 Estimates of the diagnostic specificity (Sp) and sensitivity (Se) of the field IMS-LFD and laboratory-based IMS-qPCR and IMS-culture tests for *M. bovis* in faeces from 100 live captured badgers and 30 live captive badgers relative to live diagnostic test results, obtained using McNemar's test (95% confidence intervals are indicated in parentheses)

Test result	Putative TB infected	Putative Non-infected	Total	Diagnostic sensitivity, Se	Diagnostic specificity, Sp
IMS-LFD +	5	5	10	0.081	0.926
IMS-LFD -	57	63	120	(0.027–0.178)	(0.837–0.976)
	62	68	130		
IMS-qPCR +	36	20	56	0.581	0.706
IMS-qPCR -	26	48	74	(0.449–0.705)	(0.583–0.811)
	62	68	130		
IMS-culture +	27	14	41	0.436	0.794
IMS-culture -	35	54	89	(0.310–0.567)	(0.678–0.882)
	62	68	130		

of ~250 mg faeces per 80 µl bead sample applied to the LFD after IMS in the field, ~5 mg faeces per IMS-qPCR reaction, and ~80 mg faeces per IMS-culture (assuming no losses during sample processing), so the higher volume of sample used for the IMS-LFD assay may explain the few extra samples which tested positive by the field IMS-LFD test (Fig. 3a). That said, we estimated in preliminary studies [25] the $LOD_{50\%}$ of IMS-qPCR to be 1.7×10^4 *M. bovis* cells/ml of faeces homogenate (or 1.7×10^5 *M. bovis* cells/g faeces), indicating that the IMS-qPCR method should theoretically have greater detection sensitivity than the field IMS-LFD assay (which was found to have an $LOD_{50\%}$ of 2.8×10^5 *M. bovis* cells/ml of faecal homogenate or 2.8×10^6 *M. bovis* cells/g faeces). This being the case, more *M. bovis* positive faecal samples should have been detected by IMS-qPCR than by IMS-LFD, which was the situation during this study. Furthermore, differently sized magnetic beads were used in the field and laboratory tests, because only the smaller (300 nm) coated beads would pass along the LFD. Despite being coated with the same *M. bovis*-specific binders, we know that the 300 nm Ademtech beads have slightly less capture capability than the 1 µm MyOne Tosylactivated Dynabeads; this may also have influenced results obtained for the field IMS-LFD test compared to the laboratory IMS-based tests. We also suspect, but cannot demonstrate, that various environmental, logistical and practical considerations may have influenced the faecal sample preparation and IMS capture steps in the field, potentially leading to non-optimal performance of the IMS-LFD test. Some or all of these factors may have contributed to, and hence explain, the lack of agreement between field IMS-LFD and laboratory IMS-based test results. Test results for badger faeces collected from latrines at setts have demonstrated for the first time that the novel LFD is capable of detecting *M. bovis* cells in naturally contaminated badger faeces. However, due to the lack of agreement between results of the different IMS-based tests (Table 1A), with the lowest number of *M. bovis* positive samples being detected by IMS-LFD, results suggest that the novel IMS-LFD assay would be of limited use for badger TB surveillance purposes. Although the LFD was shown to have unique specificity for *M. bovis* (Fig. 2), the analytical sensitivity indicated by the $LOD_{50\%}$ of the combined IMS-LFD assay (2.8×10^5 *M. bovis* cells/ml faecal homogenate) means that only badgers shedding high numbers of *M. bovis* in their faeces would be detected, and infected badgers shedding lower numbers of *M. bovis* would test negative by the IMS-LFD assay. Given its reasonably high $LOD_{50\%}$, the novel IMS-LFD test may be more suited for applications where high numbers of *M. bovis* would be encountered, such as confirming the isolation of *M. bovis* from animal tissues in liquid cultures in the veterinary diagnostic laboratory context. This possibility is currently being investigated.

The ability of a novel diagnostic test to correctly identify infected and non-infected animals is an important consideration, so in order to determine the relative diagnostic sensitivity and specificity of the novel IMS-LFD assay, we tested 130 faeces samples from badgers for which independent diagnostic test results were available. Of these, the IMS-LFD tested positive in 10 (7.7%) cases, whilst 56 (43.0%) and 41 (31.5%) samples tested positive by IMS-qPCR and IMS-culture, respectively (Fig. 3a). Test results for the subset of 30 faeces samples from putative TB negative captive badgers indicated that all samples were IMS-LFD, IMS-qPCR and IMS-culture negative; thus providing evidence of the high relative specificity of the novel IMS-LFD test, and indeed the other two IMS-based tests. The IMS-LFD test was found to have high diagnostic Sp (0.926) but low diagnostic Se (0.018), relative to the comparator live animal diagnostic tests, indicating an inability to detect low numbers of *M. bovis* cells in faeces, whereas IMS-qPCR and IMS-culture had lower diagnostic Sp (0.706 and 0.794, respectively) but higher diagnostic Se (0.581 and 0.436, respectively). It is acknowledged that potential mis-classification of the TB infection status of the badgers in our study due to false negative live animal test results may have impacted our estimates of the sensitivity and specificity of IMS-based tests (Table 2), so the latter should be treated with caution and only as relative measures of test performance.

The percentages of badger faeces samples from Woodchester Park testing *M. bovis* positive by IMS-qPCR and IMS-culture reported here appear relatively high. However 62 of the 100 faeces samples we tested were from putative 'TB infected' badgers with at least one previous positive live animal test result. Hence the 8.1%, 58% and 43.5% which tested IMS-LFD, IMS-qPCR and IMS-culture positive, respectively, could be considered as the percentage of *M. bovis* faecal positives amongst putative 'TB infected' badgers only. However, it is notable that the presence of *M. bovis* was also indicated by one or more of the IMS-based tests in 25 (65.8%) of 38 faeces samples from putative 'non-infected' badgers (Fig. 4). This was unexpected since faecal shedding of *M. bovis* by badgers has been generally associated with advanced disease [9], and may be intermittent and heterogeneous [12]. It is possible that some of these putative 'non-infected' badgers were misclassified as such owing to limitations in live test performance [31]. Also, in the cases of the IMS-LFD and IMS-qPCR tests, positive results could have arisen from the detection of dead *M. bovis* cells originating from the environment and not indicative of infection, although an IMS-culture test positive result requires mycobacterial growth and so indicates the presence of live viable bacteria. In conclusion, the present study was not designed to provide estimates of the proportion of badgers shedding viable *M. bovis* in their faeces, rather to test the performance of novel non-invasive tests, nevertheless our results suggest that further investigation of the extent of faecal shedding in badgers is warranted.

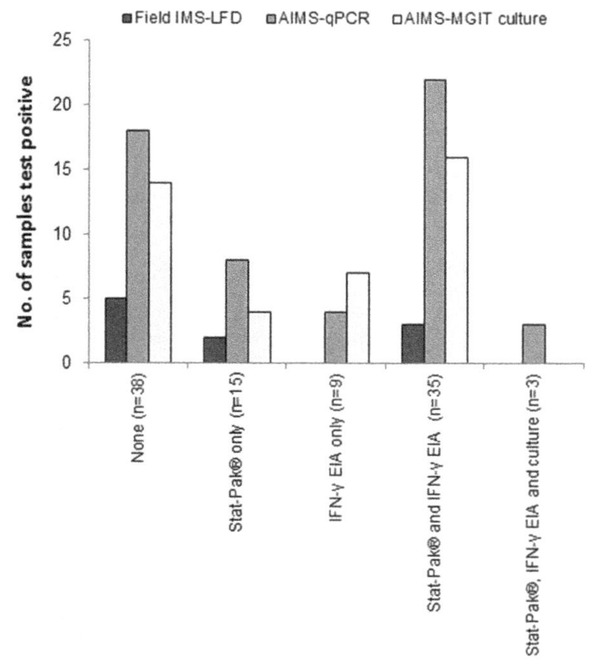

Fig. 4 Relationships between the IMS-based test results for 100 faeces samples from badgers in the Woodchester Park study area and the *M. bovis* infection status of these badgers as indicated by results of contemporaneous or previous Stat-Pak®, culture and Interferon-gamma tests

In this study, *M. bovis* cells were concentrated and selectively captured by IMS from several millilitres of an homogenate of approximately 1 g faeces in PBS in advance of detection by LFD, qPCR and culture during this study; a testing approach that has never been used before on badger faeces. The traditional badger faeces testing approach would be to decontaminate faecal suspensions in PBS with 0.75% cetylpyridinium chloride overnight prior to culture in liquid and/or solid media [10] or to extract total community DNA from approximately 0.1 g faeces prior to *M. bovis*-specific qPCR [12]. By testing a larger quantity of faeces, selectively isolating *M. bovis* cells prior to DNA extraction as well as separating them from PCR inhibitors by IMS, and not employing chemical decontamination which is known to have an adverse impact on the viability of *M. bovis* cells [32, 33], the chances of detection/isolation of *M. bovis* from faeces were likely to have been improved. The three IMS-based methods do not have equivalent detection sensitivity, so it is not surprising that the least sensitive test (IMS-LFD assay) detected lower numbers of *M. bovis* positive faecal samples than both IMS-qPCR and IMS-culture (Fig. 3a and b). Stewart et al. [22] previously reported that IMS-qPCR and IMS-culture improved detection rates of *M. bovis* in cattle lymph nodes compared to direct qPCR and chemical decontamination and culture. Results of the present study suggest that a similar boost in *M. bovis* detection rates has generally been observed by applying these IMS-based methods to test badger faeces. IMS applied to faeces samples in advance of application to the LFD should in theory have improved the detection sensitivity of the LFD, since *M. bovis* cells were concentrated from 6 ml faecal homogenate into 200 ul before testing. In reality, despite the fact that smaller (300 nm) paramagnetic beads were employed, samples after field IMS on faeces samples did not always run easily along the LFD due to bead aggregation. Consequently, detection sensitivity actually decreased and this was not simply due to a sample matrix effect. Results of a subsequent ring trial study to compare IMS-LFD and direct LFD with other methods for detecting *M. bovis* in badger faeces showed that fewer positive results were obtained after IMS than by direct LFD testing [34].

Conclusions

A novel prototype *M. bovis*-specific LFD was successfully developed which, in combination with IMS, was shown to be capable of detecting *M. bovis* cells in some badger faeces samples tested during this study. However, there was generally little agreement between results of field IMS-LFD and laboratory-based IMS-qPCR and IMS-culture tests; the IMS-LFD assay detected the lowest percentage of *M. bovis*-infected badger faecal samples, reflective of its higher $LOD_{50\%}$. The novel IMS-LFD test was shown to have relatively high diagnostic Sp (0.926, 95% CI: 0.837–0.976) but low diagnostic sensitivity (0.081, 95% CI: 0.027–0.178), relative to a suite of other live animal diagnostic tests. In light of these findings, the potential of the novel IMS-LFD test for *M. bovis* in badger faeces as a non-invasive field test for badger surveillance purposes would appear to be potentially limited to detecting badgers shedding high numbers of *M. bovis* ($\geq 10^5$ CFU/g) in their faeces. Alternative applications for the novel *M. bovis*-specific LFD are currently being explored.

Abbreviations

95% CI: 95% Confidence Interval; CFU: Colony-forming units, expressed per ml or g; C-line: Control line on LFD; DNA: Deoxyribonucleic acid; IFN-γ EIA: Interferon Gamma Enzyme Immuno Assay; IgG: Immunoglobulin G; IMS: Immunomagnetic Separation; IMS-LFD: Immunomagnetic separation followed by lateral flow device test; IMS-culture: Immunomagnetic separation followed by culture in BD MGIT culture medium; IMS-qPCR: Immunomagnetic separation followed by quantitative PCR; LFD: Lateral flow device; $LOD_{50\%}$: 50% limit of detection; Mab: Monoclonal antibody; Pab: Polyclonal antibody; PBS: Phosphate buffered saline, pH 7.2; PBS-T: PBS containing 0.05% Tween 20; PCR: Polymerase chain reaction; qPCR: Quantitative PCR; RTA: Road traffic accidents; Se: Diagnostic sensitivity; Sp: Diagnostic specificity; TB: Tuberculosis, in this case bovine tuberculosis; T-line: Test line on LFD

Acknowledgements

We would wish to thank Dr. Jim McNair, Veterinary Sciences Division, Agri-Food and Biosciences Institute for Northern Ireland, for providing access to one of the antibodies evaluated as part of this study, all the Northern Ireland farmers/landowners who permitted access to their land for collection of badger faeces, and the field team of the National Wildlife Management Centre at Woodchester Park for the live capture and sampling of badgers in their study area.

Funding

This research study was funded by the Department of Environment, Food and Rural Affairs (Defra), United Kingdom (Project SE3271). Neil Reid was supported by the Natural Heritage Research Partnership between the Northern Ireland Environment Agency and *Quercus*, Queen's University Belfast. We also thank Defra for funding the Woodchester Park study.

Authors' contributions

LDS processed faecal samples for IMS-qPCR and IMS-culture. NT and PM developed the prototype LFD using reagents supplied by LDS and IRG. JMA collected badger faeces samples from NI setts and performed field IMS-LFD. NR and WIM advised JMA on locations of badger setts throughout NI and sample collection. RN assisted LDS to perform qPCR on all samples. RJD and RA contributed faecal samples from badgers and associated live animal test results. NR and IRG performed statistical analysis of results. LDS and IRG conceived and designed the study, prepared tables and figures, and wrote the manuscript. All authors contributed to the final version of the manuscript.

Competing interests

We declare no competing interests, financial or otherwise.

Consent for publication

Not applicable.

Ethics approval

Ethics approval was not required for Northern Ireland part of the study, as only badger faeces not live badgers were involved. The capture of wild badgers at Woodchester Park is undertaken under licence from Natural England, and sampling under anaesthesia is conducted under a UK Home Office Project Licence. All live animal work was approved by the Animal and Plant Health Agency (APHA) Animal Welfare Ethical Review Process. All captive animal procedures were covered by licenses issued by the UK Home Office under the Animals (Scientific Procedures) Act 1986, and also approved by the Animal Welfare and Ethical Review Board at APHA.

Author details

[1]Institute for Global Food Security, School of Biological Sciences, Queen's University Belfast, Belfast, Northern Ireland, UK. [2]Forsite Diagnostics Limited (now Abingdon Health), National Innovation Campus, Sand Hutton, York, UK. [3]Quercus, School of Biological Sciences, Belfast, Northern Ireland, UK. [4]National Wildlife Management Centre, Animal and Plant Health Agency, Woodchester Park, Nympsfield, Gloucestershire, UK. [5]Animal and Plant Health Agency, Weybridge, New Haw, Addlestone, Surrey, UK.

References

1. Gallagher J, Clifton-Hadley RS. Tuberculosis in badgers: a review of the disease and its significance for other animals. Res Vet Sci. 2000;69:203–17.
2. Wilson GJ, Carter SP, Delahay RJ. Advances and prospects for management of TB transmission between badgers and cattle. Vet Microbiol. 2011;151:43–50.
3. Independent Study Group on Cattle TB. Bovine TB: The Scientific Evidence. 2007. [http://www.bovinetb.info/docs/final_report.pdf]. Accessed 8 May 2017.
4. Wright DM, Reid N, Montgomery WI, Allen AR, Skuce RA, Kao RR. Herd-level bovine tuberculosis risk factors: assessing the role of low-level badger population disturbance. Sci Rep. 2015;5:13062.
5. Skuce RA, Neill SD. Molecular epidemiology of *Mycobacterium bovis*: exploiting molecular data. Tuberculosis. 2001;81:169–75.
6. Haddad N, Masselot M, Durand B. Molecular differentiation of *Mycobacterium bovis* isolates: review of main techniques and applications. Res Vet Sci. 2004;76:1–18.
7. Olea-Popelka FJ, Flynn O, Costello E, McGrath G, Collins JD, O'Keeffe J, Kelton DF, Berke O, Martin SW. Spatial relationship between *Mycobacterium bovis* strains in cattle and badgers in four areas in Ireland. Prev Vet Med. 2005;71:57–70.
8. Little TWA, Naylor PF, Wilesmith JW. Laboratory study of *Mycobacterium bovis* infection in badgers and calves. Vet Rec. 1982;111:550–7.
9. Clifton-Hadley RS, Wilesmith JW, Stuart FA. *Mycobacterium bovis* in the European badger (*Meles meles*): epidemiologic findings in tuberculous badgers from a naturally infected-population. Epidemiol Infect. 1993;111:9–19.
10. Corner LAL, O'Meara D, Costello E, Lesellier S, Gormley E. The distribution of *Mycobacterium bovis* infection in naturally infected badgers. Vet J. 2012;194:166–72.
11. Hutchings MR, Service KM, Harris S. Defecation and urination patterns of badgers *Meles meles* at low density in south west England. Acta Theriol. 2001;46:87–96.
12. King HC, Murphy A, James P, Travis E, Porter D, Hung Y-J, Sawyer J, Cork J, Delahay RJ, Gaze W, Cortenay O, Wellington EM. The variability and seasonality of the environmental reservoir of *Mycobacterium bovis* shed by wild European badgers. Sci Rep. 2015;5:12318.
13. Wellington EM, Courtenay O. Badgers and bovine TB: how can environmental microbiology help? Microbiol Today. 2014;41:143–4.

14. Young JS, Gormley E, Wellington EMH. Molecular detection of *Mycobacterium bovis* and *Mycobacterium bovis* BCG (Pasteur) in soil. Appl Environ Microbiol. 2005;71:1946–52.
15. Courtenay O, Reilly LA, Sweeney FP, Hibberd V, Bryan S, Ul-Hassan A, Newman C, Macdonald DW, Delahay RJ, Wilson GJ, Wellington EMH. Is *Mycobacterium bovis* in the environment important for the persistence of bovine tuberculosis? Biol Lett. 2006;2:460–2.
16. Cheeseman CL, Wilesmith JW, Stuart FA. Tuberculosis: the disease and its epidemiology in the badger: a review. Epidemiol Infect. 1989;103:113–25.
17. Abernethy DA, Denny GO, Menzies FD, McGuckian P, Honhold N, Roberts AR. The Northern Ireland programme for the control and eradication of *Mycobacterium bovis*. Vet Microbiol. 2006;112:231–7.
18. Abernethy DA, Walton E, Menzies F, Courcier E, Robinson P. *Mycobacterium bovis* surveillance in European badgers (*Meles meles*) killed by vehicles in Northern Ireland: an epidemiological evaluation. 2011. [https://www.daera-ni.gov.uk/sites/default/files/publications/dard/m-bovis-surveillance-european-badgers-rta-epi-eval.pdf]. Accessed 8 May 2017.
19. Krebs J, Anderson R, Clutton-Brock T, Morrison I, Young D, Donnelly C. Bovine Tuberculosis in cattle and badgers.Report by the Independent Scientific Review Group. Ministry of Agriculture, Fisheries and Food, London. 1997. [http://www.bovinetb.info/docs/krebs.pdf]. Accessed 8 May 2017.
20. Delahay RJ, Walker N, Smith GS, Wilkinson D, Clifton-Hadley RS, Cheeseman CL, Tomlinson AJ, Chambers MA. Long-term temporal trends and estimated transmission rates for *Mycobacterium bovis* infection in an undisturbed high density badger population. Epidemiol Infect. 2013;141:1445–56.
21. Stewart LD, McNair J, McCallan L, Thompson S, Kulakov L, Grant IR. Production and evaluation of antibodies and phage display-derived peptide ligands for immunomagnetic separation of *Mycobacterium bovis*. J Clin Microbiol. 2012;50:1598–605.
22. Stewart LD, McNair J, McCallan L, Grant IR. Improved detection rates of *Mycobacterium bovis* infection in bovine lymph node tissue using immunomagnetic separation (IMS)-based methods. PLoS One. 2013;8:e58374.
23. AOAC International. Final report and executive summaries from the AOAC International. Presidential Task Force on Best Practices in Microbiological Methodology 2006. [http://www.fda.gov/downloads/Food/FoodScienceResearch/UCM088702.pdf]. Accessed 8 May 2017.
24. Department of Environment, Food and Rural Affairs.EVID4 Final Report on Defra Project SE3271: Development and field validation of a rapid immunomagnetic separation-lateral flow (IMS-LF) test for detecting *Mycobacterium bovis* infection in badgers and/or badger setts. 2014. [http://randd.defra.gov.uk/Document.aspx?Document=13141_SE3271.pdf]. Accessed 8 May 2017.
25. Reid N, Etherington TR, Wilson G, Montgomery WI, McDonald RA. Monitoring and population estimation of the European badger *Meles meles* in Northern Ireland. Wildlife Biol. 2011;18:46–57.
26. Sweeney FP, Courtenay O, Hibberd V, Hewinson RG, Reilly LA, Gaze WH, Wellington EMH. Environmental monitoring of *Mycobacterium bovis* in badger feces and badger sett soil by real-time PCR, as confirmed by immunofluorescence, immunocapture, and cultivation. Appl Environ Microbiol. 2007;73:7471–3.
27. Travis ER, Gaze WH, Pontiroli A, Sweeney FP, Porter D, Mason S, Keeling MJC, Jones RM, Sawyer J, Aranaz A, Castellanos Rizaldos E, Cork J, Delahay RJ, Wilson GJ, Hewinson RG, Courtenay O, Wellington EMH. An inter-laboratory validation of a real time PCR assay to measure host excretion of bacterial pathogens, particularly of *Mycobacterium bovis*. PLoS One. 2011;6:e27369.
28. Zumárraga MJ, Meikle V, Bernardelli A, Abdala A, Tarabla H, Romano MI, Cataldi A. Use of touch-down polymerase chain reaction to enhance the sensitivity of *Mycobacterium bovis* detection. J Vet Diag Invest. 2005;17:232–8.
29. Dalley D, Dave D, Lesellier S, Palmer S, Crawshaw T, Hewinson RG, Chambers M. Development and evaluation of a gamma-interferon assay for tuberculosis in badgers (*Meles meles*). Tuberculosis. 2008;88:235–43.
30. Landis JR, Koch GG. The measurement of observer agreement for categorical data. Biometrics. 1977;33:159–74.
31. Drewe JA, Tomlinson A, Walker NJ, Delahay RJ. Diagnostic accuracy and optimal use of three tests for tuberculosis in live badgers. PLoS One. 2010; 5(6):e11196.
32. Corner LAL, Trajstmann AC. An evaluation of 1-hexadecylpyridinium chloride as a decontaminant in the primary isolation of *Mycobacterium bovis* from bovine lesions. Vet Microbiol. 1988;18:127–34.
33. Ambrosio SR, de Deus Oliveira EM, Rosales Rodriguez CA, Ferreira Neto JS, Amaku M. Comparison of three decontamination methods for *Mycobacterium bovis* isolation. Braz J Microbiol. 2008;39:241–4.
34. Department of Environment, Food and Rural Affairs. Final Project Report SE3289: A study to comparatively assess diagnostic methods for detection of *M. bovis* in badger faeces. London: Department for Environment, Food and Rural Affairs; 2015. [http://randd.defra.gov.uk/Document.aspx?Document=13243_SE3289.pdf]. Accessed 8 May 2017.

17

Bovine respiratory syncytial virus seroprevalence and risk factors in non-vaccinated dairy cattle herds in Brazil

Ingrid Bortolin Affonso Lux Hoppe[1*], Andréa Souza Ramos de Medeiros[1], Clarice Weis Arns[2] and Samir Issa Samara[1]

Abstract

Background: The cattle industry is one of the most important Brazilian agribusiness sectors and is a strong contributor to the national economy. Annually about 44.6 million calves are bred, which makes the optimal management of these animals extremely important. Several diseases can affect the initial stages of the bovine production chain, being the bovine respiratory syncytial virus (BRSV) one of the most relevant pathogens. This study aimed to characterize the epidemiology of BRSV infection in dairy cattle herds of São Paulo State, Brazil, using serological and risk factors analyses. For that, 1243 blood samples were collected of animals from 26 farms and a questionnaire about possible risk factors for BRSV prevalence was performed. The obtained blood sera were analyzed using virus neutralization test (VNT).

Results: VNT results showed high BRSV prevalence in dairy cattle herds, reaching 79.5% of seropositivity. The BRSV seroprevalence among studied farms ranged from 40 to 100%. The analysis of risk factors indicated that the age group and the occurrence of coinfection with bovine herpesvirus 1 (BoHV-1) and bovine viral diarrhea virus 1 (BVDV-1) should be associated with a higher prevalence of BRSV, while natural suckling was considered a protective factor.

Conclusions: The study showed that adult animals over 1 year old are an important risk factor for the high seroprevalence of BRSV in herds. The high BRSV prevalence associated with BoHV-1 and BVDV-1 suggests that biosecurity measures should be applied in order to reduce viral dissemination. Additionally, the natural suckling may be an important management to protect calves from high BRSV seroprevalence.

Keywords: Bovine respiratory syncytial virus, Seroprevalence, Risk factors, Dairy cattle herds

Background

Bovine respiratory syncytial virus (BRSV) is an economically significant pathogen in cattle production [1], as it is one of the most important causes of lower respiratory tract infections in calves [2]. In dairy cattle, BRSV infection usually occurs in young calves aged between 2 weeks and 9 months [3]. Adult animals with subclinical infection are the main source of infection, since reinfections are common in the herds [1, 4, 5].

* Correspondence: ibaffonso@gmail.com
[1]Faculdade de Ciências Agrárias e Veterinárias (FCAV), Departamento de Medicina Veterinária Preventiva e Reprodução Animal, Univ Estadual Paulista – UNESP, Via de Acesso Prof. Paulo Donato Castellane, km 05, Jaboticabal, São Paulo CEP: 14.884-900, Brazil
Full list of author information is available at the end of the article

BRSV, bovine herpesvirus 1 (BoHV-1), bovine viral diarrhea virus (BVDV) and bovine parainfluenza type-3 (PI-3) are considered primary agents involved in the bovine respiratory complex. Additionally, secondary infection by *Pasteurella multocida*, *Histophilus somni* and mycoplasmas contribute to the aggravation of the disease [6]. Clinical signs are characterized by respiratory symptoms, initially with moderated intensity, such as nasal and ocular discharges which can be aggravated leading to pneumonia. However, mainly in calves, an acute and severe onset is also observed, due to maternal antibodies not effectively protect against BRSV infection [3].

Considering the high prevalence of the disease, several studies determined risk factors involved in the epidemiology of BRSV. In Europe, risk factors were mainly attributed to herd size, herd density, purchasing of new animals, geographic location of the farms, herd type and concomitant BVDV infection [7–11]. Similar studies have also been performed in some Latin American countries and they showed that most of the animals probably have already been exposed to the virus with consequent high BRSV prevalence in cattle herds. In these countries, herd size, age group, presence of bordering farms, herd type and geographic location of the farms were the main risk factors associated with BRSV infection [12–16].

In Brazil, BRSV was first diagnosed in calves in the state of Rio Grande do Sul [17] and some studies have shown that BRSV infection is widespread in Southern and Southeastern Brazil, with high serological prevalence rates [18–20]. Nevertheless, research has not been conducted in order to verify possible risk factors involved in BRSV epidemiology. Due to this, the current study aimed to determine antibody prevalence against BRSV and investigate some risk factors associated with BRSV seroprevalence in herds of an important milk producing region in São Paulo State, Brazil.

Methods

Study area and sample collection

The study was performed on 26 dairy cattle herds in 12 municipalities in the Northern region of the São Paulo State, Southeastern Brazil. This region produces about 10 million liters of milk annually [21]. The evaluated herds had between 6 and 150 animals and no animals were vaccinated against the pathogens associated with respiratory diseases. The farms were located in a region classified as Aw by the climatic classification of Koeppen, characterized by dry winter with average temperature higher than 18 °C in the coldest month and precipitation below 60 mm in the driest month. The altitude of these areas was 440 to 617 m above sea level [22].

Sampling of each farm was calculated [23] with an expected BRSV prevalence of 80% [19] with acceptable error of 5% and confidence level of 95%. After setting the number of samples, bovines of all categories and age group were randomly selected. According to the management adopted in the herds, the age group was defined as ≤12 months old "calf" and > 12 months old "adult". In some farms, the number of samples collected was higher than that suggested by the mathematical calculation, once it was also used for serodiagnosis of BoHV-1 and BVDV-1. On farms with a small herd size, up to 30 animals, all of them were sampled.

The samples from 1243 animals were collected from April 2012 to June 2012 as shown in Table 1. Blood samples were collected by jugular or coccygeal vein puncture using disposable needles and vacuum tubes. Samples remained at room temperature for 1 h for coagulation and after being transported refrigerated to the laboratory, they were centrifuged at 1080×*g* for 10 min to obtain the sera. The sera were aliquoted in 1.5 mL identified microtubes that were stored in freezer at − 20 °C until analyses.

Table 1 Total of blood samples collected in 26 dairy cattle herds in the Northern region of the São Paulo State, Southeastern Brazil

Dairy cattle herds	Total number of animals	Number of blood samples		Total of samples
		Adult	Calf	
1	75	47	25	72
2	38	21	14	35
3	88	50	23	73
4	55	31	20	51
5	50	25	19	44
6	120	41	25	66
7	7	5	2	7
8	9	9	0	9
9	120	85	16	101
10	150	81	37	118
11	36	24	12	36
12	120	83	36	119
13	80	59	18	77
14	40	28	3	31
15	40	26	9	35
16	15	10	5	15
17	26	20	6	26
18	15	12	3	15
19	60	37	13	50
20	100	61	27	88
21	16	11	5	16
22	6	6	0	6
23	52	37	11	48
24	22	19	3	22
25	62	44	17	61
26	22	19	3	22
Total		**891**	**352**	**1243**

Virus neutralization test

The presence of antibodies to BRSV was tested by virus neutralization test (VNT). Serum samples were thawed, inactivated in water bath at 56 °C for 30 min, and diluted in duplicates from 1:2 to 1:1024 in 96-well microplates with 50 μL of 200 $TCID_{50}$ BRSV suspended in Eagle's minimum essential medium (DIFCO E-MEM®). The viral strain was previously titrated [24]. Following incubation at 37 °C in 5% CO_2 atmosphere for 1 h, 50 µL of Madin & Darby Bovine Kidney (MDBK) cells suspension, in E-MEM and 10% bovine fetal serum solution were added to the wells. Then, the plates were re-incubated in similar conditions for 96 h. Each test included a back titration and cell culture control. Samples were positive when cytopathic effect was inhibited at 1:2 dilution, and the titration was expressed as the inverse of the dilution, as geometric mean.

Risk factors

During the sample collection, a questionnaire was administered to the owner or manager of each farm with the purpose of identifying potential risk factors related to epidemiology of BRSV. Thus, the questionnaire was designed according to data of risk factors described in the literature [8, 10, 15, 16] in addition to the information of the management adopted in dairy farms of São Paulo State. The variables explored were: herd size (≤75, > 75 animals), herd density (≤5, > 5 animals/hectare), age group (≤12 months old "calf", > 12 months old "adult"), breed (Holstein, mixed), type of reproduction (natural mating, artificial insemination), purchase of animals (last 6 months: yes, no), cleaning of facilities (often, rarely), historical of respiratory disease (last 6 months: yes, no), quarantine (yes, no), abortions (yes, no), BoHV-1 infection (serodiagnosis: yes, no), BVDV-1 infection (serodiagnosis: yes, no), type of calves housing (individual, collective), type of calves feeding (natural suckling, artificial), presence of others domestic animals (yes, no), presence of wild ruminant animals (yes, no).

The variables "herd size" and "herd density" were based on the average data; "age group" was defined from the management adopted on the farms; "quarantine" refers to the isolation of purchased animals before adding them to the herd. The serodiagnosis of BoHV-1 and BVDV-1 was performed at the same time as BRSV (unpublished data). The variables "disinfection of the umbilical cord" and "colostrum feeding" were not analyzed because these practices were applied in all dairy farms visited. Additionally, the data related to climatic classification and altitude were not included in the analysis because they were similar in all 26 farms.

Statistical analysis

The chi-square tests were employed to compare the BRSV, BoHV-1 and BVDV-1 seropositivity and also with "age group". Fisher's exact test was used to compare BRSV status according to the expected prevalence of 80% (≥80%, "high"; < 80%, "low") and the other variables. Only the variables with $p < 0,2$ (two-tailed Fisher) were analyzed by a logistic regression model. The analyses were performed using the Epi Info™ program v. 7.0.

Results

Serum samples from 1243 animals belonging to 26 dairy cattle herds were taken and tested by VNT, in which 988 (79.5%) were seropositive to BRSV. Regarding the age group, 87% (767/ 891) of the serum samples were positives for adult animals while the prevalence rate in calves was 62.8% (352/221). Antibodies to BRSV were detected in all cattle herds, with prevalence rates ranging from 40 to 100%. The mean antibody titers for adult animals was 2 to 512, and for calves, 2 to 32. Therefore, prevalence of BRSV both in herds and animals was considered high.

The chi-square test showed association of BRSV seropositivity with "age group" and animals tested seropositives to BoHV-1 and BVDV-1 (Table 2). Nevertheless, the Fisher's exact test only detected statistical difference with the variable "type of calves feeding" (Table 3). In this case, the relative risk (RR) value was less than one, i.e., the factor "natural suckling" was considered protective. Logistic regression (values of $p < 0.2$, two-tailed Fisher) did not show significant results, suggesting that the variables analyzed were not risk factors for the high seroprevalence of BRSV in the studied population.

Discussion

This is the first epidemiological study to assess risk factors for BRSV seroprevalence carried out in Brazil. Even though BRSV prevalence of 79.5% in the animals sampled was similar to that estimated, the prevalence in adult animals was higher than that expected, reaching 87% of samples. In calves, the seroprevalence was lower than that found in adult animals (62.8%) and could be even lower once VNT does not allow the distinction between antibodies from colostrum and natural infection. Thus, this study demonstrated that the prevalence of BRSV antibodies was higher in adult animals, as previously reported in other countries [13, 16].

Adult animals are associated with high seroprevalence of BRSV as consequence of a repeated exposure to the virus infection throughout their life and possibility of reinfections. Similarly, the highest antibody titers were associated with non-vaccinated adult cattle, probably due to the exposure to successive viral reinfections, which results in a booster effect on antibody titers [25]. Other factor related to high antibody titers is recent BRSV infections, which can be confirmed only by paired serology, antibody screening in calves after the period of colostral antibody detection or viral detection by direct methods. As respiratory disease was not reported in half of the herds studied, it is indicative that BRSV infection can be subclinical. This is consistent with previous reports [2]. Herds can remain free of clinical BRSV infection for many years even in areas of high prevalence of the virus [26].

Table 2 Risk factors associated with BRSV in 1243 animals from 26 dairy cattle herds in São Paulo State, Brazil

Factor		BRSV		Relative risk (RR)	Confidence interval (CI) (95%)		*p* value
		Positive	Negative		Limit inferior	Limit superior	
Age group	> 12 months (adult)	775	116	1.44	1.32	1.57	< 0.0001
	≤12 months (calf)	213	139				
BoHV-1	Seropositive	565	85	1.22	1.15	1.29	< 0.0001
	Seronegative	423	170				
BVDV-1	Seropositive	298	33	1.19	1.13	1.25	< 0.0001
	Seronegative	690	222				

The presence of other pathogens is also associated with the prevalence of BRSV [8, 11, 14, 16]. This information explains the association of BRSV serological prevalence with the prevalences of BoHV-1 and BVDV-1. The infection by these viral agents is also reported in Brazilian herds, with high prevalences [27, 28]. BVDV infection can cause impairment of the animal's immune function and thereby decrease resistance to other infections [8]. The synergistic effects of BVDV with other respiratory pathogens have been observed [29, 30]. Thus, health status of the herds may also be affected indirectly by BVDV control measures [8].

Table 3 Risk factors associated with high and low bovine respiratory syncytial virus prevalence at herd level in 26 dairy cattle herds in São Paulo State, Brazil

Factor	Condition	BRSV status		RR	CI (95%)		*p* value
		High	Low		Limit inferior	Limit Superior	
Herd size (> 75 animals)	Yes	3	2	1.40	0.59	3.34	0.422
	No	9	12				
Herd density (> 5 animals/ha)	Yes	5	4	1.34	0.60	3.05	0.387
	No	7	10				
Breed (Holstein)	Yes	7	7	1.20	0.51	2.81	0.488
	No	5	7				
Type of reproduction (natural mating)	Yes	2	8	0.32	0.09	1.17	0.420
	No	10	6				
Purchasing of animals (last six months)	Yes	6	10	0.63	0.28	1.41	0.237
	No	6	4				
Cleaning of facilities (rarely)	Yes	7	9	0.88	0.38	2.01	0.536
	No	5	5				
Historical of respiratory disease (last six months)	Yes	7	6	1.40	0.60	3.28	0.347
	No	5	8				
Quarantine (absence)	Yes	10	11	1.19	0.37	3.81	0.578
	No	2	3				
Abortions	Yes	5	6	0.97	0.42	2.26	0.632
	No	7	8				
Type of calves housing (collective)	Yes	9	14	0.39	0.24	0.65	0.085
	No	3	0				
Type of calves feeding (natural suckling)	Yes	3	10	0.33	0.12	0.96	0.023
	No	9	4				
Presence of others domestic animals	Yes	11	13	0.92	0.21	3.92	0.720
	No	1	1				
Presence of wild ruminant animals	Yes	5	9	0.61	0.26	1.43	0.224
	No	7	5				

Dairy cattle herds in São Paulo State usually have poor biosecurity measures, such as the lack of quarantine of newly purchased animals, lack of diagnosis of respiratory diseases (particularly for BRSV) and vaccination is rarely performed against these viruses. Therefore, we hypothesized that risk factors for the seroprevalence of BoHV-1, BVDV-1 and BRSV in the studied population likely to overlap.

Despite the logistic regression not confirming "type of calves feeding" variable as a risk factor for high prevalence of BRSV, the Fisher's exact test detected "natural suckling" as a protective factor. "Natural suckling" would be important as it may be able to reduce the risk of calves becoming infected by BRSV. Weaning can be stressful and results in impaired immune function, which may further exacerbate a BRSV exposure. Suckling reduces the occurrence of diarrhea, prevents the abnormal behavior of cross-suckling of other calves and improves animal health [31, 32]. Prior to the current study there have been no report about "natural suckling" and its relationship with BRSV seroprevalence or its role as a protective factor, therefore, based on the results presented, it has the potential to decrease seroprevalence to BRSV.

Similarities were observed among the results found at the present study and those previously obtained by others conducted in Brazil [18–20]. In Latin America countries, equivalents prevalences of BRSV have also been reported [12, 14–16], as well as difficulties in detecting the risk factors involved in the dissemination of the agent, even using different forms of sampling and analyzing a considerable number of variables. Thus, the dynamics of infection may differ even in a particular country or geographic area [26].

The high serological prevalence of BRSV found in this study shows the importance to know more about this infection since it is not considered important in the country, mainly due to the lack of diagnosis. The awareness of the risk factors involved in the BRSV dissemination can allow understanding its mechanisms, even though, as in other studies, these factors were not very clear. Thereby, further studies as a complement to the current one should be performed until concrete information has been found.

Conclusions

Adult animals over 1 year old can present high seroprevalences of BRSV and are an important risk factor for the virus maintenance in herds. Additionally, the concomitant seroprevalence of BoHV-1 and BVDV-1 leads us to suggest that biosecurity measures to reduce viral dissemination could be applied. Non-stressful management, like keeping calves with their mothers promoting natural suckling, may constitute a practical management strategy to reduce the seroprevalence of BRSV in Brazilian dairy herds.

Abbreviations

BoHV-1: Bovine herpesvirus type-1; BRSV: Bovine respiratory syncytial virus; BVDV: Bovine viral diarrhea virus; CI: Confidence interval; MDBK: Madin & Darby Bovine Kidney; PI-3: Bovine parainfluenza type-3; RR: Relative risk; VNT: virus neutralization test

Acknowledgments

The authors thank Coordenadoria de Assistência Técnica Integral (CATI/SAASP) for providing the dairy cattle herds for the study, Dr. Estevam G. Lux Hoppe and Andressa de Souza Pollo for assistance with manuscript revision.

Funding

This work was supported by Fundação de Amparo à Pesquisa do Estado de São Paulo, FAPESP (financial grant 2010/15912-7 and doctoral scholarship 2010/06950-2).

Authors' contributions

IBALH and ASRM performed the experiment. IBALH analyzed the data and prepared the manuscript. IBALH, CWA and SIS designed the study and revised the manuscript. All authors read and approved the final manuscript.

Consent for publication

Not applicable.

Competing interests

The authors declare that they have no competing interests.

Author details

[1]Faculdade de Ciências Agrárias e Veterinárias (FCAV), Departamento de Medicina Veterinária Preventiva e Reprodução Animal, Univ Estadual Paulista - UNESP, Via de Acesso Prof. Paulo Donato Castellane, km 05, Jaboticabal, São Paulo CEP: 14.884-900, Brazil. [2]Instituto de Biologia, Universidade Estadual de Campinas - UNICAMP, Cidade Universitária, Caixa-postal: 6109, Campinas, São Paulo CEP: 13.083-970, Brazil.

References

1. Baker JC, Frey M. Bovine respiratory syncytial virus. Vet Clin North Am Food Anim Pract. 1985;1:259–72.
2. Larsen LE. Bovine respiratory syncytial virus (BRSV): a review. Acta Vet Scand. 2000;41:1–24.
3. Baker JC, Ames TR, Belknap EB, Dubovi EJ, Bryson DG, Kelling CLBRSV. (Bovine respiratory syncytial virus) infection: its pathogenesis, diagnosis, prevention and treatment. Vet Med. 1993;88:880–906.
4. Baker JC, Ames TR, Markham RJF. Seroepizootiologic study of bovine respiratory syncytial virus in a dairy herd. Am J Vet Res. 1986;47:240–5.
5. Stott EJ, Taylor G. Respiratory syncytial virus: brief review. Arch Virol. 1985;84:1–52.
6. Juaréz F, Trigo F, Chávez G, Vargas R. Identificación de agentes virales por inmunohistoquímica en enfermedades respiratórias de bovinos en corral de engorda. Vet Mexico. 2003;34:1–12.

7. Elvander M. Severe respiratory disease in dairy cows caused by infection with bovine respiratory syncytial virus. Vet Rec. 1996;138:101–5.
8. Luzzago C, Bronzo V, Salvetti S, Frigerio M, Ferrari N. Bovine respiratory syncytial virus seroprevalence and risk factors in endemic dairy cattle herds. Vet Res Commun. 2010;34:19–24.
9. Norstöm M, Skjerve E, Jarp J. Risk factors for epidemic respiratory disease in Norwegian cattle herds. Prev Vet Med. 2000;44:87–96.
10. Ohlson A, Heuer C, Lockhart C, Travén M, Emanuelson U, Alenius S. Risk factors for seropositivity to bovine coronavirus and bovine respiratory syncytial virus in dairy herds. Vet Rec. 2010;167:201–6.
11. Yesilbag K, Güngör B. Seroprevalence of bovine respiratory viruses in North-Western Turkey. Trop Anim Health Prod. 2008;40:55–60.
12. Costa M, García L, Yunus AS, Rockemann DD, Samal SK, Cristina J. Bovine respiratory syncytial virus: first serological evidence in Uruguay. Vet Res. 2000;31:241–6.
13. Figueroa-Chávez D, Segura-Correa JC, García-Márquez LJ, Pescador-Rubio A, Valdivia-Flores AG. Detection on antibodies and risk factors for infection with bovine respiratory syncytial virus and parainfluenza virus 3 in dual purpose farms in Colima, Mexico. Trop Anim Health Prod. 2012;44:1417–21.
14. Obando RC, Hidalgo M, Merza M, Montoya A, Klingeborn B, Moreno LJ. Seroprevalence to bovine virus diarrhoea virus and other viruses of the bovine respiratory complex in Venezuela (Apure state). Prev Vet Med. 1999; 41:271–8.
15. Saa LR, Perea A, Jara DV, Arenas AJ, Garcia-Bocanegra I, Borge C, Carbonero A. Prevalence of and risk factors for bovine respiratory syncytial virus (BRSV) infection in non-vaccinated dairy and dual-purpose cattle herds in Ecuador. Trop Anim Health Prod. 2012;44:1423–7.
16. Solís-Calderón JJ, Segura-Correa JC, Aguilar-Romero F, Segura-Correa VM. Detection of antibodies and risk factors for infections with bovine respiratory syncytial vírus and parainfluenza virus-3 in beef cattle of Yucatan, Mexico. Prev Vet Med. 2007;82:102–10.
17. Gonçalvez IPD, Simanke AT, Jost HC, Hötzel I, Dal Soglio A, Moojen V. Detection of bovine respiratory syncytial virus in calves of Rio Grande do Sul, Brazil. Cienc Rural. 1993;23:389–90.
18. Affonso IB, Gatti SP, Alexandrino B, Oliveira MC, Medeiros ASR, Buzinaro MG, Samara SI. Detection of antibodies against bovine respiratory syncytial virus (BRSV) in dairy cattle with different prevalences of bovine herpesvirus type 1 (BHV-1) in São Paulo State, Brazil. Semin: Cien Agrar. 2011;32:295–300.
19. Arns CW. Vírus respiratório sincicial dos bovinos (BRSV): Situação no Brasil. In: 1° Simpósio Pfizer sobre doenças infecciosas e vacinas para bovinos; 1996; Guarulhos, Brasil.
20. Campalans J, Arns CW. Serological evidence of bovine respiratory syncytial virus in Brazil. Virus Rev Res. 1997;2:50–6.
21. IBGE. Instituto Brasileiro de Geografia e Estatística. Produção da Pecuária Municipal, 2016, Brasil. 2016. https://biblioteca.ibge.gov.br/visualizacao/periodicos/84/ppm_2016_v44_br.pdf Acessed 10 Jan 2018.
22. CEPAGRI. Centro de Pesquisas Meteorológicas e Climáticas Aplicadas à Agricultura. Campinas: UNICAMP; 2017. http://www.cpa.unicamp.br. Accessed 14 Feb 2017
23. Astudillo VM. Encuestas por muestreo para estudios epidemiologicos en poblaciones animales. Rio ce Janeiro: Centro Panamericano de Fiebre Aftosa, 1979. 60p. (Serie de Manuales Didacticos, 12).
24. Reed LJ, Muench HA. Simple method of estimating 50 per cent end point. Am J Hyg. 1938;27:493–7.
25. Van der Poel WH, Kramps JA, Middel WG, Van Oirschott JT, Brand A. Dynamics of bovine respiratory syncytial virus infections: a longitudinal epidemiological study in dairy herds. Arch Virol. 1993;133:309–21.
26. Ohlson A, Alenius S, Travén M, Emanuelson U. A longitudinal study of the dynamics of bovine corona virus and respiratory syncytial virus infections in dairy herds. Vet J. 2013;197:395–400.
27. Del Fava C, Pituco EM, D'Angelino JL. Herpesvirus bovino tipo 1 (HVB-1): revisão e situação atual no Brasil. Rev Educ Contin CRMV-SP. 2002;5:300–12.
28. Flores EF, Weiblen R, Vogel FSF, Roehe PM, Alfieri AA, Pituco EM. A infecção pelo vírus da diarreia viral bovina (BVDV) no Brasil – histórico, situação atual e perspectivas. Pesqui Vet Bras. 2005;25:125–34.
29. Liu L, Lehmkuhl HD, Kaeberle ML. Synergistic effects of bovine respiratory syncytial virus and noncytopathic bovine viral diarrhea virus infection on selected bovine alveolar macrophage functions. Can J Vet Res. 1999;63:41–8.
30. Loneragan GH, Thomson DU, Montgomery DL, Mason GL, Larson RL. Prevalence, outcome and health consequences associated with persistent infection with bovine viral diarrhoea virus in feedlot cattle. J Am Vet Med Assoc. 2005;226:595–601.
31. Flower FC, Weary DM. The effects of early separation on the dairy cow and calf. Anim Welf. 2003;12:339–48.
32. Wagenaar JP, Langhout J. Practical implications of increasing natural living through suckling systems in organic dairy calf rearing. NJAS Wagening J Life Sci. 2007;54:375–86.

18

The effectiveness of colostral antibodies for preventing bovine leukemia virus (BLV) infection in vitro

Misako Konishi[1], Hiroshi Ishizaki[2], Ken-ichiro Kameyama[3], Kenji Murakami[4] and Takehisa Yamamoto[1*]

Abstract

Background: Bovine leukemia virus (BLV) is the causative agent of enzootic bovine leukosis (EBL). The incidence of EBL in Japan is increasing annually; and the cases of EBL in cattle younger than 2 years old has been reported. Therefore, it is vital to find a method to control BLV infection, especially in young calves. In this study, to evaluate the protective ability of colostral antibodies against BLV infection, as well as the potential for BLV infection mediated by colostrum/milk, we investigated temporal fluctuations in the anti-BLV antibody titer and BLV proviral load (PVL) in colostrum/milk and peripheral blood of six infected dams during lactation. The association between PVL and antibody titer in colostrum and peripheral blood was then investigated using samples from a further twenty-seven cattle. Antibody concentrations were measured with a Syncytium-induction Inhibition Assay using colostral/milk whey and serum. PVL in peripheral blood and colostrum was measured by real-time PCR.

Results: Colostral antibodies showed high inhibitory activity until day 3 of lactation. The antibody titer and PVL in peripheral blood showed lesser changes than those in colostrum/milk throughout lactation. The colostral antibody titer was significantly higher than the serum antibody titer in all samples, whereas the colostrum PVL was significantly lower than the blood PVL. The blood PVL showed a significant correlation with serum antibody titer, colostrum PVL, and colostral antibody titer. However, there were no major correlations between the serum and colostral antibody titers.

Conclusions: This is the first report investigating the temporal changes in colostral antibody titer in terms of inhibiting BLV infection in vitro. The results of antibody detection by Syncytium-induction Inhibition Assay suggested that the protective activity of the colostral antibodies against BLV infection would be conferred by anti-BLV gp51 antibody. The high antibody titer of colostral whey suggests that colostral whey could be a potential source of antibodies with a low risk of infection in neonatal calves.

Keywords: Bovine leukemia virus, Colostral antibody, Proviral load, Prevention

Background

Bovine leukemia virus (BLV), a member of the family *Retroviridae*, is the causative agent of enzootic bovine leukosis (EBL). BLV infection is highly endemic in Japan [1]; despite of the low incidence of EBL (0.1–10% of BLV-infected cattle), the number of cattle diagnosed with EBL has increased in recent years. A nationwide investigation of the seroprevalence of BLV from 2009 to 2011 revealed that more than 20% of dairy cattle were already infected with BLV at less than 1 year old [1]. Although tumors caused by BLV are typically seen in animals over 3 years of age [2], infected calves have the potential to be affected by EBL at a younger age. Recently, several cases of EBL in cattle younger than 2 years old were reported in Japan [3]. The loss of young successor or fattening cattle can cause major economic damage to farms. Even if they are not affected by EBL, these animals would shed the virus within the farm for a longer time than cows infected at an older age. Therefore, preventing BLV infection in calves is vital for preventing the spread of the virus and reducing its

* Correspondence: mtbook@affrc.go.jp
[1]Epidemiology Unit, Division of Viral Disease and Epidemiology, National Institute of Animal Health, NARO 3-1-5 Kannondai, Tsukuba, Ibaraki 305-0856, Japan
Full list of author information is available at the end of the article

economic impact. The target cells of BLV in cattle are B lymphocytes; thus, the blood, colostrum, and milk of infected cattle are known to be the major sources of infection [2, 4, 5]. On the other hand, several studies reported that anti-BLV antibodies found in the colostrum of BLV-infected cattle could protect newborn calves from BLV infection, both in vivo by experimentally infecting calves with BLV and through prospective studies without artificially infecting calves [6–9]. However, the mechanism of protection in the colostrum from infected dam is not clear, and its importance as an infection source has never been examined in vitro. Thus, the applicability of colostrum from infected dams to prevent BLV infection in neonatal calves remains controversial. In this study, to evaluate the protective ability of colostral antibodies against BLV infection, as well as the potential for BLV infection mediated by colostrum/milk, we investigated the fluctuations in the antibody titer and proviral load (PVL) in the colostrum/milk and peripheral blood of infected dams during the lactation period. Moreover, the association between PVL and the antibody titer in the colostrum and peripheral blood were investigated.

Results

Fluctuations in BLV antibody titer and PVL in colostrum/milk

The changes in antibody titer, somatic cells (SCs) count (SCC), and PVL in cattle colostrum/milk in experiment 1 are presented in Fig. 1. The antibody titer was highest at day 1 and 3 of lactation, decreased drastically from day 5, and became undetectable from day 7 until the end of sampling. SCC also achieved a peak at day 1 and 3 of lactation in three of six infected cattle and three of four non-infected cattle; levels were maintained at under 4.5×10^6 cells/ml from day 5 in all cattle, except one infected cow, which showed levels of almost 2.0×10^6 cells/ml at 1 month into the lactation period. Low levels of BLV proviral DNA were detected in infected cattle until day 7 of lactation, but concentrations were undetectable or 0.9–1 copy/10 ng DNA from day 14 until the end of the sampling period. The non-infected cattle all showed negative results for both Syncytium-induction Inhibition Assay (SIIA) and real-time PCR.

Fluctuations in BLV antibody titer and PVL in blood

The changes in the antibody titer, PVL, and number of lymphocytes in the blood of cattle in experiment 1 are presented in Fig. 2. The antibody titers in the sera of infected cattle ranged from 16 to 512 throughout the study period; no major decreases or increases were observed. The number of lymphocytes was approximately constant in each sample throughout the study period, ranging from $28.8–121.1 \times 10^2$ /μl in infected cattle, and $21.7–47.7 \times 10^2$ /μl in non-infected cattle. Fluctuations were observed in blood PVL, but levels were maintained at $0.7–3.1 \times 10^3$ copies/10 ng DNA throughout the study period. The non-infected cattle all showed negative results for both SIIA and real-time PCR.

Antibody titer and PVL in colostrum and blood samples

The colostral antibody titers from the twenty-seven infected cattle in experiment 2 ranged from 64 to 1024 (mean value: 644.7), whereas the serum antibody titers ranged from 16 to 512 (mean value: 134.5). The antibody titer in colostrum was significantly higher than that in blood ($p < 0.05$) (Fig. 3a). Proviral DNA was detected in 74.1% (20/27) of cattle in experiment 2. The PVL in colostrum ranged from 0 (not detected) to 254.6 copies/10 ng DNA (mean value: 21.6 copies/10 ng DNA), while that in blood ranged from 0.1 to 4363.3 copies/10 ng DNA (mean value: 1166.1 copies/10 ng DNA). The PVL in colostrum was significantly lower than that in blood ($p < 0.05$) (Fig. 3b).

Correlation between PVL and antibody titer in blood and colostrum

The correlations between PVL and antibody titer in blood and colostrum are presented in Fig. 4. Statistical analysis indicated that PVL in the blood showed a significant correlation with serum antibody titer, colostral antibody titer, and PVL in colostrum ($p < 0.05$). The correlation coefficients (r) between blood PVL and serum antibody titer, colostral antibody titer, and colostrum PVL were 0.69, 0.59, and 0.53, respectively. However, a significant correlation was not found between colostral antibody titer and serum antibody titer ($r = 0.37$, $p = 0.06$), and PVL in colostrum ($r = 0.57$, $p = 0.06$).

Discussion

To evaluate the protective ability and infectivity of colostrum/milk from cattle infected with BLV, the temporal changes in antibody titer and PVL in colostrum/milk were investigated. Performing SIIA with whey samples allowed us to quantitatively measure the antibody titer in colostrum/milk. Although previous studies measured the antibody levels in colostrum and milk using ELISA [10, 11], we chose to use SIIA to measure antibody titers because one of the aims of this study was to determine the protective mechanism of colostral antibodies against BLV infection. Thus, this is the first report to investigate the temporal changes in the colostral antibody titer in terms of its protective ability against BLV infection in vitro. The results of antibody detection by SIIA revealed that colostrum from infected cattle inhibited syncytium induction caused by BLV infection. Syncytium formation results from cell-to-cell fusion caused by BLV gp51, an outer membrane

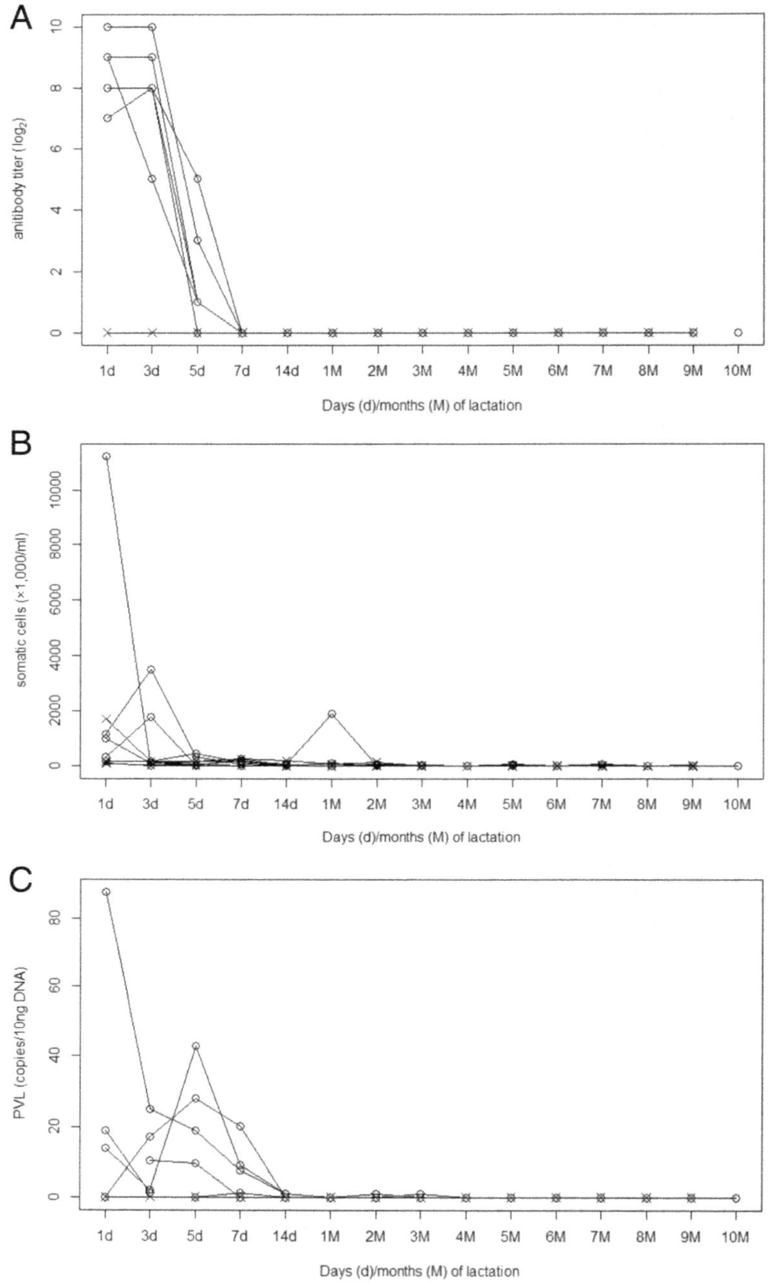

Fig. 1 Temporal changes in anti-BLV antibody titer, somatic cell counts, and PVL in colostrum/milk. The temporal changes in (**a**) antibody titer; (**b**) somatic cell counts (SCC); and (**c**) PVL in colostrum/milk of BLV-infected cattle (o) and non-infected cattle (×)

glycoprotein [12, 13]. Previous studies showed the complement-dependent cytotoxicity of anti-gp51 antibody [14, 15], and previous studies hypothesized that the protective effect of BLV infection mediated by immunoglobulin (Ig) G would be conferred by anti-glycoprotein antibodies [16]. Thus, it can be concluded that the protective effect of colostral antibodies in BLV-infected cattle against BLV infection was conferred by anti-gp51 antibody, as has been observed in serum.

The results of experiment 1 revealed the chronological changes in PVL and antibody titer in both colostrum/milk and peripheral blood. The colostral antibody titer peaked at day 3 of lactation and rapidly decreased beginning on day 5. It is known that the total Ig levels in milk

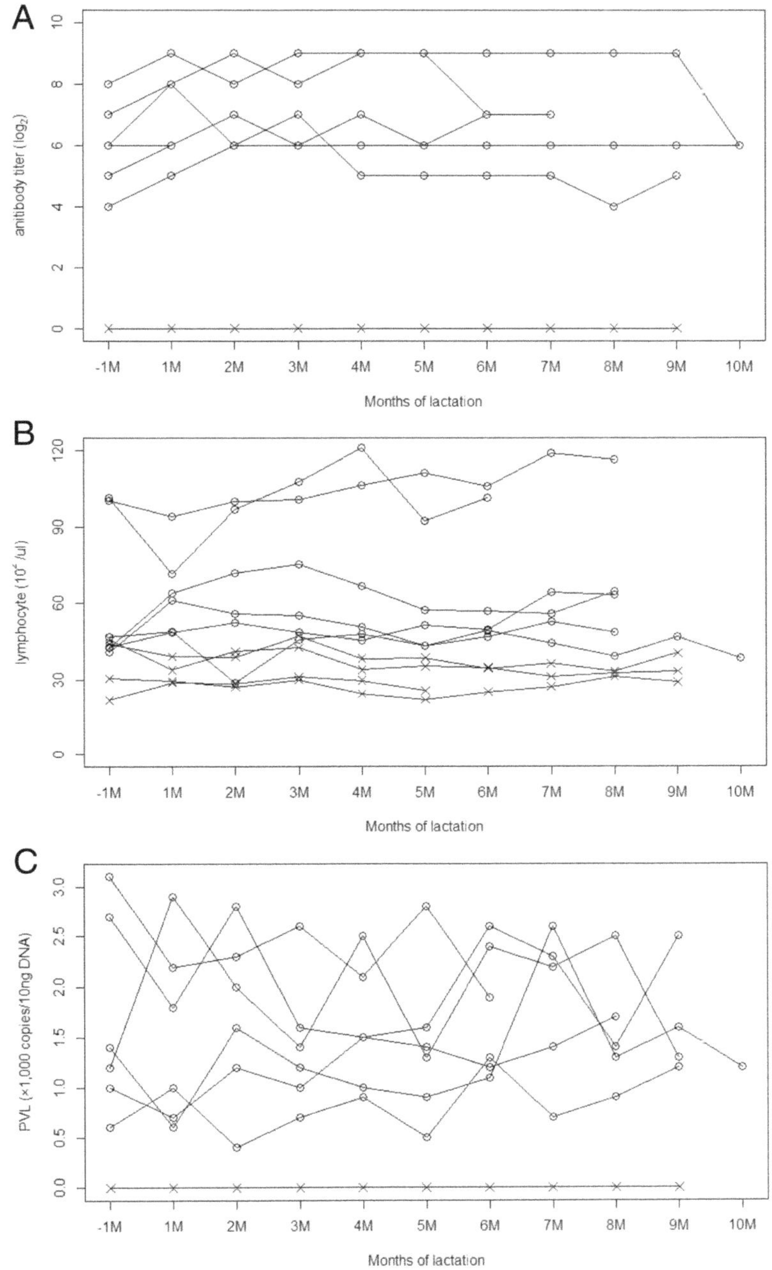

Fig. 2 Fluctuations in anti-BLV antibody titer, lymphocyte counts, and peripheral blood PVL. Fluctuations in (**a**) antibody titer; (**b**) lymphocyte count; and (**c**) PVL in peripheral blood of BLV-infected cattle (○) and non-infected cattle (×). All measurements were taken from 1 month before the delivery date

decline rapidly during the first 5 days after delivery [17, 18]. Thus, the decrease in anti-BLV antibody reflected the decrease in Igs during the transition from colostrum to mature milk. On the other hand, PVL in colostrum was lower than that in blood, and gradually decreased after day 5 of lactation. Most samples were negative for PVL after day 14 of lactation. These decreases in PVL in colostrum/milk seemed consistent with observed decreases in SCC. Since a portion of SCs were infected with BLV, a decrease in SCC would cause a decrease in PVL in colostrum/milk. Under normal circumstances, maternal antibodies and leukocytes contained in colostrum are absorbed through the intestinal epithelial cells of neonatal calves and delivered into their blood circulation. This capacity for absorption only lasts until 48 h after birth [19, 20]. Considering the low PVL in mature milk detected in this study and the decreased absorptive capacity of

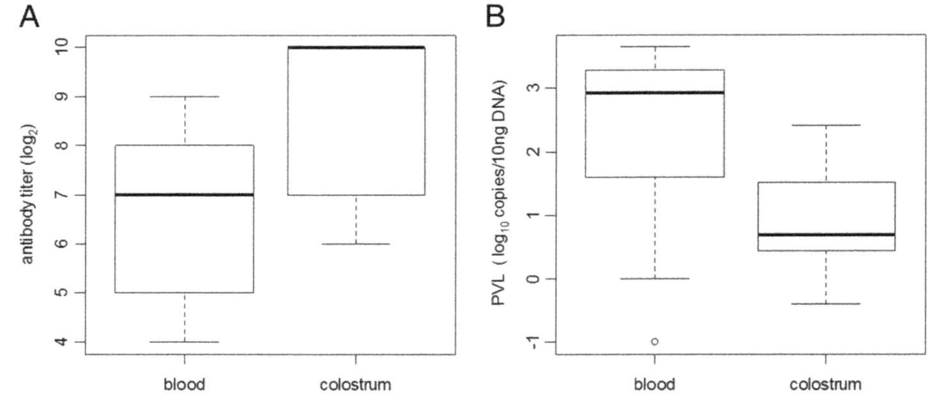

Fig. 3 Comparison of anti-BLV antibody titer and PVL in colostrum and blood of infected cattle. The distribution of (**a**) anti-BLV antibody titers and (**b**) PVL between colostrum and peripheral blood

calf intestinal epithelial cells, it is possible that the role of mature milk from infected dams as a source of infection is not a major one. However, although the stage of lactation was unknown, a previous study detected BLV proviral DNA in the milk of infected cattle by quantitative real-time PCR [11]. Thus, the PVL in milk would vary with individual, and feeding milk with high PVL to calves without maternal antibodies could cause BLV infection to the calves. Since the infection threshold of PVL in milk remains unknown, the risk of BLV infection via ingesting raw milk should be evaluated in future studies.

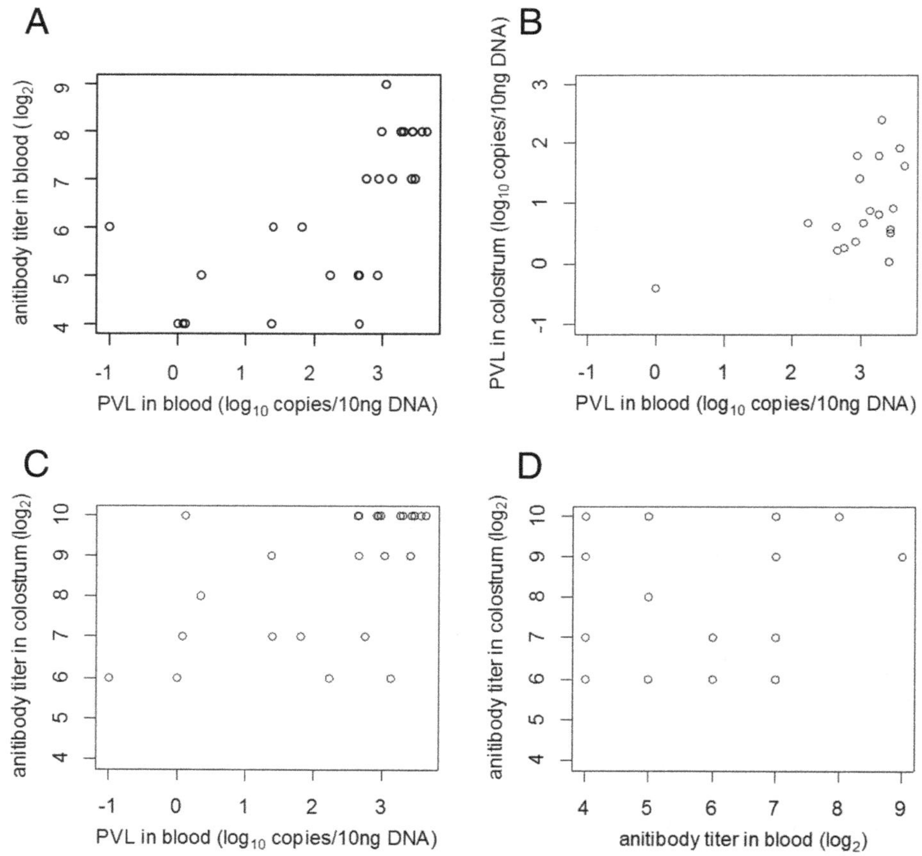

Fig. 4 Relationship between PVL of BLV and antibody titer in blood and colostrum. Correlation between (**a**) PVL in bloo\\\\\d and serum antibody; (**b**) PVL in blood and PVL in colostrum; (**c**) PVL in blood and colostral antibody; and (**d**) serum antibody and colostral antibody

The results of experiment 2 revealed that the antibody titer in colostrum was significantly higher than that in blood. Igs accumulate in the mammary gland during the prepartum dry period. Many different Igs, including IgG1, the predominant Ig in cattle, are selectively accumulated from blood circulation into the colostrum. It is known that this process causes 5- to 10-fold increases in the concentration of IgG1 in colostrum compared to maternal serum [17, 18]. Although the Ig class of the anti-gp51 antibody detected in this study was not investigated, we hypothesized that the increased antibody titer in colostrum compared to that in serum was the result of the selective accumulation of IgG1. On the other hand, PVL in colostrum was significantly lower than that in blood. In healthy cattle, the amount of PBL, SCC in colostrum, and SCC in mature milk of cattle are 4.9–12.0 × 10^3 /μl, 1.0–3.0 × 10^6 cells/ml, and 2.0 × 10^5 cells/ml, respectively [19, 21, 22]. The predominant cell type in colostrum/milk is macrophages, whereas that in PBL is lymphocytes [19, 22]. Recent studies showed that the fraction of lymphocytes in bovine PBL is ~ 50% [23, 24]. On the other hand, the percentage of lymphocytes in colostrum SCs has been reported as 22–25%; in contrast, B lymphocytes, the target cells of BLV, account for less than 5% of the total lymphocytes [19, 21]. We therefore concluded that the low levels of PVL in colostrum were caused by the smaller proportion of B lymphocytes in colostrum than in blood.

A significant correlation between PVL in blood and serum antibody titer, PVL in colostrum, and colostral antibody titer were found in this study. Our findings are consistent with previous studies reporting that the anti-BLV antibody titer in serum should reflect PVL in blood [10, 25]. As described above, leucocytes and antibodies in colostrum were transferred from the blood. Thus, PVL in colostrum should be consistent with the level of PVL in blood. However, there were no significant correlations between antibody titer in blood and that in colostrum even though colostral antibodies were also accumulated from maternal blood. Some infected cattle had high colostral antibody titers despite their low serum antibody titers. The selective accumulation of Igs in colostrum would cause a major increase in the colostral antibody titer in these cattle and might be a cause of the unclear relationship between antibody titer in the blood and colostrum. In addition, we observed that 33.3% (9/27) of colostral samples completely inhibited syncytium induction at 1024-fold dilution, the highest dilution limit in this study; therefore, we may have underestimated the antibody titers in these samples. The selective accumulation of Igs in colostrum and the possibility of higher than expected antibody titers may also be a cause of the non-significant correlation between colostral antibody titer and PVL in colostrum.

In this study, a strong protective ability of colostral whey against BLV infection was found in vitro. This result suggests that colostral whey has potential use as a source of anti-BLV antibodies in neonatal calves. A notable advantage of colostral whey as source of anti-BLV antibodies is the low risk of BLV infection. Since milk whey does not contain SCs, cell-to-cell BLV infection would not occur. Moreover, cell-free virus particles in the whey could be inactivated by heat treatment. Kono et al. [16] parenterally administrated an IgG solution derived from the sera of sheep experimentally infected with BLV to non-infected sheep. They then inoculated the sheep with 50 μl whole blood from BLV-infected sheep several days after administration. Sheep with a passive antibody titer of 64 or more (determined by an agar gel immunodiffusion test) were not infected with BLV by the inoculation [16]. Based on those results, we hypothesized that colostral whey antibodies could become a source of passive antibodies in calves by feeding them with colostral whey immediately after birth. However, breastfeeding is known as one of the major routes of mother-to-child transmission of HTLV-1, the related virus of BLV, even though maternal antibodies are present in breast milk [26]. Therefore, the actual protective ability of colostral antibodies must be evaluated in vivo. Moreover, the relationship between the dosage of antibodies in colostrum and passive antibody titers in neonatal sera, the relationship between serum antibody titer and its subsequent protective effects, the duration of antibody effectiveness, and the absence of transmission by heat-inactivated colostrum whey must be investigated in vivo in order to verify the utility and safety of colostral whey as an antibody source in BLV-infected cattle. It is necessary to find donor cattle with high colostral antibody titers to prepare sufficient doses of colostral antibody; a high blood PVL would be a useful index for the selection of donor cattle before delivery.

Conclusions

In this study, a strong protective activity of colostral antibodies against BLV infection was found in vitro. We considered that the protective effect of colostral antibodies in BLV-infected cattle against BLV infection was conferred by anti-gp51 antibody, as has been observed in serum. This result suggests that colostral whey has potential use as a source of anti-BLV antibodies in neonatal calves.

Methods

Animals and sample collection

In experiment 1, to investigate the temporal fluctuations in anti-BLV antibody titer in colostrum/milk and serum over the lactation period, colostrum/milk and blood samples were collected from six BLV-infected cattle and four non-infected cattle raised in a BLV-infected farm in Japan in 2014–2015. Blood samples were collected once a month from 1 month before the estimated date of delivery until the dry period; serum and peripheral blood leukocytes (PBL) were then extracted from the samples. Colostrum/milk samples were collected on day 1, 3, 5, 7, and 14 of lactation, and once a month from 1 month after the start of lactation until the dry-off date.

In experiment 2, twenty-seven BLV-infected cattle from a different BLV-infected farm in Japan were tested to examine the correlation between antibody titer and PVL. Colostrum was sampled at day 1 of lactation for each cow. In accordance with the owner's intention, blood collection from all cattle in experiment 2 was conducted on the same day. The time between blood collection and colostrum collection ranged from 0 to 6 months (mean: 2.7 months).

All cattle in this study were tested for BLV infection using a commercial Enzyme-linked immunosorbent assay (ELISA) kit (JNC, Tokyo, Japan) and real-time PCR. Cattle that were positive for both tests were classified as infected, and cattle that were negative for both tests were classified as non-infected. Real-time PCR was performed as described below. Serum and milk whey separation, as well as the isolation of PBL and SCs, were performed within 2 days after sampling. Then, each sample was stored at – 20 °C for further experiments.

Preparation of somatic cells and milk whey

Colostrum/milk samples (40 ml) were centrifuged at 3000 rpm for 20 min at 4 °C. The fat layer was removed using a micro-spatula, and milk whey was transferred to a new container. The precipitate was collected to isolate SCs and suspended in 1 ml phosphate-buffered saline (PBS). After the cells were counted using a TC20 automated cell counter (Bio-Rad Laboratories, Hercules, CA, USA), the cell suspension was centrifuged at 2000 rpm for 5 min at 4 °C. PBS was removed and cells were stored at – 20 °C until DNA extraction. Whey samples were prepared by centrifuging 12 ml milk whey at 30,000 rpm for 60 min at 4 °C. The whey samples were stored at – 20 °C until antibody titration, described below.

Leukocyte count

The number of leukocytes and lymphocytes in peripheral blood were counted using a veterinary hematology analyzer (Celltac Alpha, MEK-6450; Nihon-Kohden, Tokyo, Japan).

PBL isolation

PBL was isolated from 5 ml EDTA-treated blood according to the method previously described by Asfaw et al. [27].

DNA extraction

DNA was extracted from SCs and PBL using a commercial DNA extraction kit (DNeasy Blood & Tissue Kit; Qiagen, Hilden, Germany) according to the manufacturer's instructions.

Quantification of BLV PVL

To detect and quantify BLV proviral DNA, real-time PCR was performed using a TaqMan probe. Primers and probes were designed to target the BLV *tax* gene according to the complete BLV proviral sequence obtained via GenBank (accession No. K02120). Primers and probe were as follows: sense primer (BLVCG-tax-8008F), 5'-CCAT GTGACCGGTTACACGTAT-3′ (nucleotides [nt] 8008–8029); antisense primer (BLVCG-tax-8093R), 5'-ACCA ATTCGGACCAGGTTAGC-3′ (nt 8073–8093); and TaqMan MGB probe (BLVCGtax8034T_F), 5'-FAM-CAGT CCTCAGGCCTT-MGB-3′ (nt 8034–8048). A synthetic 186-bp DNA fragment was used as a positive control. The fragment, identical to nt 7958–8143 (K02120), was synthesized using GeneArt Strings DNA (Thermo Fisher Scientific, Waltham, MA, USA). Serial 10-fold dilutions of the positive control, ranging from 10 to 10^6 copies/5 µl, were used to draw a standard quantification curve. PCR was carried out using the QuantStudio 3 Real-time PCR System (Thermo Fisher Scientific) with the Premix EX-Taq (Perfect Real Time) kit (Takara Bio Inc., Shiga, Japan) according to the manufacturer's instructions at a final reaction volume of 25 µl. Each reaction mixture contained 0.25 µM each primer 0.1 µM TaqMan MGB probe, and 5 µl DNA sample. The concentration of DNA in each sample was measured using a NanoDrop ND-1000 (Thermo Fisher Scientific), and the amount of DNA in each well was adjusted to less than 100 ng/well. Amplification was performed according to the following conditions: initial denaturation at 95 °C for 30 s, followed by forty-two cycles of denaturation at 95 °C for 5 s and annealing at 60 °C for 34 s. The measured value was divided by the amount of DNA in each well, and PVL was expressed as copies/10 ng DNA.

Cell culture

CC81 cells, a feline cell line with high susceptibility to BLV, as well as fetal lamb kidney cells persistently infected with BLV (FLK-BLV), were used to measure the anti-BLV antibody titers as described below. CC81 cells were grown in Eagle's minimal essential medium (MEM) with 5% fetal bovine serum (FBS) and 10% tryptose phosphate broth. FLK-BLV cells were grown in Eagle's MEM with 5% FBS.

SIIA

SIIA was performed based as previously described by Kono et al. [14]. A rabbit complement (Standard Rabbit complement; Cedarlane Laboratories, Burlington, Canada) that had no inhibitory effects on syncytium formation in CC81 cells by FLK-BLV was used at a 1:10 dilution. FLK-BLV cells were adjusted to a concentration of 2×10^5 cells/ml, and CC81 cells were adjusted to a concentration of 1×10^6 cells/ml. Sera and whey samples were heated for 30 min at 56 °C and 60 °C, respectively. For the dilution of samples and complement, as well as cell suspension, MEM supplemented with 2% FBS (2% growth medium [GM]) was used. Equal volumes (25 µl) of serial twofold dilutions (1:2–1:1024) of samples, FLK-BLV cell suspensions, and rabbit complement were mixed in 96-well plates and incubated at 37 °C for 1 h in a CO_2-rich environment. Then, 25 µl CC81 cell suspension was added to each well and the plates were incubated for a further 2 days. Samples were tested in duplicate, and as a syncytium-positive control, 2% GM was added to eight wells instead of samples. As a syncytium-negative control, 2% GM was added to a further eight wells instead of the FLK-BLV cell suspension. The culture was stained with Giemsa and examined microscopically. Wells containing no syncytium were classified as anti-BLV antibody-positive. The antibody titer was expressed as the reciprocal of the highest serum dilution that showed a positive reaction. The antibody titer of samples that showed complete inhibition of syncytium induction in both wells of the 1024-fold dilution was designated as 1024.

Statistical analysis

Associations of the anti-BLV antibody titer and PVL with colostrum and blood were evaluated using the Wilcoxon signed rank test. Correlations between PVL in blood and antibody titer in blood and colostrum, as well as PVL in colostrum, were evaluated by Pearson's product-moment correlation coefficient. A value of $p < 0.05$ was considered statistically significant in all analyses. All statistical analyses were performed using R version 3.3.1 [28].

Abbreviations

BLV: Bovine leukemia virus; EBL: Enzootic bovine leukosis; ELISA: Enzyme-linked immunosorbent assay; FBS: Fetal bovine serum; GM: Growth medium; Ig: Immunoglobulin; MEM: Minimal essential medium; PBL: Peripheral blood leukocytes; PBS: Phosphate-buffered saline; PVL: Proviral load; SCC: Somatic cell count; SCs: Somatic cells; SIIA: Syncytium-induction Inhibition Assay

Acknowledgements

The authors thank the owners of the farms where the samples were obtained, as well as the staff of Nasu Operations Unit, Technical Support Center, Institute of Livestock and Grassland Science, NARO for their kindness and patience in sample collection; we also thank Ms. Miwa Sawai, Ms. Yuriko Taguchi, Dr. Yuka Okuwa (Prefectural government of Ishikawa), and Dr. Tomoko Kobayashi (Prefectural government of Tottori) for their technical support; finally, we thank Dr. Hiroshi Sentsui (Nihon University) for his helpful discussions.

Funding

This work was supported by Grants-in-Aid for Young Scientists (B) (Grant Number 26850203) from the Japan Society for the Promotion of Science (JSPS).

Authors' contributions

MK designed the study and wrote the initial draft of the manuscript. HI and KK participated in sample collection and processing. KM designed the real-time PCR experiments. TY performed statistical analysis, supervised the study, and reviewed the manuscript. All authors have read and approved the final manuscript.

Ethics approval and consent to participate

All animal experiments and protocols were reviewed and approved by the Institutional Animal Care and Use Committees of the National Institute of Animal Health, NARO (Permit Numbers: 14–030, 14–033, and 14,112,051).and Institute of Livestock and Grassland Science, NARO (Permit Numbers: 15112044). We explained about the aim and plan of the current study to the owners in advance of application for permission to Institutional Animal Care and Use Committees, and we obtained verbal informed consent from the owners of cattle sampled for this study.

Consent for publication

Not applicable.

Competing interests

The authors declare that they have no competing interests.

Author details

[1]Epidemiology Unit, Division of Viral Disease and Epidemiology, National Institute of Animal Health, NARO 3-1-5 Kannondai, Tsukuba, Ibaraki 305-0856, Japan. [2]Grazing Animal Unit, Division of Grassland Farming, Institute of Livestock and Grassland Science, NARO. 768 Senbonmatsu, Nasushiobara, Tochigi 329-2793, Japan. [3]National Institute of Animal Health, NARO, Exotic Diseases Research Station Josuihoncho, Kodaira, Tokyo 187-0022, Japan. [4]Cooperative Department of Veterinary Medicine, Iwate University Faculty of Agriculture, 3-18-8 Ueda, Morioka, Iwate 020-8550, Japan.

References

1. Murakami K, Kobayashi S, Konishi M, Kameyama KI, Tsutsui T. Nationwide survey of bovine leukemia virus infection among dairy and beef breeding cattle in Japan from 2009-2011. J Vet Med Sci. 2013;75:1123–6.
2. World Organisation For Animal Health (2018) the Manual of Diagnostic Tests and Vaccines for Terrestrial Animals 2018 Chapter 2. 4. 10. Enzootic bovine leukosis. http://www.oie.int/fileadmin/Home/eng/Health_standards/tahm/2.04.10_EBL.pdf. Accessed 30 Aug 2018.
3. Oguma K, Suzuki M, Sentsui H. Enzootic bovine leukosis in a two-month-old calf. Virus Res. 2017;233:120–4.
4. Romero CH, Cruz GB, Rowe CA. Transmission of bovine leukaemia virus in milk. Trop Anim Health Prod. 1983;15:215–8.
5. Chung YS, Prior HC, Duffy PF, Rogers RJ, Mackenzie AR. The effect of pasteurisation on bovine leucosis virus-infected milk. Aust Vet J. 1986;63:379–80.
6. Ferrer JF, Piper CE. Role of colostrum and milk in the natural transmission of the bovine leukemia virus. Cancer Res. 1981;41:4906–9.
7. Lassauzet ML, Johnson WO, Thurmond MC, Stevens F. Protection of colostral antibodies against bovine leukemia virus infection in calves on a California dairy. Can J Vet Res. 1989;53:424–30.
8. Van Der Maaten MJ, Miller JM, Schmerr MJ. Effect of colostral antibody on bovine leukemia virus infection of neonatal calves. Am J Vet Res. 1981;42:1498–500.
9. Nagy DW, Tyler JW, Kleiboeker SB. Decreased periparturient transmission of bovine leukosis virus in colostrum-fed calves. J Vet Intern Med. 2007;21:1104–7.
10. Gutiérrez G, Lomonaco M, Alvarez I, Fernandez F, Trono K. Characterization of colostrum from dams of BLV endemic dairy herds. Vet Microbiol. 2015;177:366–9.

11. Jaworski JP, Porta NG, Gutierrez G, Politzki RP, Álvarez I, Galarza R, Abdala A, Calvinho L, Trono KG. Short communication: relationship between the level of bovine leukemia virus antibody and provirus in blood and milk of cows from a naturally infected herd. J Dairy Sci. 2016;99:5629–34.
12. Zarkik S, Defrise-Quertain F, Portetelle D, Burny A, Ruysschaert JM. Fusion of bovine leukemia virus with target cells monitored by R18 fluorescence and PCR assays. J Virol. 1997;71:738–40.
13. Graves DC, Jones LV. Early syncytium formation by bovine leukemia virus. J Virol. 1981;38:1055–63.
14. Kono Y, Irishio W, Sentsui H. Syncytium-induction inhibition test with complement for detection of antibodies against bovine leukemia virus. Can J Comp Med. 1983;47:328–31.
15. Portetelle D, Bruck C, Bex F, Burny A, Dekegel D, Mammerickx M. Detection of complement-dependent lytic antibodies in sera from bovine leukemia virus-infected animals. Arch Int Physiol Biochim. 1978;86:955–6.
16. Kono Y, Arai K, Sentsui H, Matsukawa S, Itohara S. Protection against bovine leukemia virus infection in sheep by active and passive immunization. Nippon Juigaku Zasshi. 1986;48:117–25.
17. Gapper LW, Copestake DE, Otter DE, Indyk HE. Analysis of bovine immunoglobulin G in milk, colostrum and dietary supplements: a review. Anal Bioanal Chem. 2007;389:93–109.
18. Korhonen H, Marnila P, Gill HS. Milk immunoglobulins and complement factors. Br J Nutr. 2000;84(Suppl 1):S75–80.
19. Chase CC, Hurley DJ, Reber AJ. Neonatal immune development in the calf and its impact on vaccine response. Vet Clin North Am Food Anim Pract. 2008;24:87–104.
20. Langel SN, Wark WA, Garst SN, James RE, McGilliard ML, Petersson-Wolfe CS, Kanevsky-Mullarky I. Effect of feeding whole compared with cell-free colostrum on calf immune status: the neonatal period. J Dairy Sci. 2015;98:3729–40.
21. Li N, Richoux R, Boutinaud M, Martin P, Gagnaire V. Role of somatic cells on dairy processes and products: a review. Dairy Sci Technol. 2014;94:517–38.
22. Roland L, Drillich M, Iwersen M. Hematology as a diagnostic tool in bovine medicine. J Vet Diagn Investig. 2014;26:592–8.
23. George JW, Snipes J, Lane VM. Comparison of bovine hematology reference intervals from 1957 to 2006. Vet Clin Pathol. 2010;39:138–48.
24. Kim YM, Lee JA, Jung BG, Kim TH, Lee BJ, Suh GH. Reference ranges of hematology and lymphocyte subsets in healthy Korean native cattle (Hanwoo) and Holstein dairy cattle. Anim Sci J. 2016;87:796–801.
25. Kono Y, Sentsui H, Miyamoto T, Morozumi K, Sakamoto Y. Changes in antibody titers in cattle infected clinically and subclinically with bovine leukemia virus. Int J Cancer. 1982;30:655–7.
26. Percher F, Jeannin P, Martin-Latil S, Gessain A, Afonso PV, Vidy-Roche A, Ceccaldi PE. Mother-to-child transmission of HTLV-1 epidemiological aspects, mechanisms and determinants of mother-to-child transmission. Viruses. 2016. https://doi.org/10.3390/v8020040.
27. Asfaw Y, Tsuduku S, Konishi M, Murakami K, Tsuboi T, Wu D, Sentsui H. Distribution and superinfection of bovine leukemia virus genotypes in Japan. Arch Virol. 2005;150:493–505.
28. Kanda Y. Investigation of the freely available easy-to-use software 'EZR' for medical statistics. Bone Marrow Transplant. 2013;48:452–8.

19

Genetic diversity of Bovine Viral Diarrhea Virus from cattle in Chile between 2003 and 2007

Astrid Donoso, Felipe Inostroza, María Celedón and José Pizarro-Lucero*

Abstract

Background: *Bovine Viral Diarrhea Virus* causes significant economic losses in cattle. BVDV has high genomic diversity, with two species, BVDV-1 and BVDV-2, and at least twenty-one subgenotypes for BVDV-1 and four subgenotypes for BVDV-2. Vaccines are important tools to reduce the economic losses caused by this virus. However, vaccine strains must correspond to the antigenic profile of the viruses present in the region where the vaccine is applied. A restricted phylogenetic study with 14 viruses isolated from cattle between 1993 and 2001 showed that the genetic profile of BVDV in Chile consisted of viruses of both species and sub-genotypes 1a, 1b, 1c (currently 1j) and 2a. To determine more accurately the genetic profile of BVDV in Chile, in this study a larger number of viruses obtained from bovines between 2003 and 2007 were typed.

Results: The study was performed using partial sequences from the 5′ noncoding region (5′UTR) and E2 coding region of the viral genome of thirty-five Chilean viruses isolated from geographic regions that have 84.6% of the Chilean cattle. All tested viruses belonged to species BVDV-1. Eighteen viruses belonged to BVDV-1j subgenotype (51.4%), twelve belonged to BVDV-1b (34.3%) and five belonged to BVDV-1a (14.3%). The Chilean BVDV-1j viruses showed low genetic diversity, both among themselves and with the BVDV-1j present in other regions of the world. This could be explained by a relatively recent introduction of this viral subgenotype in cattle, which agrees with its low geographical distribution worldwide. Otherwise, Chilean BVDV-1b viruses grouped into a single cluster, different even than the viruses present in Argentina and Brazil, countries geographically close to Chile, a process of local evolution that could generate antigenic differences between the Chilean viruses and the viruses used as vaccine strains.

Conclusions: The high presence of viruses of the BVDV-1j subgenotype, which show major antigenic differences with BVDV-1a and BVDV-1b subgenotypes used in the commercial vaccines, suggest that BVDV-1j viruses could be an emergent subgenotype of BVDV in cattle in South America and suggest evaluating an update of the vaccines used in Chile.

Keywords: *Bovine viral diarrhea virus*, *Pestivirus*, BVDV, Genetic diversity, 5′UTR, E2

Background

The *Bovine Viral Diarrhea Virus* (BVDV) is a virus of worldwide distribution, which causes a wide variety of clinical symptoms in cattle, being recognized as the viral agent that causes the main economic losses in the global cattle industry [1, 2].

In immunocompetent animals, BVDV usually is associated with respiratory and gastrointestinal diseases of different severity, hemorrhagic syndrome, and reproductive problems, such as infertility. BVDV also causes immunosuppression, which increases the severity of diseases caused by other pathogens. The virus is able to cross the placenta infecting the fetus, causing embryonic reabsorption, fetal mummification, abortion and congenital malformations, especially of the central nervous system. Fetal infection with a non-cytopathic virus in the first trimester of pregnancy causes persistently infected

* Correspondence: jpizarro@uchile.cl
Laboratory of Animal Virology, Department of Animal Preventive Medicine, Faculty of Livestock and Veterinary Sciences, University of Chile, Av. Santa Rosa, 11735 Santiago, Chile

animals with BVDV (PI), which are the main source of infection of susceptible animals in the herd. Superinfection of PI animals with a cytopathic BVD virus very close antigenically with the non-cytopathic BVD virus produces the fatal bovine viral diarrhea-mucosal disease (BVD-MD) [3–6].

Bovine Viral Diarrhea Virus (BVDV) is a member of the genus *Pestivirus*, family *Flaviviridae*, which includes four specie: *Bovine Viral Diarrhea Virus 1* (BVDV-1), *Bovine Viral Diarrhea Virus 2* (BVDV-2), *Classical Swine Fever Virus* and *Border Disease Virus* [7]. The genome of BVDV is a single-stranded RNA of positive polarity, approximately 12.3 Kb in length. The genome contains a single open reading frame that encodes 11–12 viral proteins, flanked by a 5 'and 3' untranslated region [7]. Genetic typing has classified the BVDV isolates into two species, *Bovine Viral Diarrhea Virus 1* (BVDV-1) and *Bovine Viral Diarrhea Virus 2* (BVDV-2), with at least 21 subgenotypes of BVDV-1 (1a-1u) and four subgenotypes of BVDV-2 (2a-2d) [7–14]. BVDV-2 strains were initially isolated from acute hemorrhagic disease outbreaks in North America, but later it could be established that both viral species of BVDV cause similar clinical symptoms. BVDV-1 strains are distributed worldwide, while the BVDV-2 strains are present mainly in the United States, Canada and South America, with few reports of their presence in Europe and Japan [10, 15–20]. Recently, an atypical pestivirus (HoBi-like) isolated from cattle and water buffaloes has been proposed as a new species (BVDV-3) based on phylogenetic analyzes [8, 21].

BVDV infection is widespread among Chilean cattle, with a serological prevalence ranging from 59.7 to 69.2% in unvaccinated animals from different regions of the country [22, 23]. To design an effective vaccination strategy against the BVDV virus in Chile, the vaccine strains must match the genetic profile of the viruses that infect Chilean cattle for optimal protection [24, 25]. In 2006, a phylogenetic study with 14 viruses isolated from cattle between 1993 and 2001 showed that the genetic profile of BVDV in Chile consisted of viruses of both species and subgenotypes 1a, 1b, 1c (currently 1j) and 2a, with a high prevalence of sub-type 1b (42.9%) [20]. The objective of this study was to determine more precisely the genetic profile of BVDV in Chile, with a greater number of viruses obtained from bovines between 2003 and 2007.

Methods

Samples

The thirty-five viruses included in this study were obtained from sera of calves and adult cattle and tissue of bovine fetuses from different regions of central and southern Chile from 2003 to 2007. Twenty-five viruses were isolated from sera of asymptomatic calves and adult cattle or those suffering enteric, respiratory or reproductive problems in the Metropolitana, Maule, Bio-Bio, Araucanía, De Los Rios and De Los Lagos Regions, which have 84.6% of the Chilean cattle [26]. Ten viruses were isolated from organ suspensions of bovine fetuses in the Metropolitana and Araucanía Regions. The list of the BVDV viruses examined in this study is shown in Table 1.

The viruses were propagated on monolayers of MDBK cells line (ATCC CCL-22), determined to be free of BVDV and grown in Eagle's Minimum Essential Medium supplemented with 10% equine serum. All infections were monitored by direct immunofluorescence (DIF) assay. DIF was performed in acetone-fixed cells, using a FITC-conjugated anti-BVDV polyclonal serum (Central Veterinary Laboratory, Addlestone, Surrey, UK). All viruses were of the non-cytopathic biotype.

Primers

The 5'UTR region corresponding to positions 108 to 395 according to the NADL genome sequence was amplified using the panpestivirus-specific primers 324/326 [27]. This pair of primers is highly sensitive for BVDV-1 and BVDV-2 viruses, but it is less sensitive for HoBi-like viruses, which may limit the detection of Hobi-like viruses in this study [21].

To confirm the data in 5'UTR, a 700 bp DNA fragment corresponding to positions 2754 to 3453 of the E2 region, according to the NADL genome sequence, was amplified with the primers E2F (5'-ACTTTGAAT TTGGACTYTGCC-3′, nucleotides 2754–2774 of the NADL genome) and E2R (5'-TCCAGGTCAAACCAR-TATTG-3′, nucleotides 3453–3434 of the NADL genome) for selected viruses.

RT-PCR

Total RNA was obtained from infected cells using Trizol LS (Invitrogen) according to the manufacturer's instructions. The RNA was suspended in 50 μl DEPC-treated water. Amplification of viral RNA by RT-PCR was carried out in a SuperScript III One-Step RT-PCR System with Platinum Taq DNA Polymerase (Invitrogen), according to the manufacturer's instructions, under the following conditions: 1) 5'-UTR Region: 12.5 μl 2x Reaction Mix, 0.2 mM dNTP, 2 mM $MgSO_4$, 10 pmol each primer 324 and 326, 5 μl heat-denatured RNA (2 min at 94 °C), and 1 μl SuperScript III RT / Platinum Taq Mix. Synthesis of cDNA was performed in 25 μl final volume for 30 min at 55 °C. After reverse transcription, the reaction was heated in a thermocycler for 3 min at 94 °C and then submitted to 30 cycles of amplification. The amplification conditions were 30 s at 94 °C, 1 min at 55 °C and 1 min at 68 °C. 2) E2 Region: 12.5 μl 2x Reaction Mix, 0.2 mM dNTP, 1.6 mM $MgSO_4$, 10 pmol each primer E2F and E2R, 5 μl heat-denatured

Table 1 Chilean BVDV field isolates studied in this work

Isolate	Year	Sample	Region	Clinical symptoms	Accession number		Type
					5'UTR	E2	
CHL/914	2005	LN	Araucanía	Abortion	JF759955	JF776638	BVDV-1b
CHL/916	2003	Serum	de los Ríos	PI	JF759940	JF776639	BVDV-1a
CHL/917	2003	Serum	de los Lagos	PI	JF759946	JF776640	BVDV-1b
CHL/918	2003	Serum	de los Lagos	PI	JF759944	JF776641	BVDV-1b
CHL/919	2003	Serum	de los Lagos	PI	JF759945	JF776642	BVDV-1b
CHL/920	2003	Serum	de los Lagos	PI	JF759947	JF776643	BVDV-1b
CHL/921	2003	Serum	de los Lagos	PI	JF759941	JF776644	BVDV-1a
CHL/927	2006	Serum	Bío-Bío	RD	JF759926	MH078039	BVDV-1j
CHL/928	2006	Serum	Bío-Bío	RD	JF759932	MH078040	BVDV-1j
CHL/939	2006	Serum	Bío-Bío	RD	JF759931	–	BVDV-1j
CHL/958	2006	Serum	Bío-Bío	RD	JF759928	MH078041	BVDV-1j
CHL/971	2006	Serum	Bío-Bío	RD	JF759937	–	BVDV-1j
CHL/972	2006	Serum	Bío-Bío	RD	JF759930	MH078042	BVDV-1j
CHL/992	2006	Serum	Bío-Bío	RD	JF759956	MH078043	BVDV-1j
CHL/1014	2006	Serum	Bío-Bío	RD	JF759929	–	BVDV-1j
CHL/1025	2007	Serum	Metropolitana	RD	JF759948	JF776645	BVDV-1b
CHL/1061	2007	Serum	Metropolitana	RD	JF759949	–	BVDV-1b
CHL/1068	2007	Serum	Metropolitana	RD	JF759942	JF776646	BVDV-1a
CHL/1071	2003	Serum	Araucanía	Diarrhea	JF759950	–	BVDV-1b
CHL/1076	2007	Serum	Araucanía	None	JF759951	–	BVDV-1b
CHL/1078	2007	Serum	Araucanía	Abortion	JF759936	MH078044	BVDV-1j
CHL/1086	2007	Serum	Araucanía	None	JF759954	–	BVDV-1b
CHL/1087	2007	Serum	Maule	None	JF759935	MH078045	BVDV-1j
CHL/1091	2007	Serum	Bío-Bío	None	JF759922	JF776648	BVDV-1a
CHL/1092	2007	Serum	Maule	Abortion	JF759952	–	BVDV-1b
CHL/1109	2007	Serum	Bío-Bío	None	JF759953	–	BVDV-1b
CHL/P22	2006	Lung	Metropolitana	None	JF759923	–	BVDV-1j
CHL/P23	2006	Lung	Metropolitana	None	JF759927	–	BVDV-1j
CHL/P24	2006	Lung	Metropolitana	None	JF759934	–	BVDV-1j
CHL/P26	2006	Lung	Metropolitana	None	JF759938	–	BVDV-1j
CHL/P28	2006	Lung	Metropolitana	None	JF759943	–	BVDV-1a
CHL/P30	2006	Lung	Metropolitana	None	JF759939	MH078046	BVDV-1j
CHL/P31	2006	Lung	Metropolitana	None	JF759933	–	BVDV-1j
CHL/P32	2006	Lung	Metropolitana	None	JF759924	–	BVDV-1j
CHL/P33	2006	Lung	Metropolitana	None	JF759925	–	BVDV-1j

LN Lymph Node, *PI* Persistent Infection, *RD* Reproductive Disorder

RNA (2 min at 94 °C), and 1 μl SuperScript III RT/Platinum Taq Mix. Synthesis of cDNA was performed in 25 μl final volume for 30 min at 50 °C. After reverse transcription, the reaction was heated in a thermocycler for 3 min at 94 °C and then submitted to 30 cycles of amplification. The amplification conditions were 30 s at 94 °C, 1 min at 50 °C and 1 min at 68 °C. Amplified products were visualized by electrophoresis in 2% agarose gel run in 90 mM Tris, 90 mM boric acid, 2 mM EDTA at 18 V/cm of gel and stained with ethidium bromide.

Genes sequencing and genetic analysis

The amplified products were purified using the QIAquick PCR purification kit (Qiagen) and DNA sequencing was performed on an ABI-310 automated sequencer using dideoxy-sequencing chemistry utilizing the Big Dye Terminator Cycle Sequencing with Ampli Taq DNA polymerase (Applied Biosystems). Both strands of each PCR product were sequenced in triplicate from amplified products obtained from individual amplifications.

Phylogenetic reconstructions for genetic typing were compiled using a 230 nucleotide region of the 5'-UTR (nucleotides 142–371 of the NADL genome) and a 420 nucleotide region of E2 (nucleotides 2879–3298 of the NADL genome). Nucleotide sequences from representative isolates of previously identified phylogenetic groups of BVDV were included in the phylogenetic analysis.

The nucleotide sequences obtained from each region were aligned using the MUSCLE program [28], then a matrix of distances for Kimura's two-parameter model was generated, and the phylogenetic analysis was performed using the maximum likelihood method from the MEGA version 7 program [29]. The robustness of the phylogenetic analysis and significance of the branching order were determined by a bootstrap analysis carried out on 1000 replicates, which showed only bootstrap values of ≥50%. Sequence Demarcation Tool (SDT) v1.2 software was used to calculate pairwise identities using MUSCLE alignments for E2 nucleotide sequences of some viruses [30], and shown in matrix format. To analyze the differences at the molecular level of the E2 glycoprotein of the Chilean BVDV isolates with viruses of BVDV-1a, BVDV-1b and BVDV-1j subgenotypes from Argentina, Brazil and other regions of the world, the deduced amino acid sequences were aligned using MUSCLE and the pattern of amino acid substitutions near Domain C (amino acids 843 to 870), an important antigenic site of BVDV, was analyzed.

Results

The 5'UTR phylogenetic tree was constructed using the nucleotide sequences of the 35 Chilean BVDV viruses of this study and BVDV reference strains from GenBank (Fig. 1). The accession numbers of the sequences obtained during this study are given in Table 1.

On the basis of phylogenetic analysis of 5'UTR, all 35 BVDV isolates belonged to species BVDV-1. The percentage identities (PID) among all the Chilean BVDV-1 viruses were 88–100%. Eighteen Chilean viruses grouped in the BVDV-1j subgenotype (51.4%), at a confidence level of 98% by bootstrap analysis. The PID among the Chilean BVDV-1j viruses were 97–100%. The BVDV-1j subgenotype was subdivided into two clusters. All the Chilean viruses grouped together with the Argentinean isolates 2B and 17P (cluster 1j-SAM). The other cluster was composed of BVDV-1j viruses isolated in Europe, Africa and Asia (cluster 1j-INT). Twelve Chilean viruses grouped in BVDV-1b subgenotype (34.3%), at a confidence level of 78% by bootstrap analysis. The PID among the Chilean BVDV-1b viruses were 96–100%. This subgenotype was subdivided into two clusters. All the Chilean viruses of this study were grouped with the viruses CHL/113, CHL/170, CHL/226, CHL/481 and CHL/615, also isolated from bovines in Chile [20], and the CHL/Pudu/Zoo isolated from pudú (*Pudu puda*), an indigenous deer of Chile from a Chilean Zoo, [31], forming a cluster only with Chilean viruses (cluster 1b-CHL). By contrast, the Chilean BVDV-1b viruses CHL/184, CHL/379, CHL/565 [20] and the CHL/Pudu-Chillan isolated from a free-ranging pudú [32] grouped in a different cluster with BVDV-1b viruses from other regions of the world (European, American, Argentinean, Brazilian) (cluster 1b-INT). Five Chilean viruses grouped in the BVDV-1a subgenotype (14.3%) with PID among them of 92–100%. The CHL/1091 virus showed a sequence identity of 100% with the NADL strain in the analyzed region of 5'UTR. There was no obvious association of any subgenotype with geographical location.

To confirm the phylogenetic analysis obtained with the 5'UTR region, E2 genes of eighteen Chilean viruses of this study belonging to the different subgenotypes were sequenced, and the E2 phylogenetic tree was constructed using the nucleotide sequences of BVDV reference strains from GenBank (Fig. 2). The accession numbers of the sequences obtained are given in Table 1.

The results obtained with the E2 phylogenetic analysis showed the same classification as that observed using the 5'UTR nucleotide sequences, with the viruses conserving their type. The Chilean BVDV-1j, BVDV-1b, and BVDV-1a viruses grouped at a confidence level of 99%, 99%, and 78%, respectively, by bootstrap analysis. Chilean BVDV-1b viruses were grouped in a cluster only with Chilean viruses (cluster 1b-CHL) clearly apart from Brazilian and Argentinean viruses, with bootstrap values of 99% and 68%, respectively.

The pairwise identity matrix of selected E2 nucleotide sequences was calculated using SDT v1.2 software (Fig. 3). The matrix showed that the sequence identity among the Chilean BVDV-1a viruses isolated in this study ranged from 87 to 100%, between the Chilean BVDV-1b viruses ranged from 93 to 100%, and between the Chilean BVDV-1j viruses ranged from 98 to 100%. The sequence identity of BVDV-1j viruses, when viruses from other regions of the world were included (KS86ncp, 190CP and Deer-GB1), ranged between 97 and 100%. The sequence identity between the Chilean BVDV-1b viruses with the Brazilian BVDV-1b viruses ranged from 83 to 86%, and the sequence identity between the Chilean BVDV-1b viruses and the Argentinean BVDV-1b viruses ranged from 81 to 86%.

To analyze the differences of the E2 glycoprotein of the Chilean isolates at the molecular level, the deduced amino acid sequences were aligned and the substitution

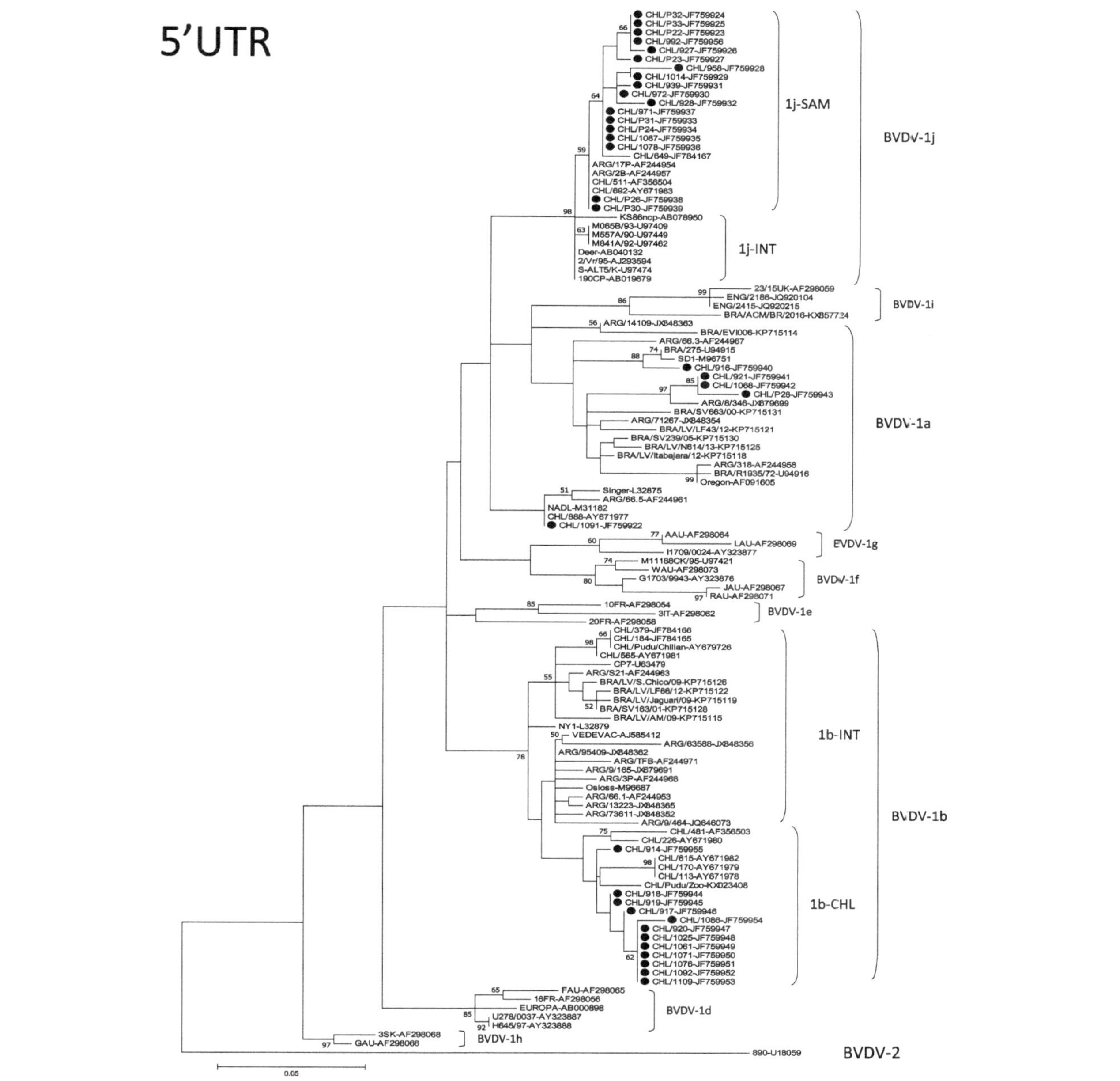

Fig. 1 Phylogenetic analysis of Chilean BVDV isolates based on partial 5'-Untranslated Region (5'UTR). The phylogenetic tree were prepared using the Maximum Likelihood method and numbers over branches indicate the percentage of 1000 bootstrap replicates that support each phylogenetic branch. The GenBak accession numbers are indicated after the name of the BVDV strains. The Chilean viruses of this study are marked with circles

patterns in or near Domain C (nDomC), an important antigenic region of BVDV located between amino acid positions 843 and 870 of the NADL polyprotein sequence were analyzed (Fig. 4).

The pattern of amino acid substitutions (PAAS) showed that viruses BVDV/1091, BVDV/921 and BVDV/1068 had the same amino acid sequences in Domain C, and zero or one amino acid substitution in the nDomC of the E2 protein, but these viruses showed three amino acid substitutions in Domain C and seven or eight amino acid substitutions in the nDomC of the E2 protein with respect to the BVDV/916 strain. The PAAS between the Chilean BVDV-1b viruses of this study showed zero or three amino acid substitutions in Domain C, and between zero and five amino acid substitutions in the nDomC of the E2 protein. The PAAS between the Chilean and Brazilian BVDV-1b viruses showed eight or ten amino acid substitutions in the

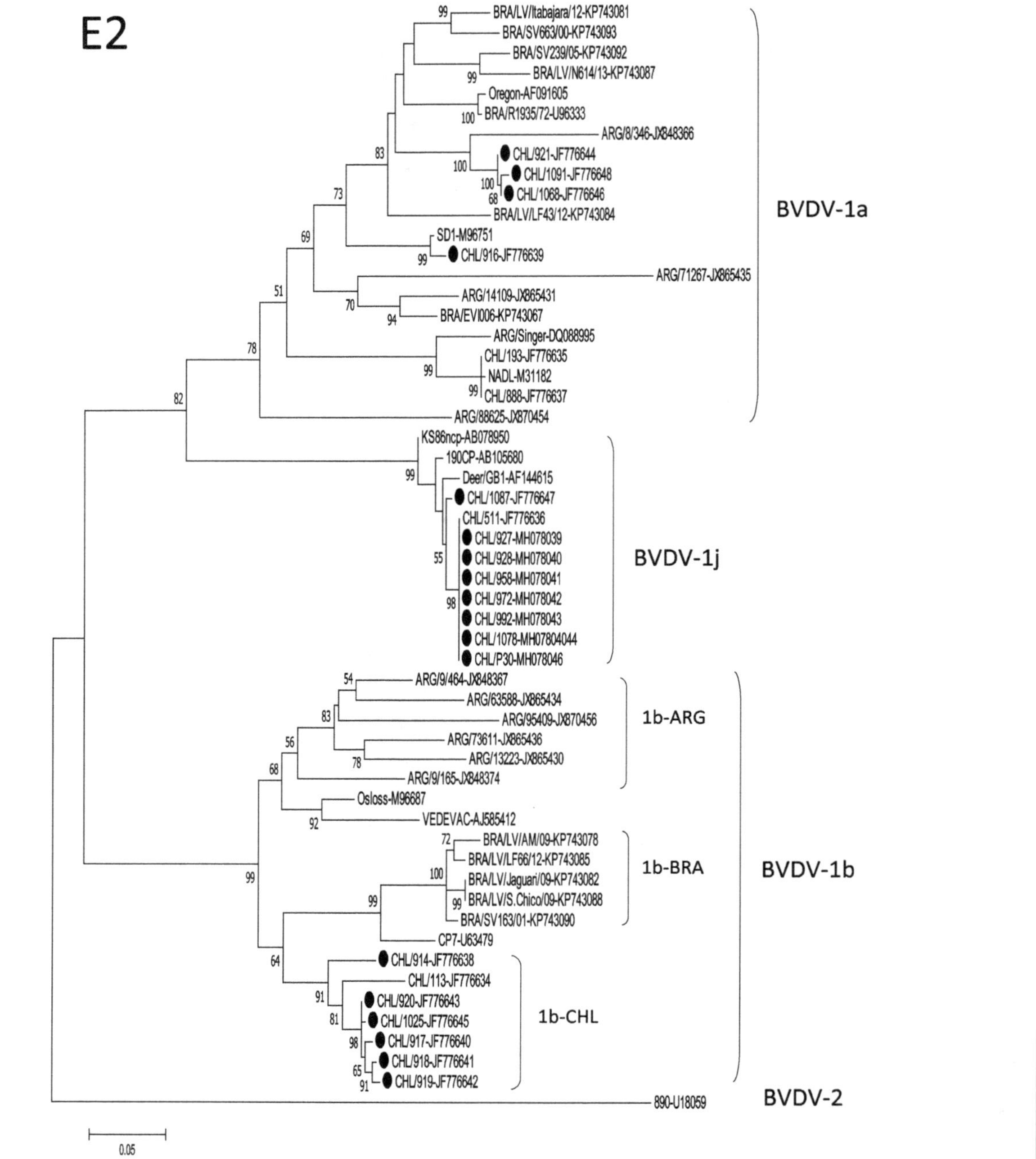

Fig. 2 Phylogenetic analysis of Chilean BVDV isolates based on partial E2 coding region (E2). The phylogenetic tree was prepared using the Maximum Likelihood method and numbers over branches indicate the percentage of 1000 bootstrap replicates that support each phylogenetic branch. The GenBak accession numbers are after the name of the BVDV strains. The Chilean viruses of this study are marked with circles

nDomC, and seven to sixteen amino acid substitutions in the nDomC between the Chilean and Argentinean BVDV-1b viruses. The PAAS between the Chilean BVDV-1j viruses of this study showed zero or one amino acid substitutions in Domain C, and between zero and three amino acid substitutions in the nDomC of the E2 protein, and the PAAS between the Chilean BVDV-1j viruses and BVDV-1j viruses from other countries was also very similar, with zero to two amino acid substitutions in Domain C, and between zero and five amino acid substitutions in the nDomC of the E2 protein.

Discussion

Bovine Viral Diarrhea Virus is widely spread in Chilean cattle, with a serological prevalence ranging from 59.7 to 69.2% [22, 23], and although an official control of BVDV

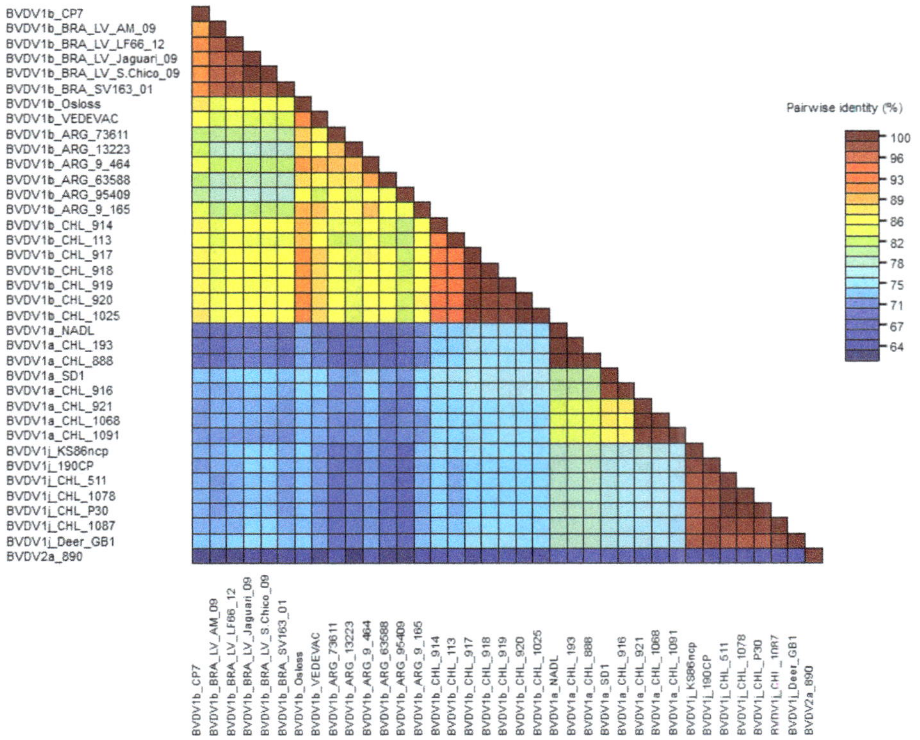

Fig. 3 SDT matrix of pairwise identity scores generated by alignment of a 420 bp fragment of the E2 gene for 37 BVDV viruses. Each colored cell represents the percentage of identity between two nucleotide sequences, one horizontally and the other vertically, that intersect in the cell. A figure indicating the correspondence between pairwise identities and the colors is included

is not applied in Chile many farmers are using vaccines in order to reduce economic losses. Nevertheless, an effective vaccination strategy against BVDV requires that vaccines reflect the genetic and antigenic types of viruses that infect Chilean cattle.

A survey of the genetic diversity of 35 field isolates infecting cattle in Chile between 2003 and 2007 was conducted by determining the nucleotide sequences of the 5'-UTR. The results showed that three subgenotypes were circulating in Chilean cattle: BVDV-1a (5/35; 14.3%), BVDV-1b (12/35; 34.3%), and BVDV-1j (18/35; 51.4%), with BVDV-1b and BVDV-1j as the predominant subgenotypes. Surprisingly, BVDV-2 was not detected, even though it had been previously detected in Chile [20]. In the study published by Pizarro-Lucero in 2006 [20], phylogenetic analysis from 14 isolates obtained between 1993 and 2001 showed the presence of viruses belonging to subgenotypes BVDV-1a (1/14; 7.1%), BVDV-1b (6/14; 42.9%), BVDV-1c (currently classified as BVDV-1j viruses) (2/14; 14.3%) and BVDV-2a (5/14; 35.7%).

The results of this study showed that the genetic composition of BVDV viruses infecting cattle in Chile has changed over the years. The BVDV-1b subgenotype has been maintained as a predominant subgenotype in the Chilean cattle, and the subgenotype BVDV-1a is present in low number. Nevertheless, BVDV-1j viruses were isolated more frequently in the samples obtained between 2003 and 2007 (51.4%) in comparison with the samples isolated between 1993 and 2001 (14.3%), and BVDV-2 was not circulating in Chilean cattle, or is present in a very low number that was not detected in this study. Furthermore, considering that all the BVDV-1j viruses analyzed except for African isolate M1515A/90 have lost the restriction site for the Xho I enzyme (data not shown), only 2/33 viruses isolated between 1993 and 2001 in Chile belonged to subgenotype BVDV1j (6.1%).

These differences could be a result of immune selection, because it has been described that BVDV-1j viruses showed significant antigenic differences with BVDV-1a and BVDV-1b viruses, mainly used as vaccine strains [12, 20, 33]. In this study, nine of eighteen BVDV-1j viruses were isolated from cattle showing reproductive problems, but the pathogenicity of the BVDV-1j subgenotype was not clear yet. Otherwise, the high similarity shown between the Chilean and Argentinean BVDV-1j viruses (cluster 1j-SAM) suggests a common ancestor for these viruses. The non-obvious association of any subgenotype with geographical location was expected due to the absence of a national control program that

```
                           843      Domain C        870
                           ----------------------------
SD-1 BVDV1a         CMLANRDTLDTAVVRTYRRSVPFPYRQGCITQKTLGEDLYDCALGGNWTCVTGDQSRYTG
NADL                .TSF.M...A.T........K...H........N.....HN.I........P...LL.K.
SINGER              ..SF.M...A.T.I......K...H..............HN.I........P..MLL.K.
ARG/88625           .....K...N.T.....K..K........V...I........T.......I..E.LT...
ARG/71267           .L.V.K.P.SPT.L......N........T...IV.G..FY.............IL.FS.
ARG/14109           .........S.T..................I..N......G.............ILQ...
ARG/8/346           .........N..LI......R................N..N.E............LT...
BRA/EVI006          .........S.T..................I.........G.............ML....
BRA/LV/LF43/12      ...............V.T.QK...................N.D............LQ...
BRA/SV663/00        ....................K........T...I......N..............LQ...
BRA/SV239/05        .V..................K............I......N.D............L....
CHL/888             .TSF.M...A.T........K...H........N.....HN.I........P...LL.K.
CHL/916             ............................................................
CHL/921             .............IQ.....R...................N.E............LQ...
CHL/1068            .............IQ.....R...................N.E........I...LQ...
CHL/1091            .............IQ.....R...................N.E........I...LQ...

CP7 BVDV1b          CTLANKDTLATIVVRTYKRVRPFPYRQDCVTQKTIGEDLYDCALGGNWTCVPGDALRYVA
Osloss              .HWS......MT.......H....F..G.I...V..G.................I....D
VEDEVAC             .HWP......LT.....T.HQ...F..G.I..........N.D.......I...Q....D
ARG/13223           .A.......DVT.L...M.LK......G.T..........N.........I...E....G
ARG/63588           .A...E...HMT.....M.LK......G.I..........N.E...............AE
ARG/73611           .A.......DVT....NT.LK......S.IS.........N.........I...I....E
ARG/95409           .A.......DGT.....T.LK........I....V..N..N.SF.......L..V....E
ARG/9/165           .A.......EVTI......LK......G.I............N.......I...Q....D
ARG/9/464           .A.......DVT.....T.L.......G.T..........N.D.......I........E
BRA/LV/AM/09        ...........T...............Y...........HN.I...........Q.....
BRA/LV/LF66/12      ...........T...............Y...........HN.I...........Q.....
BRA/LV/Jaguari/09   ...........T...............Y...H.......H..I...........Q.....
BRA/LV/S.Chico/09   ...........T...............Y...H.......H..I...........Q.....
BRA/SV163/01        ...........T...............Y...........H..I..........VQ....S
CHL/113             ...........T.......NK......G.I........................Q.Q..D
CHL/914             ...........A........K......G.I...I.........M..........Q....D
CHL/917             ...........T.......YK......G.I............V...........Q....D
CHL/918             ...........T.......YK......G.I........................Q....D
CHL/919             ...........T.......YK......G.I........................Q....D
CHL/920             ...........T.......YK......G.I........................Q....D
CHL/1025            ...........T.......YK......G.I........................Q....D

190cp BVDV1j        CVLANEDTLETTVVLTYIRSRPFPHRQGCITHKILGEDLHDCILGGNWTCVAGEQLQYAG
KS86ncp             .................M..........................................
Deer-GB1            ..............Q..R.........................F................
CHL/511             ..............M...........................S..........D......
CHL/958             ..............M...........................S..........D......
CHL/992             ..............M...........................S..........D......
CHL/1078            ..............M...........................S..........D......
CHL/1087            ............................................................
CHL/P30             ..............M...........................S..........D......
```

Fig. 4 Alignment of partial amino acid sequences of E2 of BVDV-1a, BVDV-1b and BVDV-1j subgenotypes of BVDV. The aligned sequences correspond to amino acids from 832 to 891. Dots represent identical amino acids to the standard sequence of the corresponding subgenotype (BVDV-1a: SD-1, BVDV-1b: CP7, and BVDV-1j: 190cp). Uppercase letters represent an amino acid substitution. Domain C (amino acids 843 to 870) is indicated

could limit the free movement of the BVDV infected animals around the country.

The E2 phylogenetic analysis showed the same typing obtained with the 5'UTR region. Analyzing the phylogenetic tree of E2 (Fig. 2) and the sequence identity of the viruses of the subgenotypes present in Chile (Fig. 3), three different situations can be observed: a) the Chilean BVDV-1a viruses showed greater genetic diversity between them than the viruses of the other subgenotypes. This may be explained by continuous reintroductions of these viruses to national cattle, probably through commercial vaccines, since the viral strains NADL and SD-1 are frequently used as vaccine strains; b) the Chilean BVDV-1j viruses showed low genetic diversity both among themselves and with the BVDV-1j present in other regions of the world, which is expressed in a relatively compact cluster of these viruses in the phylogenetic tree and high sequence identity between them. This low genetic diversity in the most variable protein of the virus between strains isolated from such diverse regions of the world (Chile, Japan, United Kingdom) could be explained by a relatively recent introduction of this viral subgenotype in cattle, which agrees with its low geographic distribution worldwide; and c) the Chilean BVDV-1b viruses of this study grouped into a single cluster, different even from viruses genetically representatives of the viruses that had been circulating in similar period of time in Argentina and Brazil (2001–2009 and 2006–2010, respectively) [34, 35], countries geographically close to Chile. These results could be explained by the presence of BVDV-1b viruses in the Chilean cattle for a long period of time, which would have allowed a process of local evolution. This process of local evolution could generate important antigenic differences between viruses of the BVDV-1b subgenotype but with different evolutionary histories, as reported by Pecora et al., 2014 [34]. This suggests performing studies on the antigenic diversity of the BVDV-1b viruses present in different regions of the world and evaluating the relevance of generating vaccines with local strains of this viral subgenotype.

The pattern of amino acid substitutions in or near Domain C (nDomC) in the E2 region of Chilean viruses of the different subgenotypes showed that most amino acid changes occurred in the same positions, and usually with the same amino acids in viruses of equal subgenotype (Fig. 4).

The Chilean BVDV-1a viruses BVDV/921, BVDV/1068 and BVDV/1091 showed a very similar amino acid sequence, and larger differences with BVDV/916, that showed an identical amino acid sequence with the SD-1 strain. This is similar to the CHL/888 strain that showed identical amino acid sequence with the NADL strain. These results support those observed with molecular phylogeny and pairwise identity matrix, that some of these viruses can be the result of isolation of vaccine strains. The Chilean BVDV-1b viruses showed a very similar amino acid sequence among them and with the viral strain CP7 (USA), and clearly different with the Brazilian BVDV-1b viruses (obtained between 2001 and 2012) and the Argentinean BVDV-1b viruses (obtained between 2006 and 2010). This high variability in and near Domain C, an important antigenic region of BVDV in E2, the immunodominant protein of BVDV, could cause important changes in the antigenicity of these viruses. The Chilean BVDV-1j viruses showed very similar amino acid sequences between them, and also with BVDV-1j viruses not present in Chile (KS86, 190CP and Deer-GB), but clearly different than the viruses that belong to BVDV-1a and BVDV-1b subgenotypes. These results supports those shown previously, that BVDV-1j viruses have very similar antigenicity between them, but have important antigenic differences with viruses of the BVDV-1a, BVDV-1b and BVDV-2 subgenotypes [12, 20, 33].

The results of this study showed that the genetic profile of the BVDV viruses prevalent in Chile is quite different from the virus diversity reported in South America, Europe and North America [9, 17, 34–42]. The high presence of viruses that belong to subgenotype BVDV-1j in Chile and the increase shown over time makes a significant difference with the genetic profile of the virus reported in other countries of the world, including South America, that lead us to consider viruses of the BVDV-1j subgenotype as a possible emergent group of BVDV viruses in cattle.

Although an official control of BVDV is not yet applied in Chile, vaccines are used in many farms, and the current commercial BVDV vaccines are mainly based on BVDV-1a, BVDV-1b or BVDV-2a strains. Nevertheless, although all BVDVs share epitopes of a common pestiviral antigen, antigenic differences have been demonstrated among BVDV types [43], and this is particularly true between BVDV-1a/BVDV-1b and BVDV-1j strains, which have shown major antigenic differences [12, 20, 33].

Further studies should be done to assess if the predominance of BVDV-1j strains in Chile has been maintained over time, reduces the effectiveness of vaccination campaigns, and the need to include BVDV-1j viruses when designing a vaccine for future use in Chile.

Conclusions

The results of this study showed that the genetic profile of BVDV in Chilean cattle is composed of the subgenotypes BVDV-1a, BVDV-1b, and BVDV-1j, with BVDV-1b and BVDV-1j as the predominant subgenotypes.

The Chilean BVDV-1b viruses grouped into a single cluster, apart from the viruses present in Argentina and Brazil, countries geographically close to Chile. This process of local evolution may have generated antigenic differences between the Chilean BVDV-1b viruses and the viruses used in vaccines.

The high increase shown over time of BVDV-1j viruses in Chile, and the low genetic diversity in the E2 gene, the most variable protein of the virus, both among Chilean BVDV-1j viruses and with BVDV-1j viruses present in other regions of the world, suggests that BVDV-1j is an emergent group of viruses in cattle in Chile, and since they show important antigenic differences with BVDV-1a and BVDV-1b viruses used in commercial vaccines, their inclusion in the vaccines used in Chile should be evaluated.

Abbreviations

5'UTR: 5' Untranslated Region; ATCC: American type culture collection; BVDV: *Bovine Viral Diarrhea Virus*; BVDV-1: *Bovine Viral Diarrhea Virus* species 1; BVDV-1a: *Bovine Viral Diarrhea Virus* subgenotype 1a; BVDV-1b: *Bovine Viral Diarrhea Virus* subgenotype 1b; BVDV-1j: *Bovine Viral Diarrhea Virus* subgenotype 1j; BVDV-2: *Bovine Viral Diarrhea Virus* species 2; DEPC: Diethyl pyrocarbonate; DIF: Direct immunofluorescence; E2: Glycoprotein E2; FITC: Fluorescein isothiocyanate; MDBK: Madin-Darby bovine kidney cell; nDomC: Near Domain C; PAAS: Pattern of amino acid substitutions; PCR: Polymerase Chain Reaction; PI: Persistently infected; PID: Percentage identities; RT-PCR: Reverse transcription polymerase chain reaction

Acknowledgements

We are grateful to Dr. Sagar Goyal (University of Minnesota, USA) for providing the MDBK cell line.

Funding
This study was funded by the Comisión Nacional de Investigación Científica y Tecnológica (CONICYT) from the Chilean Government, project FONDECYT-Regular 1060581, granted to José Pizarro-Lucero.

Authors' contributions
AD: Collected samples, performed experiments, and analyzed data. FI: Collected samples, performed experiments, and analyzed data. MC: Performed experiments, analyzed data, and supervised the study. JPL: Performed experiments, analyzed data, wrote the manuscript, and supervised and supported the study. All authors read and approved the manuscript.

Consent for publication
Not applicable

Competing interests
The authors declare that they have no competing interests.

References

1. Baker JC. Bovine viral diarrhea virus: a review. J Am Vet Med Assoc. 1987; 190:1449–57.
2. Brownlie J, Clarke MC, Howard CJ, Pocock DH. Pathogenesis and epidemiology of bovine virus diarrhoea virus infection of cattle. Ann Rech Vet. 1987;18:157–66.
3. Radostits OM, Littlejohns IR. New concepts in the pathogenesis, diagnosis and control of disease caused by the bovine viral diarrhea virus. Can Vet J. 1988;29:513–28.
4. Rebhun WC, French TW, Perdrizet JA, Dubovi EJ, Dill SG, Karcher LF. Thrombocytopenia associated with acute bovine virus diarrhea infection in cattle. J Vet Intern Med. 1989;3:42–6.
5. Corapi WV, Elliott RD, French TW, Arthur DG, Bezek DM, Dubovi EJ. Thrombocytopenia and hemorrhages in veal calves infected with bovine viral diarrhea virus. J Am Vet Med Assoc. 1990;196:590–6.
6. Pellerin C, Hurk JVD, Lecomte J, Tijssen P. Identification of a new group of bovine viral diarrhea virus strains associated with severe outbreaks and high mortalities. Virology. 1994;203:260–8.
7. Simmonds P, Becher P, Bukh J, Gould EA, Meyers G, Monath T, Muerhoff S, Pletnev A, Rico-Hesse R, Smith DB. Stapleton JT and ICTV report consortium. ICTV virus taxonomy profile: Flaviviridae. J Gen Virol. 2017;98:2–3.
8. Yeşilbağ K, Alpay G, Becher P. Variability and global distribution of subgenotypes of bovine viral diarrhea virus. Viruses. 2017;9(6):E128. https://doi.org/10.3390/v9060128.
9. Vilcek S, Paton DJ, Durkovic B, Strojny L, Ibata G, Moussa A, Loitsch A, Rossmanith W, Vega S, Scicluna MT, Palfi V. Bovine viral diarrhoea virus genotype 1 can be separated into at least eleven genetic groups. Arch Virol. 2001;146:99–115.
10. Flores EF, Gil LHGV, Botton SA, Weiblen R, Ridpath JF, Kreutz LC, Pilati C, Driemeyer D, Moojen V, Wendelstein AC. Clinical, pathological and antigenic aspect of bovine viral diarrhea (BVDV) type 2 isolates identified in Brazil. Vet Microbiol. 2000;77:175–83.
11. Jackova A, Novackova M, Pelletier C, Audeval C, Gueneau E, Haffar A, Petit E, Rehby L, Vilcek S. The extended genetic diversity of BVDV-1: typing of BVDV isolates from France. Vet Res Commun. 2008;32:7–11.
12. Nagai M, Hayashi M, Itou M, Fukutomi T, Akashi H, Kida H, Sakoda Y. Identification of new genetic subtypes of bovine viral diarrhea virus genotype 1 isolated in Japan. Virus Genes. 2008;36(1):135–9.
13. Xue F, Zhu YM, Li J, Zhu LC, Ren XG, Feng JK, Shi HF, Gao YR. Genotyping of bovine viral diarrhea viruses from cattle in China between 2005 and 2008. Vet Microbiol. 2010;143(2–4):379–83.
14. Giammarioli M, Ceglie L, Rossi E, Bazzucchi M, Casciari C, Petrini S, De Mia GM. Increased genetic diversity of BVDV-1: recent findings and implications thereof. Virus Genes. 2015;50:147–51.
15. Wolfmeyer A, Wolf G, Beer M, Strube W, Hehnem HR, Schmeer N, Kaaden OR. Genomic (5'UTR) and serological differences among German BVDV field isolates. Arch Virol. 1997;142:2049–57.
16. Nagai M, Sato M, Nagano H, Pang H, Kong X, Murakami T, Ozawa T, Akashi H. Nucleotide sequence homology to bovine viral diarrhea virus 2 (BVDV 2) in the 5' untranslated region of BVDVs from cattle with mucosal disease or persistent infection in Japan. Vet Microbiol. 1998;60: 271–6.
17. Jones LR, Zandomeni R, Webwe EL. Genetic typing of bovine viral diarrhea virus isolates from Argentina. Vet Microbiol. 2001;81:367–75.
18. Couvreur B, Letellier C, Collard A, Quenon P, Dehan P, Hamers C, Pastoret PP, Kerkhofs P. Genetic and antigenic variability in bovine viral diarrhea virus (BVDV) isolates from Belgium. Virus Res. 2002;85:17–28.
19. Vilcek S, Greiser-Wilke I, Durkovic B, Obritzhauser W, Deutz A, Kofer J. Genetic diversity of recent bovine viral diarrhoea viruses from the southeast of Austria (Styria). Vet Microbiol. 2003;91:285–91.
20. Pizarro-Lucero J, Celedón M-O, Aguilera M, de Calisto A. Molecular characterization of pestiviruses isolated from bovines in Chile. Vet Microbiol. 2006;115:208–17.
21. Bauermann FV, Ridpath JF. HoBi-like viruses – the typical 'atypical bovine pestivirus'. Anim Health Res Rev. 2015;16(1):64–9.
22. Celedón MO, Vargas C, Salinas A, Casanova A, Ibarra L, Berríos P. Prevalencias serológicas para el virus diarrea viral bovina y de la rinotraqueitis infecciosa bovina en predios lecheros de la Región Metropolitana de Chile. Av Cs Vet. 1996;11:75–80.
23. Celedón MO, Palacios L, Pizarro J, Ibarra L. Prevalencia de anticuerpos seroneutralizantes para el virus de la diarrea viral bovina en ganado de carne de la región Metropolitana de Chile. Av Cs Vet. 1997;12:98–100.
24. Mahony TJ, McCarthy FM, Gravel JL, Corney B, Young PL, Vilcek S. Genetic analysis of bovine viral diarrhoea viruses from Australia. Vet Microbiol. 2005;106(1–2):1–6.
25. OIE. Manual of Diagnostic Tests and Vaccines for Terrestrial Animals 2017. Chapter 24.7. http://www.oie.int/fileadmin/Home/eng/Health_standards/tahm/2.04.07_BVD.pdf. Accessed 02 March 2018.
26. INE. http://www.ine.cl/estadisticas/censos/censo-agropecuario-y-forestal-2007. Accessed 30 March 2018.
27. Vilcek S, Herring AJ, Herring JA, Nettleton PF, Lowings JP, Paton DJ. Pestiviruses isolated from pigs, cattle and sheep can be allocated into at least three genogroups using polymerase chain reaction and restriction endonuclease analysis. Arch Virol. 1994;136:309–23.
28. Edgar RC. MUSCLE: multiple sequence alignment with high accuracy and high throughput. Nucleic Acids Res. 2004;32:1792–7.
29. Kumar S, Stecher G, Tamura K. MEGA7: molecular evolutionary genetics analysis version 7.0 for bigger datasets. Mol Biol Evol. 2016;33:1870–4.
30. Muhire BM, Varsani A, Martin DP. SDT: a virus classification tool based on pairwise sequence alignment and identity calculation. PLoS One. 2014;9(9):e108277. https://doi.org/10.1371/journal.pone. 0108277.
31. Salgado R, Hidalgo-Hermoso E, Pizarro-Lucero J. Detection of persistent pestivirus infection in pudú (Pudu puda) in a captive population of artiodactyls in Chile. BMC Vet Res. 2018. https://doi.org/10.1186/s12917-018-1363-x.
32. Pizarro-Lucero J, Celedón MO, Navarro C, Ortega R, González D. Identification of a pestivirus isolated from a free-ranging pudu (Pudu puda) in Chile. Vet Rec. 2005;157:292–4.
33. Aguirre IM, Quezada MP, Celedón MO. Antigenic variability in bovine viral diarrhea virus (BVDV) isolates from alpaca (Vicugna pacos), llama (Lama glama) and bovines in Chile. Vet Microbiol. 2014;168:324–30.
34. Pecora A, Malacari DA, Ridpath JF, Perez Aguirreburualde MS, Combessies G, Odeón AC, Romera SA, Golemba MD, Wigdorovitz A. First finding of genetic and antigenic diversity in 1b-BVDV isolates from Argentina. Res Vet Sci. 2014;96:204–12.
35. Silveira S, Weber MN, Mósena ACS, da Silva MS, Streck AF, Pescador CA, Flores EF, Weiblen R, Driemeier D, Ridpath JF, Canal CW. Genetic diversity of brazilian bovine pestiviruses detected berween 1995 and 2014. Transbound Emerg Dis. 2017;64(2):613–23.
36. Ridpath JF. Practical significance of heterogeneity among BVDV strains: impact of biotype and genotype on U.S. control programs. Prev Vet Med. 2005;72:17–30.
37. Tajima M, Dubovi EJ. Genetic and clinical analyses of bovine viral diarrhea virus isolates from dairy operations in the United States of America. J Vet Diagn Investig. 2005;17(1):10–5.
38. Hornberg A, Fernández SR, Vogl C, Vilcek S, Matt M, Fink M, Köfer J, Schöpf K. Genetic diversity of pestivirus isolates in cattle from Western Austria. Vet Microbiol. 2009;135(3–4):205–13.

39. Arias P, Orlich M, Prieto M, Cedillo S, Thiel H-J, Alvarez M, Becher P. Genetic heterogeneity of bovine viral diarrhoea viruses from Spain. Vet Microbiol. 2003;96:327–36.
40. Tajima M. The prevalent genotypes of bovine viral diarrhea virus in Japan, Germany and the United States of America. Jpn J Vet Res. 2006;54(2–3):129–34.
41. Giammarioli M, Pellegrini C, Casciari C, Rossi E, De Mia GM. Genetic diversity of bovine viral diarrhea virus 1: Italian isolates clustered in at least seven subgenotypes. J Vet Diagn Investig. 2008;20(6):783–8.
42. Canal CW, Strasser M, Hertig C, Masuda A, Peterhans E. Detection of antibodies to bovine viral diarrhea virus (BVDV) and characterization of genomes of BVDV from Brazil. Vet Microbiol. 1998;63:85–97.
43. Becher P, Avalos-Ramirez R, Orlich M, Rosales SC, Konig M, Schweizer M, Stalder H, Schirrmeier H, Thiel H-J. Genetic and antigenic characterization of novel pestivirus genotypes: implications for classification. Virology. 2003;311:96–104.

20

Measuring antigen-specific responses in *Mycobacterium bovis*-infected warthogs (*Phacochoerus africanus*) using the intradermal tuberculin test

Eduard O. Roos[1], Francisco Olea-Popelka[2], Peter Buss[3], Guy A. Hausler[1], Robin Warren[1], Paul D. van Helden[1], Sven D. C. Parsons[1], Lin-Mari de Klerk-Lorist[4] and Michele A. Miller[1*]

Abstract

Background: Bovine tuberculosis (bTB) caused by *Mycobacterium bovis* has previously been diagnosed in warthogs and infection can be highly prevalent (> 30%) in endemic areas. Thus, warthogs could potentially be an important species to consider as sentinels for disease surveillance. However, disease surveillance is dependent on availability of accurate diagnostic assays and only a few diagnostic tests have been investigated for warthogs. Furthermore, the tests that have been used in this species require laboratory equipment and trained personnel to obtain results. Therefore, this study investigated the use of the intradermal tuberculin test (ITT) to screen warthogs for bTB, which can be done with minimal equipment and under field conditions by most veterinarians and other qualified professionals. Changes in skin fold thickness measurements at the bovine purified protein derivative (PPD) administration site, between 0 and 72 h, were compared with differential changes between the bovine and avian PPD sites, for 34 warthogs, to evaluate the performance when different interpretation criteria for the ITT was used.

Results: Using an increase of 1.8 mm or more at the bovine PPD site as a cut-off for positive responders, 69% of 16 *M. bovis* culture-positive warthogs had a positive test result, with 100% of the 18 culture-negative warthogs considered as test negative. When a differential of 1.2 mm or more in skin fold thickness at the bovine PPD compared to the avian PPD site was used as a cut-off for the comparative ITT, 81% of culture-positive warthogs were considered as test positive, with 100% of culture-negative warthogs considered as test negative.

Conclusion: The findings in this study suggest that the ITT is a promising tool to use when screening warthogs for *M. bovis* infection.

Keywords: Bovine tuberculosis, Screening test, *Mycobacterium bovis*, Intradermal tuberculin test, Warthog, Wildlife

Background

The primary cause of bovine tuberculosis (bTB) is an acid-fast bacterium, *Mycobacterium bovis*, which has been reported to infect more than 17 wildlife species in South Africa [1]. The disease has become endemic in some nature reserves and private game farms within South Africa [2]. Furthermore, cases of bTB have been reported in threatened or endangered species, such as lions (*Panthera leo*) and rhinoceros (*Ceratotherium simum* and *Diceros bicornis*) [3, 4]. Certain wildlife species have become maintenance hosts of the disease in South Africa including the African buffalo (*Syncerus caffer*) [5]. Warthogs are also known to become infected with *M. bovis* and could potentially act as a maintenance host in endemic areas [6, 7]. This species is capable of crossing fences and other man-made barriers, which could lead to dissemination of disease, as is the case for wild boar (*Sus scrofa*), a bTB maintenance host in the Iberian Mediterranean ecosystem [1, 8]. Moreover,

* Correspondence: miller@sun.ac.za
[1]NRF-DST Centre of Excellence for Biomedical Tuberculosis Research, South African Medical Research Council Centre for Tuberculosis Research, Division of Molecular Biology and Human Genetics, Faculty of Medicine and Health Sciences, Stellenbosch University, PO Box 241, Cape Town 8000, South Africa
Full list of author information is available at the end of the article

similar to feral pigs, warthogs may serve as a good sentinel as they are highly susceptible to this infection [9].

Accurate diagnostic tests are needed for disease surveillance. However, only a limited number of assays are available for bTB diagnosis in African wildlife species. A lack of approved laboratory facilities and logistical difficulties in getting samples to laboratories from disease controlled and remote areas also limits wildlife testing. One available method for field detection of bTB is to euthanase animals, identify granulomatous lesions on necropsy, and confirm the diagnosis using mycobacterial culture. However, it can take 6–8 weeks before culture results become available. Therefore, there is a need to have an accurate field-friendly ante-mortem assay for bTB screening of species such as warthogs, which can be readily performed by veterinarians.

The Intradermal Tuberculin Test (ITT) has been used for bTB detection in a range of species including domestic cattle, wild boar, white-tailed deer (*Odocoileus virginianus*), elk (*Cervus canadensis*), African buffalo, and lions [10–15]. The ITT is readily available to veterinarians and can be performed in the field, providing a result within 72 h. The objective of this study was to investigate the utility and test performance of the ITT for detection of *M. bovis* infection in warthogs.

Results

The ITT was measured for all 34 warthogs and individuals divided into two study cohorts based on mycobacterial culture results (Table 1). *M. bovis*-infection was confirmed by mycobacterial culture in 16 of the 34 warthogs. The SFT measurements from warthogs infected with NTMs were not significantly different from that of *M. bovis* culture-negative warthogs, for both PPD sites, and therefore grouped as culture-negative ($p = 0.086$). There was no significant difference in Δ PPD_a measurements between *M. bovis* culture-positive and culture-negative warthogs ($p = 0.650$, Additional file 1: Figure S1, Table 2). However, Δ PPD_b measurements were significantly greater for culture-positive compared to culture-negative animals (Fig. 1, Table 2). Furthermore, in *M. bovis* culture-positive warthogs, the increase in SFT at the PPD_b site (Δ PPD_b) was significantly greater than at the PPD_a site (Δ PPD_a) ($p = 0.002$), although no differences between these measurements were seen in culture-negative warthogs ($p = 0.128$, Additional file 1: Figure S1, Table 2). The PPD_{b-a} values were significantly greater for culture-positive warthogs compared to culture-negative warthogs ($p < 0.0001$, Fig. 2, Table 2).

A warthog-specific cut-off value for the SITT was calculated as ≥1.8 mm using a ROC curve analysis (AUC = 0.91, 95% CI 0.81–1.0) (Additional file 2: Table S1). Based on this cut-off, 11 out of the 16 *M. bovis* culture-positive warthogs were SITT-positive (69%), while none of the 18 culture-negative warthogs had a positive test result (100%).

The cut-off value for the CITT was ≥1.2 mm (AUC = 0.91, 95% CI 0.79–1.0) (Additional file 3: Table S2). This cut-off value resulted in 13 of 16 culture-positive warthogs being CITT-positive (81%) and classified all 18 culture-negative warthogs as test negative (100%). No signs of oedema, heat, exudation or necrosis were observed at the PPD injection sites in any of the 34 warthogs tested.

Discussion

This study shows that the ITT could distinguish between *M. bovis* culture-positive and negative warthogs from bTB endemic regions of South Africa, using both the SITT and CITT interpretations. Warthog specific cut-off values for the SITT and CITT were calculated to be ≥1.8 mm and ≥ 1.2 mm, respectively. The optimal ITT criterion for detection of infected warthogs in this study was the ≥1.2 mm cut-off for the CITT, which resulted in correct classification of 81% of culture-positive animals as CITT-positive and 100% of culture-negative warthogs as test negative. These results suggest that the interpretation of the ITT in this species should include the reaction to avian PPD (i.e., CITT) to identify the highest number of infected animals.

Importantly, diagnostic application in each species requires optimization and standardization of the ITT, as the injection site and dose may influence the delayed-type hypersensitivity response, with variable interpretation affecting test sensitivity [11, 12, 14, 16]. In this study, a double dose of tuberculin (0.2 ml PPD) was injected intradermally, caudal to each ear in warthogs, to minimise the chance of delayed-type hypersensitivity response failure due to dose, as is the case in lions and domestic cats [11].

The choice of ITT (SITT or CITT) is dependent on the prevalence and exposure of *M. bovis* as well as the presence of sensitising NTMs in a population [10]. The SITT is a simpler test, since it consists of one injection and measurement, although it lacks the discriminatory power of the CITT, where the response to PPD_a identifies sensitisation to NTMs [10]. In this study, the response at the PPD_a site was significantly less than that at the PPD_b site, indicating that the increase in SFT at the PPD_b site was a true measure of *M. bovis* infection and not a cross-reactive response to NTMs.

In many countries the initial recommendations that were in place for the ITT suggested the use of the single intradermal cervical test as the primary bTB screening test and the CITT as an ancillary test [10]. However, most of these countries have amended their regulations, as the CITT has been shown to be a more specific test than the SITT [17]. Furthermore, our results showed

Table 1 Raw data from 34 warthogs' skinfold measurements (in mm) to PPD_b and PPD_a at time points 0 h and 72 h post-injection, the delta PPD_b and PPD_a as well as each warthogs' mycobacterial culture result

Lab no.	PPD_b 0 h	PPD_b 72 h	Δ PPD_b	PPD_a 0 h	PPD_a 72 h	Δ PPD_a	Bacterial Culture
15/137	3	3	0	3.1	3.1	0	Culture negative
15/138	3.6	4.1	0.5	3.6	4.8	1.2	Culture negative
15/262	4.2	3.8	−0.4	4.6	5	0.4	Culture negative
15/271	4.9	4.9	0	4.3	4.8	0.5	Culture negative
15/302	2.6	4	1.4	2.7	4.6	1.9	Culture negative
15/304	3	3	0	3	3.3	0.3	Culture negative
15/307	5	6.1	1.1	4	6.6	2.6	Culture negative
15/308	3.3	3.3	0	3.7	3.8	0.1	Culture negative
15/310	3	3.2	0.2	3	3.4	0.4	Culture negative
15/305	3.2	4.2	1	2.8	3.1	0.3	*M. asiaticum*
15/516	5.3	4.2	-1.1	5.5	4.7	−0.8	*M. asiaticum*
15/309	3.2	3.6	0.4	3.3	3.4	0.1	*M. avium*
15/301	2.3	2.4	0.1	2.6	2.5	−0.1	*M. intracellulare*
15/515	3.9	3.4	−0.5	3.3	3	−0.3	*M. intracellulare*
15/535	3.8	3.8	0	5.5	5.2	−0.3	*M. paraffinicum*
15/514	4.8	4.7	−0.1	4	5.2	1.2	*M. simiae*
15/534	4.6	5.3	0.7	4.8	4.2	−0.6	*M. simiae*
15/536	4.5	4.5	0	4.5	5	0.5	*M. simiae*
15/140	4.8	6.9	2.1	4.6	4.6	0	*M. bovis*
15/248	3.8	8	4.2	4	3.8	−0.2	*M. bovis*
15/249	4.4	4.4	0	4.5	4.7	0.2	*M. bovis*
15/250	3.6	7	3.4	4.3	4.1	−0.2	*M. bovis*
15/251	4.8	5.7	0.9	4.1	4	−0.1	*M. bovis*
15/263	4.1	7.2	3.1	3.9	3.8	−0.1	*M. bovis*
15/264	3.8	14	10.2	3.2	3.4	0.2	*M. bovis*
15/265	4.3	4.9	0.6	3.8	3.8	0	*M. bovis*
15/266	4.3	11.2	6.9	4.2	3.6	-0.6	*M. bovis*
15/267	3.8	6.5	2.7	4.4	4.6	0.2	*M. bovis*
15/268	3.6	6.4	2.8	3.6	4.1	0.5	*M. bovis*
15/269	3.7	4.7	1	2.9	3.5	0.6	*M. bovis*
15/270	2.8	5.9	3.1	2.9	3.2	0.3	*M. bovis*
15/300	3.6	7	3.4	3.6	4	0.4	*M. bovis*
15/306	3.3	8.1	4.8	3.8	4.6	0.8	*M. bovis*
15/513	4.8	5.1	0.3	4.6	6.2	1.6	*M. bovis*

Table 2 Median values of the skinfold increase (in mm) using different combinations of measurements for the ITT in *M. bovis* culture-positive and culture–negative warthogs

Skinfold reading	Culture Positive	Culture Negative
Δ PPD_a	0.2 mm (−0.1–0.5)	0.3 mm (−0.2–0.7)
Δ PPD_b	3.0 mm (0.9–4.0)	0.0 mm (−0.1–0.6)
PPD_b - PPD_a	2.5 mm (1.3–3.5)	-0.4 mm (− 0.5–0.1)

Interquartile ranges are shown in parentheses

that the CITT was more sensitive than the SITT (81% versus 69%, correctly identifying animals with a culture-positive result). This may be due to the more sensitive cut-off value of ≥1.2 mm for the CITT compared to the ≥1.8 mm cut-off for the SITT [10, 18, 19]. It is important to note that neither the CITT nor SITT had any false positives in this study using these criteria.

Unfortunately, no biological test is perfect (i.e. has 100% sensitivity and specificity) and the CITT could not correctly classify all *M. bovis* culture-positive warthogs

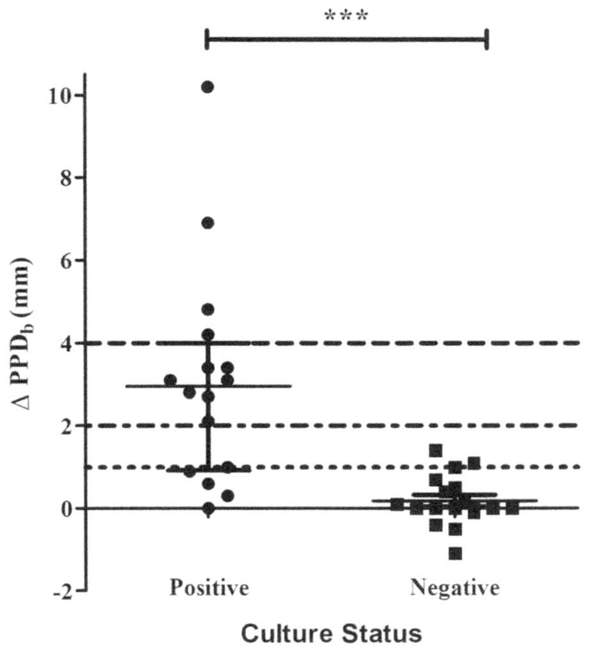

Fig. 1 Differential in skin fold thickness (Δ PPD_b) at the PPD_b injection site after 72 h in *M. bovis* culture-positive or culture-negative warthogs. Median and interquartile ranges are represented by the horizontal bars. The dotted lines represent the various published cut-off values used in other species (1, 2 and 4 mm). ** indicates $p < 0.01$, *** indicates $p < 0.001$

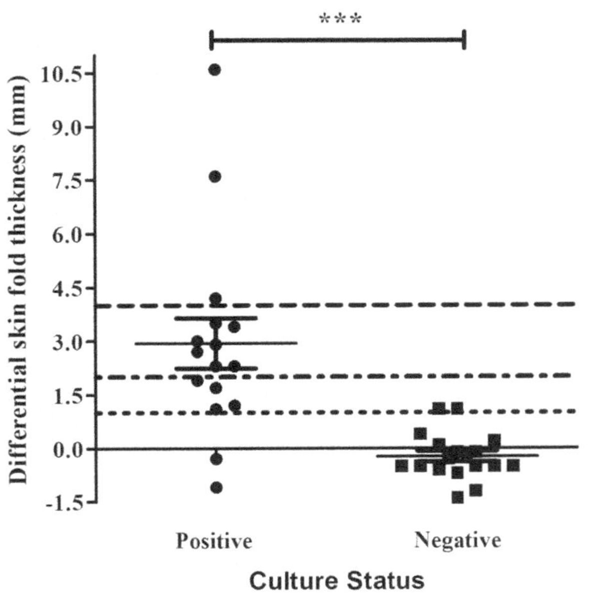

Fig. 2 Test value of the skin test for *M. bovis* infected and uninfected warthogs. Test value was calculated by subtracting the PPD_a injection sites' skin fold thickness from that of the PPD_b injection site after 72 h (PPD_b - PPD_a). Median and interquartile ranges are represented by the horizontal bars. The dotted lines represent the various published cut-off values in other species (1, 2 and 4 mm). *** indicates $p < 0.001$

as test positive and at 81%, it is comparable to the sensitivity of the CITT in cattle [20]. The sub-optimal sensitivity could be due to various factors, for example, anergy, co-infection with NTMs, immunosuppression associated with nutritional, immobilization or transport stress, operator error, faulty equipment, or tuberculin not correctly administered intradermally [10].

For disease surveillance, the cut-off value of a screening test should be set to optimize sensitivity and specificity, after considering the prevalence of disease and epidemiological factors as well as clinical and financial constraints [19, 21]. A cost-effective and logistically feasible method is required for disease surveillance in wildlife since access to laboratories may be limited. Although previous reports have shown that serological assays can be used to identify infected warthogs [6], these require laboratory equipment and techniques which may not be readily available. Therefore, the ITT may be an alternative screening test to laboratory-based assays in some situations.

One limitation of this study was that cut-off values and test specificity were determined using endemic controls rather than animals from a known *M. bovis* negative population. Therefore, future research should ideally include an unexposed population of warthogs to evaluate specificity and determine a diagnostic cut-off value for the ITT.

Conclusion

This study demonstrates that an antigen-specific in vivo response to *M. bovis* can be measured in warthogs when challenged with PPD_b, thus confirming the usefulness of the ITT for this species. Cut-off values determined by ROC curve analyses were able to distinguish between *M. bovis* culture-positive and culture-negative warthogs with good sensitivity and specificity. Interpretation of the ITT under the criteria followed for the CITT, allowed greater numbers of infected warthogs to be detected. Thus, the application of the ITT will be a valuable tool for disease surveillance in warthogs.

Methods

Animals and sampling

In 2015, warthogs were captured and culled as part of drought management in the Greater Kruger National Park area (GKNP) by park veterinarians [22]. Since bTB is endemic in the GKNP, all warthogs in this study were considered exposed to *M. bovis*. Sixteen female and eighteen male warthogs were first immobilized and held in quarantine bomas to evaluate performance of the ITT in this species, as described below. Based on physical examination at the time of capture and post-mortem evaluation, all the animals were deemed to be healthy and in good to moderate body condition. The authors did not find evidence of any condition that would result in an immunocompromised animal, when the ITT was read. After reading the ITT, immobilized warthogs were humanely euthanized using succinylcholine (25 mg/kg; Kyron Laboratories, Benrose, South Africa), saturated with potassium chloride, administered intravenous. This drug was chosen since the warthog was already unconscious, the drug was readily available, could be administered in sufficient quantities to result in rapid death to a large animal, and did not present a health hazard if meat was consumed (by scavengers or others). Since the warthogs were part of a disease surveillance program, all animals were euthanized and a full necropsy performed. Post-mortem examination and tissue sampling were performed as previously described [6]. In summary, lymph nodes were collected from all warthogs and examined for gross lesions consistent with bTB. If no visible legions were observed, samples were pooled according to anatomical site and all sets cultured.

Immobilization

All warthogs were immobilized using a drug combination of (i) zolazepam-tiletamine (Zoletil®; Virbac RSA, (Pty) Ltd., Centurion, South Africa) in combination with azaperone (Kyron Laboratories (Pty) Limited, Benrose, South Africa) or medetomidine (Kyron), or (ii) azaperone, butorphanol (Kyron), medetomidine and ketamine (Kyron) [22–24]. Immobilizations and holding conditions complied with the South African National Parks Standard Operating Procedures for the Capture, Transportation and Maintenance in Holding Facilities of Wildlife.

Intradermal tuberculin test (ITT)

The intradermal tuberculin test was performed as described elsewhere [11]. Briefly, the skin fold thickness (SFT) caudal to each ear was measured using a spring loaded Hauptner calliper with pistol grip prior to administration of the purified protein derivative (PPD; Institute for Animal Sciences, Lelystadt, Netherlands) injection (Additional file 4: Figure S2). PPD was injected intradermally at 0 h: 0.2 ml bovine PPD (30,000 IU/ml) (PPD_b) on the left and 0.2 ml avian PPD (25,000 IU/ml) (PPD_a) on the right. After 72 h, the SFT at each PPD injection site was measured and examined for signs of oedema, heat, exudation or necrosis [25]. The same experienced operator performed all measurements and PPD injections.

The ITT was interpreted in two ways. For the single intradermal tuberculin test (SITT), the SFT prior to the PPD_b injection (0 h) was subtracted from the measurement at the same site 72 h post-injection (Δ PPD_b). For the comparative intradermal tuberculin test (CITT), the 72 h SFT at the PPD_a injection site was subtracted from that at the PPD_b injection site (PPD_{b-a}). This was done since the degree of dehydration varies between individuals. Thus, only the absolute increase in response was used to calculate the PPD_b specific response. The degree of dehydration in individual animals has also been recognized by the South African Department of Agriculture, Forestry and Fisheries in TB testing of African buffaloes [26]. The Δ PPD_a was calculated in the same way as the Δ PPD_b.

Mycobacterial cultures and speciation

All tissue samples were processed using the BACTEC™ MGIT™ 960 system (BD Biosciences, New Jersey, USA) as previously described [13]. Positive cultures in the MGIT system were further analysed by Ziehl-Neelsen (ZN) staining and all ZN-positive cultures were speciated using genetic region of difference analysis [27] and 16S DNA sequencing [28]. The status of warthogs as *M. bovis*-infected or uninfected was based on culture results.

Data analysis

Statistical analyses were performed using GraphPad Prism version 5 (GraphPad Software, March 2007). The Δ PPD_b and Δ PPD_a values for *M. bovis* culture-positive and culture-negative animals were compared within and between groups using a Kruskal-Wallis statistic with a Dunn's Multiple Comparison test. The Δ PPD_a and Δ PPD_b comparisons were done to confirm the specific response of *M. bovis* culture-positive warthogs to the PPD_b injection. Evaluation of the Δ PPD_a was done to provide information as to whether non-tuberculous mycobacteria (NTM) influence the PPD_b responses. The SITT results for culture-positive and culture-negative animals were compared using a Mann Whitney test, as were results for the CITT. Warthog specific cut-off values to determine positive responders were calculated using a receiver operator characteristic (ROC) curve analysis and selected based on the Youden's index [29].

Additional files

Additional file 1: Figure S1. Differential in skin fold thickness at the PPD_b and PPD_a (Δ PPD_b and Δ PPD_a) injection site after 72 h in *M. bovis* culture-positive (CP) or culture-negative (CN) warthogs. Median and interquartile ranges are represented by the horizontal bars. ** indicates $p < 0.01$, *** indicates $p < 0.001$.

Additional file 2: Table S1. Receiver operator characteristics curve analysis data for Δ PPD_b. Warthog specific cut-off values and respective sensitivity and specificity, with 95% CI in parentheses. Youden's index for each cut-off value is also indicated.

Additional file 3: Table S2. Receiver operator characteristics curve analysis data for $PPD_b - PPD_a$. Warthog specific cut-off values and respective sensitivity and specificity, with 95% CI in parentheses. Youden's index for each cut-off value is also indicated.

Additional file 4: Figure S2. Purified protein derivative injection site for the intradermal tuberculin test, caudal to each ear. The picture shows the appropriate use of the callipers to measure the skin fold thickness (mm).

Acknowledgements
The authors wish to acknowledge and thank the following individuals for their contributions to this study: Leana Rossouw, Tebogo Manamela, Dr. Jennie Hewlett, Marius Kruger and the Veterinary Wildlife Services capture team from Kruger National Park for assistance with sample collection from the warthogs, as well as Schalk van Dyk, At Dekker, Rudi Lorist and the state veterinary Quarantine Boma Team for sample collection and general care of warthogs being housed inside the quarantine facility.

Funding
South African Medical Research Council and the National Research Foundation of South Africa [SARChI grant 86949]. The content is the sole responsibility of the authors and does not necessarily represent the official views of the funders.

Authors' contributions
EOR, L-MdK-L, SDCP and MAM conceptualised and designed the project. EOR, L-MdK-L, MAM, PB, GAH were all part of sampling and sample processing. EOR and FO-P were responsible for the data analysis and interpretation. SDCP, L-MdK-L and MAM supervised the findings and encourage EOR to investigate these. FO-P, PB, PDvH and RW supported the research with critical revision of the article. EOR, SDCP, L-MdK-L and MAM drafted the article with all authors contributed substantially to the writing and revising of the manuscript. All authors approved the final version for submission (EOR, FO-P, PDvH, GAH, RW, PDvH, SDCP, L-MdK-L and MAM).

Consent for publication
Not applicable.

Competing interests
The authors declare that they have no competing interests.

Author details
[1]NRF-DST Centre of Excellence for Biomedical Tuberculosis Research, South African Medical Research Council Centre for Tuberculosis Research, Division of Molecular Biology and Human Genetics, Faculty of Medicine and Health Sciences, Stellenbosch University, PO Box 241, Cape Town 8000, South Africa. [2]Department of Clinical Sciences, College of Veterinary Medicine and Biomedical Sciences, Colorado State University, 300 W. Drake Rd, Fort Collins, CO 80523, USA. [3]Veterinary Wildlife Services, South African National Parks, Kruger National Park, Private Bag X402, Skukuza 1350, South Africa. [4]Office of the State Veterinarian, Kruger National Park, Department of Agriculture, Forestries and Fisheries, PO Box 12, Skukuza 1350, South Africa.

References

1. Michel AL, Bengis RG, Keet DF, Hofmeyr M, De Klerk LM, Cross PC, et al. Wildlife tuberculosis in South African conservation areas: Implications and challenges. Vet Microbiol. 2006;112:91–100. Available from: http://www.sciencedirect.com/science/article/pii/S0378113505003834. [cited 19 Jan 2015].
2. Hlokwe TM, van Helden P, Michel AL. Evidence of increasing intra and inter-species transmission of *Mycobacterium bovis* in South Africa: Are we losing the battle? Prev Vet Med. 2014;115:10–7. https://doi.org/10.1016/j.prevetmed.2014.03.011.
3. Sylvester TT, Martin LER, Buss P, Loxton AG, Hausler GA, Rossouw L, et al. Prevalence and risk factors for *Mycobacterium bovis* infection in African lions (*Panthera leo*) in the Kruger National Park. J Wildl Dis. 2017;53:372–6 Available from: http://www.jwildlifedis.org/doi/10.7589/2016-07-159.
4. Miller MA, Buss PE, van Helden PD, Parsons SDC. *Mycobacterium bovis* in a free-ranging black rhinoceros, Kruger National Park, South Africa, 2016. Emerg Infect Dis. 2017;23:557–8.
5. De Vos V, Bengis RG, Kriek NP, Michel A, Keet DF, Raath JP, et al. The epidemiology of tuberculosis in free-ranging African buffalo (*Syncerus caffer*) in the Kruger National Park, South Africa. Onderstepoort J Vet Res. 2001;68:119–30.
6. Roos EO, Buss P, de Klerk-Lorist L-M, Hewlett J, Hausler GA, Rossouw L, et al. Test performance of three serological assays for the detection of *Mycobacterium bovis* infection in common warthogs (*Phacochoerus africanus*). Vet Immunol Immunopathol. 2016;182:79–84. https://doi.org/10.1016/j.vetimm.2016.10.006.
7. Renwick AR, White PCL, Bengis RG. Bovine tuberculosis in southern African wildlife: a multi-species host–pathogen system. Epidemiol Infect. 2007;135:529. Available from: http://www.pubmedcentral.nih.gov/articlerender.fcgi?artid=2870607&tool=pmcentrez&rendertype=abstract. [cited 19 Jan 2015].
8. Naranjo V, Gortazar C, Vicente J, de la Fuente J. Evidence of the role of European wild boar as a reservoir of *Mycobacterium tuberculosis* complex. Vet Microbiol. 2008;127:1–9. Available from: http://www.sciencedirect.com/science/article/pii/S0378113507004853. [cited 23 Feb 2015].
9. Roos EO, Olea-Popelka F, Buss P, de Klerk-Lorist L-M, Cooper D, van Helden PD, et al. Seroprevalence of *Mycobacterium bovis* infection in warthogs (*Phacochoerus africanus*) in bovine tuberculosis-endemic regions of South Africa. Transbound Emerg Dis. 2018;65:1182–9. Available from: http://doi.wiley.com/10.1111/tbed.12856.
10. de la Rua-Domenech R, Goodchild AT, Vordermeier HM, Hewinson RG, Christiansen KH, Clifton-Hadley RS. Ante mortem diagnosis of tuberculosis in cattle: A review of the tuberculin tests, gamma-interferon assay and other ancillary diagnostic techniques. Res Vet Sci. 2006;81:190–210. Available from: http://www.sciencedirect.com/science/article/pii/S0034528806000026. [cited 16 Jan 2015].
11. Keet DF, Michel AL, Bengis RG, Becker P, van Dyk DS, van Vuuren M, et al. Intradermal tuberculin testing of wild African lions (*Panthera leo*) naturally exposed to infection with *Mycobacterium bovis*. Vet Microbiol. 2010;144:384–91. https://doi.org/10.1016/j.vetmic.2010.01.028.
12. Jaroso R, Vicente J, Fernandez-de-Mera IG, Aranaz A, Gortazar C. Eurasian wild boar response to skin-testing with mycobacterial and non-mycobacterial antigens. Prev Vet Med. 2010;96:211–7. https://doi.org/10.1016/j.prevetmed.2010.06.011.
13. Goosen WJ, Miller MA, Chegou NN, Cooper D, Warren RM, van Helden PD, et al. Agreement between assays of cell-mediated immunity utilizing *Mycobacterium bovis*-specific antigens for the diagnosis of tuberculosis in African buffaloes (*Syncerus caffer*). Vet Immunol Immunopathol. 2014;160:133–8. Available from: http://www.sciencedirect.com/science/article/pii/S0165242714000816. [cited 5 Jan 2015].
14. Palmer MV, Whipple DL, Waters WR. Tuberculin skin testing in white-tailed deer (*Odocoileus virginianus*). J Vet Diagn Investig. 2001;13:530–3 Available from: http://www.ncbi.nlm.nih.gov/pubmed/11724147.
15. Palmer MV, Whipple DL, Payeur JB, Bolin CA. Use of the intradermal tuberculin test in a herd of captive elk (*Cervus elaphus nelsoni*) naturally infected with *Mycobacterium bovis*. J Vet Diagn Investig. 2011;23:363–6.
16. Good M, Clegg TA, Costello E, More SJ. The comparative performance of the single intradermal test and the single intradermal comparative tuberculin test in Irish cattle, using tuberculin PPD combinations of differing potencies. Vet J. 2011;190:e60–5. Available from: http://linkinghub.elsevier.com/retrieve/pii/S1090023311000128. [cited 13 June 2016].
17. Goodchild AV, Downs SH, Upton P, Wood JLNN, De La Rua-Domenech R, De Rua-domenech R. Specificity of the comparative skin test for bovine tuberculosis in Great Britain. Vet Rec. 2015;177:258.
18. Metz CE. Basic principles of ROC analysis. Semin Nucl Med. 1978;8:283–98 Available from: http://www.sciencedirect.com/science/article/pii/S0001299878800142.
19. Greiner M, Pfeiffer D, Smith RD. Principles and practical application of the receiver-operating characteristic analysis for diagnostic tests. Prev Vet Med. 2000;45:23–41.
20. Hartnack S, Torgerson PR. The Accuracy of the single intradermal comparative skin test for the diagnosis of bovine Tuberculosis-estimated from a systematic literature search. Mycobact Dis. 2012;2. Available from: https://www.omicsonline.org/the-accuracy-of-the-single-intradermal-comparative-skin-test-for-the-diagnosis-of-bovine-tuberculosis-estimated-from-a-systematic-literature-search-2161-1068.1000120.php?aid=8272. Accessed 13 June 2016.
21. van Erkel AR, Pattynama PM. Receiver operating characteristic (ROC) analysis: basic principles and applications in radiology. Eur J Radiol. 1998;27:88–94.
22. SANParks. Coordinated Policy Framework Governing Park Management Plans [Internet]. SANParks Manag. Plan Policy Framew; 2006. p. 60. Available from: https://www.sanparks.org/docs/conservation/cpfjanuary2010.pdf.

23. Hewlett J. Evaluation of a partially reversible immobilization protocol using Medetomidine, Butorphanol, Zolazepam-Tiletamine, and ketamine in free-ranging warthogs (*Phacochoeus africanus*) in Kruger National Park. University of Pretoria; 2017.
24. Moon PF, Smith LJ. General anesthetic techniques in swine. Vet Clin North Am Food Anim Pract. 1996;12:663–91. Available from: http://www.ncbi.nlm.nih.gov/pubmed/8916392.
25. OIE WO for AH. OIE. OIE Terr. Man. 2009 [Internet]. Paris; 2009. p. 1–16. Available from: http://www.oie.int/fileadmin/Home/eng/Healthstandards/tahm/2.04.07BOVINETB.pdf. Accessed 13 June 2016.
26. DAFF D of AF and F. Buffalo disease risk management [Internet]. South Africa; 2017. p. 1–15. Available from: https://www.daff.gov.za/vetweb/pamphlets&Information/Policy/Buffalo%20Disease%20Risk%20Management%20VPN%20%20ADDENDUMS_2017-02-17.pdf. Accessed 13 June 2016.
27. Warren RM, Gey van Pittius NC, Barnard M, Hesseling A, Engelke E, de Kock M, et al. Differentiation of *Mycobacterium tuberculosis* complex by PCR amplification of genomic regions of difference. Int J Tuberc Lung Dis. 2006; 10:818–22.
28. Leclerc M-C, Haddad N, Moreau R, Thorel M-F. Molecular characterization of environmental *Mycobacterium* strains by PCR-restriction fragment length polymorphism of hsp65 and by sequencing of hsp65, and of 16S and ITS1 rDNA. Res Microbiol. 2000;151:629–38. Available from: http://www.sciencedirect.com/science/article/pii/S0923250800901293. [cited 8 July 2015].
29. Youden WJ. Index for rating diagnostic tests. Cancer. 1950;3:32–5.

Development of a recombinase polymerase amplification combined with a lateral flow dipstick assay for rapid detection of the *Mycoplasma bovis*

Guimin Zhao[1], Peili Hou[1], Yanjun Huan[2], Chengqiang He[1*], Hongmei Wang[1*] and Hongbin He[1*]

Abstract

Background: *Mycoplasma bovis* (*M. bovis*) is a major etiological agent of bovine mycoplasmosis around the world. Point-of-care testing in the field is lacking owing to the requirement for a simple, robust field applicable test that does not require professional laboratory equipment. The recombinase polymerase amplification (RPA) technique has become a promising isothermal DNA amplify assay for use in rapid and low-resource diagnostics.

Results: Here, a method for specific detection of *M. bovis* DNA was established, which was RPA combined with lateral flow dipstick (LFD). First, the analytical specificity and sensitivity of the RPA primer and LF-probe sets were evaluated. The assay successfully detected *M. bovis* DNA in 30 min at 39 °C, with detection limit of 20 copies per reaction, which it was compared the real-time quantitative PCR (qPCR) assay. This method was specific because it did not detect a selection of other bacterial pathogens in cattle. Both qPCR and RPA-LFD assays were used to detect *M. bovis* 442 field samples from 42 different dairy farms in Shandong Province of China, also the established RPA-LFD assay obtained 99.00% sensitivity, 95.61% specificity, and 0.902 kappa coefficient compared with the qPCR.

Conclusions: To the author's knowledge, this is the first report using an RPA-FLD assay to visualise and detect *M. bovis*. Comparative analysis with qPCR indicates the potential of this assay for rapid diagnosis of bovine mycoplasmosis in resource limited settings.

Keywords: *Mycoplasma bovis*, Lateral flow dipstick, Recombinase polymerase amplification, Isothermal nucleic acid amplification, Rapid and visual detection

Background

Mycoplasma bovis (*M. bovis*) is a major etiological agent of bovine mycoplasmosis around the world. *M. bovis* has not only been confirmed as a major pathogen in bovine respiratory disease (BRD), but it has also causes disease in cattle of all ages, such as arthritis, otitis media, mastitis, and reproductive disorders [1]. Due to lack of effectiveness of treatments for controlling the disease in affected herds and decreasing growth rate of the cattle, it can result in serious economic losses in both dairy and beef cattle herds [2].

In 2008, a severe cattle respiratory disease was reported in Hubei Province of China, thereafter, it quickly spread to over 11 Chinese provinces. The organisms isolated from calf lungs were identified as *M. bovis* and designated strain Hubei-1. The 16S rRNA demonstrated 99.5% homology with *M. bovis* type strain PG45 [3]. Other places in China, such as Ningxia, Xinjiang, Guizhou, Chongqing, and Qingdao, later reported *M. bovis* isolated from dairy cows and beef cattle [4]. The lack of an effective control methods to prevent the rapid spread of *M. bovis* as well as its stubborn persistence on farms requires rapid and accurate diagnosis when clinical signs first appear [1].

* Correspondence: hchqiang@sdnu.edu.cn; hongmeiwang@sdnu.edu.cn; hongbinhe@sdnu.edu.cn
[1]Key Laboratory of Animal Resistant Biology of Shandong, Ruminant Disease Research Center, College of Life Science Shandong Normal University, No.88 Wenhua East Road, Lixia District, Jinan 250014, Shandong Province, China
Full list of author information is available at the end of the article

The development of simple and quick nucleic acid detection methods could greatly improve diagnostics; however, practical on-site testing is infrequently done due to the lack of availability of robustly tested methods. Detection of *M. bovis* from clinical samples by traditional culture methods is quite time-consuming and is often hampered by bacterial contamination. Although detection technology of molecular biology for nucleic acids, such as polymerase chain reaction (PCR) and real-time quantitative PCR (qPCR) has shown high sensitivity and specificity, these methods need professional diagnostic laboratories and thermal cycling device. Such facilities may be lacking in disease epidemic and poor areas, especially in developing countries, the use of rapid

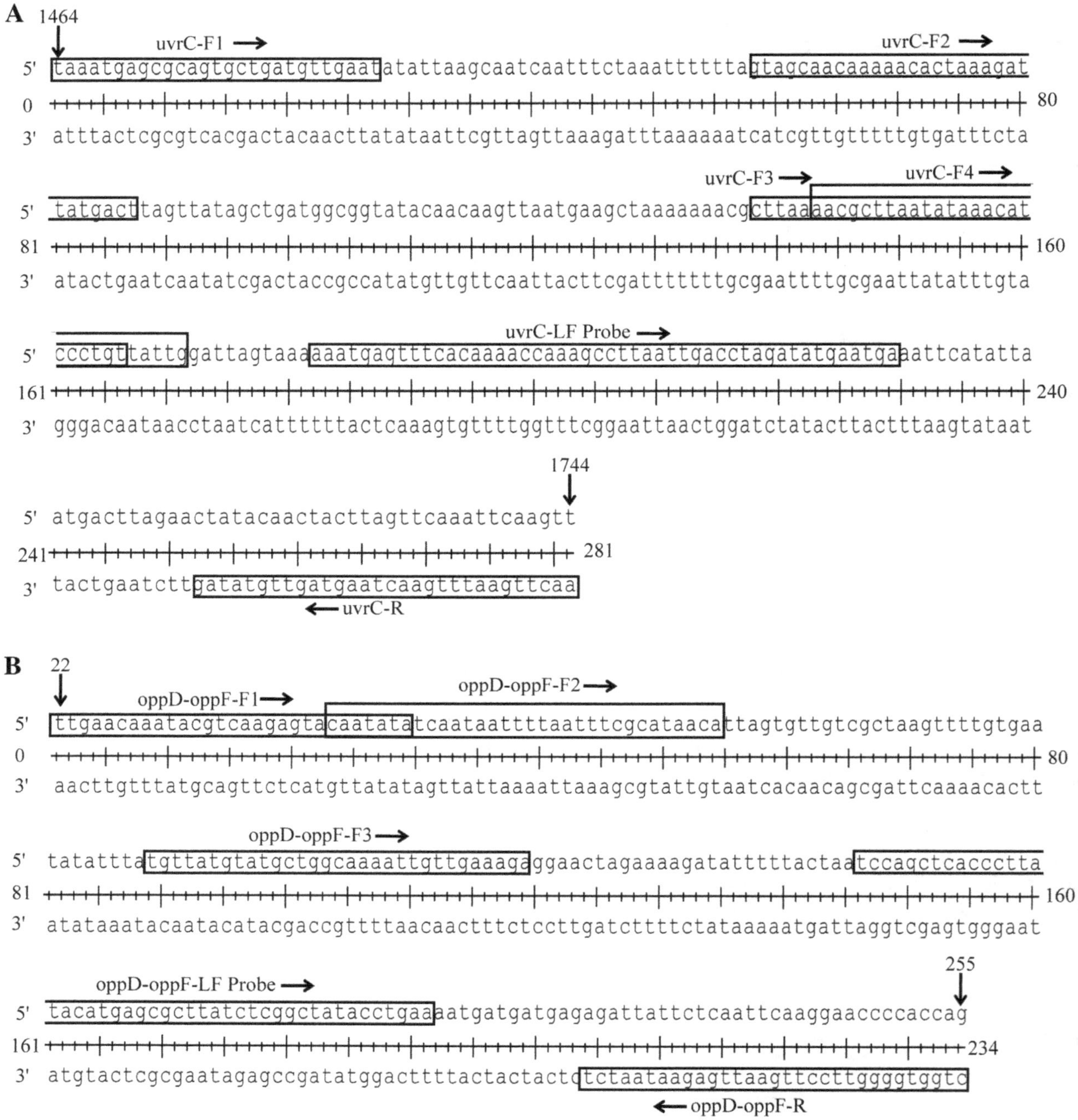

Fig. 1 Details (location and sequence) for each primer and LF probe set used in our RPA-LFD assay. **a** The target region spanned nucleotides 1464–1744 of the *uvrC* gene of *Mycoplasma bovis* (GenBank Accession: AF003959.1); **b** The target region spanned nucleotides 22–255 of the *oppD-oppF* gene of *Mycoplasma bovis* (GenBank Accession: AF130119.1)

on-site diagnostic methods would be extraordinary helpful in controlling bovine mycoplasmosis.

Recently, for DNA amplification, the recombinase polymerase amplification (RPA) technique has become a promising molecular technology for low-resource, rapid diagnostics [5]. Several types of tests have been described [6], and the RPA combined with lateral flow dipstick (LFD) appears especially suitable for point-of-care diagnosis in clinical specimens. The RPA assay has been reported for the rapid detection of Caprine arthritis-encephalitis virus, *Chlamydia trachomatis*, *Plasmodium falciparum* and other pathogens [7–9].

However, the detection of *M. bovis* using RPA-LFD assay has not yet been reported. In this study, we developed a rapid, sensitive, and on-site RPA combined with a LFD assay for the specific detection of *M. bovis* in the field.

Results

Evaluation of RPA nfo primer and probe sets

The analytical specificity of seven primers combinations with LF-probes (Fig. 1 and Table 1) was confirmed using the genomic DNA extracted from *M. bovis* reference type strain PG45. The candidate primers for the RPA-LFD assay was screened with TwistAmp nfo reactions and preliminary analysis was performed on 2% agarose gel with labeled amplicons. The result showed that primer set uvrC-F1/uvrC-R/uvrC-LF probe yielded specific amplification efficiency for the RPA assay, and produced the expected size of the product of 281 base-pairs (Fig. 2a). The RPA-LFD test line appeared more quickly, within 5 min, and was more distinct than the other sets (Fig. 2b). This set (uvrC-F1/uvrC-R/uvrC-LF probe) was selected for subsequent evaluation (Fig. 1 and Table 1).

Determination of RPA reaction temperature and time

The results showed that the RPA reaction could be determined at a wide range of temperatures from 30 to 45 °C. In addition, the test band was the brightest between 35 °C to 42 °C (Fig. 3a). Therefore, in the later the reaction of RPA-LFD assay temperature was set in 39 °C. Next, the optimum reaction time was estimated between 1 to 35 min. Results indicated that the most distinct band could be seen in the test zone position between 20 to 35 min with only weak bands seen after 10 min (Fig. 3b). According to the results, the incubation time was set at 30 min for the following RPA-LFD testing.

Specificity and sensitivity of the *M. bovis* RPA-LFD assay

RPA specificity was tested using various Mycoplasma species from cattle and other pathogens that cause respiratory disease and mastitis (Table 2). RPA-LFD revealed high specificity and no cross-reaction was observed against other Mycoplasmas (*Mycoplasma agalactiae, Mycoplasma mycoides* subsp. *mycoides, Mycoplasma bovirhinis, Mycoplasma bovoculi, Mycoplasma bovigenitalium, Mycoplasma dispar, Mycoplasma canadense, Mycoplasma alkalescens, Mycoplasma canis, Mycoplasma arginini*), respiratory bacterial pathogens (*Pasteurella multocida, Mannheimia haemolytica, Trueperella pyogenes, Histophilus somni, Klebsiella pneumoniae*) and mastitis or other pathogens (*Staphylococcus aureus, Streptococcus agalactiae, Corynebacterium bovis, Pseudomonas aeruginosa, Proteus mirabilis, Enterobacter aerogenes, Brucella abortus, Escherichia coli*) (Additional file 1: Figure S1).

The sensitivity of RPA-LFD and qPCR assay was evaluated, and the repeatability test of limits of detection was showed in Table 3 and Fig. 4. Results from the

Table 1 Primer and probe sequences used for RPA-LFD assay

Name	Sequence (5′-3′)	Genome location	Amplification size (bp)
uvrC-F1	TAAATGAGCGCAGTGCTGATGTTGAAT	1464–1490	281
uvrC-F2	GTAGCAACAAAAACACTAAAGATTATGACT	1521–1550	224
uvrC-F3	CTTAAAACGCTTAATATAAACATCCCTGT	1601–1629	144
uvrC-F4	AACGCTTAATATAAACATCCCTGTTATTG	1606–1634	139
uvrC-R	Biotin-AACTTGAATTTGAACTAAGTAGTTGTATAG	1715–1744	
uvrC-LF Probe	FAM-AAATGAGTTTCACAAAACCAAAGCCTTAAT [dSpacer]GACCTAGATATGAATGA-C3 Spacers	1645–1692	100
oppD-oppF-F1	TTGAACAAATACGTCAAGAGTACAATATA	22–50	234
oppD-oppF-F2	CAATATATCAATAATTTTAATTTCGCATAACA	44–75	212
oppD-oppF-F3	TGTTATGTATGCTGGCAAAATTGTTGAAAGA	110–140	146
oppD-oppF-R	Biotin-CTGGTGGGGTTCCTTGAATTGAGAATAATCT	225–255	
oppD-oppF-LF Probe	FAM-TCCAGCTCACCCTTATACATGAGCGCTTATC [dSpacer]CGGCTATACCTGAA-C3 Spacers	167–212	89

Abbreviations: FAM is 6-Carboxyfluorescein, dSpacer is an exonuclease site, and C3 Spacers is a polymerase extension blocking site

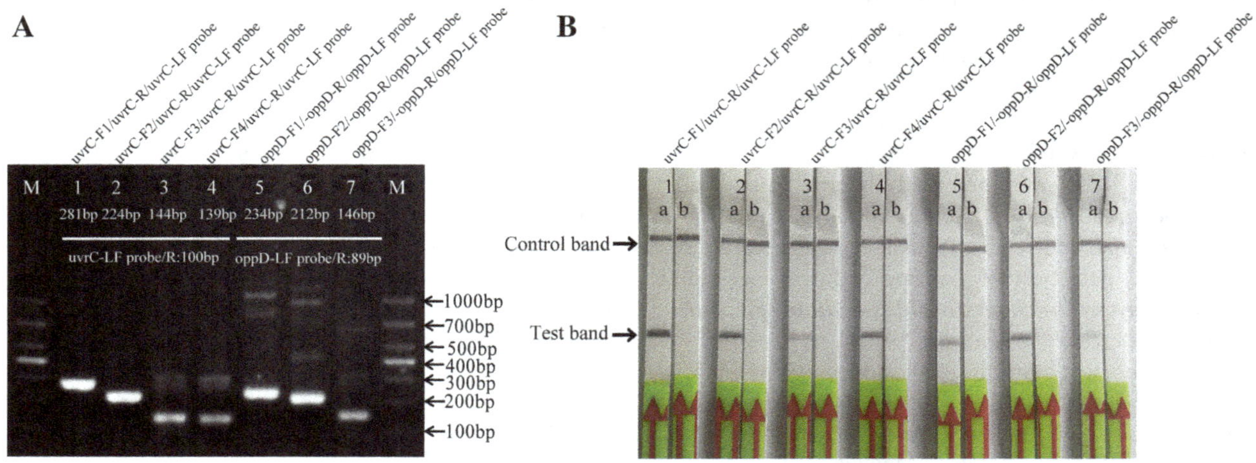

Fig. 2 Screening of *Mycoplasma bovis* recombinase polymerase amplification combined with a lateral flow dipstick (RPA-LFD) primers and probe. **a**: The results of RPA-nfo reaction were detected by agarose-gel electrophoresis from seven set of primers and probe combination; **b**: 'a' showed results of RPA-nfo reaction by LFD test, and DNA template came from extracted *Mycoplasma bovis* reference type strain PG45 colonies, and 'b' was negative control (DNase-free water) that the corresponding combination of primers and probe. Samples were tested in triplicate with one reaction displayed in figure for each triplicate

testing of serially diluted plasmid DNA showed that RPA-LFD assay was capable of detecting 20 copies/reaction standards DNA, which was 4 times more sensitive than the qPCR assay (Fig. 4).

Performance of RPA-LFD assay on clinical samples

RPA-LFD performance was analyzed using 442 clinical samples obtained from 42 different dairy farms in Shandong Province, China. The RPA-LFD and qPCR were executed in parallel. The RPA-LFD detected *M. bovis* DNA in 114 of 442 (25.79%) clinical samples while the qPCR assay found 100 (22.62%) of the same samples positive (Table 4). It indicated both assays were not significantly different using the independent-samples t test ($P > 0.05$). The established RPA-LFD assay yielded 99.00% sensitivity, 95.61% specificity, and 0.902 kappa coefficient with the qPCR (Table 5).

Discussion

Successful surveillance of bovine mycoplasmosis needs a rapid, specific and sensitive diagnostic method. The laboratory-based diagnosis techniques such as qPCR and

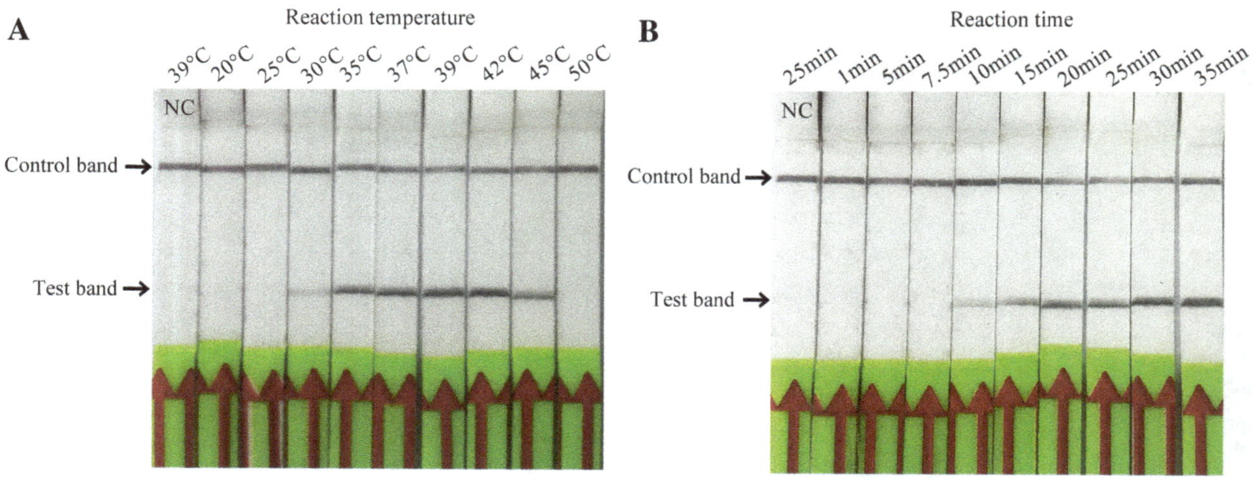

Fig. 3 Optimization of incubation temperature and reaction time for *Mycoplasma bovis* recombinase polymerase amplification combined with a lateral flow dipstick (RPA-LFD) assay. **a** The amplification performance of RPA-LFD was effectively within the range of 35 °C to 45 °C. **b** Determination of amplification time. After 10 min of amplification reaction, the test line was clearly visible on the strip. Lane NC: negative control (DNase-free water). Samples were tested in triplicate with one reaction displayed in figure for each triplicate

Table 2 *Mycoplasma bovis* and other bacterial species tested for specificity of the recombinase polymerase amplification combined with a lateral flow dipstick (RPA-LFD) assay

Number	Species	Strains/origin	RPA-LFD
1	*Mycoplasma bovis* PG45	ATCC25523[a]	Positive
2	*Mycoplasma bovis* Madison	ATCC27368[a]	Positive
3	*Mycoplasma bovis*	ATCC25025[a]	Positive
4	*Mycoplasma bovis* TJ14	Clinical separation[b]	Positive
5	*Mycoplasma bovis* SD16	Clinical separation[b]	Positive
6	*Mycoplasma agalactiae* PG2	BNCC132475[a]	Negative
7	*Mycoplasma mycoides* subsp. *mycoides*	BNCC126186[a]	Negative
8	*Mycoplasma bovirhinis* PG43	ATCC27748[b]	Negative
9	*Mycoplasma bovoculi*	ATCC29104[b]	Negative
10	*Mycoplasma bovigenitalium*	ATCC14173[b]	Negative
11	*Mycoplasma dispar*	ATCC27140[a]	Negative
12	*Mycoplasma canadense*	ATCC29418[a]	Negative
13	*Mycoplasma alkalescens*	ATCC29103[a]	Negative
14	*Mycoplasma canis* PG14	ATCC19525[a]	Negative
15	*Mycoplasma arginini*	ATCC23838[a]	Negative
16	*Pasteurella multocida* (A)	BNCC126487[a]	Negative
17	*Mannheimia haemolytica*	BNCC128674[a]	Negative
18	*Trueperella pyogenes*	Clinical separation[b]	Negative
19	*Histophilus somni*	Clinical separation[b]	Negative
20	*Klebsiella pneumoniae*	BNCC194477[b]	Negative
21	*Staphylococcus aureus*	Clinical separation[b]	Negative
22	*Streptococcus agalactiae*	BNCC185941[a]	Negative
23	*Brucella abortus* A19 vaccine strain	in our laboratory[b]	Negative
24	*Corynebacterium bovis*	BNCC131589[a]	Negative
25	*Escherichia coli* O157:H7	BNCC186579[a]	Negative
26	*Pseudomonas aeruginosa*	Clinical separation[b]	Negative
27	*Proteus mirabilis*	Clinical separation[b]	Negative
28	*Enterobacter aerogenes*	BNCC337113[a]	Negative

[a]These strains were purchased from BeNa Culture Collection biotechnology research institute (Beijing, China)
[b]These strains were preserved in our laboratory

enzyme linked immunosorbent assay (ELISA) are not able to meet the needs of a field test because the equipment required to perform them is not sufficiently portable or robust; furthermore some remote areas lack reliable power. With the development of isothermal nucleic acid amplification method, it is possible to perform on-site diagnostics in resource-limited settings. Here we established a new diagnostic assay based on RPA-LFD and evaluated its applicability to robustly and rapidly identify *M. bovis*, one of the crucial diseases affecting dairy and beef cattle herds in all over the world.

Rapid diagnostic tests for infectious diseases ordinarily use nucleic acid amplification technologies. Molecular tests for *M. bovis* have been developed based on the unique DNA sequences of the *uvrC* and *oppD/F* genes [10]. Subramaniam et al. (1998) [11] developed a PCR based on the DNA repair *uvrC* gene, which was shown to clearly differentiate between *M. bovis* and *M. agalactiae.* In this study, the analytical specificity of RPA primers and LF-probes based on *uvrC* and *oppD/F* gene was performed by agarose-gel electrophoresis. At the dSpacer position, when LF-probe is cleaved by nfo nuclease, the probe will be translated into a primer and act as priming for polymerase extension [6]. The one amplified fragment is from the different F primers and common R primers, and the other amplified fragment is LF-probe and common R primers. Therefore, the common R primers give two bands.

This paper describes a novel RPA-LFD assay based on LF-probe for *M. bovis* detection. Diagnostic specificity

Table 3 Results of *Mycoplasma bovis* plasmid DNA standards detected by real-time qPCR and recombinase polymerase amplification combined with a lateral flow dipstick (RPA-LFD) assay

standards DNA (copies/ul)	Real-time qPCR			RPA-LFD		
	Ct 1	Ct 2	Ct 3	Test 1	Test 2	Test 3
NC	40.00	40.00	40.00	–	–	–
10^0	40.00	40.00	40.00	–	+	–
10^1	40.00	37.07	40.00	+	+	+
10^2	36.76	36.79	36.41	+	+	+
10^3	33.04	32.17	32.04	+	+	+
10^4	28.63	28.02	28.30	+	+	+
10^5	25.24	25.12	24.94	+	+	+
10^6	20.30	20.76	20.71	+	+	+
10^7	17.53	17.52	17.29	+	+	+

NC negative control (DNase-free water)

showed that the assay could detect reference type strain *M. bovis* PG45 and 4 others, but not other pathogens commonly found in cattle. Sensitivity revealed that the RPA-LFD assay was 4 times more sensitive than the qPCR method. To verify the diagnostic suitability of *M. bovis* RPA-LFD assay, the same clinical sample ($n = 442$) set was confirmed by the qPCR assay and yielded 0.902 kappa coefficient with the qPCR.

For diagnostic purposes, several isothermal molecular amplification technologies have been developed in the recent decade [12]. A comparison of 11 isothermal technologies indicates that RPA has some advantages over others. Firstly, RPA reaction is rapid, and nucleic acid amplification can be completed within 10–20 min. Secondly, it operates at lower temperatures (39 °C) than all comparable techniques with the exception of rolling cycle amplification (23 °C) [13]. Several published studies have performed RPA using a simple heat source system. Lillis et al. (2014) demonstrated that incubation of the RPA HIV-1 assay via ambient temperatures or using chemical heaters yields similar results to using electrically powered devices [14]. Moreover, the capacity of RPA to catalyze nucleic acid amplification using only body heat was also demonstrated [15]. A water bath is sufficient to carry out the RPA-LFD testing in the field or in less well-equipped laboratories [16]. Thirdly, commercial availability of freeze-dried reagents makes it easier operation in outside laboratory settings and in remote areas. Moreover, the RPA-LFD provides an easy to read visual signal for clinical point-of-care diagnosis. While PCR needs rapid and accurate temperature control during the amplification cycle, RPA can tolerates temperatures ranging from 35 to 42 °C without loss of reaction efficiency. This simplifies the instrument and reduces the cost [7]. One disadvantage however is the current price of testing: in China, this is estimated to be ¥75 CNY (about 11 USD) for the RPA-LFD and about ¥15 CNY (2 USD) for the qPCR reaction. The RPA-LFD is a new technology and it is believed that the cost will become cheaper as it becomes more widely used.

Further work is clearly necessary for this technology to be taken into the field including using body heat to activate the test and simplified DNA extraction possibly using NaOH DNA extraction [17].

Conclusions

An RPA-LFD assay was developed for the rapid detection of *M. bovis* which will be suitable for on-farm testing and in particular in developing countries where sophisticated laboratory equipment is lacking. Its sensitivity and specificity were shown to be comparable to a previously published qPCR.

Methods

Strains and clinical samples

Reference type strain *M. bovis* PG45 was cultured as previously described [18], and originally purchased from BeNa culture collection biotechnology research institute (Beijing, China). A total of 442 clinical samples comprising nasal swabs ($n = 288$); fresh lungs ($n = 80$); joint fluids ($n = 32$); and bulk tank milk samples ($n = 42$) were collected between February 2015 and April 2017. Clinical samples from 400 cattle from 42 different dairy farms were examined, and the 42 farms were located in seventeen distinct geographic regions of Shandong province, China [19–21]. Bulk tank milk samples were used to estimate the apparent prevalence of *M. bovis* infection in 42 different dairy farms. A respiratory disease score was assigned and more than 6 points of cattle have at least two clinical symptoms of respiratory diseases, so they are considered sick [22]. The 288 nasal swab samples taken from all 42 dairy farms in which case suggests after BRD. The 80 fresh lung samples were sampled from postmortem cattle with BRD and the joint fluids

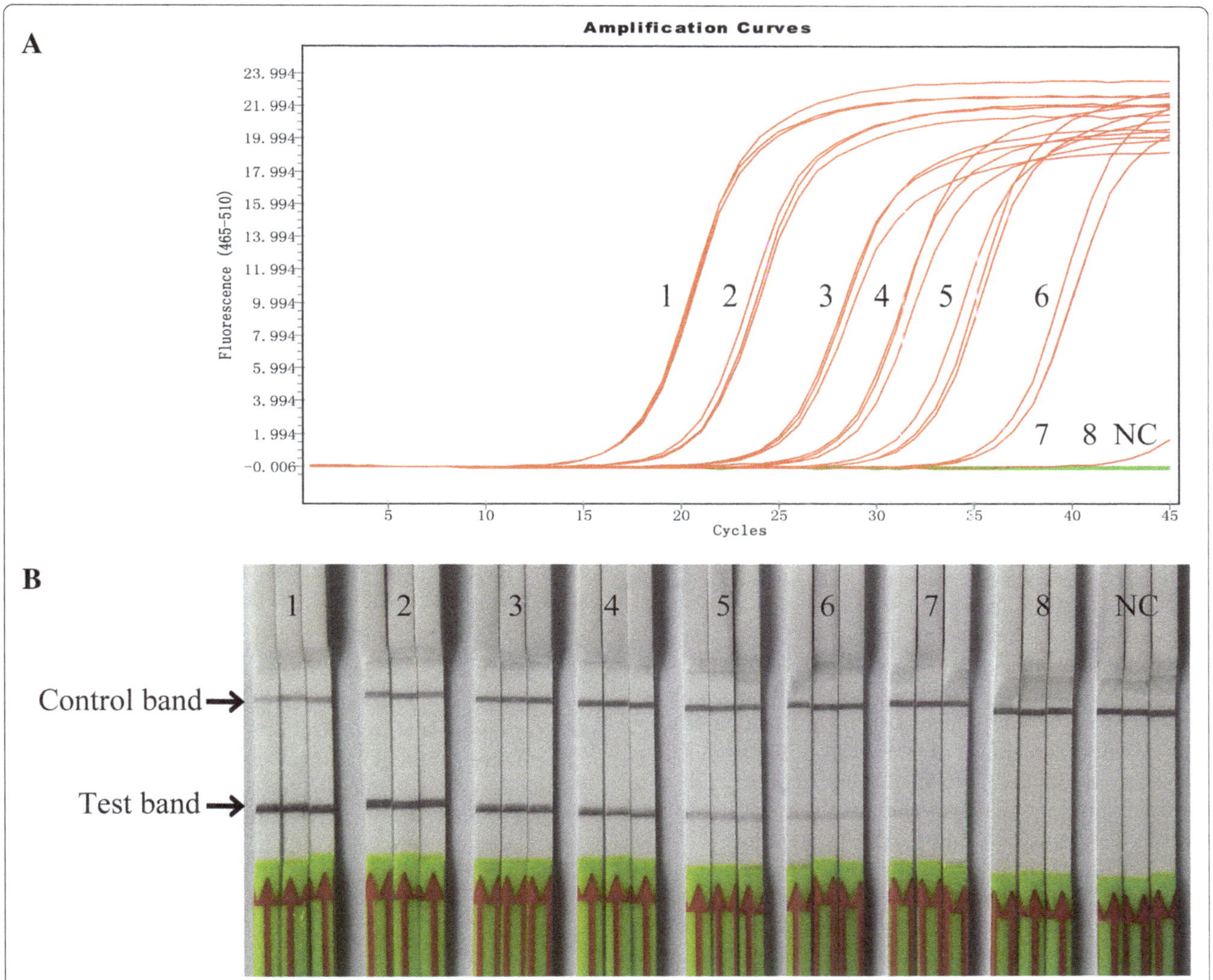

Fig. 4 Comparison of sensitivities of the recombinase polymerase amplification combined with a lateral flow dipstick (RPA-LFD) and Real-time qPCR assays. Molecular sensitivity test results of the two assays were assessed using 10-fold serially diluted DNA as template. **a** Results by Real-time qPCR (with a detection limit of 83 copies/reaction DNA standards). **b** Results by RPA-LFD (with a detection limit of 20 copies/reaction DNA standards). Lane 1 to 8: 10-fold serially diluted *Mycoplasma bovis* plasmid DNA standards from 10^7 to 10^0 copies/uL. Lane NC: negative control (DNase-free water)

Table 4 Camparision of *Mycoplasma bovis* recombinase polymerase amplification combined with a lateral flow dipstick (RPA-LFD) assay and Real-time qPCR assay on clinical samples

Samples	Number of samples	RPA-LFD			Real-time qPCR		
		Positive	Negative	Positive rate (%)	Positive	Negative	Positive rate (%)
Nasal swabs	288	72	216	25.00	61	227	21.18
Fresh lungs	80	32	48	40.00	31	49	38.75
Joint fluids	32	4	28	12.50	4	28	12.50
Bulk tanks	42	6	36	14.29	4	38	9.52
Total	442	114	328	25.79	100	342	22.62

Table 5 Specificity, sensitivity, predictive value and kappa value of recombinase polymerase amplification combined with a lateral flow dipstick (RPA-LFD) and Real-time qPCR assays for diagnosing *Mycoplasma bovis* infection

		Real-time qPCR			
		Positive	Negative	Total	
RPA-LFD	Positive	99	15	114	92.11% (PPV)
	Negative	1	327	328	98.78% (NPV)
	Total	100	342	442	
		99.00% (Sensitivity)	95.61% (Specificity)	0.902 (Kappa coefficient)	

PPV Positive predictive value, *NPV* negative predictive value

were collected from 32 calves with arthritis. These clinical samples were tested for *M. bovis* by RPA-LFD and qPCR assay, in the ruminant disease research center laboratory

DNA extraction

Approximately 2–4 colonies of the reference type strain *M. bovis* PG45 were transferred into 200 µl of sterile PBS using sterile disposable loop. The genomic DNA was extracted and eluted in 100 µl of sterile water by using bacterial genome DNA extraction kit (Tiangen Biotech Co., Ltd., Beijing, China) according to the manufacturer's instructions. Then, DNA was maintained at − 20 °C until screening of the RPA-LFD primer and LF-probe could be performed. The genomic DNA of clinical samples (nasal swabs, fresh lungs and joint fluids) was extracted using TIANamp genomic DNA kit and TIANamp swab DNA kit (Tiangen Biotech Co., Ltd., Beijing, China), specific steps carried out in accordance with the instruction book. The genomic DNA of bulk tank milk samples from the pellet was extracted using TIANamp genomic DNA kit according to reported in literature [23].

RPA primer and LF-probe design

The primers and LF-probe of the RPA reaction were used to amplify the *uvrC* gene (nucleotides 1464 to 1744 of the Genbank accession number: AF003959.1) and *oppD-oppF* gene (nucleotides 22 to 255 of the Genbank accession number: AF130119.1) sequences for *M. bovis*, and seven combinations of candidate primers (7 forward and 2 reverse) and two LF-probes were designed according to this two gene sequences. The details were shown in Fig. 1 and Table 1. The analytical specificity was performed using BLAST and no matches with other bacteria.

RPA reaction and lateral flow dipstick (LFD) assay

Each 50 µl reaction volume was performed according to manufacturer's instructions (TwistAmp nfo kit), and the volume of primer and LF-probe (10 µM) was adjusted accordingly. The following ingredients remained the same: 29.5 µl rehydration buffer, 2 µl DNA template, and 2.5 µl of 280 nM magnesium acetate. The test tubes were incubated at 39 °C for 25 min in a thermostatic water tank (Shanghai JingHong laboratory Co., Ltd., China). RPA amplification products were purified and the size of the RPA oligonucleotides was detected by 2% agarose-gel electrophoresis. Visualization of RPA amplicons was performed using LFD (HybriDetect, Milenia Biotec GmbH, Germany) according to manufacturer's instructions.

RPA conditions and optimization

To achieve optimal primers and LF-probe, different combinations were analysed for specificity and sensitivity detection. Next, the incubated temperature and time of RPA reaction were assessed according to the reagent instruction (TwistDX); temperature ranges were 20 °C to 50 °C, and time range was 1 min to 35 min.

Specificity and sensitivity of the RPA-LFD assay

The diagnostic specificity of RPA-LFD assay was confirmed with DNA from various reference bacteria strains and strains from clinical cases (Table 2). Most of bacteria species were supplied by BNCC using their recommended media. The forward primer (uvrC-F1): 5'-TAAATGAGCGCAGTGCTGATGTTGAAT-3′ and the reverse primer (uvrC-R2): 5'-AACTTGAATTTGAA CTAAGTAGTTGTATAG-3′ were used to amplify 281 bp of the *uvrC* gene of *M. bovis* (1464–1744 of Genbank accession number AF003959.1). The amplified fragment was ligated into plasmid pEASY-T3 cloning vector (Beijing TransGen Biotech Co., Ltd., Beijing, China). The DNA copy number was calculated as described in literature [24]. The analytical sensitivity of the RPA-LFD assay and qPCR assay was tested on standard plasmid DNA diluted in 10-fold serial steps from 10^7 to 1 copies/ul. For the RPA-LFD assay, in order to evaluate the repeatability limits of detection, the standard plasmid DNA dilutions were tested in duplicates, and this was repeated three times.

Real-time qPCR assay

The real-time qPCR assay for *M. bovis* was carried out to amplify a 170 bp sequences between 370 and 538 regions of *urvC* gene. The DNA molecular standard was prepared as previously described [5]. The qPCR amplification condition were as previously described [25, 26]. Briefly, the reaction was prepared as a 20 μl reaction volume containing 2 × Probe qPCR Mix, 0.8 μl of each 25 μM Mb-F: 5'-CAAAAGCAAAATGTTAAATTCAGG-3′ and Mb-R: 5'-CATATATAAGTGAGACTAACTTATT-3′, 0.8 μl of 7.5 μM probe: 5'-FAM-CAAAAGCAAAATGTTAAATTCAGG-BHQ2–3′ and 2 μl of DNA template. The thermal cycling parameters were as previously described [25, 26].

Statistical analysis

Statistical analysis was performed using SPSS 16.0 software (Chicago, IL, USA); also independent-samples *t* test was used for evaluation of the results. For all analyses, $P < 0.05$ was considered significant. The diagnostic performance of the RPA-LFD and qPCR assays was assessed as described previously [27–29]. The kappa coefficient was defined as (Po – Pe)/(1 – Pe) [28].

Additional file

Additional files 1: Figure S1. Specificity of the recombinase polymerase amplification combined with a lateral flow dipstick (RPA-LFD) assay. The specificity of the *Mycoplasma bovis* RPA-LFD assay was assessed for other bacterial pathogens genome cDNA of cattle that present similarly in the clinic. Lanes +: positive control (*Mycobacterium bovis* PG45), Lane NC: negative control (DNase-free water), Lanes 1: *Mycobacterium bovis* (Clinical separation), Lanes 2 to 23: *Mycoplasma agalactiae, Mycoplasma mycoides* subsp. *mycoides, Mycoplasma bovirhinis, Mycoplasma bovoculi, Mycoplasma bovigenitalium, Mycoplasma dispar, Mycoplasma canadense, Mycoplasma alkalescens, Mycoplasma canis, Mycoplasma arginini, Pasteurella multocida, Mannheimia haemolytica, Trueperella pyogenes, Histophilus somni, Klebsiella pneumoniae, Staphylococcus aureus, Streptococcus agalactiae, Corynebacterium bovis, Pseudomonas aeruginosa, Proteus mirabilis, Enterobacter aerogenes, Brucella abortus,* and *Escherichia coli,* respectively. Samples were tested in triplicate with one reaction displayed in figure for each triplicate.

Abbreviations

BRD: Bovine respiratory disease; ELISA: Enzyme linked immunosorbent assay; LFD: Lateral flow dipstick; PCR: Polymerase chain reaction; qPCR: Real-time quantitative PCR; RPA: Recombinase polymerase amplification

Acknowledgements

Not applicable.

Funding

This work was partially supported by grants from the earmarked fund for the Taishan Scholar and Distinguished Experts (Hongbin He), the National Natural Science Fund of China (31872490, 31672556). Shandong province Key Research & Development program Fund (2018GNC113011, 2016GNC113006).

Authors' contributions

HBH and GMZ conceived and designed the experiments. GMZ, PLH and YJH performed the experiments. HMW and CQH analyzed the data. GMZ and HBH wrote the paper. All the authors read and approved the final manuscript.

Consent for publication

Not applicable.

Competing interests

The authors declare that they have no competing interests.

Author details

[1]Key Laboratory of Animal Resistant Biology of Shandong, Ruminant Disease Research Center, College of Life Science Shandong Normal University, No.88 Wenhua East Road, Lixia District, Jinan 250014, Shandong Province, China. [2]College of Animal Science and Technology, Qingdao Agricultural University, No.700 Changcheng Road, Chengyang District. Qingdao 266109, Shandong Province, China.

References

1. Nicholas RA. Bovine mycoplasmosis: silent and deadly. Vet Rec. 2011;168: 459–62.
2. Nicholas RA, Ayling RD. Mycoplasma bovis: disease, diagnosis, and control. Res Vet Sci. 2003;74:105–12.
3. Li Y, Zheng H, Liu Y, Jiang Y, Xin J, Chen W et al. The complete genome sequence of mycoplasma bovis strain Hubei-1. PLoS One. 2011;6:e20999.
4. Sun P, Luo H, Zhang X, Xu J, Guo Y, He S. Whole-Genome Sequence of Mycoplasma bovis Strain Ningxia-1. Genome Announc. 2018;pii: e01367–e01317.
5. Hou P, Wang H, Zhao G, He C, He H. Rapid detection of infectious bovine Rhinotracheitis virus using recombinase polymerase amplification assays. BMC Vet Res. 2017;13:386.
6. Piepenburg O, Williams CH, Stemple DL, Armes NA. DNA detection using recombination proteins. PLoS Biol. 2006;4:e204.
7. Daher RK, Stewart G, Boissinot M, Bergeron MG. Recombinase polymerase amplification for diagnostic applications. Clin Chem. 2016;62:947–58.
8. Kersting S, Rausch V, Bier FF, von Nickisch-Rosenegk M. Rapid detection of plasmodium falciparum with isothermal recombinase polymerase amplification and lateral flow analysis. Malar J. 2014;13:99.
9. Tu PA, Shiu JS, Lee SH, Pang VF, Wang DC. Wang PH. Development of a recombinase polymerase amplification lateral flow dipstick (RPA-LFD) for the field diagnosis of caprine arthritis-encephalitis virus (CAEV) infection. J Virol Methods. 2017;243:98–104.
10. Caswell JL, Bateman KG, Cai HY, Castillo-Alcala F. Mycoplasma bovis in respiratory disease of feedlot cattle. Vet Clin North Am Food Anim Pract. 2010;26:365–79.
11. Subramaniam S, Bergonier D, Poumarat F, Capaul S, Schlatter Y, Nicolet J, et al. Species identification of mycoplasma bovis and mycoplasma agalactiae based on the uvrC genes by PCR. Mol Cell Probes. 1998;12:161–9.
12. James A, Macdonald J. Recombinase polymerase amplification. Emergence as a critical molecular technology for rapid, low-resource diagnostics. Expert Rev Mol Diagn. 2015;15:1475–89.
13. Fire A, Xu SQ. Rolling replication of short DNA circles. Proc Natl Acad Sci U S A. 1995;92:4641–5.
14. Lillis L, Lehman D, Singhal MC, Cantera J, Singleton J, Labarre P, et al. Non-instrumented incubation of a recombinase polymerase amplification assay for the rapid and sensitive detection of proviral HIV-1 DNA. PLoS One. 2014; 9:e108189.
15. Crannell ZA, Rohrman B, Richards-Kortum R. Equipment-free incubation of recombinase polymerase amplification reactions using body heat. PLoS One. 2014;9:e112146.
16. Yang Y, Qin X, Zhang W, Li Y, Zhang Z. Rapid and specific detection of porcine parvovirus by isothermal recombinase polymerase amplification assays. Mol Cell Probes. 2016;30:300–5.
17. Wang R, Zhang F, Wang L, Qian W, Qian C, Wu J, et al. Instant, visual, and instrument-free method for on-site screening of GTS 40-3-2 soybean based on body-heat triggered recombinase polymerase amplification. Anal Chem. 2017;89:4413–8.

18. Mustafa R, Qi JJ, Ba XL, Chen YY, Hu CM, Liu XL, et al. In vitro quinolones susceptibility analysis of Chinese mycoplasma bovis isolates and their phylogenetic scenarios based upon QRDRs of DNA topoisomerases revealing a unique transition in ParC. Pak Vet J. 2013;33:364–9.
19. Zheng S, Wu X, Zhang L, Xin C, Liu Y, Shi J, et al. The occurrence of porcine circovirus 3 without clinical infection signs in Shandong Province. Transbound Emerg Dis. 2017;64:1337–41.
20. Zheng S, Shi J, Wu X, Peng Z, Xin C, Zhang L, et al. Presence of torque Teno sus virus 1 and 2 in porcine circovirus 3-positive pigs. Transbound Emerg Dis. 2018;65:327–30.
21. He CQ, Liu YX, Wang HM, Hou PL, He HB, Ding NZ. New genetic mechanism, origin and population dynamic of bovine ephemeral fever virus. Vet Microbiol. 2016;182:50–6.
22. Lago A, McGuirk SM, Bennett TB, Cook NB, Nordlund KV. Calf respiratory disease and pen microenvironments in naturally ventilated calf barns in winter. J Dairy Sci. 2006;89:4014–25.
23. McDonald WL, Rawdon TG, Fitzmaurice J, Bolotovski I, Voges H, Humphrey S, et al. Survey of bulk tank milk in New Zealand for mycoplasma bovis, using species-specific nested PCR and culture. N Z Vet J. 2009;57:44–9.
24. Yang Y, Qin X, Wang G, Jin J, Shang Y, Zhang Z. Development of an isothermoal amplification-based assay for rapid visual detection of an Orf virus. Virol J. 2016;13:46.
25. Naikare H, Bruno D, Mahapatra D, Reinisch A, Raleigh R, Sprowls R. Development and evaluation of a novel Taqman real-time PCR assay for rapid detection of mycoplasma bovis: comparison of assay performance with a conventional PCR assay and another Taqman real-time PCR assay. Vet Sci. 2015;2:32–42.
26. Hou P, Zhao G, He C, Wang H, He H. Biopanning of polypeptides binding to bovine ephemeral fever virus G1 protein from phage display peptide library. BMC Vet Res. 2018;14:3.
27. Zhao G, Wang H, Hou P, He C, He H. Rapid visual detection of Mycobacterium avium subsp. paratuberculosis by recombinase polymerase amplification combined with a lateral flow dipstick. J Vet Sci. 2018;19:242–50.
28. Sun K, Xing W, Yu X, Fu W, Wang Y, Zou M, et al. Recombinase polymerase amplification combined with a lateral flow dipstick for rapid and visual detection of Schistosoma japonicum. Parasit Vectors. 2016;9:476.
29. Song L, Zhang H, Hou P, Wang H, Zhao G, Xia X, et al. Development and preliminary application of an indirect ELISA to detect infectious bovine Rhinotracheitis virus using recombinant glycoprotein D of IBRV strain SD. Kafkas Univ Vet Fak. 2016;22:503–9.

22

Identification of a new bovine viral diarrhea virus subtype in the Republic of Korea

Du-Gyeong Han[1†], Ji-Hyung Ryu[1†], Jinho Park[2] and Kyoung-Seong Choi[1*]

Abstract

Background: Bovine viral diarrhea virus (BVDV) is prevalent in Korean indigenous cattle leading to substantial economic losses. This study was conducted to investigate the occurrence of BVDV. In 2016, a total of 143 blood samples were collected from asymptomatic Korean indigenous calves younger than 3-months of age from six different farms in the Republic of Korea (ROK).

Results: Eighty-seven calves (60.8%, 87/143) were tested positive for BVDV as evaluated by RT-PCR analysis. Phylogenetic analysis based on the 5′-untranslated region was used to classify these cases into three subtypes: BVDV-1b, BVDV-1o, and BVDV-2a. These results showed that BVDV-1b was the predominant subtype, while 2 samples clustered with BVDV-2a. Interestingly, one sample formed a separate group as a potentially new subtype, BVDV-1o. To our knowledge, this is the first report of BVDV-1o infection in Korean native calves. The BVDV-1o subtype identified in this study was closely related to cattle isolates obtained from Japan, indicating that this subtype is a new introduction to the ROK.

Conclusions: This study provides useful information for carrying out epidemiological surveys of BVDV in the ROK and developing a vaccine for future use in the ROK, particularly for the first detection of BVDV-1o in Korean indigenous calves. Further studies are required to investigate the prevalence and pathogenicity of this BVDV-1o subtype.

Keywords: Bovine viral diarrhea virus, 5′-untranslated region, BVDV-1o

Background

Bovine viral diarrhea virus (BVDV) causes significant economic losses worldwide in the cattle industry through decreased productive performance and immunosuppression of herds [1, 2]. BVDV belongs to the genus *Pestivirus* along with classical swine fever virus and border disease virus in the family *Flaviviridae*. BVDV infects not only cattle, but also pigs, goats, sheep, and wild ruminants. BVDV includes two species, BVDV-1 and BVDV-2. Additionally, HoBi-like pestivirus has been proposed as a third new species, BVDV-3. Based on the 5′-untranslated region (UTR), BVDV-1 can be further divided into 21 subtypes (1a–1u) [3], BVDV-2 into four subtypes (2a–2d) [4, 5], and BVDV-3 into two genotypes of Brazilian and Thai origin [6]. Infection with BVDV is characterized by gastroenteritis, respiratory diseases and reproductive problems including abortion, congenital abnormalities, and the development of persistently infected (PI) calves that gain immunotolerance to BVDV through vertical transmission of the virus during early gestation [1, 7, 8].

To date, seven BVDV subtypes (1a, 1b, 1c, 1d, 1 m, 1n, and 2a) have been identified in the Republic of Korea (ROK) [9, 10]. Of these, BVDV-1b and BVDV-2a are predominant and widespread in cattle in the ROK [10–12]. The genetic diversity of BVDV must be considered when designing and constructing effective vaccination strategies against the virus. Additionally, a vaccine must accurately reflect the antigenic subtypes present in the country of use [13]. In the present study, we report a new subtype recently identified in the ROK. The results provide useful information for vaccine development.

* Correspondence: kschoi3@knu.ac.kr
†Du-Gyeong Han and Ji-Hyung Ryu contributed equally to this work.
1Department of Animal Science and Biotechnology, College of Ecology and Environmental Science, Kyungpook National University, Sangju 37224, Republic of Korea
Full list of author information is available at the end of the article

Methods

Sample collection

Blood samples were collected from 143 asymptomatic Korean indigenous calves under 3 months of age from six different farms (Gimje, Gochang, Iksan, Sancheong, Wanju, and Hoenseong) in the ROK (Fig. 1). Five milliliters of blood was collected from the jugular veins of each calf in EDTA-supplemented tubes. The samples were delivered to the lab immediately after blood collection. These calves were the offspring of cows that had not previously been vaccinated against BVDV. The collected samples were stored at −80°C until analysis.

RNA extraction, RT-PCR, and sequencing

Total RNA was extracted from 200 μL of blood using RNAiso Plus Reagent (Takara Bio, Shiga, Japan) according to the manufacturer's instructions. RNA was eluted in 20 μL of RNase-free water and stored at −80°C. The 5′-UTR and N-terminal protease (N^{pro}) regions were used to detect BVDV as previously described [4, 11]. Reverse transcription-polymerase chain reaction (RT-PCR) was performed to amplify BVDV using DiaStar™ One-Step RT-PCR Smart Mix (Solgent, Daejeon, Korea). Briefly, RT-PCR was carried out at 50°C for 30 min, followed by 94°C for 5 min, and then 30 cycles at 94°C for 30 s, 55°C for 30 s, and 72°C for 1 min, with a final extension step at 72°C for 10 min. Distilled water was used as a negative control in each PCR run. The predicted sizes of the amplified PCR products were 288 bp and 425 bp for the 5′-UTR and for N^{pro}, respectively. The amplicons were subjected to 1.5% agarose gel electrophoresis and visualized following ethidium bromide staining. The PCR products were purified using an AccuPrep® PCR Purification Kit (Bioneer, Daejeon, Korea) and cloned into the pGEM®-T Easy vector (Promega, Madison, WI, USA), which was directly sequenced (Macrogen, Inc., Seoul, Korea).

Phylogenetic analysis

For homology analysis of BVDV genes, the obtained sequence data were analyzed using the Basic Local Alignment Search Tool of the National Center for Biotechnology

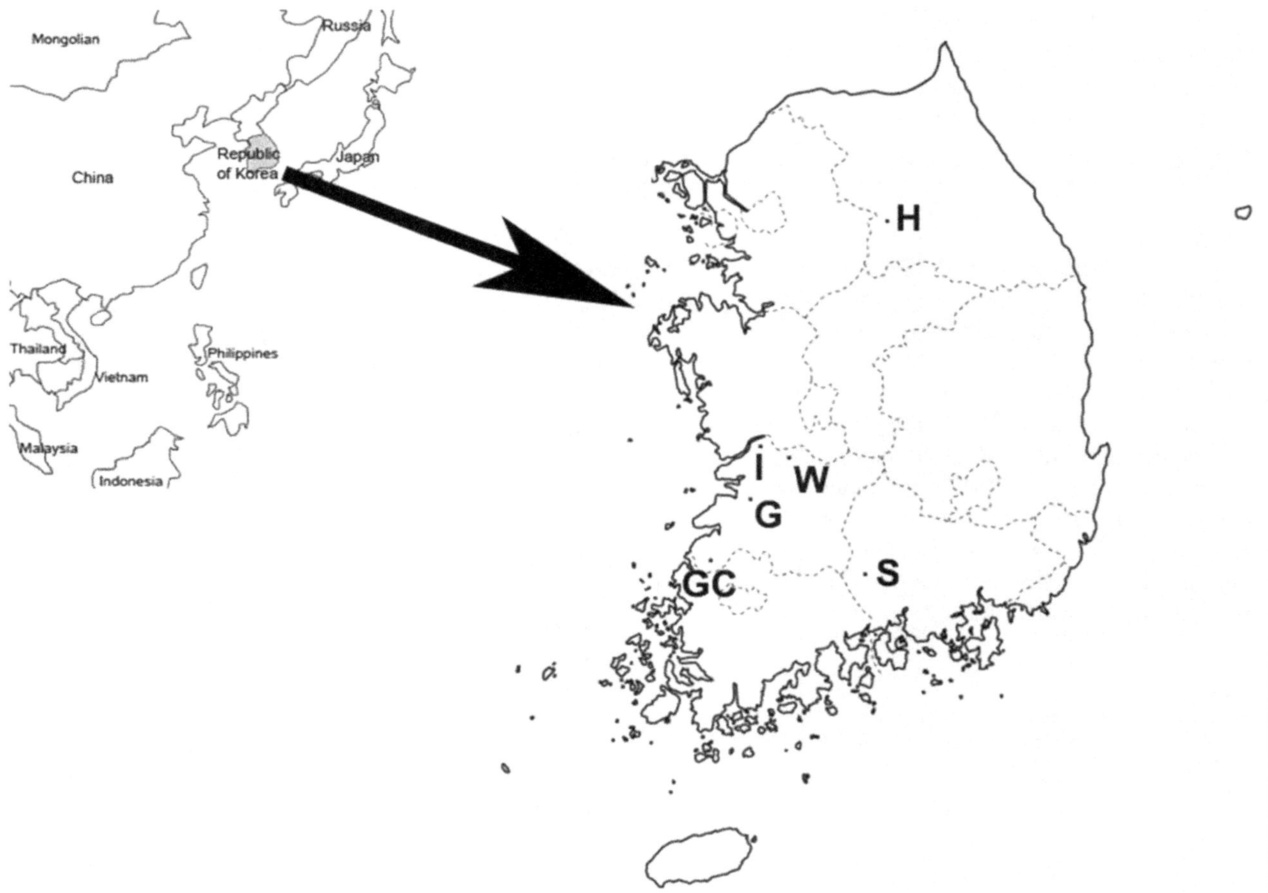

Fig. 1 Map of the Republic of Korea. Dots indicate the regions where blood samples were collected: G, Gimje; GC, Gochang: I, Iksan; W, Wanju; H, Hoengseong; and S, Sancheong

Table 1 Information in the regions where fecal samples were collected

Farm	No. of samples	BVDV positive	Subtype	Colostrum intake	Growth type
Gimje	20	14 (70.0%)	1b	Yes	Housing
Gochang	20	16 (80.0%)	1b	Yes	Housing
Wanju	62	42 (67.7%)	1b	Yes	Housing
Sancheong	14	7 (50.0%)	1b	Yes	Grazing
Hoengseong	20	8 (40.0%)	1b, 1o, 2a	No	Housing
Iksan	7	0 (0.0%)	–	No	Grazing
Total	143	87 (60.8%)			

Information database. Homologous sequences were analyzed using Chromas software (version 2.33, http://www.technelysium.com.au/chromas.html) and aligned using ClustalX (version 1.8). Construction of the phylogenetic trees based on the 5′-UTR and N^{pro} were performed using the maximum-likelihood method with a Kimura 2-parameter [14] substitution model using MEGA7 software [15]. To construct each phylogenetic tree, additional sequences were obtained from GenBank (http://www.ncbi.nlm.nih.gov). The 5′-UTR of the gene sequences obtained in this study was assigned the following accession numbers: MH355922–MH355950, MH396616, and MH396618 for BVDV-1b, and MH396617 and MH396619 for BVDV-2a. The 5′-UTR and N^{pro} for the gene sequence of BVDV-1o obtained in this study were assigned the accession numbers MF449421 and MG030482, respectively.

Statistical analysis

Statistical analysis was performed to assess the association between BVDV infection and the variables: colostrum intake and grazing. Binary univariate logistic regression models were constructed using the generalized linear mixed model in SPSS 24.0 software package (SPSS, Inc., Chicago, IL, USA), with the farm as a random effect. Odds ratios (ORs) with 95% confidence intervals (CIs) were calculated to assess the likelihood of association. A value of $P < 0.05$ was considered significant.

Results

From the analysis of 143 blood samples, BVDV was detected in 87 calves (60.8%) from five of the six farms sampled (Table 1). Data for colostrum intake and growth type from the farms in the regions where fecal samples were collected are presented in Table 1. The Korean native calves examined in this study were born to cows that were not vaccinated against BVDV. There was no significant difference between colostrum intake and BVDV infection ($P = 0.09$). In calves that had not been fed colostrum (Heongseong and Iksan), BVDV infection was reduced by grazing (Iksan). In the Iksan and Sancheong regions where animals are grazed, colostrum-fed calves (Sancheong) showed an even higher rate of BVDV infection than in Iksan, where calves had not been fed colostrum (Table 1). Our results show that grazing decreased the OR for the incidence of BVDV by 5-fold compared to housing calves (OR = 0.2; 95% CI: 0.1–0.4; $P = 0.001$). BVDV infection showed the highest prevalence (64.7%) in 1–21-day-old animals and the prevalence of BVDV infection gradually reduced with age, but remained high (Table 2).

To investigate the genetic relationship between the BVDV isolates identified in this study, we sequenced all amplicons. Of these, 34 good sequences for 5′-UTR and one sequence for N^{pro} were obtained and were included in the phylogenetic tree. Thirty-four isolates identified from Gimje, Gochang, Sancheong, Wanju, and Hoengseong were classified into 3 subtypes: BVDV-1b (31 isolates), BVDV-1o (1 isolate, new subtype), and BVDV-2a (2 isolates) based on sequence analysis of 5′-UTR (Fig. 2). Particularly, in case of Hoengseong farm, three subtypes were detected simultaneously. Phylogenetic analysis revealed genetic differences in samples derived from the same farm. Two isolates of BVDV-2a were detected in this study and were similar to those that had previously been isolated in the ROK. The BVDV-1o found in Hoengseong farm was closely related to that identified in Japanese cattle (LC089875) (Fig. 2). Another phylogenetic tree based on the N^{pro} region was constructed to confirm the subtyping of BVDV-1o. As shown in Fig. 3, the Hoengseong isolate formed the same branch as BVDV-1o as determined by the sequence of 5′-UTR. Additionally, higher similarity was observed for most isolate relationships, except for the camel isolate. Homology values between the Hoengseong isolate identified in this study and BVDV-1o

Table 2 Prevalence of BVDV infection according to age group of calves

Age group (days)	No. of examined calves	No. of BVDV positive
1–21	51	33(64.7%)
22–42	54	33 (61.1%)
43–84	38	21 (55.3%)
Total	143	87 (60.8%)

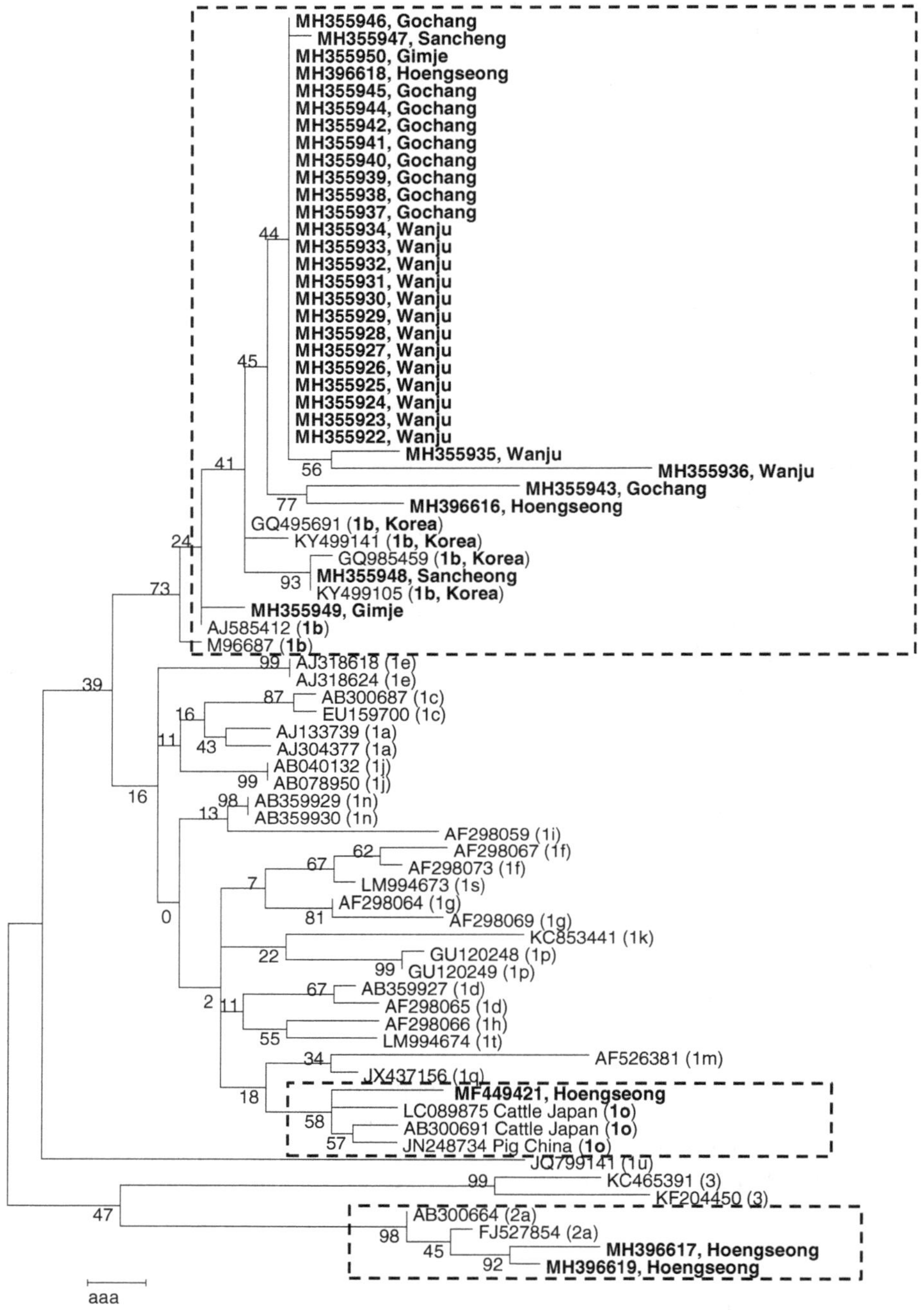

Fig. 2 Phylogenetic tree based on partial nucleotide sequences of the 5′-UTR of reference BVDV strains/isolates and Korean isolates identified in this study was constructed in MEGA7 using the maximum-likelihood (ML) method. The robustness of the tree was evaluated by bootstrapping 1000 replicates by ML. The Korean isolates identified in this study are indicated in bold

reference strains LC089875 and AB359931 were 95 and 88% for the 5′-UTR sequence and N^{pro} sequence, respectively. This is the first report of BVDV-1o infection in calves in the ROK. The results demonstrated that BVDV-1b was the most frequently detected subtype and genetic variations were evident among BVDV-1b circulating in the ROK (Fig. 2).

Discussion

In this study, we investigated the occurrence of BVDV in Korean indigenous calves. Our findings showed that the infection rate of BVDV was high, indicating the difficulty in controlling the spread of BVDV in the field. Unexpectedly, the highest rate of BVDV infection was observed in 1–21-day-old calves. Most BVDV infections

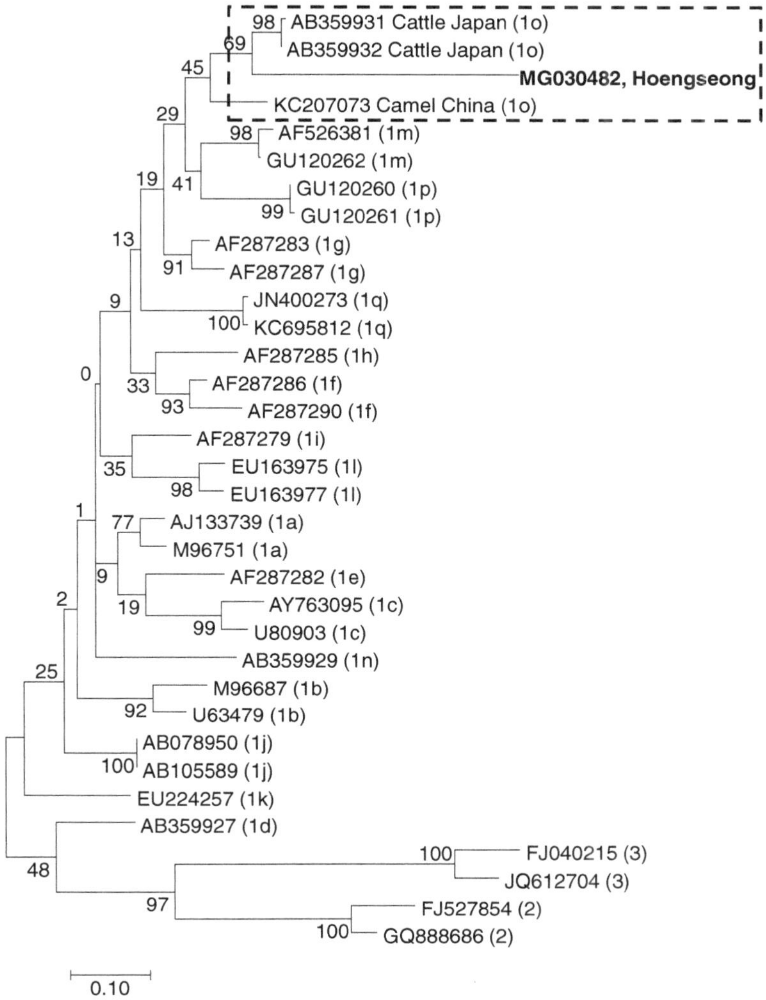

Fig. 3 Phylogenetic tree of the N^{pro} region from Korean isolate identified in this study was constructed in MEGA7 by the maximum-likelihood (ML) method. The robustness of the tree was evaluated by bootstrapping 1000 replicates by ML. The Korean isolate identified in this study is indicated in bold

in calves less than 30-days-old are likely PI. In this study, we could not examine whether these calves were PI or acutely infected because the farmers objected to a second collection of blood from the calves. Previous reports from several countries have highlighted the clinical significance of BVDV infections, particularly of PI [16, 17]. Because PI animals remain unidentified, they can contribute to the spread of BVDV to other members of the herd. Measures to prevent BVDV circulation in herds should focus on removing the PI animals. Alterations in the immune system due to BVDV infection result in an increased susceptibility to other enteric diseases in PI calves [18, 19]. Because PI animals are important for the ongoing transmission of BVDV in a population, our findings highlight the need for rapid diagnosis and elimination of PI animals.

Our findings showed that BVDV infection was not associated with colostrum intake ($P = 0.09$). However, BVDV infection significantly decreased when animals were allowed to graze in a pasture ($P = 0.001$) rather than being confined to housing. In this study, BVDV infection was not detected in the Iksan region, where animals grazed. Interestingly, on the Sancheong farm, where animals also grazed, the prevalence of BVDV was relatively higher than that on the Iksan farm (Table 1). This difference between the two farms may be related to colostrum intake. The prevalence of BVDV was high in colostrum-fed calves, supporting the possibility that cows that served as sources of colostrum were infected with BVDV or PI. Moreover, the high prevalence of BVDV in calves can be explained by the failure to vaccinate. In the ROK, vaccination of pregnant dams against BVDV is not implemented on most farms. This study highlights the importance of BVDV vaccination. Consequently, an outbreak of BVDV may commonly be associated not only with grazing but also with other factors, including cattle management systems, herd sizes, and vaccination. Further studies are necessary to determine the effects of these variables in reducing the occurrence of BVDV.

Although the number of samples was limited, our results revealed that three subtypes (BVDV-1b, BVDV-1o, and BVDV-2a) of BVDV were detected in Korean native cattle. Of these, BVDV-1b was the predominant subtype identified. Our data support those of previous studies [10, 11]. However, the BVDV isolates obtained in this study showed more genetic variation compared to those in other Korean BVDV-1b strains/isolates reported previously in the ROK. Additionally, two isolates were classified as BVDV-2a based on phylogenetic analysis. The BVDV-2a outbreak is known to be associated with severe acute infections in the ROK [12], but the isolates were detected in calves without any clinical symptoms. Recent studies demonstrated that BVDV-2c causes severe and often fatal illness in cattle in European countries [20, 21]. Thus, disease outbreaks appear to change over time. BVDV-1o was identified for the first time in the present study, and a total of eight subtypes of BVDV (1a, 1b, 1c, 1d, 1 m, 1n, 1o, and 2a) have now been found in the ROK, including BVDV-1o newly detected. This study provides useful information for constructing a vaccine for future use in the ROK, particularly for detecting the BVDV-1o subtype in Korean indigenous calves. BVDV1o was first isolated from a calf that developed a mucosal disease and from PI calves in Japan [22, 23], and has been detected in camels, goats, and pigs in China [3, 24, 25]. However, this isolate has not been detected anywhere other than Japan and China. Our results indicate that BVDV-1o is genetically heterogeneous but geographically restricted. At present, we cannot conclude how this virus spread. It is possible that trade between countries could be a possible pathway for the introduction of the new subtype into Korean cattle.

Conclusions

Our results provide evidence of the predominance of BVDV-1b in Korean native calves. Additionally, we identified the BVDV-1o subtype, which had not been previously documented in the ROK. As the number of calves examined was limited, larger epidemiological surveys are needed to investigate the prevalence of the BVDV-1o subtype as well as other subtypes. These results provide useful information for the development an effective vaccination for BVDV control.

Abbreviations

5'-UTR: 5'- untranslated region; BVDV: Bovine viral diarrhea virus; ML: Maximum-likelihood; N^{pro}: N-terminal protease; PI: Persistent infection; ROK: Republic of Korea; RT-PCR: Reverse transcription-polymerase chain reaction

Funding

This work was supported by the National Research Foundation of Korea (NRF), funded by the Korea government (MSIP) (No. 2015R1C1A2A01053080).

Authors' contributions

KSC designed this study and wrote the manuscript. DGH and JHP participated in sample collection. DGH and JHR performed the experiments, data analysis, and drafted the manuscript. All authors read and approved the final manuscript.

Consent for publication

Not applicable

Competing interests

The authors declare that they have no competing interests.

Author details

[1]Department of Animal Science and Biotechnology, College of Ecology and Environmental Science, Kyungpook National University, Sangju 37224, Republic of Korea. [2]College of Veterinary Medicine, Chonbuk National University, Iksan 54596, Republic of Korea.

References

1. Gates MC, Humphry RW, Gunn GJ, Woolhouse ME. Not all cows are epidemiologically equal: quantifying the risks of bovine viral diarrhoea virus (BVDV) transmission through cattle movements. Vet Res. 2014;45:110.
2. Pinior B, Firth CL, Richter V, Lebl K, Trauffler M, Dzieciol M, Hutter SE, Burgstaller J, Obritzhauser W, Winter P, et al. A systematic review of financial and economic assessments of bovine viral diarrhea virus (BVDV) prevention and mitigation activities worldwide. Prev Vet Med. 2017;137:77–92.
3. Mao L, Li W, Yang L, Wang J, Cheng S, Wei Y, Wang Q, Zhang W, Hao F, Ding Y, et al. Primary surveys on molecular epidemiology of bovine viral diarrhea virus 1 infecting goats in Jiangsu province, China. BMC Vet Res. 2016;12:181.
4. Vilcek S, Paton DJ, Durkovic B, Strojny L, Ibata G, Moussa A, Loitsch A, Rossmanith W, Vega S, Scicluna MT, et al. Bovine viral diarrhoea virus genotype 1 can be separated into at least eleven genetic groups. Arch Virol. 2001;146:99–115.
5. Flores EF, Ridpath JF, Weiblen R, Vogel FS, Gil LH. Phylogenetic analysis of Brazilian bovine viral diarrhea virus type 2 (BVDV-2) isolates: evidence for a subgenotype within BVDV-2. Virus Res. 2002;87:51–60.
6. Liu L, Xia H, Wahlberg N, Belak S, Baule C. Phylogeny, classification and evolutionary insights into pestiviruses. Virology. 2009;385:351–7.
7. Brownlie J, Clarke MC, Howard CJ. Experimental production of fatal mucosal disease in cattle. Vet Rec. 1984;114:535–6.
8. Polak MP, Zmudzinski JF. Experimental inoculation of calves with laboratory strains of bovine viral diarrhea virus. Comp Immunol Microbiol Infect Dis. 2000;23:141–51.
9. Joo SK, Lim SI, Jeoung HY, Song JY, Oem JK, Mun SH, An DJ. Genome sequence of bovine viral diarrhea virus strain 10JJ-SKR, belonging to genotype 1d. Genome Announc. 2013;1:4.
10. Oem JK, Chung JY, Roh IS, Kim HR, Bae YC, Lee KH, Jin YH, Lee OS. Characterization and phylogenetic analysis of bovine viral diarrhea virus in brain tissues from nonambulatory (downer) cattle in Korea. J Vet Diagn Invest. 2010;22:518–23.
11. Choi KS, Song MC. Epidemiological observations of bovine viral diarrhea virus in Korean indigenous calves. Virus Genes. 2011;42:64–70.
12. Oem JK, Hyun BH, Cha SH, Lee KK, Kim SH, Kim HR, Park CK, Joo YS. Phylogenetic analysis and characterization of Korean bovine viral diarrhea viruses. Vet Microbiol. 2009;139:356–60.
13. Mahony TJ, McCarthy FM, Gravel JL, Corney B, Young PL, Vilcek S. Genetic analysis of bovine viral diarrhoea viruses from Australia. Vet Microbiol. 2005;106:1–6.
14. Kimura M. A simple method for estimating evolutionary rates of base substitutions through comparative studies of nucleotide sequences. J Mol Evol. 1980;16:111–20.
15. Kumar S, Stecher G, Tamura K. MEGA7: molecular evolutionary genetics analysis version 7.0 for bigger datasets. Mol Biol Evol. 2016;33:1870–4.

16. Graham DA, Clegg TA, O'Sullivan P, More SJ. Influence of the retention of PI calves identified in 2012 during the voluntary phase of the Irish national bovine viral diarrhoea virus (BVDV) eradication programme on herd-level outcomes in 2013. Prev Vet Med. 2015;120:298–305.
17. Kelling CL, Steffen DJ, Cooper VL, Higuchi DS, Eskridge KM. Effect of infection with bovine viral diarrhea virus alone, bovine rotavirus alone, or concurrent infection with both on enteric disease in gnotobiotic neonatal calves. Am J Vet Res. 2002;63:1179–86.
18. Gunn GJ, Stott AW, Humphry RW. Modelling and costing BVD outbreaks in beef herds. Vet J. 2004;167:143–9.
19. Hessman BE, Fulton RW, Sjeklocha DB, Murphy TA, Ridpath JF, Payton ME. Evaluation of economic effects and the health and performance of the general cattle population after exposure to cattle persistently infected with bovine viral diarrhea virus in a starter feedlot. Am J Vet Res. 2009;70:73–85.
20. Gethmann J, Homeier T, Holsteg M, Schirrmeier H, Sasserath M, Hoffmann B, Beer M, Conraths FJ. BVD-2 outbreak leads to high losses in cattle farms in western Germany. Heliyon. 2015;1:e00019.
21. Jenckel M, Hoper D, Schirrmeier H, Reimann I, Goller KV, Hoffmann B, Beer M. Mixed triple: allied viruses in unique recent isolates of highly virulent type 2 bovine viral diarrhea virus detected by deep sequencing. J Virol. 2014;88:6983–92.
22. Nagai M, Hayashi M, Itou M, Fukutomi T, Akashi H, Kida H, Sakoda Y. Identification of new genetic subtypes of bovine viral diarrhea virus genotype 1 isolated in Japan. Virus Genes. 2008;36:135–9.
23. Sato A, Tateishi K, Shinohara M, Naoi Y, Shiokawa M, Aoki H, Ohmori K, Mizutani T, Shirai J, Nagai M. Complete genome sequencing of bovine viral diarrhea virus 1, subgenotypes 1n and 1o. Genome Announc. 2016;4:1.
24. Deng Y, Sun CQ, Cao SJ, Lin T, Yuan SS, Zhang HB, Zhai SL, Huang L, Shan TL, Zheng H, et al. High prevalence of bovine viral diarrhea virus 1 in Chinese swine herds. Vet Microbiol. 2012;159:490–3.
25. Gao S, Luo J, Du J, Lang Y, Cong G, Shao J, Lin T, Zhao F, Belak S, Liu L, et al. Serological and molecular evidence for natural infection of Bactrian camels with multiple subgenotypes of bovine viral diarrhea virus in western China. Vet Microbiol. 2013;163:172–6.

23

Molecular characterization of bovine tuberculosis strains in two slaughterhouses in Morocco

Hind Yahyaoui-Azami[1,2,3*], Hamid Aboukhassib[5], Mohammed Bouslikhane[3], Jaouad Berrada[3], Soukaina Rami[3], Miriam Reinhard[2,4], Sebastien Gagneux[2,4], Julia Feldmann[2,4], Sonia Borrell[2,4] and Jakob Zinsstag[1,2]

Abstract

Background: Bovine tuberculosis (BTB) is caused by *Mycobacterium bovis*, which belongs to the *Mycobacterium tuberculosis* complex. *Mycobacterium bovis* have been described to be responsible of most cases of bovine tuberculosis. Although *M. tuberculosis*, *M. africanum* and non-complex mycobacteria were isolated from cattle.
In Morocco, so far, no molecular studies were conducted to characterize the strains responsible of BTB. The present study aims to characterize *M. bovis* in Morocco.
The present study was conducted in slaughterhouses in Rabat and El Jadida. Samples were collected from 327 slaughtered animals with visible lesions suggesting BTB.

Results: A total of 225 isolates yielded cultures, 95% (n = 215) of them were acid-fast (AF). Sixty eight per cent of the AF positive samples were confirmed as tuberculous mycobacteria (n = 147), 99% of these (n = 146) having RD9 and among the latter, 98% (n = 143) positive while 2% (n = 3) negative for RD4
A total of 134 samples were analyzed by spoligotyping of which 14 were in cluster and with 41 different spoligotypes, ten of them were new patterns (23%). The most prevalent spoligotypes were SB0121, SB0265, and SB0120, and were already identified in many other countries, such as Algeria, Spain, Tunisia, the United States and Argentina.

Conclusion: The shared borders between Algeria and Morocco, in addition to the previous importation of cattle from Europe and the US could explain the similarities found in *M. bovis* spoligotypes. On the other hand, the desert of Morocco could be considered as an efficient barrier preventing the introduction of BTB to Morocco from West Central and East Africa. Our findings suggest a low level endemic transmission of BTB similar to other African countries. However, more research is needed for further knowledge about the transmission patterns of BTB in Morocco.

Keywords: *Mycobacterium bovis*, Bovine tuberculosis, Morocco, Cattle, Slaughterhouse, Spoligotype, PCR

Background

Bovine tuberculosis (BTB) is a chronic granulomatous caseous-necrotising inflammatory disease that mainly affects the lungs and their draining lymph nodes, it can also affect other organs, depending on the route of infection [1–3]. BTB is caused by *Mycobacterium bovis*, which belongs to the *Mycobacterium tuberculosis* complex (MTBC). *M. bovis* has the particular ability to infect a wide range of host species other than cattle (livestock, wildlife and pets) and humans, [3, 4], however, cattle remain the most important reservoir for *M. bovis* [5]. There exist important wildlife reservoirs like the badger (*Meles meles*), the Possum (*Trichosurus vulpecula*) [4].

M. bovis can be transmitted between animals by inhalation of aerosols and the ingestion of contaminated food. The transmission is enhanced by many risk factors, mostly related to intensive livestock system [6]. The transmission of *M. bovis* to humans occurs by consumption of unpasteurized infected raw milk and by the contact with infected cattle [7].

While BTB is still occurring in some developed countries in low prevalence [8–10] because of a wildlife

* Correspondence: yahyouiazamihind@gmail.com
[1]Department of Epidemiology and Public Health, Swiss Tropical and Public Health Institute, Socinstrasse 57, 4002 Basel, Switzerland
[2]University of Basel, Basel, Switzerland
Full list of author information is available at the end of the article

reservoir [11] i.e. badgers in the UK [12], this zoonosis is endemic in many of the developing countries, who lack the financial resources to control this disease. Bovine tuberculosis is highly prevalent in many African countries [13, 14], where it causes economic losses by its effects on animal health and productivity and by international trade restrictions. [15]. Bovine tuberculosis is also a zoonosis and, consequently, considered as a public health issue [1, 16, 17].

In Morocco, the agriculture sector is of key importance to the economy, representing approximately 14% of total gross domestic product (GDP) (75bn MAD/ €6.6bn) and approximately 7% of exports (2009). Livestock represents 38% of the total agriculture sector GDP [18]. Both extensive and intensive livestock production systems exist in Morocco, with local, crossbred and imported breeds, mostly Holstein. Local breeds have been shown to be more resistant to the disease [14, 19]. Bovine tuberculosis is an endemic zoonosis in Morocco. The last national survey based on skin tuberculin test was conducted in 2004 and showed an individual prevalence of 18% and a herd prevalence of 33% [20]. Furthermore, a cross-sectional tuberculin study was conducted in the Sidi Kacem area in Morocco in 2012 showing an individual prevalence of 20.4% and a herd prevalence of 57.7% [19].

Officially, skin test and slaughter is the current control strategy applied in Morocco; however this strategy is not fully applied as it is not respected; in addition, there is no systematic BTB screening of cattle at a national level [21].

In a review published by Muller et al. in 2013, the proportion of zoonotic human tuberculosis (TB) among all TB cases was estimated at 1.4% for the non-African countries, and at 2.8% in Africa [22]. The highest prevalence were found to be 13.8% and 7% respectively in Mexico [23] and in Uganda [24]. However, the World Health Organisation states a worldwide median prevalence of 3.1% of *M. bovis* among human TB patients [25]. Even if those prevalence values are mostly low, Muller et al., Pérez-Lago et al. and Navarro, and García-de-Viedma highlight the major consequences of TB due to *M. bovis* on certain groups of the population, and report a potential underestimation of the prevalence of zoonotic human TB [22, 25].

The phylogeny of MTBC showed recently that the strains found in animals belong to a single lineage which showed the deletion of the "Region of Difference" 9 (RD9) [22, 26]. Indeed, *M. bovis* is the most recent strain in his lineage showing the deletion of RD4 [27].

Molecular deletion typing had been found to be an important tool to differentiate *M. bovis* from the other strains of the MTBC [28]. Pattern of presence or absence of these RDs would allow a discrimination among MTBC strains [28–30].

Currently there is no data available in Morocco about the molecular characterization of BTB and the prevalence of MTBC among slaughtered cattle. The aim of the present study was to characterize the strains of MTBC which are responsible for BTB among the slaughtered cattle in Morocco.

Methods

Study area and sample collection

The study was conducted in two slaughterhouses in Morocco, one in Rabat and another in EL Jadida, which are two coastal cities separated by 200 km. The cattle slaughtered in these two slaughterhouses come from the rural areas surrounding the two cities and also from many other areas of the country. Individual information of every animal, such as gender, age, breed, and the possible origin were recorded in our database, as well as the date of sampling. The sample collection was performed in Rabat from March to July 2015 and in El Jadida from June 2014 to April 2015.

The samples were conveyed to the Veterinary and Agriculture Institute (IAV) in Rabat and stored in −20 °C until their treatment.

Tissue preparation, culture

Prior to treatment, samples were thawed overnight at 4 °C. Subsequently, samples were desiccated to remove adipose tissue, and 5 g of the desiccated lesions were mixed with sterilized sand and 10 ml of phenol red. The solution (7.5 ml) was placed in a 15 ml conic tube, 2.5 ml of NaOH 1 N was added at room temperature for 10 min, and then HCl 6 N was added for sample neutralization. As a final step, the tube was centrifuged for 25 min at 3500 rpm.

The supernatant was discarded and pellet was distributed in two of the four pre-tested culture media: Lowenstein-Jensen (LJ), LJ with glycerol (LJG) or pyruvate (LJP) and Herrold according to the availability in the laboratory. Cultures were incubated for 12 weeks at 37 °C and observed daily for growing colonies during the first week then weekly from the second week onwards.

All the grown cultures were deactivated by adding a loopful of mycobacterium colonies to 1 ml of sterilized water contained in small tubes. The samples were then inactivated for 1 h at 90 °C.

Determination of MTBC and deletion typing

Mycobacterium molecular characterization was performed using Multiplex polymerase chain reaction (PCR). The PCR was performed in the TB laboratory at Swiss TPH. We performed first MrpoB PCR in order to differentiate MTC and NTM as described earlier [31]. Deletion analysis by PCR was used to differentiate *M. bovis* and *M. tuberculosis* from other species of the MTBC by assessing the presence or absence of Regions of Difference 9 and 4 (RD). The analysis was carried out as previously described [13, 28].

Spoligotyping

Spoligotyping was performed as previously described [32]. Spoligotyping patterns were defined according to the SITVIT WEB database [33] and to *Mycobacterium bovis* molecular typing database [34]. All the patterns which were not found in the two databases were submitted as new patterns; new spoligotype numbers were assigned to them.

Results

Cattle information

In the present study, a total number of 8658 animals were examined. Three hundred and twenty seven animal presented gross visible lesions (3.7%) and were cultured, 66% (n = 215) of the total sampled animals were analysed by Ziehl-Neelsen(ZN), 68% (n = 147) of the latter were ZN positive and heat-killed for further molecular typing.

Figure 1 represents the geographic distribution of the samples (Fig. 1). While the age and gender distribution, in addition to the localization of the lesions sampled are shown in the Tables 1 and 2. The majority of the lesions were localised in the lymph nodes and the lungs (Table 2).

The majority of the sampled animals were males between 1 and 3 years and females more than 3 years (Table 1).

MrpoB PCR

A total of 68% (n = 147) of the 215 samples which were AF positive were confirmed as MTBC strains using MrpoB PCR. Thirty two per cent (n = 69) of animals were negative for MrpoB.

Deletion typing

The samples confirmed as MTBC strains were all positive to RD9 deletion typing and then confirmed to be not *M. tuberculosis* strains. A total of 144 (1.7%) of the samples were confirmed to be *M. bovis* as they were positive to the RD4 pcr. Three samples were negative for RD4.

Out of the total of the confirmed *M. bovis* samples, 30% were female while 70% were male. The predominant breed in the positive animals was Crossbreed prime Holstein.

Spoligotyping

A total of 136 analysed samples were lacking spacers 39 to 43. Forty one different spoligopatterns were found. The most frequent patterns were SB0121, SB0265, SB0120, with frequencies of 24.3% (n = 33). 16.9%

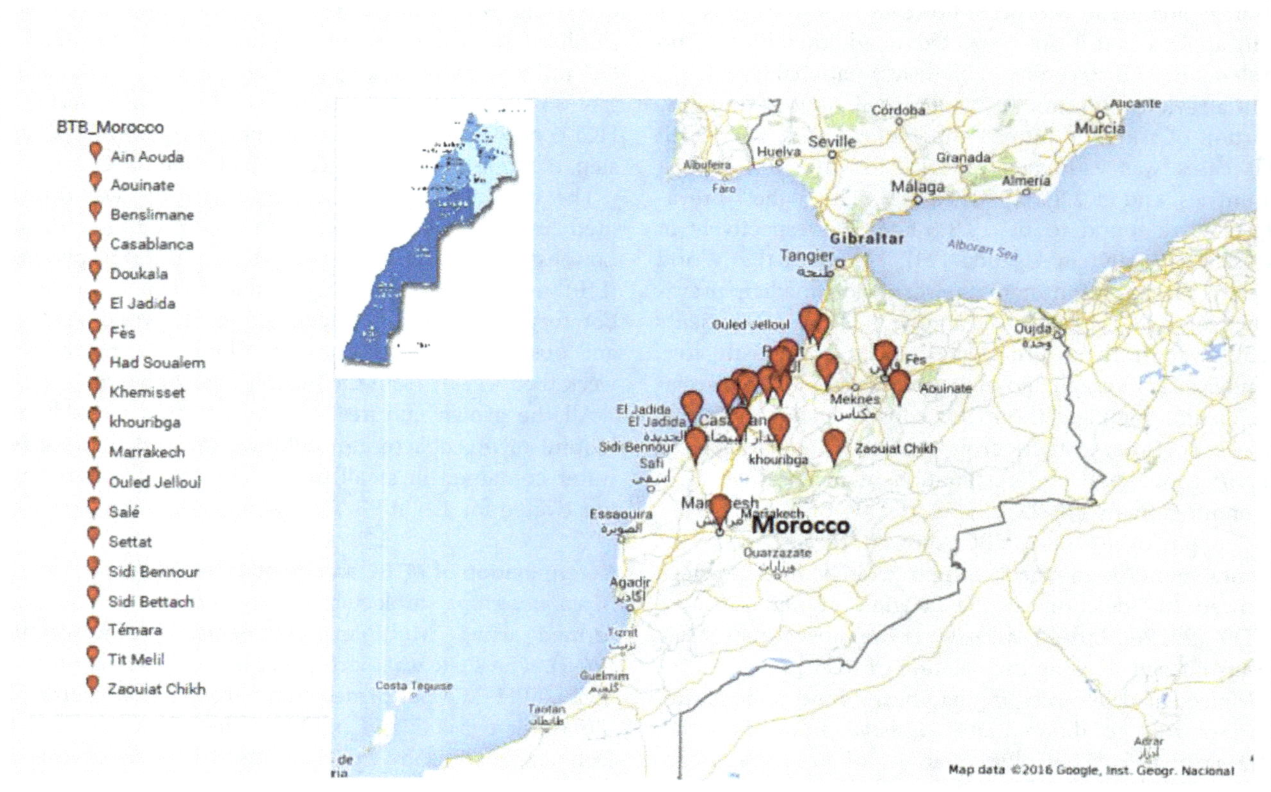

Fig. 1 Geographic distribution of the origin of the sampled animals

Table 1 Age and gender distribution of the sampled animals according to positive and negative cultures

	Male			Female			Total
	<1 year	1–3 years	>3 years	<1 year	1–3 years	>3 years	
Culture +	6	153	20	1	3	66	249
Culture -	4	40	6	2	3	23	78
Total	10	193	26	3	6	89	327

(n = 23), 9.6% (n = 13) respectively. They were shown to belong to BOV-1 family. Two other spoligotypes were found in 9 and 6 samples respectively, SB0125 and SB0869. Three spoligotype patterns had no SIT reference on the SITVIT database and were designated as orphan. Ten isolates presented nine undescribed spoligotypes, which were submitted to *M. bovis* website (www.mbovis.org) (Table 3). The discrimination power of spoligotyping, calculated using Hunter and Gaston's formula was D = 0.9057 [35].

Discussion

To our knowledge, this is the first study investigating the molecular characterization of bovine tuberculosis among cattle in Morocco. The prevalence of the gross visible lesions suggesting BTB in Rabat and El Jadida slaughterhouses (3.7%) was low compared to the prevalence found previously using tuberculin skin test in the last national survey performed in 2004 [20]. This prevalence was close to those observed in Mali (1.8%) and in Algeria (3.6%).

Surprisingly, no non-tuberculous mycobacteria was found, while in the African context, among slaughterhouse gross visible lesions, 3.3% in Mali [36], and 9% in Burkina Fasso [37] were confirmed as non-tuberculous mycobacteria. This was also observed in Chadian slaughtered cattle [38, 39].

Table 2 Localisation of the collected lesions, in addition to the specifications of the animals sampled

Lesion localisation	*n*	Gender		Breed		
		F	M	I	C	L
Liver	5	1	4	0	5	0
Lungs	4	2	2	0	4	0
Lungs and diaphragm	1	0	1	0	0	0
LN	185	45	140	67	117	8
LN and diaphragm	4	1	3	1	3	0
LN and liver	4	1	3	1	3	0
LN and lungs	70	30	40	35	35	2
LN, lungs, and diaphragm	6	1	5	4	2	0
LN, lungs, and liver	18	7	11	4	14	0
LN, lungs, liver, and diaphragm	24	4	20	21	2	1
LN, lungs, liver, and kidney	2	2	0	0	2	0
LN, lungs, pleura, and pericardium	2	2	0	0	2	0
Miliary tuberculosis	2	2	0	0	2	0
Total	327	88	229	133	191	11

LN Lymph nodes, *I* Imported, *C* Crossed, *L* Local

Almost 52.4% of the overall sample size was confirmed to be *M. bovis*, three samples were negative to RD4. While two spoligotypes were typical for the caprae family, the third sample was a new spoligotype. Studies in other Countries (e.g. Nigeria, Ethiopia) found *M. tuberculosis* in cattle [40], whereas in Morocco, remarkably, we didn't find this MTBC species in our samples.

The most predominant spoligotype pattern found in Morocco is SB0121, belonging to the family BOV 1, this spoligopattern was already reported in Algeria [41], in Tunisia [42] and in Spain [43]. The second most frequent spoligotype was SB0265 which was reported as the second most frequent in the United States from a set of strains collected between 1989 and 2013 [44], in addition, this spoligotype was isolated in Tunisia from a strain coming from Morocco [33], and was also reported in many European countries [45, 46], as well as in Taiwan [47]. The spoligopattern SB0120 had the frequency of 11.7% in our sample size and was reported previously in France from a sample originating from Morocco (SITVIT database), it was also reported in many African countries like Algeria [41], Tunisia [42] and Zambia [48] as well as in Argentina and Spain [43, 49]. Our study shows no similar spoligotype pattern with Mali, indicating that the Sahara desert and the long distance between cattle rearing areas (cattle are only kept until a Latitude of 12 degrees in Mali) seem to be an effective barrier for the transmission of *M. bovis* and/or that there is probably little trade of cattle between Morocco and Mali [36].

Two spoligotypes of three samples belonged to the *M. caprae* family, of which one was found as well in *M.bovis* database as SB0866, this spoligotype was already reported in Spain from one goat, one cattle and one pig in 2011 [50].

The similarities found in some spoligopatterns between Morocco and Algeria could be explained by the shared borders between the two countries, in addition some patterns found in Morocco were previously reported in the United States and in Argentina, two countries from where Morocco have previously imported cattle.

Table 3 The different spoligotypepatterns of the analysed samples and their relative frequencies

Spol	Nb.	Frequency	SIT	Family	SB Nb.
■■□■■■■■□■■■■■■□■■■■□■■■■■■■■■■■■■■■■■□□□□□	33	24.3	481	BOV_1	SB0121
■■□■■□■■□■■■■■■□■■■■□■■■■■■■■■■■■■■■■■□□□□□	23	16.9	684	BOV_1	SB0265
■■□■■■■■□■■■■■■□■■■■■■■■■■■■■■■■■■■■■■□□□□□	13	9.6	482	BOV_1	SB0120
■■□■■■■■□■■■■■■□■■■■□■■■■■■■■■■□□■■■■■□□□□□	9	6.6	Orphan	BOV_1	SB0125
■■□■■■■■□■■■■■■□■■■■□■■■■■■■■■■■■■□□■■□□□□□	6	4.4	1026	BOV_1	SB0869
■■□■■■■■□■■■■■■□■■■■□■■■■■■■■□□□■■■■■■□□□□□	4	2.9			SB1025
■■□■■■■■□■■■■■■□■■■■□■■■■□□□□■■■■■■■■■□□□□□	4	2.9	696	BOV_1	SB0339
■■□□□■■□□□■■■■■□■■■■■■■■■■■■■■■■■■■■■■□□□□□	3	2.2	1673	BOV	SB0136
■□□□■■■■□■■■■■■□■■■■□■■■■■□■■■■□■■■■■■□□□□□	3	2.2			SB2225
■■□■■■■■□□■■■□□□■■■■□■■■■■■■■■■■■■■■■■□□□□□	2	1.5			SB1269
■■□■■■■■□■■■■■■□■■■■□■■■■■■■■■■■■■■□■□□□□□	2	1.5	698	BOV_1	SB0295
□■□□□□□□□□□□□□□□■■■■■■■■■■■□■□□□□■■■■■□□□□□	2	1.5	646	BOV_4-CAPRAE	
■■□□□□□■□■■■■■■□■■■■□■■■■□□□□■■■■■■■■■□□□□□	2	1.5	Orphan	BOV_1	SB1145
■■□□□■■■□■■■■■■□■■■■■■■■■■■■■■■■■■■■■■□□□□□	2	1.5	665	BOV_1	SB0134
■■□■■■■■□■■■■■□□■■■■■■■■■■■■■■■■■■■■■■□□□□□	1	0.7	820	BOV	SB0856
■■□■■■■■□■■■■■□□■■■■□■■■■■■■■■■■■■■■■■□□□□□	1	0.7	695	BOV	SB0119
■■□□□■■■□■■■■■■□■■■■■□□□■■■■■■■■■■■■■■□□□□□	1	0.7			SB1888
■■□■■□■□□□□□■■■□■■■■■■■■■■■■■□□□□□□□■■□□□□□	1	0.7			SB2073
■□□□□□□□□□□□□□□□□□□□□■■■■■■■■■■■■■■■■■□□□□□	1	0.7	980	BOV	SB0152
■■□■■■■□□□□□□■■□■■■■□■■■■■■■■■■■■■■■□■□□□□□	1	0.7			SB1230
■■□■■■■■□■■■■□□□■■■■■■■■■■■■■■■■■■■■■■□□□□□	1	0.7	694	BOV	SB0127
■□□□□□□□□□□□□□□□□□□□□■■■■■■■■■■■■■■■■■□□□□□	1	0.7	980	BOV	SB0152
■■□■□□□■□■■■■■■□■■■■□■■■■■■■■■■■■■■■■■□□□□□	1	0.7	Orphan	BOV_1	SB2271
□■□□□□□□□□□□□□□□■■■■■■■■□□□□□□□□□□□□□□□□□□□	1	0.7	818	BOV_4-CAPRAE	SB0866
■■□■■■□■□■■■■■■□■■■■□■■■■■■■■■■■■■■■■■□□□□□	1	0.7			SB1361
■■□□□■■■□■■■■■□□■■■■■■■■■■■■■■■■■■■■■■□□□□□	1	0.7			SB1265
■■□□□■■■□□■■■□□□■■■■■■■■■■■■■■■■■■■■■■□□□□□	1	0.7			SB1074
□□□□□□□■□■■■■■■□■■■■□■■■■■■■■■■■■■■■■■□□□□□	1	0.7			SB2224
■■□■■■■■□■■■■■■□□□■■□■■■■■■■■■■■■■■■■■□□□□□	1	0.7			SB1993
■□□□■■■■□■■■■■■□■■■■□■■■■■■■■■■■■■□□■■□□□□□	1	0.7	650	BOV	SB0341
□□□□□□■■□■■■■■■□■■■■□■■■■■■■■■■■■■■■■■□□□□□	1	0.7	Orphan	BOV	
■■□■■■■■□□■■■■□□■■■■□■■■■■■■■■■■■■■■■■□□□□□	1	0.7			SB1333
■■□■■■■■□■■■■■■□□□□■□■■■■■■■■■■■■■■■■■□□□□□	2	1.5		New	SB2381
■□□■□■■□□□■■■□□□■■■■□□■■■■■■■■■□□■■□■■□□□□□	1	0.7		New	SB2382
□□□□□■□□□□□□■□□□□□□□□□□■■□■■□□□□□□□□□□□□□□□	1	0.7		New	SB2383
■■□■■■■■□■■■■■■□□■□■□■■■■■■■■■■■■■■■■■□□□□□	1	0.7		New	SB2384
■□□□■■■■□■■■■■■□■■■■□□□□□□□■■■■□■■■■■■□□□□□	1	0.7		New	SB2385
■■□□□■□■□■■■■■■□■□□□□□■■■■■■■■■■■■■■■■□□□□□	1	0.7		New	SB2386
■■□■■■■■□■■■■■□□■■■■□■■■■■■■■■■□□■■■■■□□□□□	1	0.7		New	SB2387
■□□■□■■□□□■■■□□□■■■■□□■■■□□□□■■□□■■□■■□□□□□	1	0.7		New	SB2388
■□□□■■■■□■■■■■■□■■■■□■■□□□□■■■■□■■■■■■□□□□□	1	0.7		New	SB2389

Spoligotypes of African 1 and African 2 clonal complexes were not found among our characterized isolates [51, 52]. African 1 is localized in West and Central Africa, and African 2 is localized in East Africa, consequently, the desert of Morocco could be considered as a potential efficient barrier preventing the introduction of BTB to Morocco from West, Central and East Africa.

The relatively low prevalence of proven *M. bovis* infection in two Moroccan abattoirs has to be interpreted with caution. Firstly, the abattoir prevalence reflects more the prevalence in young bulls and old cows rather than the whole population. Secondly, not all granuloma yielded a bacteriological isolate, hence the true prevalence may be much higher than the one observed. Overall, our findings reflect rather the epidemiological situation of a low level endemic transmission similar to other African countries rather than the one of a peri-urban intensive system [53, 54]. More research is needed to further characterize the ongoing transmission patterns of bovine tuberculosis in view of the development of a locally adapted elimination strategy of bovine tuberculosis in Morocco [55].

Conclusion

This study presents the first molecular characterization of BTB isolates from Moroccan cattle. *M. bovis* represented a high amount of granulomatous lesions detected in the abattoirs of Rabat and El Jadida. Spoligotype suggests a link of Moroccan BTB to Europe, rather than to Africa, highlighting then the potential of the Moroccan desert barrier for BTB introduction to Morocco from sub-Saharan Africa. Further investigations of BTB strains using new molecular techniques such as whole genome sequencing are needed to clarify more the potential links between Moroccan BTB strains and those of Europe and other African countries.

Abbreviations

BTB: Bovine tuberculosis; LJ: Lowenstein Jensen; LJG: Lowenstein Jensen with glycerol; LJP: Lowenstein Jensen with pyruvate; MTBC: Mycobacterium tuberculosis complex; NTM: Non-tuberculous mycobacteria; PCR: Polymerase chain reaction; RD: Region of difference; TB: Tuberculosis; ZN: Ziehl-Neelsen

Acknowledgements

We would like to acknowledge the veterinarians in the two slaughterhouses of El Jadida and Rabat, for their help and collaboration.

Funding

This study was supported by the EU FP7 ICONZ program (grant agreement n ° 221,948), by the local government of Basel-Stadt, Switzerland, and by the IFS scholarship B 5643.

Authors' contributions

HYA: Participated to the acquisition of a part of the funds (IFS grant), participated in the conception and design of the study, culture of Mycobacteria, molecular analysis, statistical analysis, writing of the manuscript. HA: Participated in sample collection. MB: Participated in the conception and design of the study, acquisition of funds, principle supervision in Morocco and intellectual contributions. JB: Participated in the conception and design of the study, Principle supervision of the laboratory work in Morocco (culture of mycobacteria). SR: Participated to the laboratory work in Morocco (culture of mycobacteria). MR: supervision of the molecular analysis in the tuberculosis laboratory in the Swiss TPH. SG: Supervision of the laboratory work in the Swiss TPH, important intellectual contribution. JF: Supervision of the molecular analysis in the tuberculosis laboratory in the Swiss TPH. SB: Supervision of the molecular analysis, and participated to the conception and the design of the study. JZ: Principal supervision of the project, Principle acquisition of the funds, important intellectual contribution. All the authors have read and approved the final version of the manuscript.

Consent for publication

Not applicable.

Competing interests

The authors declare that they have co competing interests.

Author details

[1]Department of Epidemiology and Public Health, Swiss Tropical and Public Health Institute, Socinstrasse 57, 4002 Basel, Switzerland. [2]University of Basel, Basel, Switzerland. [3]Department of Pathology and Veterinary Public Health, Hassan II Agronomy and Veterinary Institute, Rabat, Morocco. [4]Département de Biologie, Equipe Physiopathologies Nutritionnelles et Toxicologie, Faculté des Sciences UCD, El Jadida, Morocco. [5]Office Nationale de Sécurité Sanitaire des produits Alimentaires, Rabat, Morocco.

References

1. Ayele WY, Neill SD, Zinsstag J, Weiss MG, Pavlik I. Bovine tuberculosis: an old disease but a new threat to Africa. Int J Tuberc Lung Dis Off J Int Union Tuberc Lung Dis. 2004;8(8):924–37.
2. Domingo M, Vidal E, Marco A. Pathology of bovine tuberculosis. Res Vet Sci. 2014;97(Suppl):S20–9.
3. Pesciaroli M, Alvarez J, Boniotti MB, Cagiola M, Di Marco V, Marianelli C, et al. Tuberculosis in domestic animal species. Res Vet Sci. 2014;97(Suppl):S78–85.
4. Palmer MV. Mycobacterium Bovis: characteristics of wildlife reservoir hosts. Transbound Emerg Dis. 2013;60(Suppl 1):1–13.
5. Amanfu W. The situation of tuberculosis and tuberculosis control in animals of economic interest. Tuberculosis. 2006;86(3–4):330–5.
6. Goodchild AV, Clifton-Hadley RS. Cattle-to-cattle transmission of Mycobacterium Bovis. Tuberc Edinb Scotl. 2001;81(1–2):23–41.
7. Dankner WM, Davis CE. Mycobacterium Bovis as a significant cause of tuberculosis in children residing along the United States-Mexico border in the Baja California region. Pediatrics. 2000;105(6):E79.
8. Aranaz A, Liébana E, Mateos A, Dominguez L, Vidal D, Domingo M, et al. Spacer oligonucleotide typing of Mycobacterium Bovis strains from cattle and other animals: a tool for studying epidemiology of tuberculosis. J Clin Microbiol. 1996;34(11):2734–40.
9. Haddad N, Ostyn A, Karoui C, Masselot M, Thorel MF, Hughes SL, et al. Spoligotype diversity of Mycobacterium Bovis strains isolated in France from 1979 to 2000. J Clin Microbiol. 2001;39(10):3623–32.
10. Smith NH, Dale J, Inwald J, Palmer S, Gordon SV, Hewinson RG, et al. The population structure of Mycobacterium Bovis in great Britain: clonal expansion. Proc Natl Acad Sci U S A. 2003;100(25):15271–5.
11. Collins JD. Tuberculosis in cattle: strategic planning for the future. Vet Microbiol. 2006;112(2–4):369–81.
12. Delahay RJ, Walker N, Smith GC, Smith GS, Wilkinson D, Clifton-Hadley RS, et al. Long-term temporal trends and estimated transmission rates for Mycobacterium Bovis infection in an undisturbed high-density badger (Meles Meles) population. Epidemiol Infect. 2013;141(7):1445–56.
13. Mwakapuja RS, Makondo ZE, Malakalinga J, Moser I, Kazwala RR, Tanner M. Molecular characterization of Mycobacterium Bovis isolates from pastoral livestock at Mikumi-Selous ecosystem in the eastern Tanzania. Tuberc Edinb Scotl. 2013;93(6):668–74.
14. Moiane I, Machado A, Santos N, Nhambir A, Inlamea O, Hattendorf J, et al. Prevalence of bovine tuberculosis and risk factor assessment in cattle in rural livestock areas of Govuro District in the southeast of Mozambique. PLoS One. 2014;9(3):e91527.
15. Palmer MV. Mycobacterium bovis Infection in Animals and Humans, 2nd Edition. Emerg Infect Dis. 2006;12(8):1306. https://dx.doi.org/10.3201/eid1208.060526.
16. Cosivi O, Grange JM, Daborn CJ, Raviglione MC, Fujikura T, Cousins D, et al. Zoonotic tuberculosis due to Mycobacterium Bovis in developing countries. Emerg Infect Dis. 1998;4(1):59–70.
17. Thoen C, Lobue P, de Kantor I. The importance of Mycobacterium Bovis as a zoonosis. Vet Microbiol. 2006;112(2–4):339–45.
18. Samuelle C. Livestock sector in Morocco. Bord Bia Ir Food Board [Internet]. 2014 [cited 2015 Oct 2]; Available from: http://www.bordbia.ie/industry/manufacturers/insight/alerts/Pages/LivestocksectorinMorocco.aspx?year=2014&wk=28.
19. Yahyaoui Azami H, Ducrotoy M, Bouslikhane M, Hattendorf J, Thrusfield M, Conde-Alvarez R, et al. The prevalence of ruminant brucellosis and bovine tuberculosis in Sidi Kacem area in Morocco. Press. 2016.
20. FAO. Principales réalisations depuis l'ouverture de la Représentation de la FAO à Rabat en 1982. 2011 Juillet.
21. Tuberculose bovine [Internet]. 2016 [cited 2016 Mar 1]. Available from: http://www.onssa.gov.ma/fr/index.php?option=com_content&view=article&id=181&Itemid=122.
22. Müller B, Dürr S, Alonso S, Hattendorf J, Laisse CJM, Parsons SDC, et al. Zoonotic Mycobacterium Bovis-induced tuberculosis in humans. Emerg Infect Dis. 2013 19(6):899–908.

23. Pérez-Guerrero L, Milián-Suazo F, Arriaga-Díaz C, Romero-Torres C, Escartín-Chávez M. Molecular epidemiology of cattle and human tuberculosis in Mexico. Salud Pública México. 2008;50(4):286–91.
24. Oloya J, Opuda-Asibo J, Kazwala R, Demelash AB, Skjerve E, Lund A, et al. Mycobacteria causing human cervical lymphadenitis in pastoral communities in the Karamoja region of Uganda. Epidemiol Infect. 2008; 136(5):636–43.
25. Pérez-Lago L, Navarro Y, García-de-Viedma D. Current knowledge and pending challenges in zoonosis caused by Mycobacterium Bovis: a review. Res Vet Sci. 2014;97(Suppl):S94–100.
26. Smith NH, Kremer K, Inwald J, Dale J, Driscoll JR, Gordon SV, et al. Ecotypes of the mycobacterium tuberculosis complex. J Theor Biol. 2006;239(2):220–5.
27. Smith NH, Gordon SV, de la Rua-Domenech R, Clifton-Hadley RS, Hewinson RG. Bottlenecks and broomsticks: the molecular evolution of Mycobacterium Bovis. Nat Rev Microbiol. 2006;4(9):670–81.
28. Brosch R, Gordon SV, Marmiesse M, Brodin P, Buchrieser C, Eiglmeier K, et al. A new evolutionary scenario for the mycobacterium tuberculosis complex. Proc Natl Acad Sci U S A. 2002;99(6):3684–9.
29. Mostowy S, Cousins D, Brinkman J, Aranaz A, Behr MA. Genomic deletions suggest a phylogeny for the mycobacterium tuberculosis complex. J Infect Dis. 2002;186(1):74–80.
30. van Ingen J, de Zwaan R, Dekhuijzen R, Boeree M, van Soolingen D. Region of difference 1 in Nontuberculous mycobacterium species adds a Phylogenetic and taxonomical character. J Bacteriol. 2009;191(18):5865–7.
31. Malla B, Stucki D, Borrell S, Feldmann J, Maharjan B, Shrestha B, et al. First Insights into the Phylogenetic Diversity of Mycobacterium tuberculosis in Nepal. PLoS ONE [Internet]. 2012 ;7(12). [cited 2016 Jan 13]; Available from: http://www.ncbi.nlm.nih.gov/pmc/articles/PMC3530561/.
32. Kamerbeek J, Schouls L, Kolk A, van Agterveld M, van Soolingen D, Kuijper S, et al. Simultaneous detection and strain differentiation of mycobacterium tuberculosis for diagnosis and epidemiology. J Clin Microbiol. 1997;35(4):907–14.
33. SITVIT WEB - M. tuberculosis genotyping WorldWide Database Online Consultation : Description [Internet]. 2016 [cited 2016 Jan 13]. Available from: http://www.pasteur-guadeloupe.fr:8081/SITVIT_ONLINE/tools.jsp.
34. Mycobacterium bovis molecular typing database [Internet]. 2016 [cited 2016 Jan 13]. Available from: http://www.mbovis.org/.
35. Hunter PR, Gaston MA. Numerical index of the discriminatory ability of typing systems: an application of Simpson's index of diversity. J Clin Microbiol. 1988;26(11):2465–6.
36. Müller B, Steiner B, Bonfoh B, Fané A, Smith NH, Zinsstag J. Molecular characterisation of Mycobacterium Bovis isolated from cattle slaughtered at the Bamako abattoir in Mali. BMC Vet Res. 2008;4(1):1.
37. Sanou A, Tarnagda Z, Kanyala E, Zingué D, Nouctara M, Ganamé Z, et al. Mycobacterium Bovis in Burkina Faso: epidemiologic and genetic links between human and cattle isolates. PLoS Negl Trop Dis. 2014;8(10):e3142.
38. Diguimbaye-Djaibe C, Hilty M, Ngandolo R, Mahamat HH, Pfyffer GE, Baggi F, et al. Mycobacterium Bovis isolates from tuberculous lesions in Chadian zebu carcasses. Emerg Infect Dis. 2006;12(5):769–71.
39. Ngandolo BNR, Müller B, Diguimbaye-Djaïbe C, Schiller I, Marg-Haufe B, Cagiola M, et al. Comparative assessment of fluorescence polarization and tuberculin skin testing for the diagnosis of bovine tuberculosis in Chadian cattle. Prev Vet Med. 2009;89(1):81.
40. Gumi B, Schelling E, Berg S, Firdessa R, Erenso G, Mekonnen W, et al. Zoonotic transmission of tuberculosis between pastoralists and their livestock in south-East Ethiopia. EcoHealth. 2012;9(2):139–49.
41. Sahraoui N, Müller B, Guetarni D, Boulahbal F, Yala D, Ouzrout R, et al. Molecular characterization of Mycobacterium Bovis strains isolated from cattle slaughtered at two abattoirs in Algeria. BMC Vet Res. 2009;5:4.
42. Lamine-Khemiri H, Martínez R, García-Jiménez WL, Benítez-Medina JM, Cortés M, Hurtado I, et al. Genotypic characterization by spoligotyping and VNTR typing of Mycobacterium Bovis and Mycobacterium Caprae isolates from cattle of Tunisia. Trop Anim Health Prod. 2014;46(2):305–11.
43. Navarro Y, Romero B, Copano MF, Bouza E, Domínguez L, de Juan L, et al. Multiple sampling and discriminatory fingerprinting reveals clonally complex and compartmentalized infections by M. Bovis in cattle. Vet Microbiol. 2015;175(1):99–104.
44. Tsao K, Robbe-Austerman S, Miller RS, Portacci K, Grear DA, Webb C. Sources of bovine tuberculosis in the United States. Infect Genet Evol. 2014;28:137–43.
45. Rodriguez-Campos S, Aranaz A, de Juan L, Sáez-Llorente JL, Romero B, Bezos J, et al. Limitations of Spoligotyping and variable-number tandem-repeat typing for molecular tracing of Mycobacterium Bovis in a high-diversity setting. J Clin Microbiol. 2011;49(9):3361–4.
46. Matos F, Cunha MV, Canto A, Albuquerque T, Amado A, Botelho A. Snapshot of Mycobacterium Bovis and Mycobacterium Caprae infections in livestock in an area with a low incidence of bovine tuberculosis. J Clin Microbiol. 2010;48(11):4337–9.
47. Chang J-R, Chen Y-Y, Huang T-S, Huang W-F, Kuo S-C, Tseng F-C, et al. Clonal expansion of both modern and ancient genotypes of mycobacterium tuberculosis in southern Taiwan. PLoS One. 2012;7(8):e43018.
48. Malama S, Johansen TB, Muma JB, Mwanza S, Djønne B, Godfroid J. Isolation and molecular characterization of Mycobacterium Bovis from Kafue lechwe (Kobus Leche Kafuensis) from Zambia. Trop Anim Health Prod. 2014;46(1):153–7.
49. Shimizu E, Macías A, Paolicchi F, Magnano G, Zapata L, Fernández A, et al. Genotyping Mycobacterium Bovis from cattle in the central pampas of Argentina: temporal and regional trends. Mem Inst Oswaldo Cruz. 2014; 109(2):236–45.
50. Rodríguez S, Bezos J, Romero B, de Juan L, Álvarez J, Castellanos E, et al. Mycobacterium Caprae infection in livestock and wildlife. Spain Emerg Infect Dis. 2011;17(3):532–5.
51. Müller B, Hilty M, Berg S, Garcia-Pelayo MC, Dale J, Boschiroli ML, et al. African 1, an epidemiologically important clonal complex of Mycobacterium Bovis dominant in Mali, Nigeria, Cameroon, and Chad. J Bacteriol. 2009; 191(6):1951–60.
52. Berg S, Garcia-Pelayo MC, Müller B, Hailu E, Asiimwe B, Kremer K, et al. African 2, a clonal complex of Mycobacterium Bovis epidemiologically important in East Africa. J Bacteriol. 2011;193(3):670–8.
53. Tschopp R, Hattendorf J, Roth F, Choudhoury A, Shaw A, Aseffa A, et al. Cost estimate of bovine tuberculosis to Ethiopia. In: One Health: The Human-Animal-Environment Interfaces in Emerging Infectious Diseases. Springer; 2012(ISBN: 978-3-642-36888-2). p. 249–268. ; Available from: http://link.springer.com/chapter/10.1007/82_2012_245.
54. Tschopp R, Schelling E, Hattendorf J, Young D, Aseffa A, Zinsstag J. Repeated cross-sectional skin testing for bovine tuberculosis in cattle kept in a traditional husbandry system in Ethiopia. Vet Rec. 2010;167(7):250–6.
55. Abakar MF, Yahyaoui Azami H, Justus Bless P, Crump L, Lohmann P, Laager M, et al. (2017) Transmission dynamics and elimination potential of zoonotic tuberculosis in morocco. PLoS Negl Trop Dis 11(2):e0005214. https://doi.org/10.1371/journal.pntd.0005214.

Cyto-adherence of *Mycoplasma mycoides* subsp. *mycoides* to bovine lung epithelial cells

Racheal Aye[1*], Martin Kiogora Mwirigi[1], Joachim Frey[2], Paola Pilo[2], Joerg Jores[1,2] and Jan Naessens[1]

Abstract

Background: *Mycoplasma mycoides* subsp. *mycoides* (*Mmm*) is the causative agent of contagious bovine pleuropneumonia (CBPP), a respiratory disease of cattle, whereas the closely related *Mycoplasma mycoides* subsp. *capri* (*Mmc*) is a goat pathogen. Cyto-adherence is a crucial step in host colonization by mycoplasmas and subsequent pathogenesis. The aim of this study was to investigate the interactions between *Mmm* and mammalian host cells by establishing a cyto-adherence flow cytometric assay and comparing tissue and species specificity of *Mmm* and *Mmc* strains.

Results: There were little significant differences in the adherence patterns of eight different *Mmm* strains to adult bovine lung epithelial cells. However, there was statistically significant variation in binding to different host cells types. Highest binding was observed with lung epithelial cells, intermediate binding with endothelial cells and very low binding with fibroblasts, suggesting the presence of effective adherence of *Mmm* on cells lining the airways of the lung, which is the target organ for this pathogen, possibly by high expression of a specific receptor. However, binding to bovine fetal lung epithelial cells was comparably low; suggesting that the lack of severe pulmonary disease seen in many infected young calves can be explained by reduced expression of a specific receptor.

Conclusions: *Mmm* bound with high efficiency to adult bovine lung cells and less efficiently to calves or goat lung cells. The data show that cyto-adherence of *Mmm* is species- and tissue- specific confirming its role in colonization of the target host and subsequent infection and development of CBPP.

Keywords: *Mycoplasma mycoides* subsp. *mycoides*, Contagious bovine pleuropneumonia, Cyto-adherence, Epithelial cells

Background

Mycoplasma species (class *Mollicutes*) are widespread parasites of man, animals, plants and insects that are considered typical surface parasites [1]. *Mycoplasma* species have a small genome and are the smallest self-replicating organisms [2]. Owing to their limited biosynthetic capabilities, most *Mycoplasma* species exhibit strict host and tissue specificities [2]. Due to lack of a cell wall, mycoplasmal adhesins must be part of their cell membrane allowing for direct contact between the mycoplasmal cell membrane and specific receptors on the host cell membrane [3]. This close interaction probably creates a micro-environment which allows for the uptake of important nutrients and accumulation of mycoplasmal metabolic end products causing damage to host cell membranes [1]. Adhesion mechanisms of *M. pneumoniae* [4] and *M. genitalium* [5] are the best studied among *Mycoplasma* species. In *M. genitalium* defective mutants of the adhesions P1 and P30 have been shown to be avirulent, hence considering them as major virulence factors, [6]. For *M. conjunctivae*, adhesion was shown to depend on the RGD motif (Arg-Gly-Asp) of Lipoprotein T (LppT), a protein belonging to the α-integrin binding lectin family that includes fibronectin, vibronectin, fibrillin and von Willebrand factor [7]. No adhesion molecules of *Mycoplasma mycoides* subsp. *mycoides* (*Mmm*) have been described yet.

Mmm is the causative agent of contagious bovine pleuropneumonia (CBPP), a severe, highly contagious respiratory disease of cattle. The disease has also been reported in Italian buffaloes (*Bubalus bubalis*) [8], American bison (*Bison bison*) and Asian yak (*Bos grunniens*), but never in African buffalo (*Syncerus caffer*) [9]. CBPP is transmitted via aerosols of infected animals and

* Correspondence: racheal.aye@gmail.com
[1]International Livestock Research Institute, P. O. Box 30709-00100, Nairobi, Kenya
Full list of author information is available at the end of the article

is characterized by severe inflammatory, exudative lesions at lung and pleural membranes. In calves however, infection of *Mmm* results mainly in swollen painful limbs (arthritis) and associated lameness, but rarely in pulmonary lesions [9]. *Mmm* belongs to the closely related *M. mycoides* cluster [10] which includes four other species and subspecies, namely *M. mycoides* subsp. *capri* (*Mmc*), *M. capricolum* subsp. *capripneumoniae*, *M. capricolum* subsp. *capricolum*, and *M. leachii*. Although *Mmc* and *Mmm* are phylogenetically closely related [11], they greatly differ in host tropism [12]. Unlike *Mmm*, *Mmc* affects small ruminants causing clinical signs including mastitis, arthritis, kerato-conjonctivitis, pneumonia and septicemia, abbreviated as 'MAKePS' [13]. *Mmm* has been isolated from sheep and goats [14] however there is no indication that it can cause disease in these species. Likewise, *Mmc* has also been isolated from cattle [15], but has not been reported to cause disease in cattle.

A previous study [16] demonstrated the adherence of *Mmm* to embryonic calf nasal epithelial (ECaNEp) cells using realtime PCR assays. Flow cytometric assays have been previously described to measure cyto-adherence of other *Mycoplasma* species [17,18]. The aim of this study was to set up a novel flow cytometry (FCM)-based high throughput adhesion screening for *Mmm* and utilize this model for characterization of adhesion among different ruminant cell lines and a panel of *M. mycoides* strains. This approach might reveal an *in vitro* binding pattern that correlates with disease outcomes observed in young and adult cattle.

Methods

Cell culture

Primary epithelial and endothelial cells were cultured from adult bovine tissues including accessory lung lobe epithelial cells (BoLEC) and aorta endothelial cells (BoAEC), bovine fetal lung epithelial cells (BoFLEC) and caprine lung epithelial cells (CaLEC) were cultured from bovine fetuses and goat lungs respectively. Additionally, previously established immortal bovine skin fibroblasts (IBoSF) were used in this study [19].

BoLEC and CaLEC were cultured using the protease digestion technique as described elsewhere [20]. Briefly, tissues were digested using 1% protease XIV (Sigma, St Louis, USA) at 4°C overnight before collecting cells. BoAEC were cultured using the same technique as described above however tissues were digested in 0.25% collagenase (Sigma, St Louis, USA) [21]. BoFLEC were cultured according to a method described by Schweizer and Peterhans (1999) [22] with slight modifications. Fetal lung tissue was digested in trypsin-EDTA (0.025%: 0.01%) in PBS at 37°C for 1 h with shaking (200 rpm). All cell lines were maintained in Dulbecco's minimum essential medium (DMEM) supplemented with 10% inactivated fetal bovine serum (Sigma, St Louis, USA), 200 IU/ml penicillin, 150 μg/ml streptomycin, 1 μ g/ml nystatin, 2 mM L-glutamine and 0.15 M 2-mercaptoethanol.

Mycoplasma culture preparations

Mmm and *Mmc* strains used in this study (Table 1) were cultured in 20 ml "pleuropneumonia -like organism" (PPLO) medium (Becton Dickinson, Park, USA) supplemented with 10% horse serum (Sigma, St Louis, USA), 0.9 g/l yeast extract, 0.5% glucose and 0.03% penicillin G at 37°C for 48 and 18 h to a density of 10^8 and 10^9 cfu/ml respectively. Each *Mycoplasma* strain concentration was determined by the Spearman–Karber formula [23] before centrifugation. The mycoplasmas were harvested by centrifugation at 6,000 × g at 4°C for 30 min, washed once in DMEM without supplements and suspended in 10 ml of the same media. Final *Mycoplasma* titers were calculated using optical density at OD650 and readings plotted on a standard curve based on correspondence between OD650 and *Mmm* numbers as determined by TaqMan Real Time PCR.

Polyclonal rabbit antibody production

The production of rabbit polyclonal antibodies was approved by the institutional animal care and use committee (IACUC reference number 2008.14). *Mmm* strain Afadé was cultured as described above and the proteins prepared by ultra-sonication, and protein concentration determined by the micro BCA according to the manufacturer's instructions. One six weeks old rabbit was immunized twice with 1 mg of whole cell lysate at an interval of eight weeks. The rabbit was immunized by giving two immunizations with heat inactivated (60°C for 10 min) whole cell lysate (500 μl) mixed with the same volume of complete Freund's adjuvant in the first immunization or the same volume of incomplete Freund's adjuvant in the boost. At each immunization half of the antigen-adjuvant mixture was administered intradermally (500 μl) and half subcutaneously (500 μl). Pre-immunization serum was collected two weeks before initial immunization. Post-immunization serum was collected four weeks after the second immunization, heat inactivated at 56°C for 30 min, aliquoted and stored at -20°C until use.

The rabbit serum was validated using dot blot for all the *Mycoplasma* strains used in this study. Briefly, 2 μl of proteins from each *Mycoplasma* strain was dotted on to nitrocellulose membrane (0.45 μm pore size, Bio-rad), and allowed to dry at room temperature for 30 min. Unspecific binding sites on the blot were blocked in 5% BSA-PBS for 1 hr at room temperature. The blot was then incubated for 1 hr at room temperature with the rabbit serum diluted at 1:2,500. After 3 washes in PBS-Tween 20, the blots were incubated for 1 hr at room

Table 1 *Mycoplasma* strains used in this study*

Species		Strain name	Other name**	Date of isolation	Country of isolation	Host	Provider+
Mycoplasma mycoides subsp *mycoides* (*Mmm*)		Afade	DL 06/06	1968	Cameroon	Cattle/lung	FLI
		B237	DL 04/09	1997	Kenya		KARI
		B66		2000		Cattle	
		T144	DL 12/06	1951	Tanzania	Cattle/vaccine strain	CIRAD
		V5	DL 641/08	1936	Australia		FLI
		Gladysdale	008/06	1953		Cattle	
		Madrid	636/08	1993	Spain		
		L2	008/07	1993	Italy	Cattle/lung	
Mycoplasma mycoides subsp *capri* (*Mmc*)	*Mmc* serovar	PG3	R 88	1950	Turkey	Goat/type strain	
		Capri-L	402/97	1975	France	Goat	
	Mmm LC serovar	83/93	387/94	1993	Spain		
		136/93	383/94	1993			
		171/93	388/94	1993			
		152/93	385/94	1993			
		My325	64/97	1986	Croatia		
		G1313.94	211/94	1994	Germany	Sheep	
		G1255.94	209/94	1994			

*Strain selection was done to include a wide geographical location, varied years of isolation and different virulence.
+FLI-Friedrich Loeffler Institute; KARI- Kenya Agricultural Research Institute; CIRAD- Centre de coopération internationale en recherche agronomique pour le développement.
**All other names are FLI names.

temperature with anti-rabbit IgG (whole molecule)-alkaline phosphatase antibody produced in goat (Sigma) at a dilution of 1:5000. After three washes, blots were developed with 5-bromo-4-chloro-3-indolyl phosphate/nitro blue tetrazolium (BCIP/NBT, Sigma) in alkaline phosphatase buffer (100 mM NaCl, 5 mM $MgCl_2$, 100 mM Tris, pH 9.5).

Indirect immunofluorescent microscopy

1×10^5 BoLEC resuspended in 500 µl complete DMEM were seeded into a six cell well plate (Corning, New York, USA) containing sterile glass cover slips (Thermo Scientific) and cultured for 2-3 days at 37°C in 5% CO_2. Cover slips were collected and washed three times in DMEM without supplements. *Mmm* strain Afadé was cultured as described above and 200 µl (approximately 1.5×10^8 mycoplasmas) was added to the cell culture and incubated for two hours. Unbound mycoplasmas were washed off three times using 500 µl DMEM without supplements, prewarmed to 37°C. Cells were fixed in 3% paraformaldehyde for 15 min at room temperature. Cyto-adherent mycoplasmas were indirectly stained using anti-*Mmm* Afadé polyclonal rabbit serum (100 µl, 1:100 dilution) for 1 hour on ice, followed by washing thrice with 500 µl cold DMEM without supplements and 1 hour incubation with goat anti-rabbit FITC (Sigma, St Louis, USA; 100 µl, 1:500 dilution). Cover slips were air dried and images acquired using a fluorescent microscope (Axio Imager, Carl Zeiss AG, Gottingen, Germany) at a magnification of 400x. A control experiment was done as described above only that mycoplasmas were omitted and the cells were counter stained with 4′, 6 –Diamidino-2-phenylindole (DAPI).

Flow cytometry analysis of cyto-adherence

Cell lines were cultured in 24 well plates to a density of approximately 1.5×10^5 cells per well. To determine the optimum minimum concentration of mycoplasmas for cyto-adherence, all the *Mycoplasma* strains used in this study were ten-fold serially diluted. The cyto-adherence assay was performed as described above. Unbound mycoplasmas were washed off thrice with 500 µl prewarmed DMEM without supplements. Cells with bound mycoplasmas were detached from the culture plates with 250 µl PBS/EDTA buffer and the reaction stopped after 3 min by adding 500 µl prewarmed DMEM without supplements, transferred to 1.5 ml eppendorf tubes and centrifuged at 1,000 g for 10 min. The supernatant was discarded and the cells transferred to 96 round bottom well plates (Corning, New York, USA). Experiments were performed three times in duplicate. Staining was done as described above (100 µl/well, 1:100 dilution), followed by washing thrice with 200 µl of cold DMEM without supplements and centrifugation for 2 minutes at

1000 g. Cells were incubated with goat anti- rabbit FITC (Sigma, St Louis, USA; 100 μl/well, 1:250 dilution) for 1 hour on ice. After the final wash, cells were suspended in 100 μl of FACS medium (PBS, 2% horse serum, 0.2% sodium azide and 2% formalin). Cells were analysed by flow cytometry (FACS canto II, Becton Dickinson Co., San Jose, USA) in 5 ml falcon tubes according to the manufacturer's instructions. Three thousand signals were acquired and the results presented as dot plots. To calculate the percentage of positive cells, fluorescence threshold was set such that unstained cells without mycoplasmas would have 0% fluorescence. This threshold was kept the same for all samples of each experiment and reset for each cell type. Percentage of cells with bound mycoplasmas and mean fluorescence intensity (MFI) were calculated using flow jo software [24]. Statistical analysis of the cells with bound mycoplasmas was done using ANOVA.

Results

Specificity and kinetics of cyto-adherence

Rabbit serum directed against whole cell antigens of *Mmm* reacted to both *Mmm* and *Mmc* with similar efficiency (see Additional file 1: Figure S1), which justified its subsequent use for the detection of both *Mycoplasma* subspecies.

Microscopic analysis of adherent *Mmm* to BoLEC showed uneven distribution of *Mmm* on the cell surface. The adherent mycoplasmas appeared as aggregated bright fluorescent spots on the surface of the cells (Figure 1). Due to the small size of *Mmm*, it was not possible to visualize individual *Mycoplasma* cells under the conditions used.

Mmm cyto-adherence kinetics were analyzed using an indirect flow cytometry assay with appropriate controls using unstained lung epithelial cells without adherent mycoplasmas to set the fluorescence cut-off level (Figure 2). In all subsequent experiments the MFI was used to compare binding of *Mmm* to target cells, as this was a more representative parameter of the relative average number of mycoplasmas bound per cell. Saturation of *Mmm* binding to BoLEC and *Mmc* to CaLEC occurred 2 hours post infection (Figure 3A) at approximately 10^8 and 10^9 mycoplasmas per 1.5×10^5 cells (Figure 3B and C). In all subsequent experiments, mycoplasmas from each strain were used at saturating numbers.

Cell lines from different host tissues were cultured to assess the binding specificity of a panel of eight *Mmm* strains (Table 1). Maximum binding of all *Mmm* strains occurred on BoLEC, whereas intermediate binding occurred with BoAEC ($p = 0.006$) and low binding with BoFLEC ($p = 2.12 \times 10^{-10}$) and IBoSF ($p = 7.24 \times 10^{-11}$) (Figure 4).

Cyto-adherence of *Mmm* and *Mmc* to specific host cells was assessed by testing the binding ability of both *Mycoplasma* species to goat and cattle cells. We demonstrated a statistically significant difference between the cyto-adherence capacities of *Mmm* to BoLEC and CaLEC ($p = 1.11 \times 10^{-12}$), with *Mmm* binding more efficiently to BoLEC than CaLEC (Figure 5). On the other hand, *Mmc* bound more efficiently to CaLEC than BoLEC (Figure 6) however the difference was less apparent than in the case of *Mmm* but statistically significant ($p = 0.006$).

Intraspecies variation of cyto-adherence capacity

The different strains of *Mmm* did not show much variation in the ability to adhere to BoLEC although some small statistical differences of cyto-adherence capacities could be detected for certain strains; in particular with strain Madrid which seemed to have a higher binding capacity compared to the other strains (Figure 5; see Additional file 2: Table S1). *Mmc* on the other hand

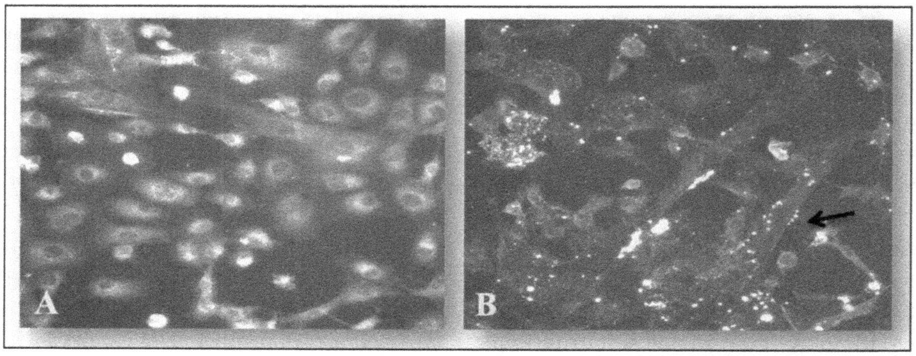

Figure 1 Indirect immunofluorescent staining of *Mycoplasma mycoides* subsp. *mycoides* (*Mmm*) bound to bovine lung epithelial cells (BoLEC). **A** shows BoLEC without *Mmm* stained with anti-*Mmm* (Afade) + anti-rabbit FITC and counter stained with DAPI. **B** shows BoLEC with adherent *Mmm* stained with anti-*Mmm* (Afade) + anti-rabbit FITC and counter stained without DAPI. The arrow indicates bright fluorescent patches of *Mycoplasma* clusters on the surface of an epithelial cell.

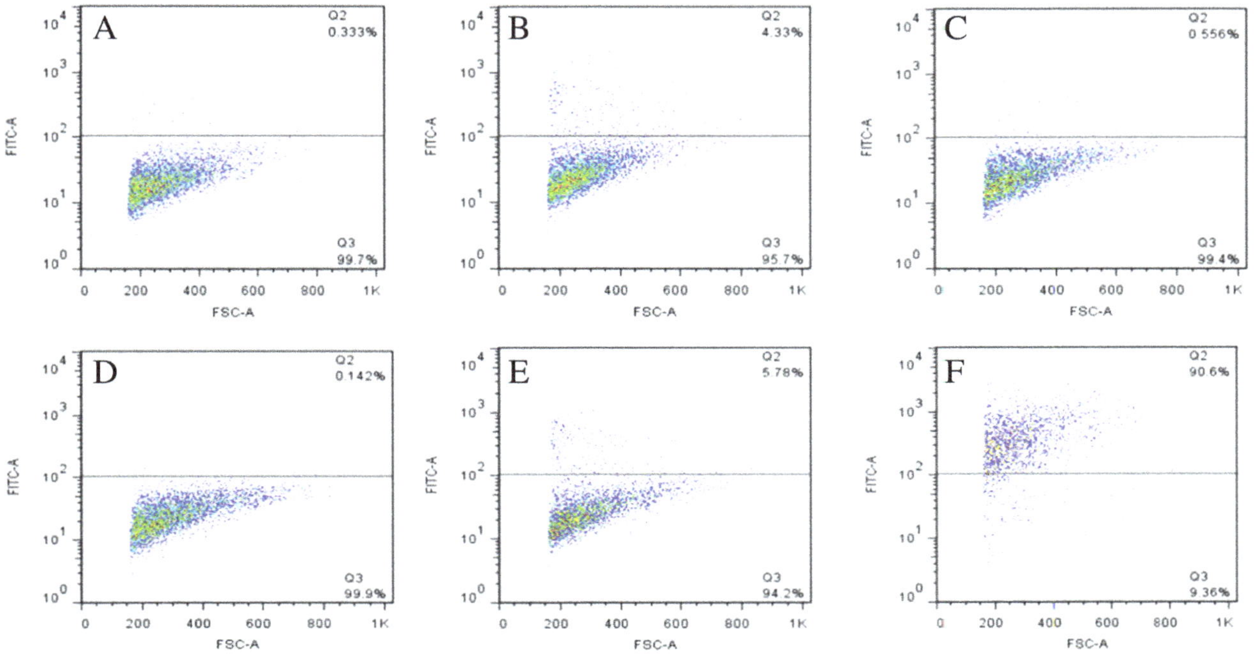

Figure 2 Flow cytometric analysis of *Mycoplasma mycoides* subsp. *mycoides* (*Mmm* strain Afade) attachment to bovine lung epithelial cells (BoLEC). Adherent *Mmm* was detected by specific rabbit anti-*Mmm* serum followed by FITC-conjugated goat anti-rabbit-Ig **(A)** unstained BoLEC without *Mmm*; **(B)** stained BoLEC without *Mmm*; **(C)** BoLEC + *Mmm* without anti-*Mmm* rabbit serum; **(D)** BoLEC + *Mmm* + anti-*Mmm* rabbit serum without goat anti- rabbit FITC; **(E)** BoLEC + *Mmm* + pre-immunization rabbit serum + goat anti-rabbit FITC; **(F)** BoLEC + *Mmm* + anti-*Mmm* rabbit serum + goat anti-rabbit FITC. Vertical axis: relative fluorescence intensity. Horizontal axis: forward light scatter.

showed relatively high intra-species variation in its capacity to adhere to CaLEC with strains PG3, Capri-L and My325 binding weakly to the cells (Figure 6; see Additional file 3: Table S2).

Discussion

The aim of this study was to set up a novel flow cytometry (FCM)-based high throughput screening for adhesion of *Mmm* and to utilize the model for characterization of adhesion of various strains of *M. mycoides* subsp. *mycoides* and *M. mycoides* subsp. *capri* to different ruminant cell lines. In our study, specks of fluorescence could be detected that varied in size, suggesting that *Mmm* were often present as clusters or aggregates of different sizes. A previous study also showed a heterogeneous distribution of *M. bovis* on the surface of host cells [20]. Using the flow cytometric assay we determined a statistical difference in the binding of *Mmm* to various bovine host tissues; the highest binding was detected with BoLEC, intermediate binding with BoAEC and low binding with IBoSF and BoFLEC. High binding to BoLEC is expected as the main lesions and pathology caused by *Mmm* are found in the lung of adult cattle [25] suggesting that there might be a receptor for *Mmm* on lung cells that allows for this interaction. Low adherence of *Mmm* to fetal lung epithelial cells may suggest a lack or low abundance of a receptor for *Mmm*, which may be acquired through activation of the corresponding genes later in life. This result probably explains why neonatal calves that are infected with *Mmm* do not develop severe lung lesions [9]. This also correlates with epidemiological observations showing that CBPP generally affects adult cattle [9,12]. In a previous study, binding of *Mmm* to embryonic calf nasal epithelial cells (ECaNEp) was measured in order to analyze the differences in the adhesion capacity of *Mmm* strains with diverse degrees of virulence, as ECaNEp cells were used as a model for cytotoxicity. However, this study did not compare host cells of animals of various ages and hence measurements have been done at a relatively low range of binding capacity [16].

Moderate binding to endothelial cells might correlate with pathology seen in capillaries and lymph vessels. *Mmm* has been isolated from the lymph nodes of cattle with CBPP [25] and vasculitis is a common occurrence in heavily infected animals. An interaction between mycoplasmas and endothelial cells may contribute to the vasculitis. Subcutaneous inoculation of mycoplasma often causes serious necrotic edema, but not in lymphatic-poor areas, such as nose or tail tip [26] however this method of inoculation does not result in typical clinical CBPP.

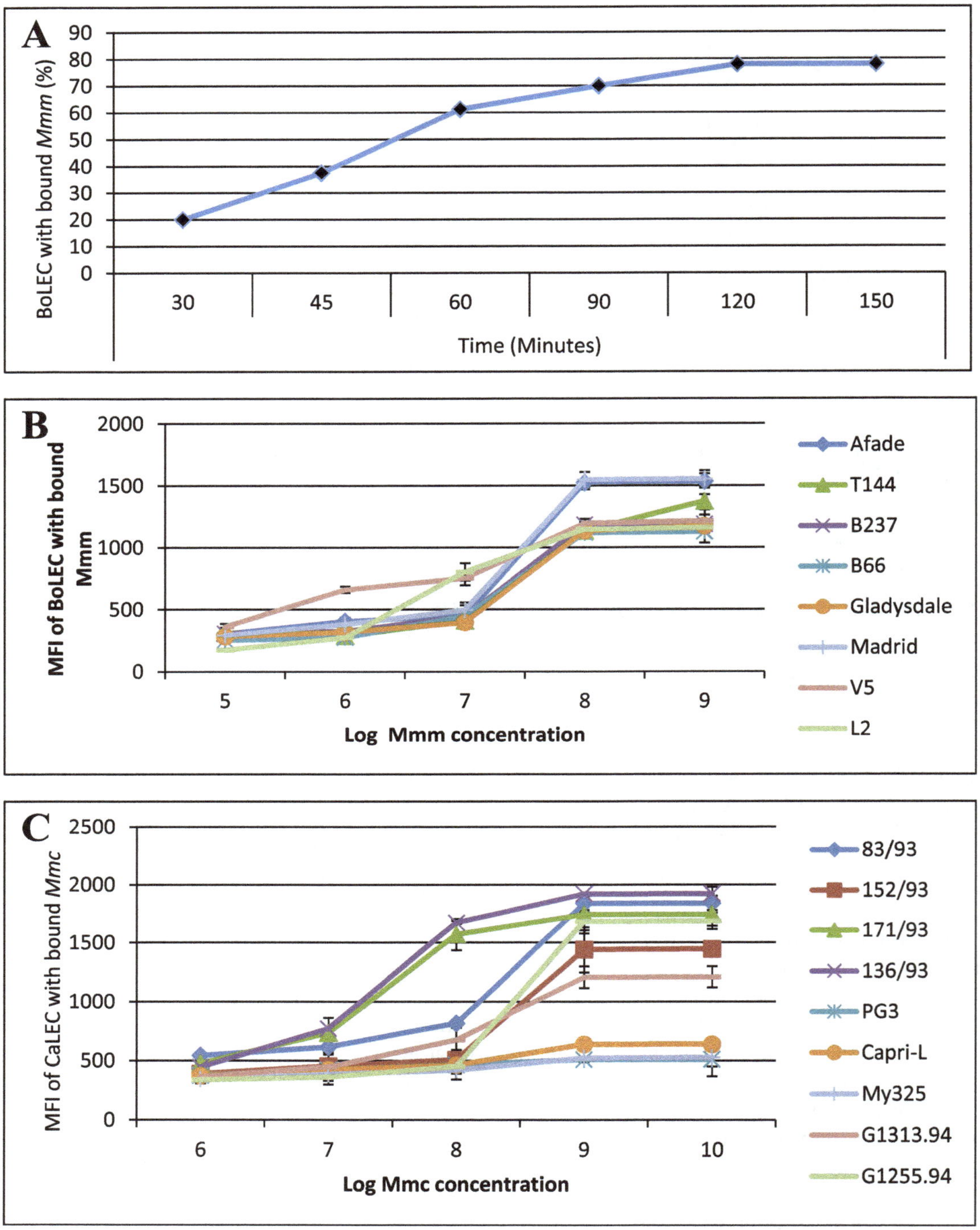

Figure 3 Cyto-adhesion kinetics of *Mycoplasma* strains used in this study. (A) Adherence of *Mycoplasma mycoides* subsp. *mycoides* (*Mmm*) strain Afade to cattle lung epithelial cells (BoLEC) as a function of incubation time. **(B)** Serial dilution (1:10) of *Mmm* strains and adherence to BoLEC. **(C)** Serial dilution (1:10) of *Mycoplasma mycoides* subsp. *capri* (*Mmc*) strains and adherence to caprine lung epithelial cells (CaLEC).

According to our results, there was little significant statistical difference between the adherence capacities of the different *Mmm* strains tested, which suggests that all strains used expressed the relevant adhesion ligands and the differences in the virulence among these strains is not due to variation in their adhesins. This is also probably due to the fact the *Mmm* strains exhibit very little genetic diversity [11]. The caprine *Mycoplasma* (*Mmc*) on the other hand showed more variation in cyto-adherence patterns among strains, which could correlate

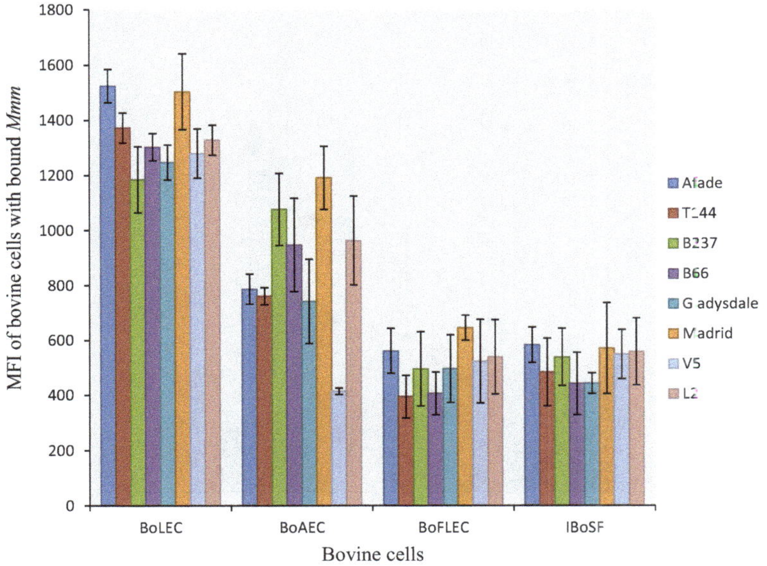

Figure 4 **Cyto-adherence capacity of different *Mycoplasma mycoides* subsp. *mycoides* (*Mmm*) strains to different cattle cell lines, expressed as mean fluorescence intensity (MFI) of cells with bound *Mycoplasma*.**

with their broader genetic diversity [11]. But the clinical signs of *Mmc* are not confined to lung, as there are many other manifestations, abbreviated as 'MAKePS' [13]. Adherence to other cell types might show different patterns and assessing the correlations between cyto-adherence of *Mmc* strains and different cell types needs further investigation. Furthermore, there is a possibility that the rabbit anti-Mmm serum used in this study might have reacted differently with individual *Mmc* strains. *Mmm* cyto-adherence assays revealed relevant host species specificity: *Mmm* adheres to bovine lung epithelial cells, but very little to caprine lung epithelial

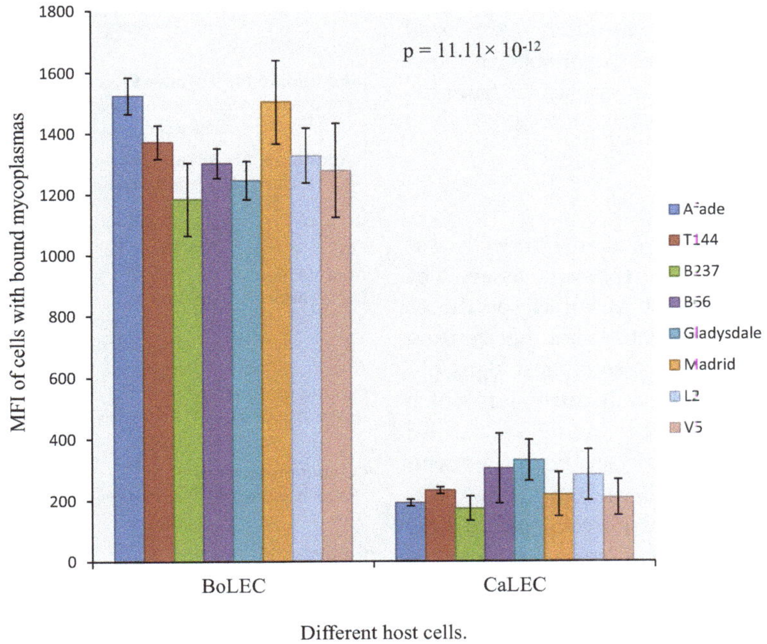

Figure 5 **Cyto-adherence capacity of different *Mycoplasma mycoides* subsp. *mycoides* (*Mmm*) strains to lung epithelial cells from cattle (BoLEC) and goats (CaLEC), expressed as mean fluorescence intensity (MFI) of cells with bound *Mycoplasma*.**

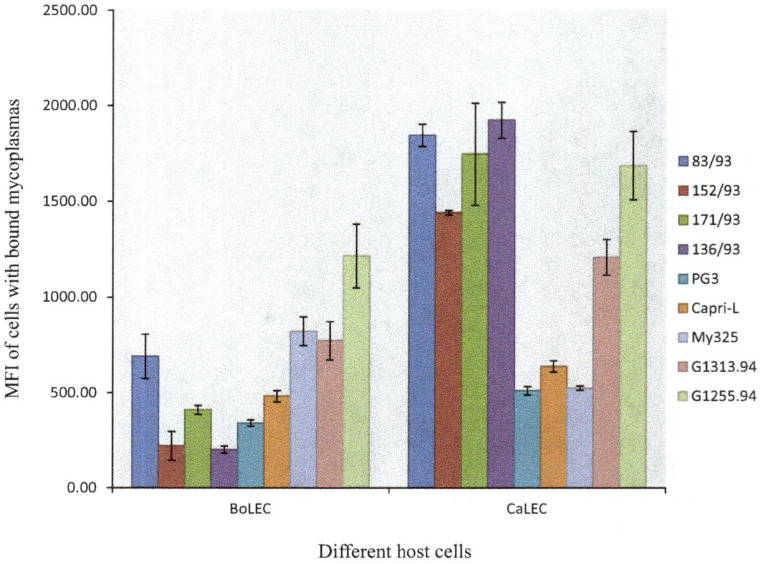

Figure 6 Cyto-adherence of different *Mycoplasma mycoides* subsp. *capri* (*Mmc*) strains to lung epithelial cells from cattle (BoLEC) and goats (CaLEC), expressed as mean fluorescence intensity (MFI) of cells with bound *Mycoplasma*.

cells. This suggests a correlation between the capacity to adhere to target cells, in this case to cattle cells, and the development of disease specifically in cattle, suggesting the presence of host specific adhesion factors. However, *Mmc* binds to lung cells from both species. This needs further investigation since *Mmc* has never been reported as causing disease in cattle [15] but other factors may influence the disease outcome. The cyto-adherence of *Mmm* supports previous reports from other *Mycoplasma* species that adherence is tissue and organ specific; however it is not uncommon to isolate mycoplasmas from tissues or hosts other than their natural habitats [27].

Conclusion

Cyto-adherence of *Mmm* to mammalian host cells was studied using an indirect, flow cytometric assay. The data show that strong binding of *Mmm* is specific to lung epithelial cells from adult cattle, but not fetuses. This correlates with the severe *in vivo* clinical signs observed in lung tissue of infected, adult cattle, but which are mostly absent in infected, very young calves. An intermediate binding to endothelial cells correlates with pathological signs detected in capillaries and lymph vessels. Binding was weak to other tissue cells and to lung cells from goats, suggesting that a strong binding of *Mmm* with their target cells might be the basis of the species and tissue specificity of CBPP, and be a requisite step in the development of the disease. Blocking adhesion *in vivo* might represent a valuable target to prevent colonization of the lung by *Mmm*.

Additional files

Additional file 1: Figure S1. Dot blot analysis of the ability of rabbit serum to recognize all the strains used in this study. 1. Blank control. No. 2-9. *Mycoplasma mycoides* subsp. *mycoides* strains including Afade, T144, B237, B66, Gladysdale, Madrid, V5 and L2 respectively. Numbers 10-18 are *Mycoplasma mycoides* subsp. *capri* strains including 83/83, 152/93, 171/93, 136/93, PG3, Capri-L, My325, G1313.94 and G1255.94 respectively. Membrane stained with *Mmm* specific rabbit serum raised against strain Afade (1:2500) and goat anti-rabbit alkaline phosphatase conjugated (1:500) (Sigma) and visualized by 5-bromo-4-chloro-3-indolyl phosphate/nitro blue tetrazolium (BCIP/NBT, Sigma).

Additional file 2: Table S1. Statistical analysis of cyto-adherence capacity of *Mycoplasma mycoides* subsp. *mycoides* (*Mmm*) strains to bovine lung epithelial cells (BoLEC).

Additional file 3: Table S2. Statistical analysis of *Mycoplasma mycoides* subsp. *capri* (*Mmc*) strains cyto-adherence to goat lung epithelial cells (CaLEC).

Abbreviations

BoAEC: Bovine aortic endothelial cells; BoFLEC: Bovine fetal lung epithelial cells; BoLEC: Bovine (adult) lung epithelial cells; CaLEC: Caprine lung epithelial cells; CBPP: Contagious bovine pleuropneumonia; IBoSF: Immortalized (bovine) skin fibroblast; Mmm: *Mycoplasma mycoides* subsp. *mycoides*; Mmc: *Mycoplasma mycoides* subsp. *capri*; DMEM: Dulbecco's minimum essential medium; DAPI: 4', 6-Diamidino-2- phenylindole; ECaNEp: Embryonic calf nasal epithelial cells.

Competing interests

The authors declare that they have no competing interests.

Authors' contributions

AR established the primary cell lines, performed the adhesion assays, performed statistical analysis and drafted the manuscript. MM helped with binding assay and flow cytometric analysis. JJ produces the polyclonal rabbit antibody. JN, JJ and AR designed the study and did analysis of results; JF and PP provided guidance in the adhesion assay and helped with interpretation of data. All authors helped to draft the manuscript and approved the final interpretation of data.

Acknowledgements

The project was financed by German Federal Ministry for Economic Cooperation and (Contract No. 81121408, Project No. 09.7860.1-001.00) and the CGAR research program on Livestock and Fish. Racheal Aye was also supported by a grant from the German Academic Exchange Service (DAAD), in-region scholarship.

Author details

[1]International Livestock Research Institute, P. O. Box 30709-00100, Nairobi, Kenya. [2]Institute of Veterinary Bacteriology, University of Bern, Bern, Switzerland.

References

1. Razin S. Adherence of pathogenic mycoplasmas to host cells. BiosciRep. 1999;19(5):367–72.
2. Pilo P, Frey J, Vilei EM. Molecular mechanisms of pathogenicity of *Mycoplasma mycoides* subsp. *mycoides* SC. Vet J. 2007;174(3):513–21.
3. Baseman JB, Tully JG. Mycoplasmas: sophisticated, reemerging, and burdened by their notoriety. Emerg Infect Dis. 1997;3(1):21–32.
4. Chourasia BK, Chaudhry R, Malhotra P. Delineation of immunodominant and cytadherence segment(s) of *Mycoplasma pneumoniae* P1 gene. BMC Microbiol. 2014;14:108.
5. Zeng Y, Liu L, He J, Liu Y, Zhu C, You X, et al. Screening and identification of the mimic epitope of the adhesion protein of *Mycoplasma genitalium*. Can J Microbiol. 2012;58(7):898–908.
6. Burgos R, Pich OQ, Ferrer-Navarro M, Baseman JB, Querol E, Piñol J. *Mycoplasma genitalium* P140 and P110 cytadhesins are reciprocally stabilized and required for cell adhesion and terminal-organelle development. J Bacteriol. 2006;188(24):8627–37.
7. Zimmermann L, Peterhans E, Frey J. RGD Motif of lipoprotein T, involved in adhesion of *Mycoplasma conjunctivae* to lamb synovial tissue cells. J Bacteriol. 2010;192:3773–9.
8. Santini FG, D'Angelo AR, Scacchia M, Di Giannatale E, Visaggio MC, Farinelli G, et al. Sequestro polomonare in unbufalo domestico da *M. mycoides* subsp. *mycoides* SC: isolamento, quadro anatomo-stopatologico ed immunoistochemico. Vet Ital. 1992;4:4–10.
9. OIE. Contagious bovine pleuropneumonia. 2014. http://www.oie.int/fileadmin/Home/eng/Health_standards/tahm/2.04.09_CBPP.pdf.
10. Manso-Silvan L, Vilei EM, Sachse K, Djordjevic SP, Thiaucourt F, Frey J. *Mycoplasma leachii* sp. nov. as a new species designation for *Mycoplasma* sp. bovine group 7 of Leach, and reclassification of *Mycoplasma mycoides* subsp. *mycoides* LC as a serovar of *Mycoplasma mycoides* subsp. *capri*. IJSEM. 2009;59:1353–8.
11. Fischer A, Shapiro B, Muriuki C, Heller M, Schnee C, Bongcam-Rudloff E, et al. The origin of the '*Mycoplasma mycoides* Cluster' coincides with domestication of ruminants. PLoS One. 2012;7(4):e36150.
12. Thiaucourt F, Manso-Silvan L, Salah W, Barbe V, Vacherie B, Jacob D, et al. *Mycoplasma mycoides*, from "*mycoides* Small Colony" to "capri": a microevolutionary perspective. BMC Genomics. 2011;12(1):114.
13. Thiaucourt F, Bölske G. Contagious caprine pleuropneumonia and other pulmonary mycoplasmoses of sheep and goats. Rev Sci Tech. 1996;15(4):1397–414.
14. Kusiluka LJ, Ojeniyi B, Friis NF, Kokotovic B, Ahrens P. Molecular analysis of field strains of *Mycoplasma capricolum* subspecies *capripneumoniae* and *Mycoplasma mycoides* subspecies *mycoides*, small colony type isolated from goats in Tanzania. Vet Microbiol. 2001;82:27–37.
15. Kapoor PK, Garg DN, Mahajan SK. Isolation of *Mycoplasma mycoides* subsp. *mycoides* (LC variant, Y goat) from naturally aborted bovine fetuses. Theriogenology. 1989;32:683–91.
16. Bischof DF, Janis C, Vilei EM, Bertoni G, Frey J. Cytotoxicity of *Mycoplasma mycoides* subsp. *mycoides* small colony type to bovine epithelial cells. Infect Immun. 2008;76(1):263–9.
17. Leigh SA, Wise KS. Identification and Functional Mapping of the *Mycoplasma fermentans* P29 Adhesin. Infect Immun. 2002;70(9):4925–35.
18. Schurwanz N, Jacobs E. Strategy to create chimeric proteins derived from functional adhesin regions of *Mycoplasma pneumoniae* for vaccine development. Infect Immun. 2009;77(11):5007–15.
19. Graham SP, Pellé R, Yamage M, Mwangi DM, Honda Y, Mwakubambanya RS, et al. Characterization of the fine specificity of bovine CD8 T-cell responses to defined antigens from the protozoan parasite *Theileria parva*. Infect Immun. 2008;76(2):685–94.
20. Thomas A, Sachse K, Farnir F, Dizier I, Mainil J, Linden A. Adherence of *Mycoplasma bovis* to bovine bronchial epithelial cells. Microb Pathog. 2003;34(3):141–8.
21. Ryan US. Isolation and culture of pulmonary endothelial cells. Environ Health Perspect. 1984;56:103–14.
22. Schweizer M, Peterhans E. Oxidative stress in cells infected with bovine viral diarrhoea virus: a crucial step in the induction of apoptosis. J Gen Virol. 1999;80(5):1147–55.
23. Litamoi J-K, Palya V-J, Sylla D, Rweyemamu M-M. Quality controls testing of contagious bovine pleuropneumonia live attenuated vaccine-standard operating procedures. Rome: FAO Animal Production and Health Paper 128, FAO; 1996. http://www.fao.org/docrep/003/v9952e/V9952E00.htm#TOC.
24. FLOWJO. Version 7.6.3. 2014. http://company.flowjo.com.
25. John B, Bashiruddin JB, de Santis P, Persson A, Regalla J. Detection of *Mycoplasma mycoides* subspecies *mycoides* SC in bovine lung and lymph node tissues by culture, sandwich ELISA and polymerase chain reaction systems. Res Vet Sci. 2005;78:199–205.
26. Wesonga HL, Manso Silvan L, Thiaucourt F. Towards sustainable CBPP control programmes for Africa: CBPP vaccine strain T1 44: possible reversion to virulence. Rome: FAO Animal Production and Health Division, FAO-OIE-AU/IEAR-IAEA Consultative Group on CBPP; 2003. http://www.fao.org/3/a-y5510e/y5510e0i.htm
27. Razin S. 1992. *Mycoplasma* taxonomy and ecology. In: Maniloff J, McElhaney RN, Finch LR, Baseman JB, editors. Mycoplasmas: molecular biology and pathogenesis. Washington, D.C: American Society for Microbiology; 1993. p. 3–22.

Permissions

All chapters in this book were first published in VR, by BioMed Central; hereby published with permission under the Creative Commons Attribution License or equivalent. Every chapter published in this book has been scrutinized by our experts. Their significance has been extensively debated. The topics covered herein carry significant findings which will fuel the growth of the discipline. They may even be implemented as practical applications or may be referred to as a beginning point for another development.

The contributors of this book come from diverse backgrounds, making this book a truly international effort. This book will bring forth new frontiers with its revolutionizing research information and detailed analysis of the nascent developments around the world.

We would like to thank all the contributing authors for lending their expertise to make the book truly unique. They have played a crucial role in the development of this book. Without their invaluable contributions this book wouldn't have been possible. They have made vital efforts to compile up to date information on the varied aspects of this subject to make this book a valuable addition to the collection of many professionals and students.

This book was conceptualized with the vision of imparting up-to-date information and advanced data in this field. To ensure the same, a matchless editorial board was set up. Every individual on the board went through rigorous rounds of assessment to prove their worth. After which they invested a large part of their time researching and compiling the most relevant data for our readers.

The editorial board has been involved in producing this book since its inception. They have spent rigorous hours researching and exploring the diverse topics which have resulted in the successful publishing of this book. They have passed on their knowledge of decades through this book. To expedite this challenging task, the publisher supported the team at every step. A small team of assistant editors was also appointed to further simplify the editing procedure and attain best results for the readers.

Apart from the editorial board, the designing team has also invested a significant amount of their time in understanding the subject and creating the most relevant covers. They scrutinized every image to scout for the most suitable representation of the subject and create an appropriate cover for the book.

The publishing team has been an ardent support to the editorial, designing and production team. Their endless efforts to recruit the best for this project, has resulted in the accomplishment of this book. They are a veteran in the field of academics and their pool of knowledge is as vast as their experience in printing. Their expertise and guidance has proved useful at every step. Their uncompromising quality standards have made this book an exceptional effort. Their encouragement from time to time has been an inspiration for everyone.

The publisher and the editorial board hope that this book will prove to be a valuable piece of knowledge for researchers, students, practitioners and scholars across the globe.

List of Contributors

Anitsi Loaiza, María D. Carretta, María A. Hidalgo and Rafael A. Burgos
Instituto de Farmacología, Facultad de Ciencias Veterinarias, Universidad Austral de Chile, Valdivia, Chile

Anja Taubert and Carlos Hermosilla
Institute of Parasitology, Faculty of Veterinary Medicine, Justus Liebig University Giessen, Giessen, Germany

Damien Barrett
Department of Agriculture, Food and the Marine, SAT Division, Admin Building, Backweston, Celbridge, Co. Kildare, Ireland

John Fagan
Department of Agriculture, Food and the Marine, Athlone RVL, Co. Westmeath, Athlone, Ireland

Alan Johnson
Department of Agriculture, Food and the Marine, Limerick RVL, Limerick Co. LimerickIreland

David Kenny and Mervyn Parr
Teagasc, Grange, Dunsany, Trim, Co. Meath, Ireland

Michael Diskin
Teagasc, Mellows College, Athenry, Co. Galway, Ireland

Jamie Tratalos
Centre for Veterinary Epidemiology and Risk Analysis, University College Dublin, Belfield, Dublin 4, Ireland

Francis Lively
Agri-Food and Biosciences Institute, 18a Newforge Lane, Belfast, Co Antrim BT9 5PX, Northern Ireland

J. Detilleux
Fundamental and Applied Research for Animals and Healh, Sustainable Animal Production, Faculty of Veterinary Medicine, University of Liège, Quartier Vallée 2, Avenue de Cureghem, 6, 4000 Liège, Belgium

Peili Hou, Hongmei Wang, Guimin Zhao, Chengqiang He and Hongbin He
Key Laboratory of Animal Resistant Biology of Shandong, Ruminant Diseases Research Center, College of Life Sciences, Shandong Normal University, No. 88 East Wenhua Road, Jinan City, Shandong Province, China

Jordon Graham, Craig Brown, Aoibheann Donaghy, Maria Guelbenzu-Gonzalo, Jim McNair, Robin Skuce, Adrian Allen and Stanley McDowell
Agri-food and Biosciences Institute, Veterinary Science Division, Stormont, Belfast, Northern Ireland BT43SD, UK

Andrew W. Byrne
Agri-food and Biosciences Institute, Veterinary Science Division, Stormont, Belfast, Northern Ireland BT43SD, UK
School of Biological Sciences, Queen's University Belfast, Belfast, Northern Ireland, UK

Jenner K P Reis
Laboratório de Retroviroses, Departamento de Medicina Veterinária Preventiva, Escola de Veterinária, Universidade Federal de Minas Gerais, Avenida Antônio Carlos 6627, Belo Horizonte, Minas Gerais, Brazil

Cairo H S De Oliveira
Laboratório de Retroviroses, Departamento de Medicina Veterinária Preventiva, Escola de Veterinária, Universidade Federal de Minas Gerais, Avenida Antônio Carlos 6627, Belo Horizonte, Minas Gerais, Brazil
Setor de Medicina Veterinária Preventiva, Escola de Veterinária e Zootecnia, Universidade Federal de Goiás, Goiânia, Goiás, Brazil

Rômulo C Leite
Laboratório de Retroviroses, Departamento de Medicina Veterinária Preventiva, Escola de Veterinária, Universidade Federal de Minas Gerais, Avenida Antônio Carlos 6627, Belo Horizonte, Minas Gerais, Brazil
Hospital Veterinário de Grandes Animais, Instituto de Medicina Veterinária, Universidade Federal do Pará, Castanhal, Pará, Brazil

Carlos MC Oliveira and José D Barbosa
Hospital Veterinário de Grandes Animais, Instituto de Medicina Veterinária, Universidade Federal do Pará, Castanhal, Pará, Brazil

Karine A Damasceno and Geovanni D Cassali
Laboratório de Patologia Comparada, Instituto de Ciências Biológicas, Universidade Federal de Minas Gerais, Belo Horizonte, Minas Gerais, Brazil

Limei Zhang, Jian Gao, Tariq Ali, Gang Liu, Youtian Deng and Bo Han
College of Veterinary Medicine, China Agricultural University, Yuan Ming Yuan West Road No. 2, Haidian District, Beijing 100193, People's Republic of China

Herman W. Barkema, Sohail Naushad and John P. Kastelic
Department of Production Animal Health, Faculty of Veterinary Medicine, University of Calgary, Calgary, AB T2N 4N1, Canada

Leíse Gomes Fernandes, Amanda Rafaela Alves Maia, Carolina de Sousa Américo Batista Santos, Clebert José Alves and Sérgio Santos de Azevedo
Laboratory of Transmissible Diseases, Academic Unit of Veterinary Medicine, Center of Rural Technology and Health, Federal University of Campina Grande, Patos, PB 58700-970, Brazil

Edviges Maristela Pituco, Adriana Hellmeister de Campos Nogueira Romaldini and Eliana De Stefano
Laboratory of Bovidae Viruses, Biological Institute, São Paulo, SP 04014-900, Brazil

Inácio José Clementino
Department of Veterinary Medicine, Federal University of Paraíba, Areia, PB 58397-000, Brazil

Phillip Senzo Mtshali
Department, National Zoological Gardens of South Africa, Pretoria 0001, South Africa

Moses Sibusiso Mtshali
Department, National Zoological Gardens of South Africa, Pretoria 0001, South Africa
Parasitology Research Programme, Department of Zoology and Entomology, University of the Free State, QwaQwa Campus, Phuthaditjhaba 9866, South Africa

Takehisa Yamamoto, Sota Kobayashi, Kiyokazu Murai and Toshiyuki Tsutsui
Viral Disease and Epidemiology Research Division, National Institute of Animal Health, National Agriculture and Food Research Organization, 3-1-5 Kannondai, Tsukuba, Ibaraki 305-0856, Japan

Sachiko Moriguchi
Viral Disease and Epidemiology Research Division, National Institute of Animal Health, National Agriculture and Food Research Organization, 3-1-5 Kannondai, Tsukuba, Ibaraki 305-0856, Japan
Department of Environmental Science Graduate School of Science and Technology, Niigata University, Niigata, Japan

Tohru Yanase
Kyushu Research Station, National Institute of Animal Health, National Agriculture and Food Research Organization, Kagoshima, Japan

Yoshiki Nitta
Yaeyama Livestock Hygiene Service Center, Okinawa Prefectural Government, Okinawa, Japan

Yoko Hayama and Moemi Suzuki
Yaeyama Livestock Hygiene Service Center, Okinawa Prefectural Government, Okinawa, Japan
Okinawa Prefectural Institute of Animal Health, Okinawa, Japan

Tsuyoshi Niwa and Kazufumi Ikemiyagi
Okinawa Prefectural Institute of Animal Health, Okinawa, Japan

Heng Wang, Yinjie Wang, Jun Sun, Xia Meng and Jianji Li
College of Veterinary Medicine, Yangzhou University, Yangzhou 225009, Jiangsu, China
Jiangsu Co-innovation Center for Prevention and Control of Important Animal Infectious Diseases and Zoonoses, Yangzhou 225009, Jiangsu, China

Chongliang Bi
College of Veterinary Medicine, Yangzhou University, Yangzhou 225009, Jiangsu, China
Jiangsu Co-innovation Center for Prevention and Control of Important Animal Infectious Diseases and Zoonoses, Yangzhou 225009, Jiangsu, China
College of Agriculture Forestry Science, Linyi University, Linyi 276000, Shandong, China

Xia Sun, Lianfeng Jin, Guangpu Yu, Qingzhang Li, Xuejun Gao and Chunmei Wang
Key Laboratory of Dairy Science of Education Ministry, Northeast Agricultural University, Harbin, Heilongjiang 150030, People's Republic of China

Yingjun Cui
Key Laboratory of Dairy Science of Education Ministry, Northeast Agricultural University, Harbin, Heilongjiang 150030, People's Republic of China
College of Life Science, Northeast Agricultural University, Harbin, Heilongjiang 150030, People's Republic of China

Jinxia Ao
College of Life Science, Northeast Agricultural University, Harbin, Heilongjiang 150030, People's Republic of China

Bernadette Earley, Paul Cormican, David Anthony Kenny, Sinead Mary Waters and Matthew Sean McCabe
Animal and Bioscience Research Department, Animal & Grassland Research and Innovation Centre, Teagasc Grange, Dunsany, Co. Meath, Ireland

Dayle Johnston
Animal and Bioscience Research Department, Animal & Grassland Research and Innovation Centre, Teagasc Grange, Dunsany, Co. Meath, Ireland
School of Agriculture Food Science and Veterinary Medicine, University College Dublin, DublinBelfield, Dublin 4, Ireland

Alan Kieran Kelly
School of Agriculture Food Science and Veterinary Medicine, University College Dublin, DublinBelfield, Dublin 4, Ireland

Gerard Murray
Department of Agriculture, Food and the Marine, Regional Veterinary Laboratory, Sligo, Co. Sligo, Ireland

Mark McGee
Livestock Systems Research Department, Animal & Grassland Research and Innovation Centre, Teagasc Grange, Dunsany, Co. Meath, Ireland

Edyta Kaczorek, Joanna Małaczewska, Roman Wójcik and Andrzej Krzysztof Siwicki
Department of Microbiology and Clinical Immunology, Faculty of Veterinary Medicine, University of Warmia and Mazury in Olsztyn, Oczapowskiego 13, 10-719 Olsztyn, Poland

Linda D. Stewart, Jose M. Argudo, Ruramayi Nzuma and Irene R. Grant
Institute for Global Food Security, School of Biological Sciences, Queen'sUniversity Belfast, Belfast, Northern Ireland, UK

Neil Reid and W. Ian Montgomery
Institute for Global Food Security, School of Biological Sciences, Queen's University Belfast, Belfast, Northern Ireland, UK
Quercus, School of Biological Sciences, Belfast, Northern Ireland, UK

Nuria Tort and Paul Meakin
Forsite Diagnostics Limited (now Abingdon Health), National Innovation Campus, Sand Hutton, York, UK

Richard J. Delahay
National Wildlife Management Centre, Animal and Plant Health Agency, Woodchester Park, Nympsfield, Gloucestershire, UK

Roland Ashford
Animal and Plant Health Agency, Weybridge, New Haw, Addlestone, Surrey, UK

Ingrid Bortolin Affonso Lux Hoppe, Andréa Souza Ramos de Medeiros and Samir Issa Samara
Faculdade de Ciências Agrárias e Veterinárias (FCAV), Departamento de Medicina Veterinária Preventiva e Reprodução Animal, Univ Estadual Paulista - UNESP, Via de Acesso Prof. Paulo Donato Castellane, km 05, Jaboticabal, São Paulo CEP: 14.884-900, Brazil

Clarice Weis Arns
Instituto de Biologia, Universidade Estadual de Campinas - UNICAMP, Cidade Universitária, Caixa-postal: 6109, Campinas, São Paulo CEP: 13.083-970, Brazil

Misako Konishi and Takehisa Yamamoto
Epidemiology Unit, Division of Viral Disease and Epidemiology, National Institute of Animal Health, NARO 3-1-5 Kannondai, Tsukuba, Ibaraki 305-0856, Japan

Hiroshi Ishizaki
Grazing Animal Unit, Division of Grassland Farming, Institute of Livestock and Grassland Science, NARO 768 Senbonmatsu, Nasushiobara, Tochigi 329-2793, Japan

Ken-ichiro Kameyama
National Institute of Animal Health, NARO, Exotic Diseases Research Station Josuihoncho, Kodaira, Tokyo 187-0022, Japan

Kenji Murakami
Cooperative Department of Veterinary Medicine, Iwate University Faculty of Agriculture, 3-18-8 Ueda, Morioka, Iwate 020-8550, Japan

Astrid Donoso, Felipe Inostroza, María Celedón and José Pizarro-Lucero
Laboratory of Animal Virology, Department of Animal Preventive Medicine, Faculty of Livestock and Veterinary Sciences, University of Chile, Av. Santa Rosa, 11735 Santiago, Chile

Eduard O. Roos, Guy A. Hausler, Robin Warren, Paul D. van Helden, Sven D. C. Parsons and Michele A. Miller
NRF-DST Centre of Excellence for Biomedical Tuberculosis Research, South African Medical Research Council Centre for Tuberculosis Research, Division of Molecular Biology and Human Genetics, Faculty of Medicine and Health Sciences, Stellenbosch University, Cape Town 8000, South Africa

Francisco Olea-Popelka
Department of Clinical Sciences, College of Veterinary Medicine and Biomedical Sciences, Colorado State University, 300 W. Drake Rd, Fort Collins, CO 80523, USA

Peter Buss
Veterinary Wildlife Services, South African National Parks, Kruger National Park, Skukuza 1350, South Africa

Lin-Mari de Klerk-Lorist
Office of the State Veterinarian, Kruger National Park, Department of Agriculture, Forestries and Fisheries, Skukuza 1350, South Africa

Guimin Zhao, Peili Hou, Chengqiang He, Hongmei Wang and Hongbin He
Key Laboratory of Animal Resistant Biology of Shandong, Ruminant Disease Research Center, College of Life Science Shandong Normal University, No.88 Wenhua East Road, Lixia District, Jinan 250014, Shandong Province, China

Yanjun Huan
College of Animal Science and Technology, Qingdao Agricultural University, No.700 Changcheng Road, Chengyang District, Qingdao 266109, Shandong Province, China

Du-Gyeong Han, Ji-Hyung Ryu and Kyoung-Seong Choi
Department of Animal Science and Biotechnology, College of Ecology and Environmental Science, Kyungpook National University, Sangju 37224, Republic of Korea

Jinho Park
College of Veterinary Medicine, Chonbuk National University, Iksan 54596, Republic of Korea

Jakob Zinsstag
Department of Epidemiology and Public Health, Swiss Tropical and Public Health Institute, Socinstrasse 57, 4002 Basel, Switzerland
University of Basel, Basel, Switzerland

Hind Yahyaoui-Azami
Department of Epidemiology and Public Health, Swiss Tropical and Public Health Institute, Socinstrasse 57, 4002 Basel, Switzerland
University of Basel, Basel, Switzerland
Department of Pathology and Veterinary Public Health, Hassan II Agronomy and Veterinary Institute, Rabat, Morocco

Miriam Reinhard, Sebastien Gagneux, Julia Feldmann and Sonia Borrell
University of Basel, Basel, Switzerland
Département de Biologie, Equipe Physiopathologies Nutritionnelles et Toxicologie, Faculté des Sciences UCD, El Jadida, Morocco

Mohammed Bouslikhane, Jaouad Berrada and Soukaina Rami
Department of Pathology and Veterinary Public Health, Hassan II Agronomy and Veterinary Institute, Rabat, Morocco

Hamid Aboukhassib
Office Nationale de Sécurité Sanitairedes produits Alimentaires, Rabat, Morocco

Index